The Cure of Imperfect Sight by
Treatment *Without Glasses*

By
W. H. BATES, M.D.

Dr. William H. Bates,
Ophthalmologist, M.D.
Eye, Ear, Nose & Throat.
Discovered the Principles
of Eye Function-Natural
Eyesight Improvement.

CENTRAL FIXATION PUBLISHING CO.
210 MADISON AVENUE, NEW YORK CITY

Perfect Sight Without Glasses

Advertised in Better Eyesight Magazine, Sept., 1919 Issue as;
The Cure Of Imperfect Sight By Treatment Without Glasses

Doctor Bates First Edition, Original Book

PERFECT SIGHT WITHOUT GLASSES

BATES

Doctor W. H. Bates

Copyright ©

The Cure Of Imperfect Sight By Treatment Without Glasses - Natural Vision Improvement (Perfect Sight Without Glasses) By Ophthalmologist William Horatio Bates. Year 1920. Central-Fixation Publishing Co. New York City, USA. Reprinted May 20, 2016. IBSN; 978-1530651177 by Clearsight Publishing Co., www.cleareyesight-batesmethod.info Articles, training added by Emily C. A. Lierman/Bates (Dr. Bates' wife, assistant) and other Bates teachers. William H. Bates' Books, 132 Issues of Better Eyesight Magazine are included in 20 Free PDF E-books. (Download from website.) Copyright by Clark Night is for assembly and preservation of this book, history/introduction to Ophthalmologist William H. Bates, his book, Better Eyesight Magazine, Medical Articles, extra pictures and training by Clark Night and other author's Antique books in the 20 E-books.

All Rights Reserved

The Author allows this Paperback and the E-Book copies to be distributed <u>free</u> to the public; Blind, Braille, Guide Dog Schools, People that need Vision Improvement, all Libraries, Schools, Colleges, Nursing Homes, Hotels, Military Bases, Veterans, Indian Reservations... CD, Paper copies only. No download, electronic transmission on the Internet from websites, businesses selling their products, books... No videos of the books. The Author/publisher does not allow this book to be sold, including sales, given free as a way to sell people medical and other treatments, including chiropractic. Read dangers of chiropractic in the PDF's, videos on the website; it can cause stroke, impair eyesight, hearing...

DISCLAIMER & DIRECTIONS

Read the entire Disclaimer, Directions on the final pages of this book.
    Contact lenses must not be worn before, during, after practicing Natural Eyesight Improvement. Contacts will not fit the eye, cornea as it changes to normal, healthy shape and function with practice of Natural Eyesight Improvement. The contacts can scrape, infect, scar the cornea. This can occur even without practice of Natural Eyesight Improvement because the eye, cornea naturally change shape. Stop use of contacts before practicing and do not return to them. The contact lens drops, solutions are also unhealthy.
    Natural Eyesight Improvement normalizes the eyes pressure, improves eye health. If there is any eye condition, glaucoma, surgery.., check with your eye doctor <u>first</u> before practicing The Bates Method, Natural Eyesight Improvement. Eye drops, drugs, medicine, un-natural treatments for eye pressure, other treatments may need to be changed, reduced, discontinued, the eyes monitored.
    Natural Eyesight Improvement also changes the eye, cornea back to normal healthy shape and function. If eye, retina, lens, cornea... surgery, any treatment

has been applied to the eyes; check with your eye doctor first to be sure the surgery, treatment and Natural Eyesight Improvement do not conflict, interfere with eachother, with the eye shape, state the doctor has set, fit the surgery, treatment... to. Natural Eyesight Improvement may help the surgery, eye to heal or it might work against the surgery because; Natural Eyesight Improvement brings the eye, cornea to normal shape - but, the surgery may have been done to place, keep the eye in an abnormal shape, a shape it was in before the surgery or a new abnormal shape. Example; Retina surgery done on an eye that is abnormally lengthened due to advanced nearsight, many years wearing eyeglasses, may act differently if the patient practices Natural Eyesight Improvement and returns the eye to normal, round shape, normal eye pressure, normal fluid, circulation flow, normal retina shape... Will it help or knock out the surgery, treatment, 'break' it or strengthen it?

Same warning for eye cornea laser, other cornea, eye surgeries and some cataract surgeries including artificial eye lens implants containing an eyeglass prescription. This places a permanent prescription in the eye; All surgeries that place a prescription in the cornea or eye for nearsight, farsight, presbyopia, astigmatism, bifocal... cannot be changed if the eyesight improves with practice of Natural Eyesight Improvement - or becomes more impaired without practice. (Prescriptions are addictive, cause more vision impairment.) Eyesight will be unclear; like trying to look through an incorrect, too strong or too weak eyeglass prescription. Only more surgery can change an eye, lens implant prescription and all surgery has risks. (Doctors can place an artificial lens replacement without a prescription in the eyes after cataract surgery. This enables the person the option of wearing eyeglasses or practicing Natural Eyesight Improvement.)

More surgery on the cornea has a high risk and further impairs the corneas health, structure, function. Avoid elective cornea surgery, implants.

People have regained clear eyesight after some types of unsuccessful eye surgery and eye muscle surgery but always check with an eye doctor first, preferably an experienced Bates Method, Natural Eyesight Improvement Ophthalmologist, Teacher with many excellent patient references.

THE MEMORY SWING

THE memory swing relieves strain and tension as well as does the long or the short swing which has been described at various times. It is done with the eyes closed while one imagines looking over first the right shoulder then over the left shoulder when the eyeballs may be seen through the closed eyelids to move from side to side. When done properly it is just as efficient as the swing which is practiced with the eyes open whether short or long. The memory swing can be shortened by remembering the swing of a small letter, a quarter of an inch or less when the eyes are closed. The memory swing has given relief in many cases of imperfect sight from myopia, astigmatism and inflammations of the outside of the eyeball as well as inflammations of the inside of the eyeball. One advantage is the fact that it can be done without attracting the attention or making one more or less conspicuous to others. It is much easier than the swing practiced with the eyes open and secures a greater amount of relaxation or rest than any other swing. It may be done wrong just as any swing may be done wrong. When done right one does not imagine things are moving necessarily. All that is important is to move the eyes from side to side as far as possible or as far as one can move them when the eyes are open.

BETTER EYESIGHT
A MAGAZINE DEVOTED TO THE PREVENTION AND CURE OF IMPERFECT SIGHT WITHOUT GLASSES

Copyright, 1921, by the Central Fixation Publishing Company
Editor—W. H. BATES, M. D.
Publisher—CENTRAL FIXATION PUBLISHING COMPANY

Vol. VII.   MARCH, 1923   No. 9

Rest
By W. H. BATES, M. D.

THE normal eye when it has normal sight is at REST. When the normal eye has imperfect sight it is not at rest. When the diseased eye is at rest it has normal sight. When the diseased eye is not at rest the sight is imperfect. There are no exceptions to these statements. In the treatment of imperfect sight without glasses it is very important that we should understand as clearly as possible what is meant by REST. The normal eye is at REST when the sight is normal or when the individual remembers or imagines normal sight. All persons with high degrees of nearsightedness have moments when the eye is normal and when the vision is normal but these moments are so short that there is not time enough to be always conscious of the normal vision.

Clarification for the Memory Swing; Do not force, or hold the eyes to the left, right. Imagining looking left and right is done *gently*. The eyes move easy, relaxed left and right under the closed eyelids as you imagine looking over the left and right shoulders. Allow the head to move with the eyes. Imagining seeing the swing of opposite movement (as is taught in this book) when looking left, right is optional.

Avoid Un-Natural, Harmful Eyesight Methods, Dishonest Teachers

There are dishonest teachers, authors altering Dr. Bates original books, method by adding unnatural practices that impair the eyesight, eyes' health. Example; the harmful cataract, detached retina, astigmatism... producing 'Plus Lens Method'. (Also called Anti-Corrective Lenses.) It consists of forcing the eyes to look through blurry, incorrect, *too strong* close eyesight reading eyeglass + prescriptions. Avoid this! The method is addictive, it causes myopia, presbyopia, farsight to develop. It forces the ciliary-lens muscle and other inner, outer eye muscles and the lens to become stiff, immobile. Circulation in the eye is lowered, health of the eyes, lens is impaired. The eyes-lens' natural refraction, movement is blocked 'frozen'. Tense outer eye muscles press on the eye altering its shape, causes tension in the eye, retina, lens. Bleeding in the retina, blind spots develop. Notice people that wear stronger and stronger reading glasses develop cataract and are then sold surgery. All eyeglasses, - minus and + plus lenses, prisms, astigmatism... lead to addiction to stronger eyeglasses, cataract, detached retina, glaucoma and other eye problems. Also avoid the plus lens method's eye stretches; forcing the eyes to look hard to the far left, right, up, down... and *not* moving the head with the eyes. This sprains the eye muscles, causes tension in the eyes and eye, head, neck muscles resulting in injury to other parts of the eyes, torn blood vessels, injury-detachment of the vitreous, retina. The tense eye muscles cause astigmatism, unclear vision, headache. Cataract, glaucoma... are also a side effect of drugs taken for certain medical and eye conditions. Eyeglasses increase the risk.

    Another method to avoid is Artificial 3-D Fusion eye exercises. (Autostereogram, single-image stereogram, SIS, magic eyes pictures...) It creates an optical illusion of depth, distance. It consists of staring straight ahead into space before or beyond 2 objects that are placed on the left and right sides of the face-eyes (in the eyes' peripheral field) to form an illusion of a 3rd merged object of the 2 objects in front of the face between the left and right eyes. The object is not truly in the central field. This method is not natural. It blocks, impairs central-fixation, eye shifting, relaxation and normal eye-brain function. Staring is a main cause of unclear eyesight. This is not a one size fits all method! Only a Behavioral Optometrist, Ophthalmologist can apply the Artificial 3-D correct. It must be done a specific way for each individual person, their eye and brain-body condition and used only if absolutely necessary after first trying The Bates Method which is a safe, effective, truly natural method to correct strabismus. The Artificial 3-D method is often not needed when the Bates Method alone is practiced. Correcting posture of the head, neck and spine, applying brain hemisphere balancing can correct wandering, crossed eyes. The artificial 3-D pictures are amusing but they can cause strabismus, impair eye movement, cause unbalanced-uneven eyesight in the left and right eyes, double vision, astigmatism, blurry eyesight and impaired convergence, divergence, accommodation, un-accommodation when looking at close and far distances; because the false 3-D disrupts the way the brain, left and right hemispheres, visual cortex, nerves work with the eyes, eye muscles, retina, lens, depth, distance perception... 3-D video games, TV's, computer screens, electronic readers, phones produce another form of unhealthy artificial 3-D.
    Practice of the Bates Method can help reverse impairment of the visual system, eyesight that the artificial 3-D has caused.
(Avoid chiropractors. Read about dangers of chiropractic in the E-books, YouTube Videos; it can cause stroke, impair eyesight, hearing...)

People selling Dr. Bates, Emily's books, his Better Eyesight Magazine for over $500.00 tried to get our copy of Dr. Bates paperback, Kindle, PDF Better Eyesight Magazine, books and the free Better Eyesight Magazines on our website, GoogleBooks unpublished. We had to prove copyright, public domain three times. The assembler, illustrator of this book was attacked though computer hacking and other ways ten times by people trying to prevent this book and Dr. Bates Original Antique Better Eyesight Magazines from being published for a lower price than they sell for. They continue to try to delete our bookstores, website and YouTube videos. *Dr. Bates magazines, books belong to the public!*

Clearsight Publishing Co. posts the truth about these dishonest teachers, authors. Our books will never contain un-natural, harmful treatments, methods. The books include essential modern instruction for clarity, safety, perfect practice. Our mission is to preserve Dr. Bates genuine work, publish *True* Natural Eyesight Improvement for clear eyesight and healthy eyes at all ages; infant to over 100 Years.

Clearsight Publishing Co. keeps Dr. Bates book prices low. Black & white copies of the color are created for a reduced price so all people, regardless of financial level have access to Dr. Bates Method. A color, printable PDF E-book copy of this book in 'King-Size' version with more teachers, training, pictures and 20 E-books are FREE at; www.cleareyesight-batesmethod.info *Training is always free to the blind.*

If you have read this book or the free E-books; please teach it, help other people learn The Bates Method and avoid unclear eyesight, cataract, other eye-eyesight problems, addiction to eyeglasses and unnecessary eye surgeries.

Author Clark Night provides Free Natural Eyesight Improvement Training to the blind, visually disabled by Phone, Skype.., in Person, E-Books and Audio-Video. Part of the profits from paperback, Kindle, Nook book, video, audio sales is given to the blind, partially blind, Guide Dog Schools; 'The Seeing Eye' - *Morris Frank and his dog Buddy*, 'Guiding Eyes For The Blind' and 'Perkins School For The Blind'. >

Read *First Lady of The Seeing Eye* for Buddy and Morris' training, life experience, creation of the Guide Dog School. Free training in the book; Learn directly from Morris, Buddy and their Guide Dog Teachers Mrs. Dorothy Eustis, Jack Humphrey and others. The method originated in Germany, to Switzerland and then Morris and Buddy brought it to the USA; first schools were started in Nashville, Tennessee, Morristown, New Jersey. Ophthalmologist W. H. Bates was born in New Jersey!
  The *First Lady of The Seeing Eye* original book has been out of print for a long time. People might be working on getting it back in print.

http://www.cleareyesight.info/id73

Donation receipts, yearly records available to the public.

Hadley - Ten years of service

The Perkins Institution for the Blind. South Boston, c 1840
Courtesy Boston Public Library Print Department.

Thank-You for Reading a Paperback, Kindle or PDF E-Book

Contact mclearsight@aol.com, www.cleareyesight-batesmethod.info, www.cleareyesight-batesmethod.info/id148.html for the Color PDF version of this book, videos and 20 E-books.

Your purchase supports free and low cost Natural Eyesight Improvement and Donations to the Guide Dog Schools, Perkins School for the Blind, DAV at; http://cleareyesight.info/id73.html

20 PDF E-Books: Natural Eyesight (Vision) Improvement Training
Do It Yourself-Natural Eyesight Improvement-Original and Modern Bates Method

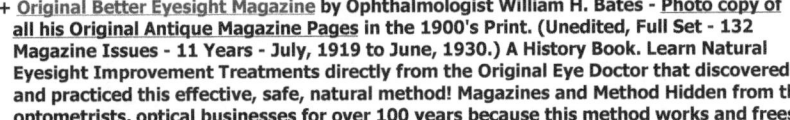

+ **A Exact Copy the Author's Natural Eyesight Improvement Website** www.cleareyesight-batesmethod.info and Dr. Bates **Better Eyesight Magazine website** in book form with all Training, Activities, Text, Pictures, Downloads and Links.
+ **Natural Eyesight Improvement Training Book** with 100+ Color Pictures. Less reading; Easy to learn steps-read the short directions on the pictures to quickly learn, apply a treatment, activity for Fast Vision Improvement. (All of Dr. Bates, Clark Night's Kindle, Paperback and PDF books are in this E-Book and the 20 E-books collection.)
+ **Better Eyesight Magazine** by Ophthalmologist William H. Bates - (Unedited, Full Set - 132 Magazine Issues - 11 Years - July, 1919 to June, 1930.) Illustrated with 500 Pictures and additional up to date Modern Natural Eyesight Improvement Training.
+ **Original Better Eyesight Magazine** by Ophthalmologist William H. Bates - **Photo copy of all his Original Antique Magazine Pages** in the 1900's Print. (Unedited, Full Set - 132 Magazine Issues - 11 Years - July, 1919 to June, 1930.) A History Book. Learn Natural Eyesight Improvement Treatments directly from the Original Eye Doctor that discovered and practiced this effective, safe, natural method! Magazines and Method Hidden from the public by eye surgeons, optometrists, optical businesses for over 100 years because this method works and frees the patient from the need to purchase eyeglasses, drugs, eye drops, unnecessary eye surgery. Yes, it can and has reversed cataracts and other eye conditions including glaucoma, various types of partial and full blindness!

Dr. Bates observes perfect light ray refraction (focus) with the glass and retinoscope as the patient sees fine print clear with relaxation.

+ **The Cure of Imperfect Sight by Treatment Without Glasses** by Dr. Bates (Photo Copy of the Original Antique Book Pages) with Pictures. Dr. Bates First, Original Book. (Text version with Modern Treatments included.) Main title, on book cover; Perfect Sight Without Glasses.
+ **Medical Articles** by Dr. Bates - with Pictures.
+ **Stories From The Clinic** by Emily C. A. Lierman/Bates. (Dr. Bates Clinic Assistant, Wife.)
+ **Use Your Own Eyes** by Dr. William B. MacCracken M.D. (Trained with Dr. Bates.)
+ **Normal Sight Without Glasses** by Dr. William B. MacCracken M.D.
+ **Strengthening The Eyes** by Bernarr MacFadden & Dr. Bates - with Pictures and Modern Training. (Trained with Dr. Bates. One of the First Physical Fitness Teachers.)
+ **EFT Training Booklet** - with Acupressure, Energy Balance, Strengthening, Positive Emotions. Easy step by step directions with Pictures.
+ **Seeing, Reading Fine Print Clear, Clear Close Vision** (Presbyopia Treatments) with Videos.
+ **Eight Correct, Relaxed Vision Habits** - A Quick Course in Natural Eyesight Improvement. (10 Steps For Clear Eyesight.)
+ **Astigmatism Removal Treatments** - Natural Eyesight Improvement with Astigmatism Swings, Eyecharts and Videos.
+ **Eyecharts Booklet** with Natural Eyesight Improvement Basic Training.
+ **Eyecharts** - 15 Large, Small & Fine Print Big C, E Charts for Close and Distant Vision, White and Black Letter Charts, Tumbling E Chart, Astigmatism Test and Removal Charts, Behavioral Optometry Charts. Eyechart Video Training.
+ **Audio Training in Every Chapter**
+ **Video Links in Training Chapters** - Learn a Treatment, Activity Quick and Easy.
+ **Videos Page;** Links to 120+ Natural Eyesight Improvement Training Videos; YouTube and on the Author's Website. Download Videos to DVD. Convert for Television. Watch YouTube Videos on Cable TV. New videos added in 2015+; https://www.youtube.com/user/ClarkClydeNight/videos

E-Book contains over 1500 pages. 650+ Color Pictures. No password; print, bind all 20 books. Read the books, watch the videos for an entire Natural Eyesight Improvement Training Course.
Check the 'New Stuff Page'; http://cleareyesight.info/id61.html for notice when new Free PDF E-Books, new Chapters, Activities are added to the E-Books. Print the pages, add them to the paperback book.

This list is limited. More books have been added; http://cleareyesight-batesmethod.info/id148.html and the GuestPage; http://naturaleyesightimprovement-batesmethod.com/GuestPage/index.php

This book and all the Author's books on Amazon included; http://www.amazon.com/Clark-Night/e/B004HU1MNS/ref=dp_byline_cont_pop_book_1 Books are in Color with Pictures. Read or listen to/record Dr. Bates Better Eyesight Magazines on the Internet at; http://www.cleareyesight.info/naturalvisionimprovementoriginalandmodernbatesmethod/

Entire Introduction, Dedication to Dr. Bates, The Bates Method of Natural Eyesight Improvement History, Original and Modern Practices, Directions and Eyecharts are placed at the end of this book.
See the pictures with short directions to quickly learn the method. Then the Ophthalmology, technical part of the book, purpose for the eye, eye muscle... experiments and each practice taught by Dr. Bates will be easy to absorb, put into immediate practice for fast eyesight improvement.

Dr. Bates' original treatments, experiments, directions with pictures in his book and *Better Eyesight Magazine* are necessary to see, understand the true method. Training directly from the mind of the original eye doctor that discovered Natural Eyesight Improvement. Books, magazine contain *True Life Stories* of the doctors, patients. Their eye/vision conditions, natural treatments and the results.

Some original practices are removed and new things added in versions of Dr. Bates' book written by new authors, publishers after 1940. There are many very effective natural treatments in Dr. Bates' original book that are not included in the new authors' editions.

Perfect Sight Without Glasses 9 editions from 1920 to 1940 are the true original editions, method. This book contains <u>all</u> of Dr. Bates' training. Nothing is removed. New treatments are added. Read the Kindle and Paperback *TextBook Edition, Better Eyesight Magazine Illustrated with 500 Pictures*, Dr. Bates' *Antique Print Better Eyesight Magazine* and his *Medical Articles* for many Original and Modern Eyesight Treatments. Blue Print in this book is by Author Clark Night to describe new practices added to a few older treatments.

The Cure of
Imperfect Sight by Treatment
WITHOUT GLASSES

By
W. H. BATES, M.D.

CENTRAL FIXATION PUBLISHING CO.
NEW YORK CITY

Ophthalmologist
William Horatio Bates

Ophthalmologist William H. Bates discovered the natural function of the eyes, Natural Eyesight Improvement. He cured thousands of patient's vision <u>without</u> eyeglasses, eye surgery, drugs; *unclear close and distant vision, astigmatism, crossed/wandering eyes, amblyopia, cataracts, cornea ulcers* and *scars, retinitis pigmentosa, glaucoma* and other conditions.

Author of; *The Cure of Imperfect Sight by Treatment Without Glasses* (subtitle of this book), *Better Eyesight Magazine* and *Medical Articles*. His wife/assistant Emily C. Lierman/Bates' book; *Stories From The Clinic.* Contact; <u>www.cleareyesight-batesmethod.info</u>, <u>mclearsight@aol.com</u> for free PDF E-book copies of these books in text and Original Antique Print.

This is Dr. Bates' original book. Later editions by other authors (after Dr. Bates' death, after his wife Emily A. Bates' final 1940 edition) are changed; Open Eyes Sunning, the Sun-Glass, Dr. Bates' experiments with pictures are removed. <u>Example</u>; Sunning (Sun-Gazing) in new editions is changed. It is done with the eyes closed. Looking at the bright sunny sky near, away from the sun with eyes open is allowed. Move 'shift' the eyes. Blink. <u>True</u> Bates teachers allow open and closed eyes sunning. When sunning; keep the head and open, closed eyes <u>moving</u>. Eyes shifting. (open eyes blink.) Shift side to side, up, down...
    Many Bates Method teachers prefer Dr. Bates' original training in *his* book and Better Eyesight Magazine. Sunning with *eyes open*, facing the sun, moving across it is practiced a specific way; time limit, with the eyes, head *constantly moving*. The eyes blink often. Many people benefit from sunning. It improves the vision, eyes' health and cures some forms of blindness.

Copyright, 1920 By W. H. BATES, M.D.,
BURR PRINTING HOUSE, NEW YORK

```
                    TO THE MEMORY
                       OF THE
               PIONEERS OF OPHTHALMOLOGY
            THIS BOOK IS GRATEFULLY DEDICATED
```

FERDINAND VON ARLT
(1812-1887)

Distinguished Austrian ophthalmologist, Professor of Diseases of the Eye at Vienna, who believed for a time that accommodation was produced by an elongation of the visual axis, but finally accepted the conclusions of Cramer and Helmholtz.

FERDINAND VON ARLT (1812-1887) Distinguished Austrian ophthalmologist, Professor of Diseases of the Eye at Vienna, who believed for a time that accommodation was produced by an elongation of the visual axis, but finally accepted the conclusions of Cramer and Helmholtz.

On a tomb in the Church of Santa Maria Maggiore in Florence was found an inscription which read: "Here lies Salvino degli Armati, Inventor of Spectacles. May God pardon him his sins.

" Nuova Enciclopedia Italiana, Sixth Edition.

CONTENTS

Preface vii

CHAPTER I
Introductory 1

Prevalence of errors of refraction—Believed to be incurable and practically unpreventable—The eye regarded as a blunder of Nature—Facts which seem to justify this conclusion—Failure of all efforts to prevent the development of eye defects—Futility of prevailing methods of treatment—Conflict of facts with the theory of incurability of errors of refraction—These facts commonly explained away or ignored—The author unable to ignore them, or to accept current explanations—Finally forced to reject accepted theories.

CHAPTER II
Simultaneous Retinoscopy 17

Retinoscopy the source of much of the information presented in this book—What the retinoscope is—Its possibilities not realized—Commonly used only under artificial conditions—Used by the author under the conditions of life on human beings and the lower animals—Thus many new facts were discovered—Conflict of these facts with accepted theories—Resulting investigations.

CHAPTER III
Evidence For the Accepted Theory of Accommodation 23

Development of the theory—Behavior of the lens in accommodation as noted by Helmholtz—General acceptance of these observations as facts—Abandonment by Arlt of the true explanation of accommodation—Inability of Helmholtz to explain satisfactorily the supposed change of form in the lens—Question still unsettled—Apparent accommodation in lenseless eyes—Curious and unscientific theories advanced to account for it—Voluntary production of astigmatism—Impossibility of reconciling it with the theory of an inextensible eyeball.

CHAPTER IV
The Truth About Accommodation As Demonstrated By Experiments on the Eye Muscles of Fish, Cats, Dogs, Rabbits and Other Animals . . 38

Disputed function of the external muscles of the eyeball—Once regarded as possible factors in accommodation—This idea dismissed after supposed demonstration that accommodation depends upon the lens—Author's experiments demonstrate that accommodation depends wholly upon these muscles—Accommodation prevented and produced at will by their manipulation—Also errors of refraction—The oblique muscles of accommodation—The recti concerned in the production of hypermetropia and astigmatism—No accommodation with one oblique cut, paralyzed, or absent—Paralysis of accommodation in experimental animals accomplished only by injection of atropine deep into the orbit, so as to reach the oblique muscles—Accommodation unaffected by removal of the lens—Fourth cranial nerve supplying superior oblique muscle a nerve of accommodation—Sources of error believed to have been eliminated in experiments.

CHAPTER V
The Truth About Accommodation As Demonstrated By a Study of Images Reflected From the Cornea, Iris, Lens and Sclera 54

Technique of Helmholtz defective—Image obtained by his method on the front of the lens not sufficiently distinct or stable to be measured—Failure of author to get reliable image with various sources of light—Success with 1,000-watt lamp, diaphragm and condenser—Image photographed—Images on cornea, iris, lens and sclera also photographed—Results confirmed earlier observations—Eyeball changes its shape during accommodation—Lens does not—Strain to see at near-point produces hypermetropia—Strain to see at distance myopia—Method of obtaining the corneal image.

CHAPTER VI
The Truth About Accommodation As Demonstrated By Clinical Observations 69

Results of experimental work confirmed by clinical observations—Atropine supposed to prevent accommodation—Conflict of facts with this theory—Normal accommodation observed in eyes under influence of atropine for long periods—Evidence of these cases against accepted theories overwhelming—Cases of accommodation in lenseless eyes observed by author—Reality of the apparent act of accommodation demonstrated by the retinoscope—Evidence from the cure of presbyopia—Harmony of all clinical observations with views of accommodation and errors of refraction presented in this book.

CHAPTER VII
The Variability of the Refraction of the Eye . . 75

Refractive states supposed to be permanent—Retinoscope demonstrates the contrary—Normal sight never continuous—Refractive errors always changing—Conditions which produce errors of refraction—Variability of refractive states the cause of many accidents—Also of much statistical confusion.

CHAPTER VIII
What Glasses Do to Us 81

The sins of Salvino degli Armati reputed inventor of spectacles—How glasses harm the eyes—Sight never improved by them to normal—Always resented at first by the eye—Objects of vision distorted by them—Disagreeable sensatoins produced—Field of vision contracted—Difficulty of keeping the glass clean—Reflection of light from lenses annoying and dangerous—Inconvenience of glasses to physically active persons—Effect on personal appearance—No muscular strain relieved by them—Apparent benefits often due to mental suggestion—Fortunate that many patients refuse to wear them—At best an unsatisfactory substitute for normal sight.

CHAPTER IX
Cause and Cure of Errors of Refraction . . . 89

All abnormal action of external muscles of the eyeball accompanied by a strain to see—With relief of this strain all errors of refraction disappear—Myopia (or lessening of hypermetropia) associated with strain to see at the distance—Hypermetropia (or lessening of myopia) associated with strain to see at the near-point—Facts easily demonstrated by retinoscope—Effect of strain at the near-point accounts for apparent loss of accommodation in the lenseless eye—Mental origin of eyestrain—Accounts for effect of civilization on the eye—Lower animals affected as man is—Remedy to get rid of mental strain—Temporary relaxation easy—Permanent relaxation may be difficult—Eyes not rested by sleep or tired by use—Rested only by resting the mind—Time required for a cure.

CHAPTER X
Strain 106

Foundation of the strain to see—Act of seeing passive—Same true of action of all sensory nerves—Their efficiency impaired when made the subject of effort—The mind the source of all such efforts brought to bear upon the eye—Mental strain of any kind produces eyestrain—This strain takes many forms—Results in production of many abnormal conditions — Circulation disturbed by strain—Normal circulation restored by mental control—Thus errors of refraction and other abnormal conditions are cured.

CHAPTER XI
Central Fixation 114

The center of sight—The eye normally sees one part of everything it looks at best—Central fixation lost in all abnormal conditions of the eye—Cause of mental strain—With central fixation the eye is perfectly at rest—Can be used indefinitely without fatigue—Open and quiet—No wrinkles or dark circles around it—Visual axes parallel—With eccentric fixation the contrary is the case—Eccentric fixation cured by any method that relieves strain—Limits of vision determined by central fixation—Organic diseases relieved or cured by it—No limit can be set to its possibilities—Relation to general efficiency and general health.

CHAPTER XII
Palming 123

Relaxation with the eyes shut—With light excluded by palms of the hands (palming)—Evidence of complete relaxation in palming—Of incomplete relaxation—Difficulties of palming—How dealt with—Futility of effort—All the sensory nerves relaxed by successful palming—Pain relieved in all parts of the body—Patients who succeed at once are quickly cured—A minority not helped and should try other methods.

^ These are pictures of the Contents pages from the Original Antique book. Free on the website in PDF E-Book. See the text version contents on the following pages for page numbers in this book.

CHAPTER XIII
Memory As an Aid to Vision 136

Memory a test of relaxation—Memory of black most suitable for the purpose—Application of this fact to treatment of functional eye troubles—Sensation not a reliable index of strain—Memory of black is—Enables the patient to avoid conditions that produce strain—Conditions favorable to memory—Retention of memory under unfavorable conditions—Quick cures by its aid—A great help to other mental processes—Tests of a perfect memory.

CHAPTER XIV
Imagination As an Aid to Vision 148

Retinal impressions interpreted by the mind—Memory or imagination normally used as an aid to sight—In imperfect sight the mind adds imperfections to the imperfect retinal image—Only a small part of the phenomena of refractive errors accounted for by the inaccuracy of the focus—Difference between the photographic picture when the camera is out of focus and the visual impressions of the mind when the eye is out of focus—Patients helped by understanding of this fact—Dependence of imagination upon memory—Coincidence of both with sight—Perfect imagination dependent upon relaxation—Therefore imagination cures—Method of using it for this purpose—Remarkable cures effected by it.

CHAPTER XV
Shifting and Swinging 159

Apparent movement of objects regarded with normal vision—Due to unconscious shifting of the eye—Impossibility of fixing a point for an appreciable length of time—lowering of vision by attempt to do so—Inconspicuousness of normal shifting—Its incredible rapidity—Staring an important factor in the production of imperfect sight—Tendency to stare corrected by conscious shifting and realization of apparent movement resulting from it—Conditions of success with shifting—The universal swing—Methods of shifting—Cures effected by this means.

CHAPTER XVI
The Illusions of Imperfect and of Normal Sight . . 172

Normal and abnormal illusions—Illusions of color—Of size—Of form—Of number—Of location—Of non-existent objects—Of complementary colors—Of the color of the sun—Blind spots—Twinkling stars—Cause of illusions of imperfect sight—Voluntary production of illusions—Illusions of central fixation—Normal illusions of color—Illusions produced by shifting—The upright position of objects regarded an illusion.

CHAPTER XVII
Vision Under Adverse Conditions a Benefit to the Eye 183

Erroneous ideas of ocular hygiene—Conditions supposedly injurious may be a benefit to the eye—No foundation for universal fear of the light—Temporary discomfort but no permanent injury from it—Benefits of sun-gazing—Of looking at a strong electric light—Not light but darkness a danger to the eye—Sudden contrasts of light may be beneficial—Advantages of the movies—Benefits of reading fine print—Reading in moving vehicles—In a recumbent posture—Vision under difficult conditions good mental training.

CHAPTER XVIII
Optimums and Pessimums 198

All objects not seen equally well when sight is imperfect—The eye has its optimums and pessimums—Some easily accounted for—Others unaccountable—Familiar objects optimums—Unfamiliar objects pessimums—Examples of unaccountable optimums and pessimums—Variability of optimums and pessimums—Test card usually a pessimum—Pessimums which the patient is not conscious of seeing—Pessimums associated with a strain to see—How pessimums may become optimums.

CHAPTER XIX
The Relief of Pain and Other Symptoms by the Aid of the Memory 202

No pain felt when the memory is perfect—All the senses improved—Efficiency of the mind increased—Operations performed without anaesthetics—Organic disorders relieved—Facts not fully explained, but attested by numerous proofs—Possible relationship of the principle involved to cures of Faith Curists and Christian Scientists.

CHAPTER XX
Presbyopia: Its Cause and Cure 210

Failure of near vision as age advances—Supposed normality of this phenomenon—Near-points expected at different ages—Many do not fit this schedule—Some never become presbyopic—Some retain normal vision for some objects while presbyopic for others—First and second of these classes of cases explained away or ignored—Third not heretofore observed—Presbyopia both preventable and curable—Due to a strain to see at the near-point—No necessary connection with age—Lens may flatten and lose refractive power with advancing years, but not necessarily—Temporary increase of presbyopia by strain at the near-point—Temporary relief by closing the eyes or palming—Permanent relief by permanent relief of strain—How the author cured himself—Other cures—Danger of putting on glasses at the presbyopic age—Prevention of presbyopia.

CHAPTER XXI
Squint and Amblyopia: Their Cause 221

Definition of squint—Theories as to its cause—Failure of these theories to fit the facts—Failure of operative treatment—State of the vision not an important factor—Amblyopia ex anopsia—Association with squint not invariable—Supposed incurability—Spontaneous recovery—Curious forms of double vision in squint—Invariable association of squint and amblyopia with strain—Invariable relief following relief of strain—Voluntary production of squint by strain.

CHAPTER XXII
Squint and Amblyopia: Their Cure 227

Squint and amblyopia purely functional troubles—Cured by any method that relieves strain—Relaxation sometimes gained by voluntary increase of squint, or production of other kinds—Remarkable cure effected in this way—Strain relieved when patient is able to look more nearly in the proper direction—Proper use of a squinting eye encouraged by covering the good eye—Children cured by use of atropine in one or both eyes—Examples of cases cured by eye education.

CHAPTER XXIII
Floating Specks: Their Cause and Cure . . . 236

Floating specks a common phenomenon of imperfect sight—Their appearance and behavior—Theories as to their origin—A fruitful field for the patent-medicine business—Examples of the needless alarm they have caused—May be seen at times by any one—Simply an illusion caused by mental strain—This strain easily relieved—Illustrative cases.

CHAPTER XXIV
Home Treatment 242

Many persons can cure themselves of defective sight—Only necessary to follow a few simple directions—How to test the sight—Children who have not worn glasses cured by reading the Snellen test card every day—Adults of the same class also benefited in a short time—Cases of adults and children who have worn glasses more difficult—Glasses must be discarded—How to make a test card—Need of a teacher in difficult cases—Qualifications of such teachers—Duty of parents.

CHAPTER XXV
Correspondence Treatment 246

Correspondence treatment usually regarded as quackery—Impossible in the case of most diseases—Errors of refraction, not being diseases, admit of such treatment—Glasses successfully fitted by mail—Less room for failure in correspondence treatment of imperfect sight without glasses—Personal treatment more satisfactory, but not always available—Examples of cases cured by correspondence—Need for the co-operation of local practitioners in such treatment.

CHAPTER XXVI
The Prevention of Myopia in Schools: Methods That Failed 251

A much debated question—Literature on the subject voluminous and unreliable—All that is certainly known—Studies of Cohn—Confirmation of his observations by other investigators in America and Europe—Increase of myopia during school life unanimously attributed to near work—Inadequacy of this theory—Failure of preventive measures based upon it—New difficulties—The appeal to heredity—To natural adaptation—Objections to these views—Why all preventive measures have failed.

Contents

CHAPTER XXVII

The Prevention and Cure of Myopia and Other Errors of Refraction in Schools: A Method That Succeeded 259

Production of eyestrain by unfamiliar objects—Relief by familiar objects—Facts furnish the means of preventing and curing errors of refraction in schools—By this means children often gain normal vision with incredible rapidity—Results in schools of Grand Forks, N. D.; New York, and other cities—Improvement in mentality of children as eyesight improved—Reformation of truants and incorrigibles—Hypermetropia and astigmatism prevented and cured—Method succeeded best when teachers did not wear glasses—Success would be greater still under a more rational educational system—Prevalence of defective sight in American children—Its results—Practically all cases preventable and curable—Inexpensiveness of method recommended—Imposes no additional burden on the teachers—Cannot possibly hurt the children—Directions for its use.

CHAPTER XXVIII

The Story of Emily 270

Cure of defective eyesight by cured patients—Cures of fellow students, parents and friends by school children—Remarkable record of Emily—An illustration of the benefits to be expected from the author's method of preventing and curing imperfect sight in school children.

CHAPTER XXIX

Mind and Vision 274

Poor sight one of the most fruitful causes of retardation in schools—More involved in it than inability to see—The result of an abnormal condition of the mind—This cannot be changed by glasses—Memory among faculties impaired when vision is impaired—Memory of primitive man may have been due to the same cause as his keen vision—A modern example of primitive memory combined with primitive keenness of vision—Correspondence between differences in the faculty of memory and differences in visual acuity—Memory and eyesight of children spoiled by the same causes—Both dependent upon interest—Illustrative cases—All the mental faculties improved when vision becomes normal—Examples of such improvement—Relief of symptoms of insanity by eye education—Facts indicate a close relation between the problems of vision and those of education.

CHAPTER XXX

Normal Sight and the Relief of Pain for Soldiers and Sailors 284

Growth of militarism in the United States—Demand for universal military training—Lack of suitable material for such training—Defective eyesight greatest impediment to the raising of an efficient army—None more easily removed—Plan for correcting defects of vision submitted to Surgeon General during the war—Not acted upon—Now presented to the public with some modifications—First requisite eye education in schools and colleges—Eye education in training camps and at the front also needed, even for those whose sight is normal—How school system might be modified for military and naval use—Soldiers should not be allowed to wear glasses—Importance of eye training to aviators—Eye training for the relief of pain.

CHAPTER XXXI

Letters from Patients 290

Army officer cures himself—A teacher's experiences—Mental effects of central fixation—Relief after twenty-five years—Search for myopia cure rewarded—Facts versus theories—Cataract relieved by central fixation.

CHAPTER XXXII

Reason and Authority 304

Inaccessibility of average mind to reason—Facts discredited if contrary to authority—Patients discredit their own experience under this influence—Cure of cataract ignored by medical profession—Expulsion of author from N. Y. Post Graduate Medical School for curing myopia—Man not a reasoning being—Consequences to the world.

LIST OF ILLUSTRATIONS

Portrait of Ferdinand von Arlt .... Frontispiece

FIG.		PAGE
1.	Patagonians	2
2.	African Pigmies	3
3.	Moros from the Philippines	6
4.	Diagram of the hypermetropic, emmetropic and myopic eyeballs	11
5.	The eye as a camera	13
6.	Mexican Indians	15
7.	Ainus, the aboriginal inhabitants of Japan	16
8.	The usual method of using the retinoscope	18
9.	Diagrams of the images of Purkinje	24
10.	Diagram by which Helmholtz illustrated his theory of accommodation	27
11.	Portrait of Thomas Young	28
12.	Portrait of Hermann Ludwig Ferdinand von Helmholtz	31
13.	Demonstration upon the eye of a rabbit that the inferior oblique muscle is an essential factor in accommodation	40
14.	Demonstration upon the eye of a carp that the superior oblique muscle is essential to accommodation	41
15.	Demonstration upon the eye of a rabbit that the production of refractive errors is dependent upon the action of the external muscles	42
16.	Demonstration upon the eye of a fish that the production of myopic and hypermetropic refraction is dependent upon the action of the extrinsic muscles	43
17.	Production and relief of mixed astigmatism in the eye of a carp	45
18.	Demonstration upon the eyeball of a rabbit that the obliques lengthen the visual axis in myopia	46
19.	Demonstration upon the eye of a carp that the recti shorten the visual axis in hypermetropia	47
20.	Lens pushed out of the axis of vision	48
21.	Rabbit with lens removed	49
22.	Experiment upon the eye of a cat, demonstrating that the fourth nerve, which supplies only the superior oblique muscle, is just as much a nerve of accommodation as the third, and that the superior oblique muscle which it supplies is a muscle of accommodation	50-51
23.	Pithing a fish preparatory to operating upon its eyes	52
24.	Arrangements for photographing images reflected from the eyeball	55
25.	Arrangements for holding the head of the subject steady while images were being photographed	56
26.	Image of electric filament on the front of the lens	57
27.	Images of the electric filament reflected simultaneously from the cornea and lens	58
28.	Image of electric filament upon the cornea	60
29.	Image of electric filament on the front of the sclera	62
30.	Images on the side of the sclera	63
31.	Multiple images upon the front of the lens	64
32.	Reflection of the electric filament from the iris	65
33.	Demonstrating that the back of the lens does not change during accommodation	67
34.	Straining to see at the near-point produces hypermetropia	90
35.	Myopia produced by unconscious strain to see at the distance is increased by conscious strain	91
36.	Immediate production of myopia and myopic astigmatism in eyes previously normal by strain to see at the distance	92-93
37.	Myopic astigmatism comes and goes according as the subject looks at distant objects with or without strain	94
38.	Patient who has had the lens of the right eye removed for cataract produces changes in the refraction of this eye by strain	96-97
39.	A family group strikingly illustrating the effect of the mind upon the vision	99
40.	Myopes who never went to school, or read in the Subway	100
41.	One of the many thousands of patients cured of errors of refraction by the methods presented in this book	104
42.	Palming	125
43.	Patient with atrophy of the optic nerve gets flashes of improved vision after palming	127
44.	Paralysis of the seventh nerve cured by palming	131
45.	Glaucoma cured by palming	133
46.	Woman with normal vision looking directly at the sun	187
47.	Woman aged 37—child aged 4, both looking directly at the sun without discomfort	189
48.	Focussing the rays of the sun upon the eye of a patient by means of a burning glass	191
49.	Specimen of diamond type	195
50.	Photographic type reduction	195
51.	Operating without anaesthetics	204
52.	Neuralgia relieved by palming and the memory of black	207
53.	Voluntary production of squint by strain to see	223
54.	Case of divergent vertical squint cured by eye education	230
55.	Temporary cure of squint by memory of a black period	232
56.	Face-rest designed by Kallmann, a German optician	254

CENTRAL FIXATION - SEE CLEAR WITH THE CENTER OF THE VISUAL FIELD

THE RETINA CONTAINS CONES AND RODS - LIGHT, ENERGY RECEPTORS.
CONES PRODUCE VERY CLEAR VISION - CLEARER THAN 20/20 AND BRIGHT COLOR.
RODS PRODUCE LESS CLEAR VISION (20/400) - RODS PERCEIVE GREY/BLACK/WHITE, LIGHT AND DARK BUT NO OTHER COLORS. RODS DETECT MOVEMENT OF OBJECTS IN THE VISUAL FIELD AND CONTINUE TO FUNCTION IN ALMOST COMPLETE DARKNESS.
THE FOVEA AND MACULA IN THE CENTER OF THE RETINA CONTAIN MANY CONES, (ONLY CONES IN THE CENTER OF THE FOVEA) AND PRODUCE VERY CLEAR VISION IN THE CENTER OF THE VISUAL FIELD.
THE PERIPHERAL FIELD OF THE RETINA AROUND, NEAR AND AWAY FROM THE FOVEA/MACULA CONTAINS LESS CONES AND MORE RODS, AND ONLY RODS (NO CONES) IN THE FAR OUTER PERIPHERAL FIELD.
THIS RESULTS IN LESS CLEAR PERIPHERAL VISION, THE FAR OUTER PERIPHERAL FIELD BEING MOST UNCLEAR.
SEE CLEAR WITH CENTRAL FIXATION - A CORRECT VISION HABIT - PLACE THE OBJECT OF VISUAL ATTENTION IN THE CENTER OF THE VISUAL FIELD.
WHEN THE EYES USE THE CENTER OF THE VISUAL FIELD, THE CENTRAL RAY FOCUS PERFECT ON THE CENTER OF THE FOVEA CENTRALIS, RAYS CLOSEST TO THE CENTRAL RAY FOCUS ON THE MACULA, AND PERIPHERAL RAYS FOCUS PERFECTLY ON THE PERIPHERAL FIELD OF THE RETINA RESULTING IN PERFECT CLEAR CENTRAL VISION, CLEARER THAN 20/20 AND MAXIMUM CLARITY AND FUNCTION OF THE PERIPHERAL FIELD. THE CLARITY OF THE ENTIRE VISUAL FIELD IMPROVES.

Video - http://www.youtube.com/watch?v=nIrKuQEJ6y4

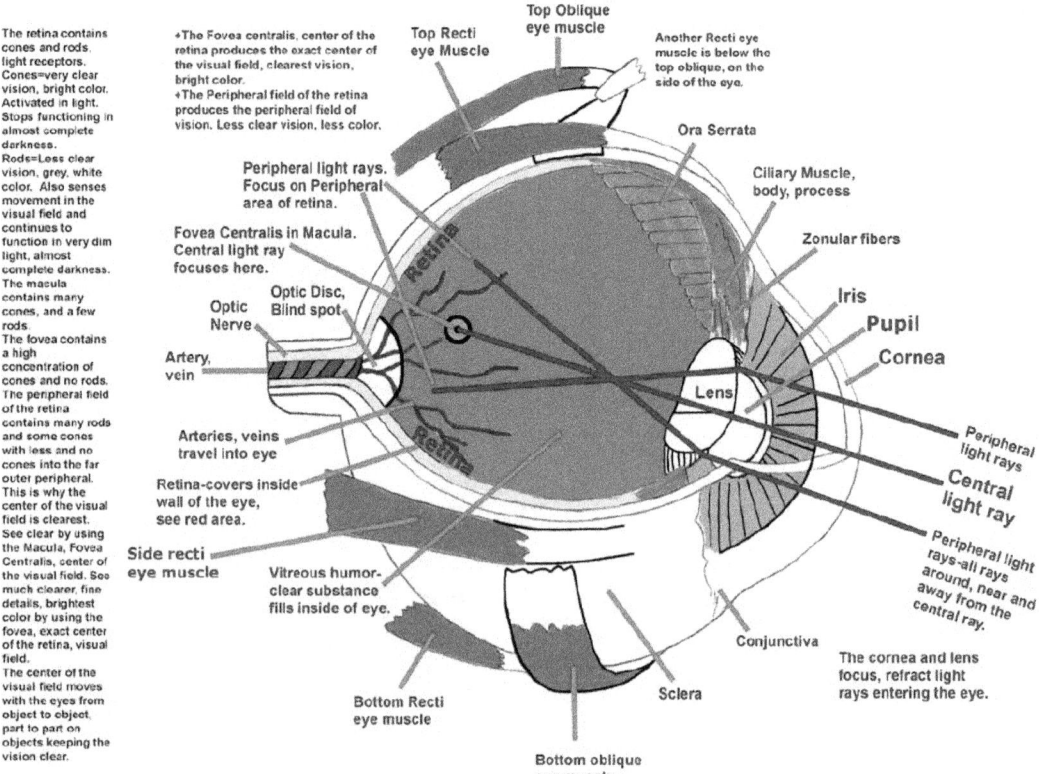

Eye socket, bones, eye, eye muscles, optic nerve.

Notice that the eye socket is composed of bone segments, aligned, grown together. These are part of the skull bones. Eye muscles attach to the skull bones in the back of the eye socket. Misalignment of the eye socket or skull bones due to accidents, birth trauma, forcep, suction delivery... can mis-align the bones, place pressure, tension on/in the eye, optic nerve, eye muscles resulting in crossed, wandering eyes, imperfect convergence, divergence, accommodation, un-accommodation, unclear vision, astigmatism and other abnormal eye conditions. Special chiropractors (Cranial, Cranio Sacral Therapy, Osteopathy) can re-align the bones of the skull if needed. Often, use of the Bates method alone can correct eye function and clarity of the vision.

Fundamentals
By
W. H. Bates, M. D.

1 - Glasses discarded permanently.

2 - Central fixation is seeing best where you are looking.
 Central-Fixation; Place the object you are looking at in the center of the eyes' visual field. The central field moves with the eyes as the eyes-vision shift (move) from part to part on an object and from object to object. The head moves with the eyes.

3 - Favorable conditions: Light may be bright or dim. The distance of the print from the eyes, where seen best, also varies with people.
 Read fine print in the sunlight daily to keep the eyesight clear in bright and dim light. Allow sunlight to shine inside the home.

4 - Shifting: With normal sight the eyes are moving all the time.

5 - Swinging: When the eyes move slowly or rapidly from side to side, stationary objects appear to move in the opposite direction.
 Oppositional Movement 'The Swing'.

6 - Long Swing: Stand with the feet about one foot apart, turn the body to the right --at the same time lifting the heel of the left foot. Do not move the head or eyes or pay any attention to the apparent movement of stationary objects. *
Now place the left heel on the floor, turn the body to the left, raising the heel of the right foot. Alternate.

 * Long Swing - Clarification; the head and eyes <u>do move</u>. They move <u>with the body, in the same direction, at the same time</u>. Synchronized; body, head, eyes moving together right, left, right, left... Easy, continual. Do NOT move the head, eyes in a direction opposite to the body's movement. Do not lock onto and try to see clearly objects that appear to swing by in the opposite direction as you move right and left. Do not try to stop the movement of the objects. Just relax and swing.
 See Dr. Bates additional directions on the right > (An alternate method allows a quick 'fraction of a second' glance-*shift* on a letter on 2 eyecharts placed on the left and right sides of the body. Swinging is not interrupted.)

LONG SWING: Stand with the feet about one foot apart. Turn the body to the right, at the same time lifting the heel of the left foot. The head and eyes move with the movement of the body. Do not pay any attention to the apparent movement of stationary objects. Now place the left heel on the floor, turn the body to the left, raising the heel of the right foot. Alternate. Pain and fatigue are relieved promptly while practicing this swing. When done correctly, relief is felt in a short time. The long swing, when done before retiring, lessens eyestrain during sleep.

7 - Drifting Swing: When using this method, one pays no attention to the clearness of stationary objects, which appear to be moving. The eyes move from point to point slowly, easily, or lazily, so that the stare or strain may be avoided.

8 - Variable Swing: Hold the forefinger of one hand six inches from the right eye and about the same distance to the right, look straight ahead and move the head a short distance from side to side. The finger appears to move.
 * Clarification for #8, Variable Swing; <u>The eyes *move*, with the head, in the same direction</u>. Look straight ahead and then; move the head and eyes together side to side. See the finger appear to move opposite the head-eyes movement.
 This can also be done with the finger 6 inches in front of the face/nose, at eye level, between the left and right eyes.

9 - Stationary Objects Moving: By moving the head and eyes a short distance from side to side, being sure to blink, one can imagine stationary objects to be moving. Oppositional Movement 'The Swing'; Stationary objects appear to move opposite of the movement 'shift' of the eyes, head. The object swings in the opposite direction. This is relaxing, improves the vision.

10 - Memory: Improving the memory of letters and other objects improves the vision for everything.

11 - Imagination: We see only what we think we see, or what we imagine. We can only imagine what we remember.
 Memory, imagination, remembering-imagining objects clear. Clear pictures stored in the mind. The brain and eyes work together; When the brain's function, memory and imagination improve; the vision improves. When the vision improves; the brain's function, memory and imagination improve. Each strengthens the other. Relaxation also works with, improves all these functions.

12 - Rest: All cases of imperfect sight are improved by closing the eyes and resting them.

13 - Palming: The closed eyes may be covered by the palm of one or both hands. (Preferably both hands.) Practice memory, imagination and relaxation with palming. Palming and other activities, correct eye-vision functions listed above are completely described with pictures in the book chapters and at the end of this book. See Better Eyesight Magazine.
14 - Blinking: The normal eye blinks, or closes and opens very frequently.

15 - Mental Pictures: As long as one is awake one has all kinds of memories of mental pictures. If these pictures are remembered easily, perfectly, the vision is benefited. Memory and imagination; remembering, imagining objects clear. Clear mental pictures. Happy thoughts, memories, imagination of places, experiences, creations, fantasies... Practice with or without palming.

Extra directions-clarifications (in Navy text) are added to Dr. Bates, Emily's books and Better Eyesight Magazine. Dr. Bates is not here to teach us in person. He included the entire instructions in his book, magazine. Five practices needed directions combined so the reader does not need to search through 2700 pages for entire description-steps; Head-Eyes, Body Moving Together when doing-seeing the Swings. Seeing the Opposite Swing on Close and Far Objects. Sunning and the Sunglass, Seeing the Glowing White Spaces between sentences and around letters 'Halos'.

The Original Method for Practicing Natural Eyesight Improvement
Described by Ophthalmologist William H. Bates

BETTER EYESIGHT
September, 1927
Perfect Sight
By William H. Bates

If you learn the fundamental principles of perfect sight and will consciously keep them in mind your defective vision will disappear. The following discoveries were made by W. H. Bates, M. D., and his method is based on them. With it he has cured so-called incurable cases:

I. Many blind people are curable.

II. All errors of refraction are functional, therefore curable.

III. All defective vision is due to strain in some form.

You can demonstrate to your own satisfaction that strain lowers the vision.
When you stare, you strain. Look fixedly at one object for five seconds or longer. What happens? The object blurs and finally disappears. Also, your eyes are made uncomfortable by this experiment. When you rest your eyes for a few moments the vision is improved and the discomfort relieved.

IV. Strain is relieved by relaxation.

To use your eyes correctly all day long, it is necessary that you:

1. Blink frequently. Staring is a strain and always lowers the vision.

2. Shift your glance constantly from one point to another, seeing the part regarded best and other parts not so clearly. That is, when you look at a chair, do not try to see the whole object at once; look first at the back of it, seeing that part best and other parts worse. Remember to blink as you quickly shift your glance from the back to the seat and legs, seeing each part best, in turn. This is central-fixation. (with shifting.)

3. Your head and eyes are moving all day long. Imagine that stationary objects are moving in the direction opposite to the movement of your head and eyes. When you walk about the room or on the street, notice that the floor or pavement seems to come toward you, while objects on either side appear to move in the direction opposite to the movement of your body.

BETTER EYESIGHT
December, 1927
INSTRUCTIONS FOR HOME TREATMENT
By William H. Bates

The most important fact is to impress upon the patient the necessity of discarding his glasses. He is told that when glasses are used temporarily a relapse always follows and the patient loses for a short time, at least, everything that has been gained. If it is impossible or unnecessary for the patient to return at regular intervals for further treatment and supervision, he is given instructions for home practice to suit his individual case, and is asked to report his progress or difficulties at frequent intervals.

The importance of practicing certain parts of the routine treatment at all times, such as blinking, central-fixation, shifting and imagining stationary objects to be moving opposite to the movement of his head and eyes, is stressed.
The normal eye does these things unconsciously, and the imperfect eye must at first practice them consciously until it becomes an <u>unconscious habit.</u>

The Natural Vision Improvement student practices 'imitates' these normal, natural eye-vision, body, mind... functions (Relaxed, Natural, Correct Vision Habits) to gently coax the eyes-vision, brain, eye muscles, body (visual system) back to normal, relaxed function with clear vision. Then; the eyes, brain, body... function correct, automatically <u>on their own</u> maintaining clear vision. All of Dr. Bates 132 Better Eyesight Magazine Issues, practices are in the E-Books. Read them; learn a variety of his techniques to obtain relaxation and movement. Choose practices that work best, easy for you. Maintain natural correct vision habits; shifting, central-fixation, movement, the opposite swing, memory-imagination, relaxed full breathing, blinking, sunlight. With practice they will become automatic, occur on their own. Sunlight will become like food; a healthy daily nourishment. Spiritual and Chi... energy improvement and Massage, posture is beneficial.

Original Fundamentals by Dr. William H. Bates, Emily Lierman from *Better Eyesight Magazine* and Emily's book *Stories From The Clinic*

Fundamentals
By
W. H. Bates, M. D.

1. Glasses discarded permanently.

2. Central Fixation is seeing best where you are looking.

3. Favorable conditions: Light may be bright or dim. The distance of the print from the eyes, where seen best, also varies with people.

4. Shifting: With normal sight the eyes are moving all the time.

5. Swinging: When the eyes move slowly or rapidly from side to side, stationary objects appear to move in the opposite direction.

6. Long Swing: Stand with the feet about one foot apart, turn the body to the right—at the same time lifting the heel of the left foot. Do not move the head or eyes or pay any attention to the apparent movement of stationary objects. Now place the left heel on the floor, turn the body to the left, raising the heel of the right foot. Alternate.

7. Drifting Swing: When practicing this swing, one pays no attention to the clearness of stationary objects, which appear to be moving. The eyes wander from point to point slowly, easily, or lazily, so that the stare or strain may be avoided.

8. **Variable Swing:** Hold the forefinger of one hand six inches from the right eye and about the same distance to the right, look straight ahead and move the head a short distance from side to side. The finger appears to move.

9. **Stationary Objects Moving:** By moving the head and eyes a short distance from side to side, being sure to blink, one can imagine stationary objects to be moving.

10. **Memory:** Improving the memory of letters and other objects improves the vision for everything.

11. **Imagination:** We see only what we think we see, or what we imagine. We can only imagine what we remember.

12. **Rest:** All cases of imperfect sight are improved by closing the eyes and resting them.

13. **Palming:** The closed eyes may be covered with the palm of one or both hands.

14. **Blinking:** The normal eye blinks, or closes and opens very frequently.

15. **Mental Pictures:** As long as one is awake one has all kinds of memories of mental pictures. If these pictures are remembered easily, perfectly, the vision is benefited.

< This is a card given to patients that have received in person vision training by Dr. Bates and Emily Lierman-Bates at their Clinic.

Entire directions for #6, 8 are placed below;

The head and eyes DO move when doing the Long Swing; The head and eyes move <u>with the body, in the same direction</u>, moving together in synchronization, swinging to the left, then to the right, then back to the left, right...

The description for #6 means;

As you swing, DO NOT turn-move the head, eyes in a direction that is *opposite* of where the body is moving, turning to. Do not move the head, eyes in any different direction. Keep them moving in the same direction with the body; head-eyes-shoulders-body all moving together. Do not stop or turn back to look at objects that appear to move 'swing by' in the opposite direction-going past the eyes, body as you swing. Avoid locking the eyes-vision on the moving objects. Let the objects move opposite.

Example of correct movement;
When moving, turning the body left <;
the eyes, head also move, turn left <.
When moving, turning the body right >;
the eyes, head also move, turn right >.

When swinging left and right the eyes can look at-shift on 'for a *fraction of a second'* a letter on eyecharts placed on the left and right sides of the body. Keep the eyes, head and body moving. Do NOT stop, do not slow down the left and right swinging. See picture in the eyecharts chapter.

Clarification for #8. Start; The head and eyes look straight ahead. Then; the head and eyes move side to side, moving <u>together</u> left and right. See the finger appear to move 'swing' in the opposite direction. A variation is to place the finger in front of the face; between the eyes, at eye level. Move the head and eyes side to side. Don't lock the eyes on the finger.

Relax, move and blink.

Memory.—When the sight is normal the mind is always perfectly at rest, and when the memory is perfect the mind is also at rest. Therefore it is possible to improve the sight by the use of the memory. Anything the patient finds it agreeable to remember is a rest to the mind, but for purposes of practice a small black object, such as a period or a letter of diamond type, is usually most convenient. The most favorable condition for the exercise of the memory is, usually, with the eyes closed and covered, but by practice it becomes possible to remember equally well with the eyes open. When patients are able, with their eyes closed and covered, to remember perfectly a letter of diamond type, it appears, just as it would if they were looking at it with the bodily eyes, to have a slight movement, while the openings appear whiter than the rest of the background. If they are not able to remember it, they are told to shift consciously from one side of the letter to another and to consciously imagine the opening whiter than the rest of the background. When they do this, the letter usually appears to move in a direction contrary to that of the imagined movement of the eye, and they are able to remember it indefinitely.

Fundamentals

1. Glasses discarded permanently.
2. Favorable conditions: Light may be bright or dim. The distance of the print from the eyes, where seen best, also varies with people.
3. Central Fixation is seeing best where you are looking.
4. Shifting: With normal sight the eyes are moving all the time. This should be practiced continuously and consciously.
5. Swinging: When the eyes move slowly or rapidly from side to side, stationary objects appear to move in the opposite direction.
6. Long Swing: Stand with the feet about one foot apart, turn the body to the right—at the same time lifting the heel of the left foot. Do not move the head or eyes or pay any attention to the apparent movement of stationary objects. Now place the left heel on the floor, turn the body to the left, raising the heel of the right foot. Alternate. This exercise can be practiced just before retiring at night fifty times or more. When done properly, it is a great rest and relieves pain, fatigue, and other symptoms of imperfect sight.
7. Stationary Objects Moving: By moving the head and eyes a short distance from side to side, one can imagine stationary objects to be moving. Since the normal eye is moving all the time, one should imagine all stationary objects to be moving. Never imagine that you see a stationary object stationary.
8. Palming: The closed eyes may be covered with the palm of one or both hands. The patient should rest the eyes and think of something else that is pleasant.
9. Blinking: The normal eye blinks, or closes and opens very frequently. If one does not blink, the vision always becomes worse.

SUGGESTIONS TO PATIENTS
The Use of the Snellen Test Card

1—Every home should have a test card.

2—It is best to place the card permanently on the wall in a good light.

3—Each member of the family or household read the card every day.

4—It takes only a minute to test the sight with the card. If you spend five minutes in the morning practicing with the card, it will be a great help during the day.

5—Place yourself ten feet from the card and read as far as you can without effort or strain. Over each line of letters are small figures indicating the distance. Over the big C at the top is the figure 50. The big C, therefore, should be read at a distance of 50 feet.

6—If you can only see the fifth line, notice that the last letter on that line is an R. Now close your eyes, cover them with the palms of the hands and remember the R. If you will remember that the left side is straight, the right side partly curved and the bottom open, you will get a good mental picture of the R with your eyes closed. This mental picture will help you to see the letter directly underneath the R, which is a T.

7—Shifting is good to stop the stare. If you stare at the letter T, you will notice that all the letters on that line begin to blur. It is beneficial to close your eyes quickly after you see the T, open them, and shift to the first figure on that line, which is a 3. Then close your eyes and remember the 3. You will become able to read all the letters on that line by closing your eyes for each letter.

8—Keep a record of each test in order to note your progress from day to day.

Clarification For Fundamentals # 6 and 7;

6 - When doing the Long Swing the head and eyes DO move; The head and eyes move with the body. The head, eyes and body move together, at the same time, in the same direction; right, left, right, left... (start direction of the swing can be left or right.)

This relaxes the mind, body, eyes and brings clear eyesight.

Dr. Bates and Emily are saying; Do NOT move the head and eyes OPPOSITE of, away from the direction the body is swinging to. Keep the eyes, head and body moving together. Do not stop to look at, see clearly stationary objects appearing to move 'swing by' in the opposite direction of the eyes, head and body's movement. Do not try to stop the movement of stationary objects. Just relax and swing.

See the previous 'Fundamentals Page' and chapters, pictures in this book for Long Swing, Sway examples, pictures.

7; The shift 'movement' of the eyes and head causes stationary objects to appear to move 'swing' past the eyes-head in the opposite direction - opposite of the direction the eyes-head (your central field of vision) are moving to. Try Dr. Bates 2 swings on the right. > The shift of the eyes causes the opposite movement. Shift left and right on the letter O. See it move in the opposite direction.

Seeing stationary objects move is a healthy illusion of the visual system. Imagining it, looking for it, inducing it helps to bring back perfect eye movement 'shifting', central-fixation and clear eyesight.

Universal Swing: The patient stands and sways the body from side to side. While the body is moving, the eyes are moving, and stationary objects nearby which have a background appear to move in the opposite direction to the movement of the head and eyes. Objects located at more distant points which have no background always appear to move in the same direction as the movement of the body. If the finger is held before the eyes while the head is moved from side to side, one may, by practice, become able to imagine that everything connected with the finger, either directly or indirectly, is moving in the opposite direction, while the background is moving in the same direction. The universal swing is very beneficial and usually prevents and cures pain, dizziness, and other nervous symptoms.

DRIFTING SWING: The patient does not think of nor regard anything longer than a fraction of a second. It is helpful in doing this for the patient to imagine himself floating down a river. He may be able to imagine the drifting movement of the boat in which he is floating, better with the eyes closed than with them open. In this case, alternate the imagination with the eyes open and with them closed. The imagination may be improved in this way. Shift continually, easy, relaxed from one object to another.

The Fundamental Principles of Treatment

Derived from Dr. Bates Better Eyesight Magazine - June, 1921 & Other Issues

HOW TO DEMONSTRATE THE FUNDAMENTAL PRINCIPLES OF TREATMENT

Experience, demonstrate that strain lowers the vision; Close the eyes and think of something disagreeable, some physical discomfort, or something seen imperfectly. When the eyes are opened, it will be found that the vision has been lowered. Next; repeat and think something pleasant, happy - open, notice clear vision.
Staring causes strain, blurred vision. Shift, blink to relax and see clear.

Closing, Resting the Eyes

Palming

Central-Fixation

Shifting and Swinging

Memory

Imagination

Flashing & Blinking

Reading Familiar Letters

Practice with the Test Card

Sun Treatment - Sunning

Shifting on Small Objects,

Shifting on, Reading Tiny Letters, Fine Print Daily

Read a variety of examples, directions for these steps in this book.
And in Dr. Bates' Better Eyesight Magazine, 2400+ pages in the PDF E-Books.

Adults can experience free Natural Eyesight Improvement Training by watching how children (that have clear vision) use their eyes-vision; relaxed, their eyes move, 'shift' often, easily, clear vision occurs effortless, automatically without thinking about-controlling their eyes and vision. Do not let the child know you are watching their eyes because this might cause them to start thinking about their eyes, clarity of vision, try to control eye function. This will interfere with completely natural, normal eye function and visual clarity. Similar to a eye doctor placing a lot of pressure on a child to see an eyechart clear. The child must be allowed to see the chart in a relaxed state, memorize the letters. Relaxation, good memory produces clear eyesight. Imitate, practice the child's correct visual system functions.

Many persons fail to secure a temporary improvement of vision by closing their eyes, because they do not keep them closed long enough. Children will seldom do this unless a grown person stands by and encourages them. Many adults also require supervision.

To demonstrate that strain lowers the vision, think of something disagreeable—some physical discomfort, or something seen imperfectly. When the eyes are opened, it will be found that the vision has been lowered. Also stare at one part of a letter on the test card, or try to see the whole letter all alike at one time. This invariably lowers the vision, and may cause the letters to disappear.

It can always be demonstrated that when the normal eye looks intently at one point the vision always becomes imperfect. The normal eye, with normal sight does not stare and to avoid the stare is continuously moving. When it moves from side to side the letter regarded appears to move in the opposite directions but usually the movement is so short, so slow, so easy that most people do not notice it. The eye with imperfect sight does not usually see things moving because it is usually staring. The eye with imperfect sight can be benefited by practicing seeing things moving. This can be done properly, successfully or it can be done wrong, without benefit. When done properly the eye is at rest, when done improperly the eye is under a strain and this strain can usually be felt by the patient when his attention is called to it. It is a great help to the cure of imperfect sight to have the patient demonstrate what is wrong. When you know what is the matter with you that makes it possible to bring about relief.

Ophthalmologist William H. Bates

One of Dr. Bates first Natural Eyesight Treatment Without Glasses Medical Articles which began in the 1800's;

New York Medical Journal, August 30, 1913, Vol. 98 - Page 410-413

MYOPIA PREVENTION BY TEACHERS.

By W. H. BATES, M. D.,
New York.

Myopia with elongation of the eyeball is incurable. It is usually acquired during school life. Acute myopia, spasm of the accommodation, or functional myopia is an early stage of incurable myopia. The cause of myopia is an effort to see distant objects.

Corroboration: 1. Myopic refraction has always been produced in man and the lower animals when regarding unfamiliar distant objects which required an effort. 2. Myopia was prevented in the

[NEW YORK MEDICAL JOURNAL]

public schools of Grand Forks, N. D., for eight years by methods which prevented an effort to see distant objects. 3. Myopia was always benefited by treatment suggested by the cause. 4. The cause suggested a method for the experimental production of myopia in rabbits, dogs, and cats. 5. Physicians, teachers, and others interested have investigated and confirmed these facts. 6. It should be emphasized that there is but *one* cause of myopia, an effort to see distant objects. There is no other cause.

Near use of the eyes is not a cause of myopia. By the aid of simultaneous retinoscopy, it was always demonstrated that an effort to see near objects lessened myopic refraction or produced hypermetropic refraction.

Prevention of diseases is usually suggested by the cause. When the cause is known, prevention may be successful, but when the cause is not known prevention is uncertain. For example: Yellow fever, twenty five years ago, was not prevented by quarantine, disinfection, or other methods until the cause was discovered, the infected mosquito. By removing the cause, yellow fever has been eliminated from Havana and Panama.

Likewise, previous efforts to prevent myopia have failed because the cause was not known. It was erroneously believed that when school children regarded, or made an effort to see, distant objects, that the eyes were at rest or that accommodation or myopic refraction did not occur. Simultaneous retinoscopy disproved this assumption. It has been repeatedly demonstrated with the aid of the retinoscope that all school children with normal eyes when regarding unfamiliar writing or figures on the blackboard, distant maps, diagrams, or pictures had myopic refraction. It was quite otherwise when they regarded a familiar distant object. The retinoscope used at the same time indicated no myopic refraction.

The Snellen test card, while being of use for testing the acuity of vision, was found also during the past ten years to be the best distant object for exercises in distant vision. It should be memorized and thus made a familiar distant object. After its daily use for half a minute or longer myopia was prevented; and, in addition the vision of many pupils with defective sight was improved for an unfamiliar Snellen card, for writing and figures on the blackboard, and for other distant objects. Furthermore, near vision was benefited by the use of the Snellen card. Many pupils stated that they could study their lessons with less or no discomfort.

Myopia prevention was introduced in Public Schools Nos. 6, 183, and 186 of New York city, January, 1912; later, Public Schools Nos. 46 and 43 tested the method.

A Snellen test card was placed permanently where all the pupils could see it from their seats. Daily the teachers recommended all the children to silently read the card with each eye separately, covering the other eye with the palm of the hand in such a way as to avoid pressure on the eyeball.

CONTENTS
PREFACE, THE FUNDAMENTAL PRINCIPLE - Pg. 12
CHAPTER I - Pg. 12

Introductory 12

Prevalence of errors of refraction—Believed to be incurable and practically unpreventable—The eye regarded as a blunder of Nature—Facts which seem to justify this conclusion—Failure of all efforts to prevent the development of eye defects—Futility of prevailing methods of treatment—Conflict of facts with the theory of incurability of errors of refraction—These facts commonly explained away or ignored—The author unable to ignore them, or to accept current explanations—Finally forced to reject accepted theories.

CHAPTER II
Simultaneous Retinoscopy 20
Retinoscopy the source of much of the information presented in this book—What the retinoscope is—Its possibilities not realized—Commonly used only under artificial conditions—Used by the author under the conditions of life on human beings and the lower animals—Thus many new facts were discovered—Conflict of these facts with accepted theories—Resulting investigations.

CHAPTER III
Evidence For the Accepted Theory of Accommodation 22
Development of the theory—Behavior of the lens in accommodation as noted by Helmholtz—General acceptance of these observations as facts—Abandonment by Arlt of the true explanation of accommodation—Inability of Helmholtz to explain satisfactorily the supposed change of form in the lens—Question still unsettled—Apparent accommodation in lensless eyes—Curious and unscientific theories advanced to account for it—Voluntary production of astigmatism—Impossibility of reconciling it with the theory of an inextensible eyeball.

CHAPTER IV
The Truth About Accommodation As Demonstrated By Experiments on the Eye Muscles of Fish, Cats, Dogs, Rabbits and Other Animals 28
Disputed function of the external muscles of the eyeball—Once regarded as possible factors in accommodation—This idea dismissed after supposed demonstration that accommodation depends upon the lens—Author's experiments demonstrate that accommodation depends wholly upon these muscles—Accommodation prevented and produced at will by their manipulation—Also errors of refraction—The oblique muscles of accommodation—The recti concerned in the production of hypermetropia and astigmatism—No accommodation with one oblique cut, paralyzed, or absent—Paralysis of accommodation in experimental animals accomplished only by injection of atropine deep into the orbit, so as to reach the oblique muscles—Accommodation unaffected by removal of the lens—Fourth cranial nerve supplying superior oblique muscle a nerve of accommodation—Sources of error believed to have been eliminated in experiments.

CHAPTER V
The Truth About Accommodation As Demonstrated By a Study of Images Reflected From the Cornea, Iris, Lens and Sclera 34
Technique of Helmholtz defective—Image obtained by his method on the front of the lens not sufficiently distinct or stable to be measured—Failure of author to get reliable image with various sources of light—Success with 1,000-watt lamp, diaphragm and condenser—Image photographed—Images on cornea, iris, lens and sclera also photographed—Results confirmed earlier observations—Eyeball changes its shape during accommodation—Lens does not—Strain to see at near-point produces hypermetropia—Strain to see at distance myopia—Method of obtaining the corneal image.

CHAPTER VI
The Truth About Accommodation As Demonstrated By Clinical Observations. 40
Results of experimental work confirmed by clinical observations—Atropine supposed to prevent accommodation—Conflict of facts with this theory—Normal accommodation observed in eyes under influence of atropine for long periods—Evidence of these cases against accepted theories overwhelming—Cases of accommodation in lensless eyes observed by author—Reality of the apparent act of accommodation demonstrated by the retinoscope—Evidence from the cure of presbyopia—Harmony of all clinical observations with views of accommodation and errors of refraction presented in this book.

CHAPTER VII
The Variability of the Refraction of the Eye 42
Refractive states supposed to be permanent—Retinoscope demonstrates the contrary—Normal sight never continuous—Refractive errors always changing—Conditions which produce errors of refraction—Variability of refractive states the cause of many accidents—Also of much statistical confusion.

CHAPTER VIII
What Glasses Do to Us . . . 44
The sins of Salvino degli Armati, reputed inventor of spectacles—How glasses harm the eyes—Sight never improved by them to normal—Always resented at first by the eye—Objects of vision distorted by them—Disagreeable sensations produced—Field of vision contracted—Difficulty of keeping the glass clean—Reflection of light from lenses annoying and dangerous—Inconvenience of glasses to physically active persons—Effect on personal appearance—No muscular strain relieved by them—Apparent benefits often due to mental suggestion—Fortunate that many patients refuse to wear them—At best an unsatisfactory substitute for normal sight.

CHAPTER IX
Cause and Cure of Errors of Refraction. . . . 47
All abnormal action of external muscles of the eyeball accompanied by a strain to see—With relief of this strain all errors of refraction disappear—Myopia (or lessening of hypermetropia) associated with strain to see at the distance—Hypermetropia (or lessening of myopia) associated with strain to see at the near-point—Facts easily demonstrated by retinoscope—Effect of strain at the near-point accounts for apparent loss of accommodation in the lensless eye—Mental origin of eyestrain—Accounts for effect of civilization on the eye—Lower animals affected as man is—Remedy to get rid of mental strain—Temporary relaxation easy—Permanent relaxation may be difficult—Eyes not rested by sleep or tired by use—Rested only by resting the mind—Time required for a cure.

CHAPTER X
Strain 54
Foundation of the strain to see—Act of seeing passive—Same true of action of all sensory nerves—Their efficiency impaired when made the subject of effort—The mind the source of all such efforts brought to bear upon the eye—Mental strain of any kind produces eyestrain—This strain takes many forms—Results in production of many abnormal conditions—Circulation disturbed by strain—Normal circulation restored by mental control—Thus errors of refraction and other abnormal conditions are cured.

CHAPTER XI
Central Fixation 57
The center of sight—The eye normally sees one part of everything it looks at best—Central fixation lost in all abnormal conditions of the eye—Cause of mental strain—With central fixation the eye is perfectly at rest—Can be used indefinitely without fatigue—Open and quiet—No wrinkles or dark circles around it—Visual axes parallel—With eccentric fixation the contrary is the case—Eccentric fixation cured by any method that relieves strain—Limits of vision determined by central fixation—Organic diseases relieved or cured by it—No limit can be set to its possibilities—Relation to general efficiency and general health.

CHAPTER XII
Palming 62
Relaxation with the eyes shut—With light excluded by palms of the hands (palming)—Evidence of complete relaxation in palming—Of incomplete relaxation—Difficulties of palming—How dealt with—Futility of effort—All the sensory nerves relaxed by successful palming—Pain relieved in all parts of the body—Patients who succeed at once are quickly cured - A minority not helped and should try other methods.

CHAPTER XIII
Memory As an Aid to Vision 67
Memory a test of relaxation—Memory of black most suitable for the purpose—Application of this fact to treatment of functional eye troubles—Sensation not a reliable index of strain—Memory of black is—Enables the patient to avoid conditions that produce strain—Conditions favorable to memory—Retention of memory under unfavorable conditions—Quick cures by its aid—A great help to other mental processes—Tests of a perfect memory.

CHAPTER XIV
Imagination As an Aid to Vision 71
Retinal impressions interpreted by the mind—Memory or imagination normally used as an aid to sight—In imperfect sight the mind adds imperfections to the imperfect retinal image—Only a small part of the phenomena of refractive errors accounted for by the inaccuracy of the focus—Difference between the photographic picture when the camera is out of focus and the visual impressions of the mind when the eye is out of focus—Patients helped by understanding of this fact—Dependence of imagination upon memory—Coincidence of both with sight—Perfect imagination dependent upon relaxation—Therefore imagination cures—Method of using it for this purpose—Remarkable cures effected by it.

CHAPTER XV
Shifting and Swinging 76
Apparent movement of objects regarded with normal vision—Due to unconscious shifting of the eye—Impossibility of fixing a point for an appreciable length of time—Lowering of vision by attempt to do so—Inconspicuousness of normal shifting—Its incredible rapidity—Staring an important factor in the production of imperfect sight—Tendency to stare corrected by conscious shifting and realization of apparent movement resulting from it—Conditions of success with shifting—The universal swing—Methods of shifting—Cures effected by this means.

CHAPTER XVI
The Illusions of Imperfect and of Normal Sight 81
Normal and abnormal illusions—Illusions of color—Of size—Of form—Of number—Of location—Of nonexistent objects—Of complementary colors—Of the color of the sun—Blind spots—Twinkling stars—Cause of illusions of imperfect sight—Voluntary production of illusions—Illusions of central fixation—Normal illusions of color—Illusions produced by shifting—The upright position of objects regarded an illusion.

CHAPTER XVII
Vision Under Adverse Conditions a Benefit to the Eye 85
Erroneous ideas of ocular hygiene—Conditions supposedly injurious may be a benefit to the eye—No foundation for universal fear of the light—Temporary discomfort but no permanent injury from it—Benefits of sun-gazing—Of looking at a strong electric light—Not light but darkness a danger to the eye—Sudden contrasts of light may be beneficial—Advantages of the movies—Benefits of reading fine print—Reading in moving vehicles—In a recumbent posture—Vision under difficult conditions good mental training.

CHAPTER XVIII
Optimums and Pessimums 91
All objects not seen equally well when sight is imperfect—The eye has its optimums and pessimums—Some easily accounted for—Others unaccountable—Familiar objects optimums—Unfamiliar objects pessimums—Examples of unaccountable optimums and pessimums—Variability of optimums and pessimums—Test card usually a pessimum—Pessimums which the patient is not conscious of seeing—Pessimums associated with a strain to see—How pessimums may become optimums.

CHAPTER XIX
The Relief of Pain and Other Symptoms by the Aid of the Memory. 92
No pain felt when the memory is perfect—All the senses improved—Efficiency of the mind increased—Operations performed without anaesthetics—Organic disorders relieved—Facts not fully explained, but attested by numerous proofs—Possible relationship of the principle involved to cures of Faith Curists and Christian Scientists.

CHAPTER XX
Presbyopia: Its Cause and Cure 95
Failure of near vision as age advances—Supposed normality of this phenomenon—Near-points expected at different ages—Many do not fit this schedule—Some never become presbyopic—Some retain normal vision for some objects while presbyopic for others—First and second of these classes of cases explained away or ignored—Third not heretofore observed—Presbyopia both preventable and curable—Due to a strain to see at the near-point—No necessary connection with age—Lens may flatten and lose refractive power with advancing years, but not necessarily—Temporary increase of presbyopia by strain at the nearpoint—Temporary relief by closing the eyes or palming—Permanent relief by permanent relief of strain—How the author cured himself—Other cures—Danger of putting on glasses at the presbyopic age—Prevention of presbyopia.

CHAPTER XXI
Squint and Amblyopia: Their Cause . . . . 100 (Strabismus, Crossed, Wandering eyes)
Definition of squint—Theories as to its cause—Failure of these theories to fit the facts—Failure of operative treatment—State of the vision not an important factor—Amblyopia ex anopsia—Association with squint not invariable—Supposed incurability—Spontaneous recovery—Curious forms of double vision in squint—Invariable association of squint and amblyopia with strain—Invariable relief following relief of strain—Voluntary production of squint by strain.

CHAPTER XXII
Squint and Amblyopia: Their Cure. . . . 102
Squint and amblyopia purely functional troubles—Cured by any method that relieves strain—Relaxation sometimes gained by voluntary increase of squint, or production of other kinds—Remarkable cure effected in this way—Strain relieved when patient is able to look more nearly in the proper direction—Proper use of a squinting eye encouraged by covering the good eye—Children cured by use of atropine in one or both eyes—Examples of cases cured by eye education.

CHAPTER XXIII
Floating Specks: Their Cause and Cure. . . . 105
Floating specks a common phenomenon of imperfect sight—Their appearance and behavior—Theories as to their origin—A fruitful field for the patent-medicine business—Examples of the needless alarm they have caused—May be seen at times by any one—Simply an illusion caused by mental strain—This strain easily relieved—Illustrative cases.

CHAPTER XXIV
Home Treatment. 108
Many persons can cure themselves of defective sight—Only necessary to follow a few simple directions—How to test the sight—Children who have not worn glasses cured by reading the Snellen test card every day—Adults of the same class also benefited in a short time—Cases of adults and children who have worn glasses more difficult—Glasses must be discarded—How to make a test card—Need of a teacher in difficult cases—Qualifications of such teachers—Duty of parents.

CHAPTER XXV
Correspondence Treatment 109
Correspondence treatment usually regarded as quackery—Impossible in the case
of most diseases—Errors of refraction, not being diseases, admit of such treatment—Glasses successfully fitted by mail—Less room for failure in correspondence treatment of imperfect sight without glasses—Personal treatment more satisfactory, but not always available—Examples of cases cured by correspondence—Need for the co-operation of local practitioners in such treatment.

CHAPTER XXVI
The Prevention of Myopia in Schools: Methods That Failed. 111
A much debated question—Literature on the subject voluminous and unreliable—All that is certainly known—Studies of Cohn—Confirmation of his observations by other investigators in America and Europe—Increase of myopia during school life unanimously attributed to near work—Inadequacy of this theory—Failure of preventive measures based upon it—New difficulties—The appeal to heredity—To natural adaptation—Objections to these views—Why all preventive measures have failed.

CHAPTER XXVII
The Prevention and Cure of Myopia and Other Errors of Refraction in Schools: A Method That Succeeded . . 114
Production of eyestrain by unfamiliar objects—Relief by familiar objects—Facts furnish the means of preventing and curing errors of refraction in schools—By this means children often gain normal vision with incredible rapidity—Results in schools of Grand Forks, N. D.; New York, and other cities—Improvement in mentality of children as eyesight improved—Reformation of truants and incorrigibles—Hypermetropia and astigmatism prevented and cured—Method succeeded best when teachers did not wear glasses—Success would be greater still under a more rational educational system—Prevalence of defective sight in American children—Its results—Practically all cases preventable and curable—Inexpensiveness of method recommended—Imposes no additional burden on the teachers—Cannot possibly hurt the children—Directions for its use.

CHAPTER XXVIII
The Story of Emily 118

Cure of defective eyesight by cured patients—Cures of fellow students, parents and friends by school children—Remarkable record of Emily—An illustration of the benefits to be expected from the author's method of preventing and curing imperfect sight in school children.

CHAPTER XXIX
Mind and Vision 120
Poor sight one of the most fruitful causes of retardation in schools—More involved in it than inability to see—The result of an abnormal condition of the mind—This cannot be changed by glasses—Memory among faculties impaired when vision is impaired—Memory of primitive man may have been due to the same cause as his keen vision—A modern example of primitive memory combined with primitive keenness of vision—Correspondence between differences in the faculty of memory and differences in visual acuity—Memory and eyesight of children spoiled by the same causes—Both dependent upon interest—Illustrative cases—All the mental faculties improved when vision becomes normal—Examples of such improvement—Relief of symptoms of insanity by eye education—Facts indicate a close relation between the problems of vision and those of education.

CHAPTER XXX
Normal Sight and the Relief of Pain for Soldiers and Sailors. . . . 124
Growth of militarism in the United States—Demand for universal military training—Lack of suitable material for such training—Defective eyesight greatest impediment to the raising of an efficient army—None more easily removed—Plan for correcting defects of vision submitted to Surgeon General during the war—Not acted upon—Now presented to the public with some modifications—First requisite eye education in schools and colleges—Eye education in training camps and at the front also needed, even for those whose sight is normal—How school system might be modified for military and naval use—Soldiers should not be allowed to wear glasses—Importance of eye training to aviators—Eye training for the relief of pain.

CHAPTER XXXI
Letters from Patients 126
Army officer cures himself—A teacher's experiences—Mental effects of central fixation—Relief after twenty-five years—Search for myopia cure rewarded—Facts versus theories—Cataract relieved by central fixation.

CHAPTER XXXII
Reason and Authority 131
Inaccessibility of average mind to reason—Facts discredited if contrary to authority—Patients discredit their own experience under this influence—Cure of cataract ignored by medical profession—Expulsion of author from N. Y. Post Graduate Medical School for curing myopia—Man not a reasoning being—Consequences to the world.

LIST OF ILLUSTRATIONS

Portrait of Ferdinand von Arlt . . . . . Frontispiece

1. Patagonians   13
2. African Pigmies   14
3. Moros from the Philippines   15
4. Diagram of the hypermetropic, emmetropic and myopic eyeballs   17
5. The eye as a camera   18
6. Mexican Indians   19
7. Ainus, the aboriginal inhabitants of Japan   19
8. The usual method of using the retinoscope   20
9. Diagrams of the images of Purkinje   22
10. Diagram by which Helmholtz illustrated his theory of accommodation   24
11. Portrait of Thomas Young   24
12. Portrait of Hermann Ludwig Ferdinand von Helmholtz   25
13. Demonstration upon the eye of a rabbit that the inferior oblique muscle is an essential factor in accommodation   29
14. Demonstration upon the eye of a carp that the superior oblique muscle is essential to accommodation   29
15. Demonstration upon the eye of a rabbit that the production of refractive errors is dependent upon the action of the external muscles   29
16. Demonstration upon the eye of a fish that the production of myopic and hypermetropic refraction is dependent upon the action of the extrinsic muscles   30

17. Production and relief of mixed astigmatism in the eye of a carp   31
18. Demonstration upon the eyeball of a rabbit that the obliques lengthen the visual axis in myopia   31
19. Demonstration upon the eye of a carp that the recti shorten the visual axis in hypermetropia   31
20. Lens pushed out of the axis of vision   32
21. Rabbit with lens removed   32
22. Experiment upon the eye of a cat, demonstrating that the fourth nerve, which supplies only the superior oblique muscle, is just as much a nerve of accommodation as the third, and that the superior oblique muscle which it supplies is a muscle of accommodation   32-33
23. Pithing a fish preparatory to operating upon its eyes   33
24. Arrangements for photographing images reflected from the eyeball   34
25. Arrangements for holding the head of the subject steady while images were being photographed   34
26. Image of electric filament on the front of the lens   35
27. Images of the electric filament reflected simultaneously from the cornea and lens   35
28. Image of electric filament upon the cornea   36
29. Image of electric filament on the front of the sclera   37
30. Images on the side of the sclera   37
31. Multiple images upon the front of the lens   38
32. Reflection of the electric filament from the iris   38
33. Demonstrating that the back of the lens does not change during accommodation   39
34. Straining to see at the near-point produces hypermetropia.   47
35. Myopia produced by unconscious strain to see at the distance is increased by conscious strain   48
36. Immediate production of myopia and myopic astigmatism in eyes previously normal by strain to see at the distance   48-49
37. Myopic astigmatism comes and goes according as the subject looks at distant objects with or without strain   49
38. Patient who has had the lens of the right eye removed for cataract produces changes in the refraction of this eye by strain   50
39. A family group strikingly illustrating the effect of the mind upon the vision   51
40. Myopes who never went to school, or read in the Subway   52
41. One of the many thousands of patients cured of errors of refraction by the methods presented in this book   53
42. Palming   63
43. Patient with atrophy of the optic nerve gets flashes of improved vision after palming   64
44. Paralysis of the seventh nerve cured by palming   65
45. Glaucoma cured by palming   66
46. Woman with normal vision looking directly at the sun   86
47. Woman aged 37-child aged 4, both looking directly at the sun without discomfort   87
48. Focusing the rays of the sun upon the eye of a patient by means of a burning glass   88
49. Specimen of diamond type   90
50. Photographic type reduction   90
51. Operating without anaesthetics   93
52. Neuralgia relieved by palming and the memory of black   94
53. Voluntary production of squint by strain to see   101
54. Case of divergent vertical squint cured by eye education   103
55. Temporary cure of squint by memory of a black period   104
56. Face-rest designed by Kallmann, a German optician   112

PREFACE

This book aims to be a collection of facts and not of theories and insofar as it is, I do not fear successful contradiction. When explanations have been offered it has been done with considerable trepidation, because I have never been able to formulate a theory that would withstand the test of the facts either in my possession at the time, or accumulated later. The same is true of the theories of every other man, for a theory is only a guess, and you cannot guess or imagine the truth. No one has ever satisfactorily answered the question, "Why?" as most scientific men are well aware, and I did not feel that I could do better than others who had tried and failed. One cannot even draw conclusions safely from facts, because a conclusion is very much like a theory, and may be disproved or modified by facts accumulated later. In the science of ophthalmology, theories, often stated as facts, have served to obscure the truth and throttle investigation for more than a hundred years. The explanations of the phenomena of sight put forward by Young, von Graefe, Helmholtz and Donders have caused us to ignore or explain away a multitude of facts which otherwise would have led to the discovery of the truth about errors of refraction and the consequent prevention of an incalculable amount of human misery.

In presenting my experimental work to the public, I desire to acknowledge my indebtedness to Mrs. E. C. Lierman, whose co-operation during four years of arduous labor and prolonged failure made it possible to carry the work to a successful issue. I would be glad, further, to acknowledge my debt to others who aided me with suggestions, or more direct assistance, but am unable to do so, as they have requested me not to mention their names in this connection.

As there has been a considerable demand for the book from the laity, an effort has been made to present the subject in such a way as to be intelligible to persons unfamiliar with ophthalmology.

THE FUNDAMENTAL PRINCIPLE

Do you read imperfectly? Can you observe then that when you look at the first word, or the first letter, of a sentence you do not see best where you are looking ; that you see other words, or other letters, just as well as or better than the one you are looking at? Do you observe also that the harder you try to see the worse you see?

Now close your eyes and rest them, remembering some color, like black or white, that you can remember perfectly. Keep them closed until they feel rested, or until the feeling of strain has been completely relieved. Now open them and look at the first word or letter of a sentence for a fraction of a second. If you have been able to relax, partially or completely, you will have a flash of improved or clear vision, and the area seen best will be smaller.

After opening the eyes for this fraction of a second, close them again quickly, still remembering the color, and keep them closed until they again feel rested. Then again open them for a fraction of a second. Continue this alternate resting of the eyes and flashing of the letters for a time, and you may soon find that you can keep your eyes open longer than a fraction of a second without losing the improved vision.

If your trouble is with distant instead of near vision, use the same method with distant letters.

In this way you can demonstrate for yourself the fundamental principle of the cure of imperfect sight by treatment without glasses.

If you fail, ask someone with perfect sight to help you.

THE CURE OF IMPERFECT SIGHT BY TREATMENT WITHOUT GLASSES
CHAPTER I
INTRODUCTORY

MOST writers on ophthalmology appear to believe that the last word about problems of refraction has been spoken, and from their viewpoint the last word is a very depressing one. Practically everyone in these days suffers from some form of refractive error. Yet we are told that for these ills, which are not only so inconvenient, but often so distressing and dangerous, there is not only no cure, and no palliative save those optic crutches known as eyeglasses, but, under modern conditions of life, practically no prevention.

It is a well-known fact that the human body is not a perfect mechanism. Nature, in the evolution of the human tenement, has been guilty of some maladjustments. She has left, for instance, some troublesome bits of scaffolding, like the vermiform appendix, behind. But nowhere is she supposed to have blundered so badly as in the construction of the eye. With one accord ophthalmologists tell us that the visual organ of man was never intended for the uses to which it is now put. Eons before there were any schools or printing presses, electric lights or moving pictures, its evolution was complete. In those days it served the needs of the human animal perfectly. Man was a hunter, a herdsman, a farmer, a fighter. He needed, we are told, mainly distant vision; and since the eye at rest is adjusted for distant vision, sight is supposed to have been ordinarily as passive as the perception of sound, requiring no muscular action whatever. Near vision, it is assumed, was the exception,

Fig. 1. Patagonians
The sight of this primitive pair and of the following groups of primitive people was tested at the World's Fair in St. Louis and found to be normal. The unaccustomed experience of having their pictures taken, however, has evidently so disturbed them that they were all, probably, myopic when they faced the camera. (see Chapter IX.)

Fig. 1. Patagonians. The sight of this primitive pair and of the following groups of primitive people was tested at the World's Fair in St. Louis and found to be normal. The unaccustomed experience of having their pictures taken, however, has evidently so disturbed them that they were all, probably, myopic when they faced the camera, (see Chapter IX.)

necessitating a muscular adjustment of such short duration that it was accomplished without placing any appreciable burden upon the mechanism of accommodation. The fact that primitive woman was a seamstress, an embroiderer, a weaver, an artist in all sorts of fine and beautiful work, appears to have been generally forgotten. Yet women living under primitive conditions have just as good eyesight as the men.

New Demands Upon the Eye

When man learned how to communicate his thoughts to others by means of written and printed forms, there came some undeniably new demands upon the eye, affecting

Fig. 2. African Pigmies. They had normal vision when tested, but their expressions show that they could not have had it when photographed.

at first only a few people, but gradually including more and more, until now, in the more advanced countries, the great mass of the population is subjected to their influence. A few hundred years ago even princes were not taught to read and write. Now we compel everyone to go to school, whether he wishes to or not, even the babies being sent to kindergarten. A generation or so ago books were scarce and expensive. To-day, by means of libraries of all sorts, stationary and traveling, they have been brought within the reach of practically everyone. The modern newspaper, with its endless columns of badly printed reading matter, was made possible only by the discovery of the art of manufacturing paper from wood, which is a thing of yesterday. The tallow candle has been but lately displaced by the various forms of artificial lighting, which tempt most of us to prolong our vocations and avocations into hours when primitive man was forced to rest, and within the last couple of decades has come the moving picture to complete the supposedly destructive process.

Was it reasonable to expect that Nature should have provided for all these developments, and produced an organ that could respond to the new demands? It is the accepted belief of ophthalmology to-day that she could not and did not, 1 and that, while the processes of civilization depend upon the sense of sight more than upon any other, the visual organ is but imperfectly fitted for its tasks.

There are a great number of facts which seem to justify this conclusion. While primitive man appears to have suffered little from defects of vision, it is safe to say that

1 The unnatural strain of accommodating the eyes to close work (for which they were not intended) leads to myopia in a large proportion of growing children. Rosenau: Preventive Medicine and Hygiene, third edition, 1917, p. 1093. The compulsion of fate as well as an error of evolution has brought it about that the unaided eye must persistently struggle against the astonishing difficulties and errors inevitable in its structure, function and circumstance. - Gould: The Cause, Nature and Consequences of Eyestrain, Pop. Sci. Monthly, Dec., 1905. With the invention of writing and then with the invention of the printing-press a new element was introduced, and one evidently not provided for by the process of evolution. The human eye which had been evolved for distant vision is being forced to perform a new part, one for which it had not been evolved, and for which it is poorly adapted. The difficulty is being daily augmented. - Scott : The Sacrifice of the Eyes of School Children, Pop. Sci. Monthly, Oct., 1907.

Military Visual Standards

of persons over twenty-one living under civilized conditions nine out of every ten have imperfect sight, and as the age increases the proportion increases, until at forty it is almost impossible to find a person free from visual defects. Voluminous statistics are available to prove these assertions, but the visual standards of the modern army 1 are all the evidence that is required.

In Germany, Austria, France and Italy the vision with glasses determines acceptance or rejection for military service, and in all these countries more than six diopters of myopia are allowed, although a person so handicapped cannot, without glasses, see anything clearly at more than six inches from his eyes. In the German Army a recruit for general service is required - or was required under the former government - to have a corrected vision of 6/12 in one eye. That is, he must be able to read with this eye at six metres the line normally read at twelve metres. In other words, he is considered fit for military service if the vision of one eye can be brought up to one-half normal with glasses. The vision in the other eye may be minimal, and in the Landsturm one eye may be blind. Incongruous as the eyeglass seems upon the soldier, military authorities upon the European continent have come to the conclusion that a man with 6/12 vision wearing glasses is more serviceable than a man with 6/24 vision (one-quarter normal) without them.

In Great Britain it was formerly uncorrected vision that determined acceptance or rejection for military service. This was probably due to the fact that previous to the recent war the British Army was used chiefly for

1 Ford : Details of Military Medical Administration, published with the approval of the Surgeon General, U. S. Army, second revised edition, 1918, pp. 498-499. 2 A diopter is the focussing power necessary to bring parallel rays to a focus at one metre.

foreign service, at such distances from its base that there might have been difficulty in providing glasses. The standard at the beginning of the war was 6/24 (uncorrected) for the better eye and 6/60 (uncorrected) for the

Fig. 3—Moros from the Philippines

Fig. 3 Moros from the Philippines. With sight ordinarily normal all were probably myopic when photographed except the one at the upper left whose eyes are shut.

poorer, which was required to be the left. Later, owing to the difficulty of securing enough men with even this moderate degree of visual acuity, recruits were accepted whose vision in the right eye could be brought up to 6/12 by correction, provided the vision of one eye was 6/24 without correction. 1

1 Tr. Ophth. Soc. U. Kingdom, vol. xxxviii, 1918, pp. 130-131.

Lowering of American Standards

Up to 1908 the United States required normal vision in recruits for its military service. In that year Bannister and Shaw made some experiments from which they concluded that a perfectly sharp image of the target was not necessary for good shooting, and that, therefore, a visual acuity of 20/40 (the equivalent in feet of 6/12 in metres), or even 20/70, in the aiming eye only, was sufficient to make an efficient soldier. This conclusion was not accepted without protest, but normal vision had become so rare that it probably seemed to those in authority that there was no use insisting upon it; and the visual standard for admission to the Army was accordingly lowered to 20/40 for the better eye and 20/100 for the poorer, while it was further provided that a recruit might be accepted when unable with the better eye to read all the letters on the 20/40 line, provided he could read some of the letters on the 20/30 line.1

In the first enrollment of troops for the European war it is a matter of common knowledge that these very low standards were found to be too high and were interpreted with great liberality. Later they were lowered so that men might be "unconditionally accepted for general military service" with a vision of 20/100 in each eye without glasses, provided that the sight of one eye could be brought up to 20/40 with glasses, while for limited service 20/200 in each eye was sufficient, provided the vision of one eye might be brought up to 20/40 with glasses. 2 Yet 21.68 per cent of all rejections in the first draft, 13 per cent more than for any other single cause, were for

1 Harvard: Manual of Military Hygiene for the Military Services of the United States, published under the authority and with the approval of the Surgeon General, U. S. Army, third revised edition, 1917, p. 195.
2 Standards of Physical Examination for the Use of Local Boards, District Boards, and Medical Advisory Boards under the Selective Service Regulations, issued through the office of the Provost Marshal General, 1918.

eye defects, 1 while under the revised standards these defects still constituted one of three leading causes of rejection. They were responsible for 10.65 per cent of the rejections, while defects of the bones and joints and of the heart and blood-vessels ran, respectively, about two and two and a half per cent higher. 2

For more than a hundred years the medical profession has been seeking for some method of checking the ravages of civilization upon the human eye. The Germans, to whom the matter was one of vital military importance, have spent millions of dollars in carrying out the suggestions of experts, but without avail; and it is now admitted by most students of the subject that the methods which were once confidently advocated as reliable safeguards for the eyesight of our children have accomplished little or nothing. Some take a more cheerful view of the matter, but their conclusions are hardly borne out by the army standards just quoted.

For the prevailing method of treatment, by means of compensating lenses, very little was ever claimed except that these contrivances neutralized the effects of the various conditions for which they were prescribed, as a crutch enables a lame man to walk. It has also been believed that they sometimes checked the progress of these conditions; but every ophthalmologist now knows that their usefulness for this purpose, if any, is very limited. In the case of myopia3 (shortsight), Dr. Sidler-Huguenin of Zurich, in a striking paper recently pub-

1 Report of the Provost Marshal General to the Secretary of War on the First Draft under the Selective Service Act, 1917. 2 Second Report of the Provost Marshal General to the Secretary of War on the Operations of the Selective Service System to December 20, 1918. 3 From the Greek myein, to close, and ops, the eye ; literally a condition in which the subject closes the eye, or blinks.

Present Methods of Treatment Futile

lished, 1 expresses the opinion that glasses and all methods now at our command are "of but little avail" in preventing either the progress of the error of refraction, or the development of the very serious complications with which it is often associated.

These conclusions are based on the study of thousands of cases in Dr. Huguenin's private practice and in the clinic of the University of Zurich, and regarding one group of patients, persons connected with the local educational institutions, he states that the failure took place in spite of the fact that they followed his instructions for years "with the greatest energy and pertinacity," sometimes even changing their professions.

I have been studying the refraction of the human eye for more than thirty years, and my observations fully confirm the foregoing conclusions as to the uselessness of all the methods heretofore employed for the prevention and treatment of errors of refraction. I was very early led to suspect, however, that the problem was by no means an unsolvable one.

Every ophthalmologist of any experience knows that the theory of the incurability of errors of refraction does not fit the observed facts. Not infrequently such cases recover spontaneously, or change from one form to another. It has long been the custom either to ignore these troublesome facts, or to explain them away, and fortunately for those who consider it necessary to bolster up the old theories at all costs, the role attributed to the lens in accommodation offers, in the majority of cases, a plausible method of explanation. According to this

1 Archiv. f. Augenh, vol. lxxix, 1915, translated in Arch. Ophth., vol. xlv, No. 6, Nov., 1916.

theory, which most of us learned at school, the eye changes its focus for vision at different distances by altering the curvature of the lens; and in seeking for an explanation for the inconstancy of the theoretically constant error of refraction the theorists hit upon the very ingenious idea of attributing to the lens a capacity for changing its curvature, not only for the purpose of normal accommodation, but to cover up or to produce accommodative errors. In hypermetropia1 - commonly but improperly called farsight, although the patient with such a defect can see clearly neither at the distance nor the nearpoint - the eyeball is too short from the front backward, and all rays of light, both the convergent ones coming from near objects, (Mis-print?: Near objects produce basically divergent light rays) and the parallel ones coming from distant objects, are focussed behind the retina, instead of upon it. In myopia it is too long, and while the divergent rays from near objects come to a point upon the retina, the parallel ones from distant objects do not reach it. Both these conditions are supposed to be permanent, the one congenital, the other acquired. When, therefore, persons who at one time appear to have hypermetropia, or myopia, appear at other times not to have them, or to have them in lesser degrees, it is not permissible to suppose that there has been a change in the shape of the eyeball. Therefore, in the case of the disappearance or lessening of hypermetropia, we are asked to believe that the eye, in the act of vision, both at the near-point and at the distance, increases the curvature of the lens sufficiently to compensate, in whole or in part, for the flatness of the eyeball. In myopia, on the

1 From the Greek hyper, over, metron. measure, and ops, the eye.

An Ingenious Theory

contrary, we are told that the eye actually goes out of its way to produce the condition, or to make an existing condition worse. In other words, the so-called "ciliary muscle," believed to control the shape of the lens, is credited with a capacity for getting into a more or less continuous state of contraction, thus keeping the lens continuously in a state of convexity which, according to the theory, it ought to assume only for vision at the near-point.

Fig. 4. Diagram of the Hypermetropic, Emmetropic and Myopic Eyeballs

* Note; Light rays from near objects are divergent. They spread outward. (Near = objects at about 19 feet and closer.) The closer the object is, the more the light rays diverge, and the more the eyes must accommodate and converge to focus the rays in the eye.)

Dr. Bates, Emily kept this page as it is here in the final 1940 original edition; *"and all rays of light, both the convergent ones coming from near objects, and the parallel ones coming from distant objects,.."*

Is the sentence a misprint or needs clarification? I have 14 copies of Dr. Bates original antique book in green, red and maroon (might be the entire 9 editions) The sentence is the same in all 14 books.

Dr. Bates might be speaking of divergent near object light rays that have been converged correctly inside a normal shaped eye with clear close and far vision by the eyeball and it's cornea, lens.

Or; he could be speaking of divergent near object light rays that have been converged incorrectly inside the farsighted eye with unclear vision by the abnormal shortened eyeball and it's cornea, lens.

Note that he states; *"divergent rays from near objects"* when speaking about myopia. When speaking about the farsighted eye, does he mean; light rays from near objects appear, act different in the farsighted eye (short) eyeball? Does he mean the rays outside or inside the eye?

The farther away a light source is (the sun...), the more parallel are the beams of light. Light rays from far objects are 'basically' considered parallel. Optometry, optics books also show far object rays with some convergence. The cornea, lens, eye converges far and close light rays in the normal eye, in the farsighted and myopia eye. See pictures next page.

Fig. 4. Diagram of the Hypermetropic, Emmetropic and Myopic Eyeballs. H, hypermetropia ; E, emmetropia; M, myopia; Ax, optic axis. Note that in hypermetropia and myopia the rays, instead of coming to a focus, form a round spot upon the retina.

These curious performances may seem unnatural to the lay mind; but ophthalmologists believe the tendency to indulge in them to be so ingrained in the constitution of the organ of vision that, in the fitting of glasses, it is customary to instill atropine - the "drops with which everyone who has ever visited an oculist is familiar - into the eye, for the purpose of paralyzing the ciliary muscle and thus, by preventing any change of curvature in the lens, bringing out "latent hypermetropia" and getting rid of "apparent myopia."

The interference of the lens, however, is believed to account for only moderate degrees of variation in errors of refraction, and that only during the earlier years of life. For the higher ones, or those that occur after forty-five years of age, when the lens is supposed to have lost its elasticity to a greater or less degree, no plausible explanation has ever been devised. The disappearance of astigmatism,[1] or changes in its character, present an even more baffling problem. Due in most cases to an unsymmetrical change in the curvature of the cornea, and resulting in failure to bring the light rays to a focus at any point, the eye is supposed to possess only a limited power of overcoming this condition ; and yet astigmatism comes and goes with as much facility as do other errors of refraction. It is well known, too, that it can be produced voluntarily. Some persons can produce as much as three diopters. I myself can produce one and a half.

Examining 30,000 pairs of eyes a year at the New York Eye and Ear Infirmary and other institutions, I observed

[1] From the Greek a, without, and stigma, a point.

Orthodox Explanations Fail

many cases in which errors of refraction either recovered spontaneously, or changed their form, and I was unable either to ignore them, or to satisfy myself with the orthodox explanations, even where such explanations were available. It seemed to me that if a statement is a truth it must always be a truth.

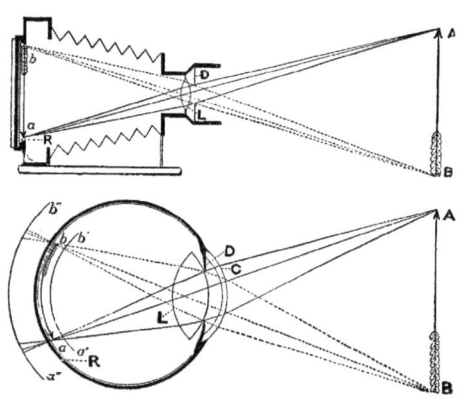

Fig. 5. The Eye As a Camera. The photographic apparatus; D, diaphragm made of circular overlapping plates of metal by means of which the opening through which the rays of light enter the chamber can be enlarged or contracted; L, lens; R, sensitive plate (the retina of the eye ; AB, object to be photographed; ab, image on the sensitive plate.

The eye: C, cornea where the rays of light undergo a first refraction; D, iris (the diaphragm of the camera); L, lens, where the light rays are again refracted; R, retina of the normal eye; AB, object of vision; ab, image in the normal or emmetropic eye; a' b', image in the hypermetropic eye; a" b", image in the myopic eye. Note that in a' b' and a" b", the rays are spread out upon the retina instead of being brought to a focus as in ab, the result being the formation of a blurred image.

There can be no exceptions. If errors of refraction are incurable, they should not recover, or change their form, spontaneously.

In the course of time I discovered that myopia and hypermetropia, like astigmatism, could be produced at will; that myopia was not, as we have so long believed, associated with the use of the eyes at the near-point, but with a strain to see distant objects, strain at the near-point being associated with hypermetropia; that no error of refraction was ever a constant condition ; and that the lower degrees of refractive error were curable, while higher degrees could be improved.

In seeking for light upon these problems I examined tens of thousands of eyes, and the more facts I accumulated the more difficult it became to reconcile them with the accepted views. Finally, about half a dozen years ago, I undertook a series of observations upon the eyes of human beings and the lower animals the results of which convinced both myself and others that the lens is not a factor in accommodation, and that the adjustment necessary for vision at different distances is affected in the eye, precisely as it is in the camera, by a change in the length of the organ, this alteration being brought about by the action of the muscles on the outside of the globe. Equally convincing was the demonstration that errors of refraction, including presbyopia, are due, not to an organic change in the shape of the eyeball, or in the constitution of the lens, but to a functional and therefore curable derangement in the action of the extrinsic muscles.

The Compulsion of Facts

In making these statements I am well aware that I am controverting the practically undisputed teaching of ophthalmological science for the better part of a century ; but I have been driven to the conclusions which they embody by the facts, and that so slowly that I am now surprised at my own blindness. At the time I was improving high degrees of myopia; but I wanted to be conservative, and I differentiated between functional myopia, which I was able to cure, or improve, and organic myopia, which, in deference to the orthodox tradition, I accepted as incurable.

Fig. 6. Mexican Indians. With normal sight when tested all the members of this primitive group are now either squinting or staring.

Fig. 7. Ainus, the Aboriginal Inhabitants of Japan. All show signs of temporary imperfect sight.

CHAPTER II
SIMULTANEOUS RETINOSCOPY

MUCH of my information about the eyes has been obtained by means of simultaneous retinoscopy. The retinoscope is an instrument used to measure the refraction of the eye. It throws a beam of light into the pupil by reflection from a mirror, the light being either outside the instrument - above and behind the subject - or arranged within it by means of an electric battery. On looking through the sight-hole one sees a larger or smaller part of the pupil filled with light, which in normal human eyes is a reddish yellow, because this is the color of the retina, but which is green in a cat's eye, and might be white if the retina were diseased. Unless the eye is exactly focussed at the point from which it is being observed, one sees also a dark shadow at the edge of the pupil, and it is the behavior of this shadow when the mirror is moved in various directions which reveals the refractive condition of the eye. If the instrument is used at a distance of six feet or more, and the shadow moves in a direction opposite to the movement of the mirror, the eye is myopic. If it moves in the same direction as the mirror, the eye is either hypermetropic or normal; but in the case of Hypermetropia the movement is more pronounced than in that of normality, and an expert can usually tell the difference between the two states merely by the nature of the movement.

Fig. 8. The Usual Method of Using the Retinoscope
The observer is so near the subject that the latter is made nervous, and this changes the refraction.

Fig. 8. The Usual Method of Using the Retinoscope. The observer is so near the subject that the latter is made nervous, and this changes the refraction.

Possibilities of Retinoscopy

In astigmatism the movement is different in different meridians. To determine the degree of the error, or to distinguish accurately between Hypermetropia and normality, or between the different kinds of astigmatism, it is usually necessary to place a glass before the eye of the subject. If the mirror is concave instead of plane, the movements described will be reversed; but the plane mirror is the one most commonly used.

This exceedingly useful instrument has possibilities which have not been generally realized by the medical profession. Most ophthalmologists depend upon the Snellen[1] test card, supplemented by trial lenses, to determine whether the vision is normal or not, and to determine the degree of any abnormality that may exist. This is a slow, awkward and unreliable method of testing the vision, and absolutely unavailable for the study of the refraction of the lower animals, of infants, and of adult human beings under the conditions of life.

The test card and trial lenses can be used only under certain favorable conditions, but the retinoscope can be used anywhere. It is a little easier to use it in a dim light than in a bright one, but it may be used in any light, even with the strong light of the sun shining directly into the eye. It may also be used under many other unfavorable conditions.

It takes a considerable time, varying from minutes to hours, to measure the refraction with the Snellen test card and trial lenses. With the retinoscope, however, it can be determined in a fraction of a second. By the

1 Herman Snellen (1835-1908). Celebrated Dutch ophthalmologist, professor of ophthalmology in the University of Utrecht and director of the Netherlandic Eye Hospital. The present standards of visual acuity were proposed by him, and his test types became the model for those now in use.

former method would be impossible, for instance, to get any information about the refraction of a baseball player at the moment he swings for the ball, at the moment he strikes it, and at the moment after he strikes it. But with the retinoscope it is quite easy to determine whether his vision is normal, or whether he is myopic, hypermetropic, or astigmatic, when he does these things; and if any errors of refraction are noted, one can guess their degree pretty accurately by the rapidity of the movement of the shadow.

With the Snellen test card and trial lenses conclusions must be drawn from the patient's statements as to what he sees ; but the patient often becomes so worried and confused during the examination that he does not know what he sees, or whether different glasses make his sight better or worse; and, moreover, visual acuity is not reliable evidence of the state of the refraction. One patient with two diopters of myopia may see twice as much as another with the same error of refraction. The evidence of the test card is, in fact, entirely subjective; that of the retinoscope is entirely objective, depending in no way upon the statements of the patient.

In short, while the testing of the refraction by means of the Snellen test card and trial lenses requires considerable time, and can be done only under certain artificial conditions, with results that are not always reliable, the retinoscope can be used under all sorts of normal and abnormal conditions on the eyes both of human beings and the lower animals; and the results, when it is used properly, can always be depended upon. This means that it must not be brought nearer to the eye than six feet; otherwise the subject will be made nervous, the refraction, for reasons which will be explained later, will be changed, and no reliable observations will be possible. In the case of animals it is often necessary to use it at a much greater distance.

Retinoscope Reveals New Facts

For thirty years I have been using the retinoscope to study the refraction of the eye. With it I have examined the eyes of tens of thousands of school children, hundreds of infants and thousands of animals, including cats, dogs, rabbits, horses, cows, birds, turtles, reptiles and fish. I have used it when the subjects were at rest and when they were in motion - also when I myself was in motion; when they were asleep and when they were awake or even under ether and chloroform. I have used it in the daytime and at night, when the subjects were comfortable and when they were excited; when they were trying to see and when they were not ; when they were lying and when they were telling the truth; when the eyelids were partly closed, shutting off part of the area of the pupil, when the pupil was dilated, and also when it was contracted to a pin-point ; when the eye was oscillating from side to side, from above downward and in other directions. In this way I discovered many facts which had not previously been known, and which I was quite unable to reconcile with the orthodox teachings on the subject. This led me to undertake the series of experiments already alluded to. The results were in entire harmony with my previous observations, and left me no choice but to reject the entire body of orthodox teaching about accommodation and errors of refraction. But before describing these experiments I must crave the reader's patience while I present a resume of the evidence upon which the accepted views of accommodation are based. This evidence, it seems to me, is as strong an argument as any I could offer against the doctrine that the lens is the agent of accommodation, while an understanding of the subject is necessary to an understanding of my experiments.

CHAPTER III
EVIDENCE FOR THE ACCEPTED THEORY OF ACCOMMODATION

THE power of the eye to change its focus for vision at different distances has puzzled the scientific mind ever since Kepler[1] tried to explain it by supposing a change in the position of the crystalline lens. Later on every imaginable hypothesis was advanced to account for it. The idea of Kepler had many supporters. So also had the idea that the change of focus was effected by a lengthening of the eyeball. Some believed that the contractive power of the pupil was sufficient to account for the phenomenon, until the fact was established, by the operation for the removal of the iris, that the eye accommodated perfectly without this part of the visual mechanism. Some, dissatisfied with all these theories, discarded them all, and boldly asserted that no change of focus took place,[2] a view which was conclusively disproven when the invention of the ophthalmoscope made it possible to see the interior of the eye.

The idea that the change of focus might be brought about by a change in the form of the lens appears to have been first advanced, according to Landolt,[3] by the

[1] Johannes Kepler (1571-1630). German theologian, astronomer and physicist. Many facts of physiological optics were either discovered, or first clearly stated, by him. [2] Donders : On the Anomalies of Accommodation and Refraction of the Eye. English translation by Moore, 1864, p. 10. Frans Cornelis Donders (1818-1889) was professor of physiology and ophthalmology at the University of Utrecht, and is ranked as one of the greatest ophthalmologists of all time. [3] Edmund Landolt (1846-) Swiss ophthalmologist who settled in Paris in 1874, founding an eye clinic which has attracted many students.

Accepted Theory of Accommodation

Jesuit, Scheiner (1619). Later it was put forward by Descartes (1637). But the first definite evidence in support of the theory was presented by Dr. Thomas Young in a paper read before the Royal Society in 1800.[1] "He adduced reasons," says Donders, "which, properly under

Fig. 9. Diagrams of the Images of Purkinje.

No. 1.—Images of a candle: a, on the cornea; b, on the front of the lens; c, on the back of the lens.
No. 2.—Images of lights shining through rectangular openings in a screen while the eye is at rest (R) and during accommodation (A): a, on the cornea; b, on the front of the lens; c, on the back of the lens (after Helmholtz).
Note that in No. 2, A, the central images are smaller and have approached each other, a change which, if actually took place, would indicate an increase of curvature in the front of the lens during accommodation.

Fig. 9. Diagrams of the Images of Purkinje. No. 1 - Images of a candle: a, on the cornea; b, on the front of the lens; c, on the back of the lens. No. 2. - Images of lights shining through rectangular openings in a screen while the eye is at rest (R) and during accommodation (A): a, on the cornea; b, on the front of the lens; c, on the back of the lens (after Helmholtz). Note that in No. 2, A, the central images are smaller and have approached each other, a change which, if actually took place, would indicate an increase of curvature in the front of the lens during accommodation.

stood, should be taken as positive proofs."[2] At the time, however, they attracted little attention.

About half a century later it occurred to Maximilian Langenbeck[3] to seek light on the problem by the aid of

[1] On the Mechanism of the Eye, Phil. Tr. Roy. Soc., London, 1801. [2] On the Anomalies of Accommodation and Refraction of the Eye, pp. 10-11. [3] Maximilian Adolf Langenbeck (1818-1877). Professor of anatomy, surgery and ophthalmology at Gottingen, from 1846 to 1851. Later settled in Hanover.

Studies of the Images of Purkinje

what are known as the images of Purkinje.1 If a small bright light, usually a candle, is held in front of and a little to one side of the eye, three images are seen: one bright and upright; another large, but less bright, and also upright; and a third small, bright and inverted. The first comes from the cornea, the transparent covering of the iris and pupil, and the other two from the lens, the upright one from the front and the inverted one from the back. The corneal reflection was known to the ancients, although its origin was not discovered till later; but the two reflections from the lens were first observed in 1823 by Purkinje; whence the trio of images is now associated with his name. Langenbeck examined these images with the naked eye, and reached the conclusion that during accommodation the middle one became smaller than when the eye was at rest. And since an image reflected from a convex surface is diminished in proportion to the convexity of that surface, he concluded that the front of the lens became more convex when the eye adjusted itself for near vision. Donders repeated the experiments of Langenbeck, but was unable to make any satisfactory observations. He predicted, however, that if the images were examined with a magnifier they would "show with certainty" whether the form of the lens changed during accommodation. Cramer,2 acting on this suggestion, examined the images as magnified from ten to twenty times, and thus convinced himself that the one reflected from the front of the lens became considerably smaller during accommodation.

1 Johannes Evangelista von Purkinje (1787-1869). Professor of physiology at Breslau and Prague, and the discoverer of many important physiological facts. 2 Antonie C. Cramer (1822-1855). Dutch ophthalmologist.

Subsequently Helmholtz, working independently, made a similar observation, but by a somewhat different method. Like Donders, he found the image obtained by the ordinary methods on the front of the lens very unsatisfactory, and in his "Handbook of Physiological Optics" he describes it as being "usually so blurred that the form of the flame cannot be definitely distinguished." 1 So he placed two lights, or one doubled by reflection from a mirror, behind a screen in which were two small rectangular openings, the whole being so arranged that the lights shining through the openings of the screen formed two images on each of the reflecting surfaces. During accommodation, it seemed to him that the two images on the front of the lens became smaller and approached each other, while on the return of the eye to a state of rest they grew larger again and separated. This change, he said, could be seen "easily and distinctly." 2 The observations of Helmholtz regarding the behavior of the lens in accommodation, published about the middle of the last century, were soon accepted as facts, and have ever since been stated as such in every text-book dealing with the subject.

"We may say," writes Landolt, "that the discovery of the part played by the crystalline lens in the act of accommodation is one of the finest achievements of medical physiology, and the theory of its working is certainly one of the most firmly established; for not only have "savans" furnished lucid and mathematical proofs of its correctness, but all other theories which have been advanced as explaining accommodation have been easily

1 Handbuch der physiologischen Optik, edited by Nagel, 1909-11, vol. i, p. 121. 2 Ibid, vol. i, p. 122.

Observations of Helmholtz Accepted

and entirely overthrown . . . The fact that the eye is accommodated for near vision by an increase in the curvature of its crystalline lens, is, then, incontestably proved." 1

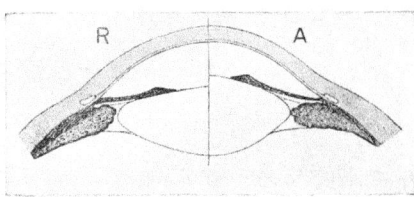

Fig. 10. Diagram by Which Helmholtz Illustrated His Theory of Accommodation

R is supposed to be the resting state of the lens, in which it is adjusted for distant vision. In A the suspensory ligament is supposed to have been relaxed through the contraction of the ciliary muscle, permitting the lens to bulge forward by virtue of its own elasticity.

Fig. 10. Diagram by Which Helmholtz Illustrated His Theory of Accommodation. R is supposed to be the resting state of the lens, in which it is adjusted for distant vision. In A the suspensory ligament is supposed to have been relaxed through the contraction of the ciliary muscle, permitting the lens to bulge forward by virtue of its own elasticity.

"The question was decided," says Tscherning, "by the observation of the changes of the images of Purkinje during accommodation, which prove that accommodation is effected by an increase of curvature of the anterior surface of the crystalline lens."[2]

1 The Refraction and Accommodation of the Eye and their Anomalies, authorized translation by Culver, 1886, p. 151. 2. Physiologic Optics, authorized translation by Weiland, 1904, p. 163. Marius Hans Erik Tscherning (1854-) is a Danish ophthalmologist who for twenty-five years was co-director and director of the ophthalmological laboratory of the Sorbonne. Later he became professor of ophthalmology in the University of Copenhagen.

Fig. 11. Thomas Young (1773-1829)

English physician and man of science who was the first to present a serious argument in support of the view that accommodation is brought about by the agency of the lens.

Fig. 11. Thomas Young (1773-1829). English physician and man of science who was the first to present a serious argument in support of the view that accommodation is brought about by the agency of the lens.

Scientific Credulity

"The greatest thinkers," says Cohn, "have mastered a host of difficulties in discovering this arrangement, and it is only in very recent times that its processes have been clearly and perfectly set forth in the works of Sanson, Helmholtz, Brticke, Hensen and Volckers."[1]

Huxley refers to the observations of Helmholtz as the "facts of adjustment with which all explanations of that process must accord,"[2] and Donders calls his theory the "true principle of accommodation."[3]

Arlt, who had advanced the elongation theory and believed that no other was possible, at first opposed the conclusions of Cramer and Helmholtz,[4] but later accepted them.[5]

Yet in examining the evidence for the theory we can only wonder at the scientific credulity which could base such an important department of medical practice as the treatment of the eye upon such a mass of contradictions. Helmholtz, while apparently convinced of the correctness of his observations indicating a change of form in the lens during accommodation, felt himself unable to speak with certainty of the means by which the supposed change was effected,[6] and strangely enough the question is still being debated. Finding, as he states, "absolutely nothing but the ciliary muscle to which accommodation could be attributed,"[7] Helmholtz concluded that the changes which he thought he had observed in the curvature of the lens must be effected by the action of this muscle; but he was unable to offer any satisfac-

1 The Hygiene of the Eye in Schools, English translation edited by Turnbull, 1886, p. 23. Hermann Cohn (1838-1906) was professor of ophthalmology in the University of Breslau, and is known chiefly for his contributions to ocular hygiene. 2 Lessons in Elementary Physiology, sixth edition, 1872, p. 231. 3 On the Anomalies of Accommodation and Refraction of the Eye,

p. 13. 4 Krankheiten des Auges, 1853-56, vol. iii, p. 219, et seq. 5 Ueber die Ursachen und die Entstehung der Kurzsichtigkeit, 1876. Vorwort. 6 Handbuch der physiologischen Optik, vol. i, pp. 124 and 145. 7 Ibid, vol. i, p. 144.

tory theory of the way it operated to produce these results and he explicitly stated that the one he suggested possessed only the character of probability. Some of his disciples, "more loyal than the king," as Tscherning has pointed out, "have proclaimed as certain what he himself with much reserve explained as probable," 1 but there has been no such unanimity of acceptance in this case as in that of the observations regarding the behavior of the images reflected from the lens. No one except the present writer, so far as I am aware, has ventured to question that the ciliary muscle is the agent of accommodation ; but as to the mode of its operation there is generally felt to be much need for more light. Since the lens is not a factor in accommodation, it is not strange that no one was able to find out how it changed its curvature. It is strange, however, that these difficulties have not in any way disturbed the universal belief that the lens does change.

When the lens has been removed for cataract the patient usually appears to lose his power of accommodation, and not only has to wear a glass to replace the lost part, but has to put on a stronger glass for reading. A minority of these cases, however, after they become accustomed to the new condition, become able to see at the near-point without any change in their glasses. The existence of these two classes of cases has been a great stumbling block to ophthalmology. The first and more numerous appeared to support the theory of the agency of the lens in accommodation; but the second was hard to explain away, and constituted at one time, as Dr. Thomas Young observed, the "grand objection" to this idea. A number of these cases of apparent change of focus

1 Physiologic Optics, p. 166.

Herman Ludwig Ferdinand von Helmholtz (1821-1894) whose observations regarding the behavior of images reflected from the front of the lens are supposed to have demonstrated that the curvature of this body changes during accommodation

Herman Ludwig Ferdinand von Helmholtz (1821-1894) whose observations regarding the behavior of images reflected from the front of the lens are supposed to have demonstrated that the curvature of this body changes during accommodation.

in the lensless eye having been reported to the Royal Society by competent observers, Dr. Young, before bringing forward his theory of accommodation, took the trouble to examine some of them, and considered himself justified in concluding that an error of observation had been made. While convinced, however, that in such eyes the "actual focal distance is totally unchangeable," he characterized his own evidence in support of this view as only "tolerably satisfactory." At a later period Donders made some investigations from which he concluded that "in aphakia 1 not the slightest trace of accommodative power remains."2 Holmholtz expressed similar views, and von Graefe, although he observed a "slight residuum" of accommodative power in lensless eyes, did not consider it sufficient to discredit the theory of Cramer and Helmholtz. It might be due, he said, to the accommodative action of the iris, and possibly also to a lengthening of the visual axis through the action of the external muscles.3

For nearly three-quarters of a century the opinions of these masters have echoed through ophthalmological literature. Yet it is to-day a perfectly well-known and undisputed fact that many persons, after the removal of the lens for cataract, are able to see perfectly at different distances without any change in their glasses. Every ophthalmologist of any experience has seen cases of this kind, and many of them have been reported in the literature.

In 1872, Professor Forster of Breslau, reported 4 a

1 Absence of the lens. 2 On the Anomalies of Accommodation and Refraction of the Eye, p. 320. 3 Archiv. f. Ophth., 1855, vol. ii, part 1, p. 187 et seq. Albrecht von Graefe (1828-1870) was professor of ophthalmology in the University of Berlin, and

is ranked with Donders and Arlt as one of the greatest ophthalmologists of the nineteenth century. 4 Klin. Montasbl. f. Augenh., Erlangen, 1872, vol. x, p. 39, et seq.

Not To Be Deputed

series of twenty-two cases of apparent accommodation in eyes from which the lens had been removed for cataract. The subjects ranged in age from eleven to seventy-four years, and the younger ones had more accommodative power than the elder. A year later Woinow of Moscow1 reported eleven cases, the subjects being from twelve to sixty years of age. In 1869 and 1870, respectively, Loring reported 2 to the New York Ophthalmological Society and the American Ophthalmological Society the case of a young woman of eighteen who, without any change in her glasses, read the twenty line on the Snellen test card at twenty feet and also read diamond type at from five inches to twenty. On October 8, 1894, a patient of Dr. A. E. Davis who appeared to accommodate perfectly without a lens consented to go before the New York Ophthalmological Society. "The members," Dr. Davis reports, 3 "were divided in their opinion as to how the patient was able to accommodate for the nearpoint with his distance glasses on"; but the fact that he could see at this point without any change in his glasses was not to be disputed.

The patient was a chef, forty-two years old, and on January 27, 1894, Dr. Davis had removed a black cataract from his right eye, supplying him at the same time with the usual outfit of glasses, one to replace the lens, for distant vision, and a stronger one for reading. In October he returned, not because his eye was not doing well, but because he was afraid he might be "straining" it. He had discarded his reading glasses after a few weeks, and had since been using only his distance glasses. Dr.

1 Archiv. f. Ophth., 1873, vol. xix, part 3, p. 107. 2 Flint: Physiology of Man, 1875, vol. v, pp. 110-111. 3 Davis : Accommodation in the Lensless Eye, Reports of the Manhattan Eye and Ear Hospital, Jan., 1895. The article gives a review of the whole subject.

Davis doubted the truth of his statements, never having seen such a case before, but found them, upon investigation, to be quite correct. With his lensless eye and a convex glass of eleven and a half diopters, the patient read the ten line on the test card at twenty feet, and with the same glass, and without any change in its position, he read fine print at from fourteen to eighteen inches. Dr. Davis then presented the case to the Ophthalmological Society but, as has been stated, he obtained no light from that source. Four months later, February 4, 1895, the patient still read 20/10 at the distance and his range at the near point had increased so that he read diamond type at from eight to twenty-two and a half inches. Dr. Davis subjected him to numerous tests, and though unable to find any explanation for his strange performances, he made some interesting observations. The results of the tests by which Donders satisfied himself that the lensless eye possessed no accommodative power were quite different from those reported by the Dutch authority, and Dr. Davis therefore concluded that these tests were "wholly inadequate to decide the question at issue." During accommodation the ophthalmometer1 showed that the corneal curvature was changed and that the cornea moved forward a little. Under scopolamine, a drug sometimes used instead of atropine to paralyze the ciliary muscle (1/10 per cent solution every five minutes for thirty-five minutes, followed by a wait of half an hour), these changes took place as before; they also took place when the lids were held up. With the possible influence of lid pressure and of the ciliary muscle eliminated, therefore, Dr. Davis felt himself bound to conclude that the changes "must

1 An instrument for measuring the curvature of the cornea.

Another Puzzling Case

have been produced by the action of the external muscles." Under scopolamine, also, the man's accommodation was only slightly affected, the range at the near point being reduced only two and a half inches.

The ophthalmometer further showed the patient to have absolutely no astigmatism. It had showed the same thing about three months after the operation, but three and a half weeks after it he had four and a half diopters.

Seeking further light upon the subject Dr. Davis now subjected to similar tests a case which had previously been reported by Webster in the "Archives of Pediatrics." 1 The patient had been brought to Dr. Webster at the age of ten with double congenital cataract. The left lens had been absorbed as the result of successive needlings, leaving only an opaque membrane, the lens capsule, while the right, which had not been interfered with, was sufficiently transparent around the edge to admit of useful vision. Dr. Webster made an opening in the membrane filling the pupil of the left eye, after which the vision of this eye, with a glass to replace the lens, was about equal to the vision of the right eye without a glass. For this reason Dr. Webster did not think it necessary to give the patient distance glasses, and supplied him with reading glasses only - plane glass for the right eye and convex 16D for the left. On March 14, 1893, he returned and stated that he had been wearing his reading glasses all the time. With this glass it was found that he could read the twenty line of the test card at twenty feet, and read diamond type easily at fourteen inches. Subsequently the right lens was removed, after which no accommodation was observed in this eye. Two years later

1 Nov.. 1893, p. 932.

March 16, 1895, he was seen by Dr. Davis, who found that the left eye now had an accommodative range of from ten to eighteen inches. In this case no change was observed in the cornea. The results of the Donders tests were similar to those of the earlier case, and under scopolamine the eye accommodated as before, but not quite so easily. No accommodation was observed in the right eye.

These and similar cases have been the cause of great embarrassment to those who feel called upon to reconcile them with the accepted theories. With the retinoscope the lensless eye can be seen to accommodate; but the theory of Helmholtz has dominated the ophthalmological mind so strongly that even the evidence of objective tests was not believed. The apparent act of accommodation was said not to be real, and many theories, very curious and unscientific, have been advanced to account for it. Davis is of the opinion that "the slight change in the curvature of the cornea, and its slight advancement observed in some cases, may, in those cases, account for some of the accommodative power present, but it is such a small factor that it may be eliminated entirely, since in some of the most marked cases of accommodation in aphakial eyes no such changes have been observed."

The voluntary production of astigmatism is another stumbling block to the supporters of the accepted theories, as it involves a change in the shape of the cornea, and such a change is not compatible with the idea of an "inextensible"1 eyeball. It seems to have given them less trouble, however, than the accommodation of the lensless

1 Inasmuch as the eye is inextensible, it cannot adapt itself for the perception of objects situated at different distances by increasing the length of its axis, but only by increasing the refractive power of its lens.- De Schweinitz: Diseases of the Eye, eighth edition, 1916, pp. 35-36.

Voluntary Production of Astigmatism

eye, because fewer of these cases have been observed and still fewer have been allowed to get into the literature. Some interesting facts regarding one have fortunately been given by Davis, who investigated it in connection with the corneal changes noted in the lensless eye. The case was that of a house surgeon at the Manhattan Eye and Ear Hospital, Dr. C. H. Johnson. Ordinarily this gentleman had half a diopter of astigmatism in each eye ; but he could, at will, increase this to two diopters in the right eye and one and a half in the left. He did this many times, in the presence of a number of members of the hospital staff, and also did it when the upper lids were held up, showing that the pressure of the lids had nothing to do with the phenomenon. Later he went to Louisville, and here Dr. J. M. Ray, at the suggestion of Dr. Davis, tested his ability to produce astigmatism under the influence of scopolamine (four instillations, 1/5 per cent solution). While the eyes were under the influence of the drug the astigmatism still seemed to increase, according to the evidence of the ophthalmometer, to one and a half diopters in the right eye and one in the left. From these facts, the influence of the lids and of the ciliary muscle having been eliminated, Dr. Davis concluded that the change in the cornea was "brought about mainly by the external muscles." What explanation others offer for such phenomena I do not know.

CHAPTER IV

THE TRUTH ABOUT ACCOMMODATION AS DEMONSTRATED BY EXPERIMENTS ON THE EYE MUSCLES OF FISH, CATS, DOGS, RABBITS AND OTHER ANIMALS

THE function of the muscles on the outside of the eyeball, apart from that of turning the globe in its socket, has been a matter of much dispute; but after the supposed demonstration by Helmholtz that accommodation depends upon a change in the curvature of the lens, the possibility of their being concerned in the adjustment of the eye for vision at different distances, or in the production of errors of refraction, was dismissed as no longer worthy of serious consideration. "Before physiologists were acquainted with the changes in the dioptic system," 1 says Donders, "they often attached importance to the external muscles in the production of accommodation. Now that we know that accommodation depends on a change of form in the lens this opinion seems scarcely to need refutation." He states positively that "many instances occur where the accommodation is wholly destroyed by paralysis, without the external muscles being the least impeded in their action," and also that "some cases are on record of paralysis of all or nearly all of the muscles of the eye, and of deficiency of the same, without diminution of the power of accommodation."2

If Donders had not considered the question settled, he

1 The refractive system. 2 On the Anomalies of Accommodation and Refraction of the Eye, p. 22.

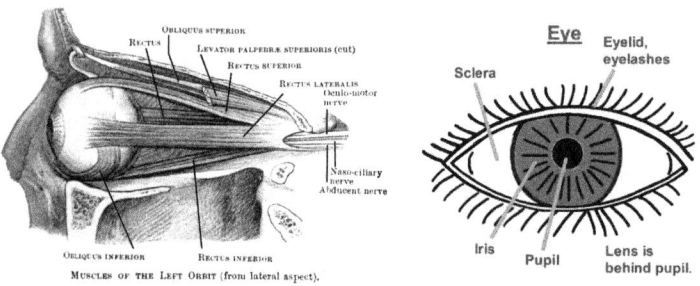

The External Muscles of the Eyeball

might have inquired more carefully into these cases, and if he had, he might have been less dogmatic in his statements ; for, as has been pointed out in the preceding chapter, there are plenty of indications that the contrary is the case. In my own experiments upon the extrinsic eye muscles of fish, rabbits, cats, dogs and other animals, the demonstration seemed to be complete that in the eyes of these animals accommodation depends wholly upon the action of the extrinsic muscles and not at all upon the agency of the lens. By the manipulation of these muscles I was able to produce or prevent accommodation at will, to produce myopia, hypermetropia and astigmatism, or to prevent these conditions. Full details of these experiments will be found in the "Bulletin of the New York Zoological Society" for November, 1914, and in the "New York Medical Journal" for May 8, 1915; and May 18, 1918; but for the benefit of those who have not the time or inclination to read these papers, their contents are summarized below.

There are six muscles on the outside of the eyeball, four known as the "recti" and two as the "obliques." The obliques form an almost complete belt around the middle of the eyeball, and are known, according to their position, as "superior" and "inferior." The recti are attached to the sclerotic, or outer coat of the eyeball, near the front, and pass directly over the top, bottom and sides of the globe to the back of the orbit, where they are attached to the bone round the edges of the hole through which the optic nerve passes. According to their position, they are known as the "superior," "inferior," "internal" and "external" recti. The obliques are the muscles of accommodation ; the recti are concerned in the production of Hypermetropia and astigmatism.

Accommodation: Experiments on Animals

In some cases one of the obliques is absent or rudimentary, but when two of these muscles were present and active, accommodation, as measured by the objective test

Fig. 13. Demonstration Upon the Eye of a Rabbit that the Inferior Oblique Muscle is an Essential Factor in Accommodation. No. 1. The inferior oblique muscle has been exposed and two sutures are attached to it. Electrical stimulation of the eyeball produces accommodation, as demonstrated by simultaneous retinoscopy. No. 2. The muscle has been cut. Electrical stimulation produces no accommodation. No. 3. The muscle has been sewed together. Electrical stimulation produces normal accommodation.

of retinoscopy, was always produced by electrical stimulation either of the eyeball, or of the nerves of accommodation near their origin in the brain. It was also produced by any manipulation of the obliques whereby their pull was increased. This was done by a tucking operation of one or both muscles, or by an advancement of the point at which they are attached to the sclerotic. When one or more of the recti had been cut; the effect of operations increasing the pull of the obliques was intensified.

Oblique Muscles Inactive: No Accommodation

Fig. 14. Demonstration Upon the Eye of a Carp That the Superior Oblique Muscle Is Essential to Accommodation.

No. 1.—The superior oblique is lifted from the eyeball by two sutures, and the retinoscope shows no error of refraction. No. 2.—Electrical stimulation produces accommodation, as determined by the retinoscope. No. 3.—The muscle has been cut. Stimulation of the eyeball with electricity fails to produce accommodation. No. 4.—The divided muscle has been reunited by tying the sutures. Accommodation follows electrical stimulation as before.

Fig. 15. Demonstration Upon the Eye of a Rabbit That the Production of the Refractive Errors Is Dependent Upon the Action of the External Muscles. The String Is Fastened to the Insertion of the Superior Oblique and Rectus Muscles

No. 1.—Backward pull. Myopia is produced.

No. 2.—Forward pull. Hypermetropia is produced.

No. 3.—Upward pull in the plane of the iris. Mixed astigmatism is produced.

Fig. 14. Demonstration Upon the Eye of a Carp That the Superior Oblique Muscle Is Essential to Accommodation. No. 1. The superior oblique is lifted from the eyeball by two sutures, and the retinoscope shows no error of refraction. No. 2. Electrical stimulation produces accommodation, as determined by the retinoscope. No. 3. The muscle has been cut. Stimulation of the eyeball with electricity fails to produce accommodation. No. 4. The divided muscle has been reunited by tying the sutures. Accommodation follows electrical stimulation as before.

Fig. 15. Demonstration Upon the Eye of a Rabbit That the Production of the Refractive Errors Is Dependent Upon the Action of the External Muscles. The String Is Fastened to the Insertion of the Superior Oblique and Rectus Muscles. No. 1. Backward pull. Myopia is produced. No. 2. Forward pull. Hypermetropia is produced. No. 3. Upward pull in the plane of the iris. Mixed astigmatism is produced.

The Extrinsic Muscles in Refractive Errors

After one or both of the obliques had been cut across, or after they had been paralyzed by the injection of atropine deep into the orbit, accommodation could never be produced by electrical stimulation; but after the effects of the atropine had passed away, or a divided muscle had been sewed together, accommodation followed electrical stimulation just as usual. Again when one oblique muscle was absent, as was found to be the case in a dogfish, a shark and a few perch, or rudimentary, as in all cats observed, a few fish and an occasional rabbit, accommodation could not be produced by electrical stimulation. But when the rudimentary muscle was strengthened by advancement, or the absent one was replaced by a suture which supplied the necessary counter-traction, accommodation could always be produced by electrical stimulation.

Fig. 16. Demonstration Upon the Eye of a Fish That the Production of Myopic and Hypermetropic Refraction Is Dependent Upon the Action of the Extrinsic Muscles. Suture tied to the insertion of the superior rectus muscle. By means of strong traction upon the suture the eyeball is turned in its socket, and by tying the thread to a pair of fixation forceps which grasp the lower jaw, it is maintained in this position. A high degree of mixed astigmatism is produced, as demonstrated by simultaneous retinoscopy. When the superior oblique is divided the myopic part of the astigmatism disappears, and when the inferior rectus is cut the hypermetropic part disappears, and the eye becomes normal-adjusted for distant vision-although the same amount of traction is maintained. It is evident that these muscles are essential factors in the production of myopia and hypermetropia.

After one or both of the oblique muscles had been cut, and while two or more of the recti were present and active,[1] electrical stimulation of the eyeball, or of the nerves of accommodation, always produced hypermetropia, while by the manipulation of one of the recti, usually the inferior or the superior, so as to strengthen its pull, the same result could be produced. The paralyzing of the recti by atropine, or the cutting of one or more of them, prevented the production of hypermetropic refraction by electrical stimulation; but after the effects of the atropine had passed away, or after a divided muscle had been sewed together, hypermetropia was produced as usual by electrical stimulation.

It should be emphasized that in order to paralyze either the recti muscles, or the obliques, it was found necessary to inject the atropine far back behind the eyeball with a hypodermic needle. This drug is supposed to paralyze the accommodation when dropped into the eyes of human

[1] In many animals, notably in rabbits, the internal and external recti are either absent or rudimentary, so that, practically, in such cases, there are only two recti, just as there are only two obliques. In others, as in many fish, the internal rectus is negligible.

Production of Astigmatism

beings or animals, but in all of my experiments it was found that when used in this way it had very little effect upon the power of the eye to change its focus.

Astigmatism was usually produced in combination with myopic or hypermetropic refraction. It was also produced by various manipulations of both the oblique and recti muscles. Mixed astigmatism, which is a combination of myopic with hypermetropic refraction, was always produced by traction on the insertion of the superior or inferior rectus in a direction parallel to the plane of the iris, so long as both obliques were present and active : but if either or both of the obliques had been cut,

Fig. 17. No. 1. Production of mixed astigmatism in the eye of a carp by pulling strings attached to the conjunctiva in opposite directions. Note the oval shape of the front of the eyeball. No. 2. With the cutting of the strings the eyeball returns to its normal shape, and the refraction becomes normal.

Fig. 18. Demonstration Upon the Eyeball of a Rabbit That the Obliques Lengthen the Visual Axis in Myopia. R, rest. The eyeball is of normal length and emmetropic-that is, perfectly adjusted for distant vision. My, myopia. The pull of the oblique muscles has been strengthened by advancement, and the retinoscope shows that myopia has been produced. It can easily be noted that the eyeball is longer. It was impossible to avoid some movement of the head between the taking of the two pictures as a result of the manipulation of the strings, but the rule shows that the focus of the camera was not appreciably changed by such movements.

The Recti in Hypermetropia

the myopic part of the astigmatism disappeared. Similarly after the superior or the inferior rectus had been cut the hypermetropic part of the astigmatism disappeared. Advancement of the two obliques, with advancement of the superior and inferior recti, always produced mixed astigmatism.

Fig. 19. Demonstration Upon the Eye of a Carp That the Recti Shorten the Visual Axis in Hypermetropia. R, rest. The eyeball is of normal length and emmetropic. Hy, hypermetropia. The pull of the external and internal recti has been strengthened by advancement, and the retinoscope shows that hypermetropia has been produced. It may easily be noted that the eyeball is shorter. The rule shows that the focus of the camera was not appreciably changed between the taking of the two pictures.

Eyes from which the lens had been removed, or in which it had been pushed out of the axis of vision, responded to electrical stimulation precisely as did the normal eye, so long as the muscles were active; but when they had been paralyzed by the injection of atropine deep into the orbit, electrical stimulation had no effect on the refraction.

Fig. 20. Lens Pushed Out of the Axis of Vision. In this experiment on the eye of a carp the lens was pushed out of the axis of vision. Accommodation took place after this displacement just as it did before. Note the point of the knife in the pupil in front of the lens.

In one experiment the lens was removed from the right eye of a rabbit, the refraction of each eye having first been tested by retinoscopy and found to be normal. The wound was then allowed to heal. Thereafter, for a

Accommodation in Aphakia

period extending from one month to two years, electrical stimulation always produced accommodation in the lensless eye precisely to the same extent as in the eye which

Fig. 21. Rabbit With Lens Removed. The animal was exhibited at a meeting of the Ophthalmological Section of the American Medical Association, held in Atlantic City, and was examined by a number of ophthalmologists present, all of whom testified that electrical stimulation of the eyeball produced accommodation, or myopic refraction, precisely as in the normal eye.

had a lens. The same experiment with the same result was performed on a number of other rabbits, on dogs and on fish. The obvious conclusion is that the lens is not a factor in accommodation.

In most text-books on physiology it is stated that accommodation is controlled by the third cranial nerve, which supplies all the muscles of the eyeball except the superior oblique and the external rectus; but the fourth cranial nerve, which supplies only the superior oblique, was found in these experiments to be just as much a nerve of accommodation as the third. When either the third or the fourth nerve was stimulated with electricity near its point of origin in the brain accommodation al-

Fig. 22. Experiment Upon the Eye of a Cat Demonstrating That the Fourth Nerve, Which Supplies Only the Superior Oblique Muscle, Is Just as Much a Nerve of Accommodation As the Third, and That the Superior Oblique Muscle Which It Supplies Is a Muscle of Accommodation.

No. 1. Both nerves have been exposed near their origin in the brain, and a strip of black paper has been inserted beneath each to render it visible. The fourth nerve is the smaller one. The superior oblique muscle has been advanced by a tucking operation, as this muscle is always rudimentary in cats, and unless its pull is strengthened, accommodation cannot be produced in these animals. Stimulation of either or both nerves by the faradic current produced accommodation.

No. 2. When the fourth nerve was covered with cotton soaked in a normal salt solution, the application of the faradic current to the cotton produced accommodation. When the cotton was soaked in a one per cent solution of atropine sulphate in a normal salt solution, such application produced no accommodation, but stimulation of the third nerve did produce it.

The Role of the Fourth Nerve

No. 3. When the third nerve was covered with cotton soaked in a normal salt solution, the application of the faradic current to the cotton produced accommodation. When the cotton was soaked with atropine sulphate in a normal salt solution, such application produced no accommodation, but the stimulation of the fourth nerve did produce it.

No. 4. When both nerves were covered with cotton soaked in atropine sulphate in a normal salt solution, the application of electricity to the cotton produced no accommodation. When the parts had been washed with a warm salt solution electrical stimulation of either nerve always produced accommodation. The nerves were alternately covered with the atropine-soaked cotton and then washed with the warm saline solution for an hour, the electricity being applied in each condition with invariably the same result. Accommodation could never be produced by electrical stimulation when the nerves were paralyzed with the atropine, but always resulted from the stimulation of either or both when they had been washed with the salt solution. The experiment was performed with the same results on many rabbits and dogs.

ways resulted in the normal eye. When the origin of either nerve was covered with a small wad of cotton soaked in a two per cent solution of atropine sulphate in a normal salt solution, stimulation of that nerve produced no accommodation, while stimulation of the unparalyzed nerve did produce it. When the origin of both nerves was covered with cotton soaked in atropine, accommodation could not be produced by electrical stimulation of either or both. When the cotton was removed and the nerves washed with normal salt solution, electrical stimulation of either or both produced accommodation just as before the atropine had been applied. This experiment, which was performed repeatedly for more

Fig. 23. Pithing a Fish Preparatory to Operating Upon Its Eyes. The object of this operation is to secure greater relaxation of the muscles of the eyes and head, which would work for hours, without external stimulus, if the brain cells were not destroyed by the probe.

than an hour by alternately applying and removing the atropine, not only demonstrated clearly what had not been known before, namely, that the fourth nerve is a nerve of accommodation, but also demonstrated that the

No Room for Doubt

superior oblique muscle which is supplied by it is an important factor in accommodation. It was further found that when the action of the oblique muscles was prevented by dividing them, the stimulation of the third nerve produced, not accommodation, but hypermetropia.

In all the experiments all sources of error are believed to have been eliminated. They were all repeated many times and always with the same result. They seemed, therefore, to leave no room for doubt that neither the lens nor any muscle inside the eyeball has anything to do with accommodation, but that the process whereby the eye adjusts itself for vision at different distances is entirely controlled by the action of the muscles on the outside of the globe.

CHAPTER V

THE TRUTH ABOUT ACCOMMODATION AS DEMONSTRATED BY A STUDY OF IMAGES REFLECTED FROM THE LENS, CORNEA, IRIS AND SCLERA

AS the conclusions in which the experiments described in the preceding chapter pointed were diametrically opposed to those reached by Helmholtz in his study of the images reflected from the front of the lens, I determined to repeat the experiments of the German investigator and find out, if possible, why his results were so different from my own. I devoted four years to this work, and was able to demonstrate that Helmholtz had erred through a defective technique, the image obtained by his method being so variable and uncertain that it lends itself to the support of almost any theory.

I worked for a year or more with the technique of Helmholtz, but was unable to obtain an image from the front of the lens which was sufficiently clear or distinct to be measured or photographed. With a naked candle as the source of light a clear and distinct image could be obtained on the cornea; on the back of the lens it was quite clear; but on the front of the lens it was very imperfect. Not only was it blurred, just as Helmholtz stated, but without any ascertainable cause it varied greatly in size and intensity. At times no reflection could be obtained at all, regardless of the angle of the light to the eye of the subject, or of the eye of the observer to that of the subject. With a diaphragm I got

How the Focus Was Changed

Fig. 24.—Arrangements for Photographing Images Reflected From the Eyeball

CM, concave mirror in which the subject may observe the images reflected from various parts of her eye; C, condenser; D, diaphragm; L, 1000-watt lamp; F, forehead rest; MP, bar which the subject grasps with her teeth for the purpose of holding her head steady; P, plane mirror upon which is pasted a letter of diamond type and in which is reflected a Snellen test card twenty feet behind the subject (the mirror is just above the letter P); CAM, camera; Pr, perimeter used to measure the angle of the light to the eye; R, plane mirror reflecting light from the 1000-watt lamp upon the eye, which otherwise would be in total darkness except for the part from which the highly condensed image of the filament is reflected; B, blue glass screen used to modify the light reflected from the mirror R. When the subject read the bottom line of the Snellen test card reflected in the mirror P, her eye was at rest, and when she saw the letter of diamond type distinctly it was accommodated ten diopters, as demonstrated by the retinoscope.

Fig. 24. Arrangements for Photographing Images Reflected From the Eyeball. CM, concave mirror in which the subject may observe the images reflected from various parts of her eye; C, condenser; D, diaphragm; L, 1000-watt lamp; F, forehead rest; MP, bar which the subject grasps with her teeth for the purpose of holding her head steady; P, plane mirror upon which is pasted a letter of diamond type and in which is reflected a Snellen test card twenty feet behind the subject (the mirror is just above the letter P); CAM, camera; Pr, perimeter used to measure the angle of the light to the eye; R, plane mirror reflecting light from the 1000- watt lamp upon the eye, which otherwise would be in total darkness except for the part from which the highly condensed image of the filament is reflected; B, blue glass screen used to modify the light reflected from the mirror R. When the subject read the bottom line of the Snellen test card reflected in the mirror P, her eye was at rest, and when she saw the letter of diamond type distinctly it was accommodated ten diopters, as demonstrated by the retinoscope.

Accommodation: Study of Images

Fig. 25. Arrangements for Holding the Head of the Subject Steady While Images Were Being Photographed. CM, concave mirror; F, forehead rest; C, condenser, MP, mouthpiece; Pr, perimeter.

Fig. 25. Arrangements for Holding the Head of the Subject Steady While Images Were Being Photographed

CM, concave mirror; F, forehead rest; C, condenser, MP, mouthpiece; Pr, perimeter.

a clearer and more constant image, but it still was not sufficiently reliable to be measured. To Helmholtz the indistinct image of a naked flame seemed to show an appreciable change, while the images obtained by the aid of the diaphragm showed it more clearly; but I was

Inconstancy of Candle Image

unable, either with a diaphragm or without it, to obtain images which I considered sufficiently distinct to be reliable.

Men who had been teaching and demonstrating Helmholtz's theory repeated his experiments for my benefit; but the images which they obtained on the front of the lens did not seem to me any better than my own. After

Fig. 26. Image of Electric Filament on the Front of the Lens. R, rest; A, accommodation. Under the magnifying glass no change can be observed in the size of the two images. The image at the right looks larger only because it is more distinct. To support the theory of Helmholz it ought to be the smaller. The comet's tail at the left of the two images is an accidental reflection from the cornea. The spot of light beneath is a reflection from the light used to illuminate the eye while the photo-graphs were being taken. It took two years to get these pictures.

studying these images almost daily for more than a year I was unable to make any reliable observation regarding the effect of accommodation upon them. In fact, it seemed that an infinite number of appearances might be obtained on the front of the lens when a candle was used as the source of illumination. At times the image became smaller during accommodation and seemed to sustain the theory of Helmholtz; but just as frequently it became larger. At other times it was impossible to tell what it did.

With a thirty-watt lamp, a fifty-watt lamp, a 250-watt lamp and a 1000-watt lamp, there was no improvement. The light of the sun reflected from the front of the lens produced an image just as cloudy and uncertain as the reflections from other sources of illumination, and just as variable in shape, intensity and size. To sum it all up, I was convinced that the anterior surface of the lens

Fig. 27. Images of the Electric Filament Reflected Simultaneously From the Cornea and Lens. R, rest; A, accommodation. The size of the images in both pictures is the same. The corneal image is so small that it has not been noticeably altered by the slight change that takes place in the cornea during accommodation. In A both images have changed their position and the end of the reflection from the lens has been cut off by the iris, but its width remains the same. The white spot between the two images of the filament is a reflection from the lamp used to illuminate the eye. Note that in A more of the sclera is visible, owing to the elongation of the eyeball during accommodation.

was a very poor reflector of light, and that no reliable images could be obtained from it by the means described.

After a year or more of failure I began to work at an aquarium on the eyes of fish. It was a long story of failure. Finally I became able, with the aid of a strong light -1000 watts - a diaphragm with a small opening and a condenser, to obtain, after some difficulty, a clear

Image on the Lens Photographed

and distinct image from the cornea of fish. This image was sufficiently distinct to be measured, and after many months a satisfactory photograph was obtained. Then the work was resumed on the eyes of human beings. The strong light, combined with the diaphragm and condenser, the use of which was suggested by their use to improve the illumination of a glass slide under the microscope, proved to be a decided improvement over the method of Helmholtz, and by means of this technique an image was at last obtained on the front of the lens which was sufficiently clear and distinct to be photographed. This was the first time, so far as published records show, that an image of any kind was ever photographed from the front of the lens. Professional photographers whom I consulted with a view to securing their assistance assured me that the thing could not be done, and declined to attempt it. I was therefore obliged to learn photography, of which I have previously known nothing, myself, and I then found that so far as the image obtained by the method of Helmholtz is concerned the professionals were right.

The experiments were continued until, after almost four years of constant labor, I obtained satisfactory pictures before and after accommodation and during the production of myopia and hypermetropia, not only of images on any surface at will without reflections from the iris, cornea, the front of the sclera (white of the eye) and the side of the sclera. I also became able to obtain images on any surface at will without reflections from the other parts. Before these results were obtained, however, many difficulties had still to be overcome.

Complicating reflections were a perpetual source of trouble. Reflections from surrounding objects were easily prevented ; but those from the sides of the globe of the electric light were difficult to deal with, and it was useless to try to obtain images on the front of the lens until they had been eliminated, or reduced to a minimum, by

Fig. 28. Image of Electric Filament Upon the Cornea. R, rest ; A, accommodation. The image is smaller in A, but the change is so slight as to be scarcely noticeable, showing that the alteration in the shape of the cornea during accommodation is very slight. For this reason the ophthalmometer, with its small image, has been thought to demonstrate that the cornea did not change during accommodation.

Fig. 28. Image of Electric Filament Upon the Cornea
R, rest; A, accommodation. The image is smaller in A, but the change is so slight as to be scarcely noticeable, showing that the alteration in the shape of the cornea during accommodation is very slight. For this reason the ophthalmometer, with its small image, has been thought to demonstrate that the cornea did not change during accommodation.

a proper adjustment of the light. The same apparent adjustment did not, however, always give similar results. Sometimes there would be no reflections for days; then would come a day when, with the light apparently at the same angle, they would reappear.

With some adjustments of the light multiple images were seen reflected from the front of the lens. Sometimes these images were arranged in a horizontal line, sometimes in a vertical one and sometimes at angles of

Unexplained Difficulties

different degrees, while their distance from each other also varied. Usually there were three of them; sometimes there were more; and sometimes there were only two. Occasionally they were all of the same size, but usually they varied, there being apparently no limit to their possibilities of change in this and other respects. Some of them were photographed, indicating that they were real reflections. Changes in the distance of the diaphragm from the light and from the condenser, and alterations in the size and shape of its opening, appeared to make no difference. Different adjustments of the condenser were equally without effect. Changes in the angle at which the light was adjusted sometimes lessened the number of images and sometimes increased them, until at last an angle was found at which but one image was seen. The images appear, in fact, to have been caused by reflections from the globe of the electric light.

Even after the light had been so adjusted as to eliminate reflections it was often difficult, or impossible, to get a clear and distinct image of the electric filament upon the front of the lens. One could, rearrange the condenser and the diaphragm and change the axis of fixation, and still the image would be clouded or obscured and its outline distorted. The cause of the difficulty appeared to be that the light was not adjusted at the best angle for the purpose and it was not always possible to determine the exact axis at which a clear, distinct image would be produced. As in the case of the reflections from the sides of the globe, it seemed to vary without a known cause. This was true, however: that there were angles of the axis of the globe which gave better images than others, and that what these angles were could not be determined with exactness. I have labored with the light for two or three hours without finding the right angle. At other times the axis would remain unchanged for days, giving always a clear, distinct image.

Fig. 29. Image of Electric Filament on the Front of the Sclera

R, rest; A, accommodation. During accommodation the front of the sclera becomes more convex, because the eyeball has elongated, just as a camera is elongated when it is focussed upon a near object. The spot of light on the cornea is an accidental reflection.

Fig. 29. Image of Electric Filament on the Front of the Sclera. R, rest; A, accommodation. During accommodation the front of the sclera becomes more convex, because the eyeball has elongated, just as a camera is elongated when it is focussed upon a near object. The spot of light on the cornea is an accidental reflection.

The results of these experiments confirmed the conclusions drawn from the previous ones, namely, that accommodation is due to a lengthening of the eyeball, and not to a change in the curvature of the lens. They also confirmed, in a striking manner, my earlier conclusions as to the conditions under which myopia and Hypermetropia are produced.1

The images photographed from the front of the lens did not show any change in size or form during accommodation. The image on the back of the lens also remained unchanged, as observed through the telescope of the ophthalmometer; but as there is no dispute about its behavior during accommodation, it was not photographed. Images photographed from the iris before

1 Bates: The Cause of Myopia, N. Y. Med. Jour., March 16, 1912.

No Change in Iris Image

and during accommodation were also the same in size and form, as was to be expected from the character of the lens images. If the lens changed during accommodation, the iris, which rests upon it, would change also.

Fig. 30. Images on the Side of the Sclera

R, rest; A, accommodation. The image in A is the larger, indicating a flattening of the side of the sclera as the eyeball elongates. My, Myopia. The eye is straining to see at the distance and the image is larger, indicating that the eyeball has elongated, resulting in a flattening of the side of the sclera. Hy, Hypermetropia. The eye is straining to see at two inches. The image is the smallest of the series, indicating that the eyeball has become shorter than in any of the other pictures, and the side of the sclera more convex. The two lower pictures confirm the author's previous observations that farsight is produced when the eye strains to see near objects and nearsight when it strains to see distant objects.

Fig. 30. Images on the Side of the Sclera. R, rest; A, accommodation. The image in A is the larger, indicating a flattening of the side of the sclera as the eyeball elongates. My, Myopia. The eye is straining to see at the distance and the image is larger, indicating that the eyeball has elongated, resulting in a flattening of the side of the sclera. Hy, Hypermetropia. The eye is straining to see at two inches. The image is the smallest of the series, indicating that the eyeball has become shorter than in any of the other pictures, and the side of the sclera more convex. The two lower pictures confirm the author's previous observations that farsight is produced when the eye strains to see near objects and nearsight when it strains to see distant objects.

A Series of Four Changes

The images photographed from the cornea and from the front and side of the sclera showed, however, a series of four well-marked changes, according to whether the vision was normal or accompanied by a strain. During accommodation the images from the cornea were smaller than when the eye was at rest, indicating elongation of the eyeball and a consequent increase in the convexity of the cornea. But when an unsuccessful effort was made to see at the near-point, the image became larger, indicating that the cornea had become less convex, a condition which one would expect when the optic axis was shortened, as in hypermetropia. When a strain was made to see at a distance the image was smaller than when the eye was at rest, again indicating elongation of the eyeball and increased convexity of the cornea.

Fig. 31. Multiple Images Upon the Front of the Lens

Fig. 31. Multiple Images Upon the Front of the Lens. This picture illustrates one of the difficulties that had to be overcome in photographing images reflected from various parts of the eyeball. Unless the light was adjusted at precisely the right angle the filament was multiplied by reflection from the sides of the globe. Usually the image was doubled, sometimes it was tripled, as shown in the picture, and sometimes it was quadrupled. Often days of labor were required to eliminate these reflections, and for reasons that were not definitely determined the same adjustment did not always give the same results. Sometimes all would go well for days, and then, without any apparent reason, the multiple images would return.

The images photographed from the front of the sclera showed the same series of changes as the corneal images, but those obtained from the side of the sclera were found to have changed in exactly the opposite manner, being larger where the former were smaller and vice versa, a

Fig. 32. Reflection of the Electric Filament From the Iris

Fig. 32. Reflection of the Electric Filament From the Iris. This picture is shown to illustrate the fact that it is possible to get a reflection from any reflecting surface of the eyeball without reflections from the other parts, although these may be exposed. This is done by changing the angle of the light to the eye. In No. 1 observations of the eye at the time the picture was taken demonstrated that the image was from the iris, not from the cornea, and the fact is also apparent in the picture. (Compare the image with the corneal reflection in Fig. 28.) In No. 2, where the image overlaps the margin of the pupil, the fact that the reflection is from the iris is manifest from the circumstance that only part of the filament is seen. If it were from the cornea, the whole of it would be reflected. Note in this picture that there is no reflection from the lens. The images on the iris did not change their size or shape during accommodation, demonstrating again that the lens, upon which the iris rests, does not change its shape when the eye adjusts itself for near vision.

difference which one would naturally expect from the fact that when the front of the sclera becomes more convex the sides must become flatter.

When an effort was made to see at a distance the image reflected from the side of the sclera was larger than the image obtained when the eye was at rest, indicating that this part of the sclera had become less convex or flatter, because of elongation of the eyeball. The image obtained during normal accommodation was also larger than when the eye was at rest, indicating again a flattening of the side of the sclera. The image obtained, however, when an effort was made to see near was much smaller than any of the other images, indicating that the sclera had become more convex at the side, a condition which one would expect when the eyeball was shortened, as in hypermetropia.

The most pronounced of the changes were noted in the images reflected from the front of the sclera. Those on the side of the sclera were less marked, and, owing to the difficulty of photographing a white image on a white background, could not always be readily seen on the photographs. They were always plainly apparent, however, to the observer, and still more so to the subject, who regarded them in a concave mirror. The alterations in the size of the corneal image were so slight that they did not show at all in the photographs, except when the image was large, a fact which explains why the ophthalmometer, with its small image, has been thought to show that the cornea did not change during accommodation. They were always apparent, however, to the subject and observer.

The corneal image was one of the easiest of the series to produce and the experiment is one which almost any

No Change in Back of Lens

Fig. 33. Demonstrating That the Back of the Lens Does Not Change During Accommodation. The filament of an electric light (L) is shining into the eye of the subject (S), and the reflection on the back of the lens can be seen by the observer (O) in the telescope (T). The subject holds in her hand, at a distance of four inches, a mirror on which is pasted a small letter, and in which is reflected a Snellen test card hung above and behind her head at a distance of twenty feet. The retinoscope reveals that when she looks at the reflection of the test card and reads the bottom line the eye is at rest, and that when she looks at the letter pasted on the mirror it accommodates. The image on the lens does not change during these changes of focus. The telescope is the telescope of the ophthalmometer, the prisms having been removed. As there is no dispute about the behavior of the back of the lens during accommodation this image was not photographed.

one can repeat, the only apparatus required being a fifty candlepower lamp - an ordinary electric globe - and a concave mirror fastened to a rod which moves back and forth in a groove so that the distance of the mirror from the eye can be altered at will. A plane mirror might also be used; but the concave glass is better, because it magnifies the image. The mirror should be so arranged that it reflects the image of the electric filament on the cornea, and so that the eye of the subject can see this reflection by looking straight ahead.

The image in the mirror is used as the point of fixation, and the distance at which the eye focuses is altered by altering the distance of the mirror from the eye. The light can be placed within an inch or two of the eye, as the heat is not great enough to interfere with the experiment. The closer it is the larger the image, and according to whether it is adjusted vertically, horizontally, or at an angle, the clearness of the reflection may vary. A blue glass screen can be used, if desired, to lessen the discomfort of the light. If the left eye is used by the subject - and in all the experiments it was found to be the more convenient for the purpose - the source of light should be placed to the left of that eye and as much as possible to the front of it, at an angle of about forty-five degrees. For absolute accuracy the light and the head of the subject should be held immovable, but for demonstration this is not essential. Simply holding the bulb in his hand the subject can demonstrate that the image changes according to whether the eye is at rest, accommodating normally for near vision, or straining to see at a near or a distant point.

In the original report were described possible sources of error and the means taken to eliminate them.

CHAPTER VI

THE TRUTH ABOUT ACCOMMODATION AS DEMONSTRATED BY CLINICAL OBSERVATIONS

THE testimony of the experiments described in the preceding chapters to the effect that the lens is not a factor in accommodation is confirmed by numerous observations on the eyes of adults and children, with normal vision, errors of refraction, or amblyopia, and on the eyes of adults after the removal of the lens for cataract.

It has already been pointed out that the instillation of atropine into the eye is supposed to prevent accommodation by paralyzing the muscle credited with controlling the shape of the lens. That it has this effect is stated in every text-book on the subject, 1 and the drug is daily used in the fitting of glasses for the purpose of eliminating the supposed influence of the lens upon refractive states.

In about nine cases out of ten the conditions resulting from the instillation of atropine into the eye fit the theory upon which its use is based; but in the tenth case they do not, and every ophthalmologist of any experience has noted some of these tenth cases. Many of them are reported in the literature, and many of them have come under my own observation. According to the theory,

1 Certain substances have the power of producing a dilation of the pupil (mydriasis), and hence are termed mydriatics. At the same time they act upon the ciliary body, diminishing and, when applied in sufficient strength, completely paralyzing the power of accommodation, thus rendering the eye for some time unalterably focussed for the farthest point. - Herman Snellen, Jr.: Mydriatics and Myotics, System of Diseases of the Eye, edited by Morris and Oliver, 1897-1900, vpl. ii, p. 30.

Accommodation: Clinical Observations

atropine ought to bring out latent hypermetropia in eyes either apparently normal, or manifestly hypermetropic, provided, of course, the patient is of the age during which the lens is supposed to retain its elasticity. The fact is that it sometimes produces myopia, or changes Hypermetropia into myopia, and that it will produce both myopia and hypermetropia in persons over seventy years of age, when the lens is supposed to be as hard as a stone, as well as in cases in which the lens is hard with incipient cataract. Patients with eyes apparently normal will, after the use of atropine, develop hypermetropic astigmatism, or myopic astigmatism, or compound myopic astigmatism, or mixed astigmatism. 1 In other cases the drug will not interfere with the accommodation, or alter the refraction in any way. Furthermore, when the vision has been lowered by atropine the subjects have often become able, simply by resting their eyes, to read diamond type at six inches. Yet atropine is supposed to rest the eyes by affording relief to an overworked muscle.

In the treatment of squint and amblyopia I have often used atropine in the better eye for more than a year, in order to encourage the use of the amblyopic eye; and at the end of this time, while still under the influence of atropine, such eyes have become able in a few hours, or less, to read diamond type at six inches (see Chapter XXII). The following are examples of many similar cases that might be cited:

A boy of ten had hypermetropia in both eyes, that of

1 In simple hypermetropic astigmatism one principal meridian is normal and the other, at right angles to it, is flatter. In simple myopic astigmatism the contrary is the case ; one principal meridian is normal and the other, at right angles to it, more convex. In mixed astigmatism one principal meridian is too flat, the other too convex. In compound hypermetropic astigmatism both principal meridians are flatter than normal, one more so than the other. In compound myopic astigmatism both are more convex than normal, one more so than the other.

Atropine Fails to Paralyze Accommodation

the left or better eye amounting to three diopters. When atropine was instilled into this eye the Hypermetropia was increased to four and a half diopters, and the vision lowered to 20/200. With a convex glass of four and a half diopters the patient obtained normal vision for the distance, and with the addition of another convex glass of four diopters he was able to read diamond type at ten inches (best). The atropine was used for a year, the pupil being dilated continually to the maximum. Meantime the right eye was being treated by methods to be described later. Usually in such cases the eye which is not being specifically treated improves to some extent with the others, but in this case it did not. At the end of the year the vision of the right eye had become normal; but that of the left eye remained precisely what it was at the beginning, being still 20/200 without glasses for the distance, while reading without glasses was impossible and the degree of the hypermetropia had not changed. Still under the influence of the atropine and still with the pupil dilated to the maximum, this eye was now treated separately; and in half an hour its vision had become normal both for the distance and the nearpoint, diamond type being read at six inches, all without glasses. According to the accepted theories, the ciliary muscle of this eye must not only have been completely paralyzed at the time, but must have been in a state of complete paralysis for a year. Yet the eye not only overcame four and a half diopters of hypermetropia, but added six diopters of accommodation, making a total of ten and a half. It remains for those who adhere to the accepted theories to say how such facts can be reconciled with them.

Equally, if not more remarkable, was the case of a little girl of six who had two and a half diopters of hypermetropia in her right or better eye, and six in the other, with one diopter of astigmatism. With the better eye under the influence of atropine and the pupil dilated to the maximum, both eyes were treated together for more than a year, and at the end of that time, the right being still under the influence of the atropine, both became able to read diamond type at six inches, the right doing it better, if anything, than the left. Thus, in spite of the atropine, the right eye not only overcame two and a half diopters of hypermetropia, but added six diopters of accommodation, making a total of eight and a half. In order to eliminate all possibility of latent hypermetropia in the left eye - which in the beginning had six diopters - the atropine was now used in this eye and discontinued in the other, the eye education being continued as before. Under the influence of the drug there was a slight return of the hypermetropia; but the vision quickly became normal again, and although the atropine was used daily for more than a year, the pupil being continually dilated to the maximum, it remained so, diamond type being read at six inches without glasses during the whole period. It is difficult for me to conceive how the ciliary muscle could have had anything to do with the ability of this patient to accommodate after atropine had been used in each eye separately for a year or more at a time.

According to the current theory, atropine paralyzes the ciliary muscle and thus, by preventing a change of curvature in the lens, prevents accommodation. When accommodation occurs, therefore, after the prolonged use of atropine, it is evident that it must be due to some factor or factors other than the lens and the ciliary muscle. The evidence of such cases against the accepted

Aphakia and Presbyopia

theories is, in fact, overwhelming; and according to these theories the other factors cited in this chapter are equally inexplicable. All of these facts, however, are in entire accord with the results of my experiments on the eye muscles of animals and my observations regarding the behavior of images reflected from various parts of the eyeball. They strikingly confirm, too, the testimony of the experiments with atropine, which showed that the accommodation could not be paralyzed completely and permanently unless the atropine was injected deep into the orbit, so as to reach the oblique muscles, the real muscles of accommodation, while hypermetropia could not be prevented when the eyeball was stimulated with electricity without a similar use of atropine, resulting in the paralysis of the recti muscles.

As has already been noted, the fact that after the removal of the lens for cataract the eye often appears to accommodate just as well as it did before is well known. Many of these cases have come under my own observation. Such patients have not only read diamond type with only their distance glasses on, at thirteen and ten inches and at a less distance, but one man was able to read without any glass at all. In all these cases the retinoscope demonstrated that the apparent act of accommodation was real, being accomplished, not by the "interpretation of circles of diffusion," or by any of the other methods by which this inconvenient phenomenon is commonly explained, but by an accurate adjustment of the focus to the distances concerned.

The cure of presbyopia (see Chapter XX) must also be added to the clinical testimony against the accepted theory of accommodation. On the theory that the lens is a factor in accommodation such cures would be manifestly impossible. The fact that rest of the eyes improves the sight in presbyopia has been noted by others, and has been attributed to the supposed fact that the rested ciliary muscle is able for a brief period to influence the hardened lens ; but while it is conceivable that this might happen in the early stages of the condition and for a few moments, it is not conceivable that permanent relief should be obtained by this means, or that lenses which are, as the saying goes, as "hard as a stone," should be influenced, even momentarily.

A truth is strengthened by an accumulation of facts. A working hypothesis is proved not to be a truth if a single fact is not in harmony with it. The accepted theories of accommodation and of the cause of errors of refraction require that a multitude of facts shall be explained away. During more than thirty years of clinical experience, I have not observed a single fact that was not in harmony with the belief that the lens and the ciliary muscle have nothing to do with accommodation, and that the changes in the shape of the eyeball upon which errors of refraction depend are not permanent. My clinical observations have of themselves been sufficient to demonstrate this fact. They have also been sufficient to show how errors of refraction can be produced at will, and how they may be cured, temporarily in a few minutes, and permanently by continued treatment.

CHAPTER VII
THE VARIABILITY OF THE REFRACTION OF THE EYE

THE theory that errors of refraction are due to permanent deformations of the eyeball leads naturally to the conclusion, not only that errors of refraction are permanent states, but that normal refraction is also a continuous condition. As this theory is almost universally accepted as a fact, therefore, it is not surprising to find that the normal eye is generally regarded as a perfect machine which is always in good working order. No matter whether the object regarded is strange or familiar, whether the light is good or imperfect, whether the surroundings are pleasant or disagreeable, even under conditions of nerve strain or bodily disease, the normal eye is expected to have normal refraction and normal sight all the time. It is true that the facts do not harmonize with this view, but they are conveniently attributed to the perversity of the ciliary muscle, or if that explanation will not work, ignored altogether.

When we understand, however, how the shape of the eyeball is controlled by the external muscles, and how it responds instantaneously to their action, it is easy to see that no refractive state, whether it is normal or abnormal, can be permanent. This conclusion is confirmed by the retinoscope, and I had observed the facts long before the experiments described in the preceding chapters had offered a satisfactory explanation for it. During thirty years devoted to the study of refraction, I have found few people who could maintain perfect sight for more than a few minutes at a time, even under the most favorable conditions; and often I have seen the refraction change half a dozen times or more in a second, the variations ranging all the way from twenty diopters of myopia to normal.

Similarly I have found no eyes with continuous or unchanging errors of refraction, all persons with errors of refraction having, at frequent intervals during the day and night, moments of normal vision, when their myopia, hypermetropia, or astigmatism, wholly disappears. The form of the error also changes, myopia even changing into hypermetropia, and one form of astigmatism into another.

Of twenty thousand school children examined in one year, more than half had normal eyes, with sight which was perfect at times; but not one of them had perfect sight in each eye at all times of the day. Their sight might be good in the morning and imperfect in the afternoon, or imperfect in the morning and perfect in the afternoon. Many children could read one Snellen test card with perfect sight, while unable to see a different one perfectly. Many could also read some letters of the alphabet perfectly, while unable to distinguish other letters of the same size under similar conditions. The degree of this imperfect sight varied within wide limits, from one-third to one-tenth, or less. Its duration was also variable. Under some conditions it might continue for only a few minutes, or less; under others it might prevent the subject from seeing the blackboard for days, weeks, or even longer. Frequently all the pupils in a classroom were affected to this extent.

Changing Refraction of Infants

Among babies a similar condition was noted. Most investigators have found babies hypermetropic. A few have found them myopic. My own observations indicate that the refraction of infants is continually changing. One child was examined under atropine on four successive days, beginning two hours after birth. A three per cent solution of atropine was instilled into both eyes, the pupil was dilated to the maximum, and other physiological symptoms of the use of atropine were noted. The first examination showed a condition of mixed astigmatism. On the second day there was compound hypermetropic astigmatism, and on the third compound myopic astigmatism. On the fourth one eye was normal and the other showed simple myopia. Similar variations were noted in many other cases.

What is true of children and infants is equally true of adults of all ages. Persons over seventy years of age have suffered losses of vision of variable degree and intensity, and in such cases the retinoscope always indicated an error of refraction. A man eighty years old, with normal eyes and ordinarily normal sight, had periods of imperfect sight which would last from a few minutes to half an hour or longer. Retinoscopy at such times always indicated myopia of four diopters or more.

During sleep the refractive condition of the eye is rarely, if ever, normal. Persons whose refraction is normal when they are awake will produce myopia, hypermetropia and astigmatism when they are asleep, or, if they have errors of refraction when they are awake, they will be increased during sleep. This is why people waken in the morning with eyes more tired than at any other time, or even with severe headaches. When the subject is under ether or chloroform, or unconscious from any other cause, errors of refraction are also produced or increased.

When the eye regards an unfamiliar object an error of refraction is always produced. Hence the proverbial fatigue caused by viewing pictures, or other objects, in a museum. Children with normal eyes who can read perfectly small letters a quarter of an inch high at ten feet always have trouble in reading strange writing on the blackboard, although the letters may be two inches high. A strange map, or any map, has the same effect. I have never seen a child, or a teacher, who could look at a map at the distance without becoming nearsighted. German type has been accused of being responsible for much of the poor sight once supposed to be peculiarly a German malady; but if a German child attempts to read Roman print, it will at once become temporarily hypermetropic. German print, or Greek or Chinese characters, will have the same effect on a child, or other person, accustomed to Roman letters. Cohn repudiated the idea that German lettering was trying to the eyes.[1] On the contrary, he always found it "pleasant, after a long reading of the monotonous Roman print, to return 'to our beloved German.' " Because the German characters were more familiar to him than any others he found them restful to his eyes. "Use," as he truly observed, "has much to do with the matter." Children learning to read, write, draw, or sew, always suffer from defective vision, because of the unfamiliarity of the lines or objects with which they are working.

A sudden exposure to strong light, or rapid or sudden changes of light, are likely to produce imperfect sight in the normal eye, continuing in some cases for weeks and months (see Chapter XVII).

[1] Eyes and School Books, Pop. Sci. Monthly, May, 1881, translated from Deutsche Rundschau.

Causes of Defective Vision in Normal Eyes

Noise is also a frequent cause of defective vision in the normal eye. All persons see imperfectly when they hear an unexpected loud noise. Familiar sounds do not lower the vision, but unfamiliar ones always do. Country children from quiet schools may suffer from defective vision for a long time after moving to a noisy city. In school they cannot do well with their work, because their sight is impaired. It is, of course, a gross injustice for teachers and others to scold, punish, or humiliate such children.

Under conditions of mental or physical discomfort, such as pain, cough, fever, discomfort from heat or cold, depression, anger, or anxiety, errors of refraction are always produced in the normal eye, or increased in the eye in which they already exist.

The variability of the refraction of the eye is responsible for many otherwise unaccountable accidents. When people are struck down in the street by automobiles, or trolley cars, it is often due to the fact that they were suffering from temporary loss of sight. Collisions on railroads or at sea, disasters in military operations, aviation accidents, etc., often occur because some responsible person suffered temporary loss of sight.

To this cause must also be ascribed, in a large degree, the confusion which every student of the subject has noted in the statistics which have been collected regarding the occurrence of errors of refraction. So far as I am aware it has never been taken into account by any investigator of the subject; yet the result in any such investigation must be largely determined by the conditions under which it is made. It is possible to take the best eyes in the world and test them so that the subject will not be able to get into the Army. Again, the test may be so made that eyes which are apparently much below normal at the beginning, may in the few minutes required for the test, acquire normal vision and become able to read the test card perfectly.

CHAPTER VIII
WHAT GLASSES DO TO US

THE Florentines were doubtless mistaken in supposing that their fellow citizen (see page v, Page 6) was the inventor of the lenses now so commonly worn to correct errors of refraction. There has been much discussion as to the origin of these devices, but they are generally believed to have been known at a period much earlier than that of Salvino degli Armati. The Romans at least must have known something of the art of supplementing the powers of the eye, for Pliny tells us that Nero used to watch the games in the Colosseum through a concave gem set in a ring for that purpose. If, however, his contemporaries believed that Salvino of the Armati was the first to produce these aids to vision, they might well pray for the pardon of his sins; for while it is true that eyeglasses have brought to some people improved vision and relief from pain and discomfort, they have been to others simply an added torture, they always do more or less harm, and at their best they never improve the vision to normal.

That glasses cannot improve the sight to normal can be very simply demonstrated by looking at any color through a strong convex or concave glass. It will be noted that the color is always less intense than when seen with the naked eye; and since the perception of form depends upon the perception of color, it follows that both color and form must be less distinctly seen with glasses than without them. <u>Even plane glass lowers the vision both for color and form, as everyone knows who has ever looked out of a window.</u> Women who wear glasses for minor defects of vision often observe that they are made more or less color-blind by them, and in a shop one may note that they remove them when they want to match samples. If the sight is seriously defective, the color may be seen better with glasses than without them.

That glasses must injure the eye is evident from the facts given in the preceding chapter. <u>One cannot see through them unless one produces the degree of refractive error which they are designed to correct.</u> But refractive errors, in the eye which is left to itself, are never constant. If one secures good vision by the aid of concave, or convex, or astigmatic lenses, therefore, it means that one is maintaining constantly a degree of refractive error which otherwise would not be maintained constantly. It is only to be expected that this should make the condition worse, and it is a matter of common experience that it does. After people once begin to wear glasses their strength, in most cases, has to be steadily increased in order to maintain the degree of visual acuity secured by the aid of the first pair. Persons with presbyopia who put on glasses because they cannot read fine print too often find that after they have worn them for a time they cannot, without their aid, read the larger print that was perfectly plain to them before. <u>A person with myopia of 20/70 who puts on glasses giving him a vision of 20/20 may find that in a week's time his unaided vision has declined to 20/200,</u> and we have the testimony of Dr. Sidler-Huguenin, of Zurich,[1] that of the thousands of myopes treated by him the majority grew steadily worse, in spite of all the skill he could apply to the fitting of glasses for them. <u>When people break their glasses and go without them for a week or two, they</u>

[1] Archiv. f. Augenh., vol. lxxix, 1915, translated in Arch. Ophth., vol. xlv, Nov. 6, 1916.

The Eye Resents Glasses

<u>frequently observe that their sight has improved.</u> As a matter of fact the sight always improves, to a greater or less degree, when glasses are discarded, although the fact may not always be noted.

That the human eye resents glasses is a fact which no one would attempt to deny. Every oculist knows that patients have to "get used" to them, and that sometimes they never succeed in doing so. Patients with high degrees of myopia and hypermetropia have great difficulty in accustoming themselves to the full correction, and often are never able to do so. The strong concave glasses required by myopes of high degree make all objects seem much smaller than they really are, while convex glasses enlarge them. These are unpleasantnesses that cannot be overcome. Patients with high degrees of astigmatism suffer some very disagreeable sensations when they first put on glasses, for which reason they are warned by one of the "Conservation of Vision" leaflets published by the Council on Health and Public Instruction of the American Medical Association to "get used to them at home before venturing where a misstep might cause a serious accident."[1] Usually these difficulties are overcome, but often they are not, and it sometimes happens that those who get on fairly well with their glasses in the daytime never succeed in getting used to them at night.

All glasses contract the field of vision to a greater or less degree. Even with very weak glasses patients are unable to see distinctly unless they look through the center of the lenses, with the frames at right angles to the line of vision; and not only is their vision lowered if they fail to do this, but annoying nervous symptoms,

[1] Lancaster: Wearing Glasses, p. 15.

such as dizziness and headache, are sometimes produced. Therefore they are unable to turn their eyes freely in different directions. It is true that glasses are now ground in such a way that it is theoretically possible to look through them at any angle, but practically they seldom accomplish the desired result.

The difficulty of keeping the glass clear is one of the minor discomforts of glasses, but nevertheless a most annoying one. On damp and rainy days the atmosphere clouds them. On hot days the perspiration from the body may have a similar effect. On cold days they are often clouded by the moisture of the breath. Every day they are so subject to contamination by dust and moisture and the touch of the fingers incident to unavoidable handling that it is seldom they afford an absolutely unobstructed view of the objects regarded.

Reflections of strong light from eyeglasses are often very annoying, and in the street may be very dangerous.

Soldiers, sailors, athletes, workmen and children have great difficulty with glasses because of the activity of their lives, which not only leads to the breaking of the lenses, but often throws them out of focus, particularly in the case of eyeglasses worn for astigmatism.

The fact that glasses are very disfiguring may seem a matter unworthy of consideration in a medical publication; but mental discomfort does not improve either the general health or the vision, and while we have gone so far toward making a virtue of what we conceive to be necessity that some of us have actually come to consider glasses becoming, huge round lenses in ugly tortoiseshell frames being positively fashionable at the present time, there are still some unperverted minds to which the wearing of glasses is mental torture and the sight of them upon others far from agreeable. Most human

Glasses to Relieve Strain

beings are, unfortunately, ugly enough without putting glasses upon them, and to disfigure any of the really beautiful faces that we have with such contrivances is surely as bad as putting an import tax upon art. As for putting glasses upon a child it is enough to make the angels weep.

Up to a generation ago glasses were used only as an aid to defective sight, but they are now prescribed for large numbers of persons who can see as well or better without them. As explained in Chapter I, the hypermetropic eye is believed to be capable of correcting its own difficulties to some extent by altering the curvature of the lens, through the activity of the ciliary muscle. The eye with simple myopia is not credited with this capacity, because an increase in the convexity of the lens, which is supposed to be all that is accomplished by accommodative effort, would only increase the difficulty; but myopia is usually accompanied by astigmatism, and this, it is believed, can be overcome, in part, by alterations in the curvature of the lens. Thus we are led by the theory to the conclusion that an eye in which any error of refraction exists is practically never free, while open, from abnormal accommodative efforts. In other words, it is assumed that the supposed muscle of accommodation has to bear, not only the normal burden of changing the focus of the eye for vision at different distances, but the additional burden of compensating for refractive errors. Such adjustments, if they actually took place, would naturally impose a severe strain upon the nervous system, and it is to relieve this strain - which is believed to be the cause of a host of functional nervous troubles - quite as much as to improve the sight, that glasses are prescribed.

It has been demonstrated, however, that the lens is not a factor, either in the production of accommodation, or in the correction of errors of refraction. Therefore under no circumstances can there be a strain of the ciliary muscle to be relieved. It has also been demonstrated that when the vision is normal no error of refraction is present, and the extrinsic muscles of the eyeball are at rest. Therefore there can be no strain of the extrinsic muscles to be relieved in these cases. When a strain of these muscles does exist, glasses may correct its effects upon the refraction, jut the strain itself they cannot relieve. On the contrary, as has been shown, they must make it worse. Nevertheless persons with normal vision who wear glasses for the relief of a supposed muscular strain are often benefited by them. This is a striking illustration of the effect of mental suggestion, and plane glass, if it could inspire the same faith, would produce the same result. In fact, many patients have told me that they had been relieved of various discomforts by glasses which I found to be simply plane glass. One of these patients was an optician who had fitted the glasses himself and was under no illusions whatever about them; yet he assured me that when he didn't wear them he got headaches.

Some patients are so responsive to mental suggestion that you can relieve their discomfort, or improve their sight, with almost any glasses you like to put on them. I have seen people with hypermetropia wearing myopic glasses with a great deal of comfort, and people with no astigmatism getting much satisfaction from glasses designed for the correction of this defect.

Landolt mentions the case of a patient who had for years worn prisms for insufficiency of the internal recti, and who found them absolutely indispensable for work, although the apices were toward the nose. The prescrip

Effects of Mental Suggestion

tion, which the patient was able to produce, called for prisms adjusted in the usual manner, with the apices toward the temples ; but the optician had made a mistake which, owing to the patient's satisfaction with the result, had never been discovered. Landolt explained the case by "the slight effect of weak prisms and the great power of imagination": [1] and doubtless the benefit derived from the glasses was real, resulting from the patient's great faith in the specialist - described as "one of the most competent of ophthalmologists" - who prescribed them.

Some patients will even imagine that they see better with glasses that markedly lower the vision. A number of years ago a patient for whom I had prescribed glasses consulted an ophthalmologist whose reputation was much greater than my own, and who gave him another pair of glasses and spoke slightingly of the ones that I had prescribed. The patient returned to me and told me how much better he could see with the second pair of glasses than he did with the first. I tested his vision with the new glasses, and found that while mine had given him a vision of 20/20 those of my colleague enabled him to see only 20/40. The simple fact was that he had been hypnotized by a great reputation into thinking he could see better when he actually saw worse ; and it was hard to convince him that he was wrong, although he had to admit that when he looked at the test card he could see only half as much with the new glasses as with the old ones.

When glasses do not relieve headaches and other nervous symptoms it is assumed to be because they were not properly fitted, and some practitioners and their patients exhibit an astounding degree of patience and

[1] Anomalies of the Motor Apparatus of the Eye, System of Diseases of the Eye, voL iv, pp. 154-155.

perseverance in their joint attempts to arrive at the proper prescription. A patient who suffered from severe pains at the base of his brain was fitted sixty times by one specialist alone, and had besides visited many other eye and nerve specialists in this country and in Europe. He was relieved of the pain in five minutes by the methods presented in this book, while his vision, at the same time, became temporarily normal.

It is fortunate that many people for whom glasses have been prescribed refuse to wear them, thus escaping not only much discomfort but much injury to their eyes. Others, having less independence of mind, or a larger share of the martyr's spirit, or having been more badly frightened by the oculists, submit to an amount of unnecessary torture which is scarcely conceivable. One such patient wore glasses for twenty-five years, although they did not prevent her from suffering continual misery and lowered her vision to such an extent that she had to look over the tops when she wanted to see anything at a distance. Her oculist assured her that she might expect the most serious consequences if she did not wear the glasses, and was very severe about her practice of looking over instead of through them.

As refractive abnormalities are continually changing, not only from day to day and from hour to hour, but from minute to minute, even under the influence of atropine, the accurate fitting of glasses is, of course, impossible. In some cases these fluctuations are so extreme, or the patient so unresponsive to mental suggestion, that no relief whatever is obtained from correcting lenses, which necessarily become under such circumstances an added discomfort. At their best it cannot be maintained that glasses are anything more than a very unsatisfactory substitute for normal vision.

CHAPTER IX

THE CAUSE AND CURE OF ERRORS OF REFRACTION

IT has been demonstrated in thousands of cases that all abnormal action of the external muscles of the eyeball is accompanied by a strain or effort to see, and that with the relief of this strain the action of the muscles becomes normal and all errors of refraction disappear. The eye may be blind, it may be suffering from atrophy of the optic nerve, from cataract, or disease of the retina; but so long as it does not try to see, the external muscles act normally and there is no error of refraction. This fact furnishes us with the means by which all these conditions, so long held to be incurable, may be cured.

It has also been demonstrated that for every error of refraction there is a different kind of strain. The study of images reflected from various parts of the eyeball confirmed what had previously been observed, namely, that myopia (or a lessening of hypermetropia) is always associated with a strain to see at the distance, while hypermetropia (or a lessening of myopia) is always associated with a strain to see at the near-point ; and the fact can be verified in a few minutes by anyone who knows how to use a retinoscope, provided only that the instrument is not brought nearer to the subject than six feet.

In an eye with previously normal vision a strain to see near objects always results in the temporary production of hypermetropia in one or all meridians. That is, the eye either becomes entirely hypermetropic, or some form

Fig. 34. Straining to See at the Near-Point Produces Hypermetropia

Patient reading fine print in a good light at thirteen inches, the object of vision being placed above the eye so as to be out of the line of the camera. Simultaneous retinoscopy indicated that the eye was focused at thirteen inches. The glass was used with the retinoscope to determine the amount of the refraction.

When the room was darkened the patient failed to read the fine print at thirteen inches and the retinoscope indicated that the eye was focused at a greater distance. When a conscious strain of considerable degree was made to see, the eye became hypermetropic.

Fig. 34. Straining to See at the Near-Point Produces Hypermetropia. Patient reading fine print in a good light at thirteen inches, the object of vision being placed above the eye so as to be out of the line of the camera. Simultaneous retinoscopy indicated that the eye was focused at thirteen inches. The glass was used with the retinoscope to determine the amount of the refraction.

When the room was darkened the patient failed to read the fine print at thirteen inches and the retinoscope indicated that the eye was focused at a greater distance. When a conscious strain of considerable degree was made to see, the eye became hypermetropic.

Voluntary Increase of Refractive Error

Fig. 35 Myopia Produced by unconscious Strain to See at the Distance is Increased by Conscious Strain.

No. 1. Normal vision.

No. 2. Same subject four years later with myopia. Note the strained expression.

No. 3. Myopia increased by conscious effort to see a distant object.

Fig. 36. Immediate Production of Myopia and Myopic Astigmatism in Eyes Previously Normal by Strain to See at the Distance.

Boy reading the Snellen test card with normal vision. Note the absence of facial strain.

The same boy trying to see a picture at twenty feet. The effort, manifested by staring, produces compound myopic astigmatism, as revealed by the retinoscope.

The same boy making himself myopic voluntarily by partly closing the eyelids and making a conscious effort to read the test card at ten feet.

The same boy making himself myopic voluntarily by partly closing the eyelids and making a conscious effort to read the test card at ten feet.

Emmetropia at the Near-Point

of astigmatism is produced of which hypermetropia forms a part. In the hypermetropic eye the hypermetropia is increased in one or all meridians. When the myopic eye strains to see a near object the myopia is lessened and emmetropia[1] may be produced, the eye being focussed for parallel rays while still trying to see at the near-point. In some cases the emmetropia may even pass over into hypermetropia in one or all meridians. All these changes are accompanied by evidences of increasing strain, in the form of eccentric fixation (see Chapter XI) and lowered vision ; but, strange to say, pain and fatigue are usually relieved to a marked degree. If, on the contrary, the eye with previously normal vision strains to see at the distance, temporary myopia is always produced in one or all meridians, and if the eye is already myopic, the myopia is increased. If the hypermetropic eye strains to see a distant object, pain and fatigue may be produced or increased; but the hypermetropia and the eccen-

[1] Emmetropia (from the Greek emmetros, in measure, and ops, the eye) is that condition of the eye in which it is focussed for parallel rays. This constitutes normal vision at the distance, but is an error of refraction when it occurs at the near-point.

tric fixation are lessened and the vision improves. This interesting result, it will be noted, is the exact contrary of what we get when the myope strains to see at the near-point. In some cases the hypermetropia is completely relieved, and emmetropia is produced, with a complete disappearance of all evidences of strain. This condition may then pass over into myopia, with an increase of strain as the myopia increases.

In other words <u>the eye which strains to see at the nearpoint becomes flatter than it was before, in one or all meridians. If it was elongated to start with, it may pass</u>

Fig. 37. Myopic Astigmatism comes and Goes According as the Subject Looks at Distant Objects With or Without Strain

No. 1.—Patient regarding the Snellen test card at ten feet without effort and reading the bottom line with normal vision.

No. 2.—The same patient making an effort to see a picture at twenty feet. The retinoscope indicated compound myopic astigmatism.

Fig. 37. Myopic Astigmatism comes and Goes According as the Subject Looks at Distant Objects With or Without Strain. No. 1 Patient regarding the Snellen test card at ten feet without effort and reading the bottom line with normal vision. No. 2. The same patient making an effort to see a picture at twenty feet. The retinoscope indicated compound myopic astigmatism.

Strain in Lensless Eyes

from this condition through emmetropia, in which it is spherical, to hypermetropia, in which it is flattened; and if these changes take place unsymmetrically, astigmatism will be produced in connection with the other conditions. The eye which strains to see at the distance, on the contrary, becomes longer than it was before in one or all meridians, and may pass from the flattened condition of hypermetropia, through emmetropia, to the elongated condition of myopia. If these changes take place unsymmetrically, astigmatism will again be produced in connection with the other conditions.

What has been said of the normal eye applies equally to eyes from which the lens has been removed. This operation produces usually a condition of hypermetropia; but when there has previously been a condition of high myopia the removal of the lens may not be sufficient to correct it, and the eye may still remain myopic. In the first case a strain to see at the distance lessens the hypermetropia, and a strain to see at the near-point increases it; in the second a strain to see at the distance increases the myopia, and a strain to see at the nearpoint lessens it. For a longer or shorter period after the removal of the lens many aphakic eyes strain to see at the near-point, producing so much hypermetropia that the patient cannot read ordinary print, and the power of accommodation appears to have been completely lost. Later, when the patient becomes accustomed to the situation, this strain is often relieved, and the eye becomes able to focus accurately upon near objects. Some rare cases have also been observed in which a measure of good vision both for distance and the near-point was obtained without glasses, the eyeball elongating sufficiently to compensate, to some degree, for the loss of the lens.

Should Have Been Impossible

No. 1.—The patient is reading the Snellen test card at twenty feet with normal vision. No. 2.—She is straining to see the test card at the same distance, and her hypermetropia is lessened by two diopters so that her glass now overcorrects it and she cannot see the card perfectly. No. 3.—With a convex reading glass of thirteen diopters the right eye is focussed accurately at thirteen inches. No. 4.—The patient is straining to see at the same distance and her hypermetropia is so increased that in order to read she would require a glass of fifteen diopters. On the basis of the accepted theory that the power of accommodation is wholly destroyed by the removal of the lens these changes in the refraction would have been impossible. The experiment was repeated several times and it was found that the error of refraction produced by straining to see varied, being sometimes more and sometimes less than two diopters.

Fig. 38. This Patient Had Had the Lens of the Right Eye Removed for Cataract and Was Wearing an Artificial Eye in the Left Socket. The Removal of the Lens created a Condition of Hypermetropia Which Was Corrected by a Convex Glass of Ten Diopters.
No. 1. The patient is reading the Snellen test card at twenty feet with normal vision. No. 2. She is straining to see the test card at the same distance, and her hypermetropia is lessened by two diopters so that her glass now overcorrects it and she cannot see the card perfectly. No. 3. With a convex reading glass of thirteen diopters the right eye is focussed accurately at thirteen inches. No. 4. The patient is straining to see at the same distance and her hypermetropia is so increased that in order to read she would require a glass of fifteen diopters. On the basis of the accepted theory that the power of accommodation is wholly destroyed by the removal of the lens these changes in the refraction would have been impossible. The experiment was repeated several times and it was found that the error of refraction produced by straining to see varied, being sometimes more and sometimes less than two diopters.

The phenomena associated with strain in the human eye have also been observed in the eyes of the lower animals. I have made many dogs myopic by inducing them to strain to see a distant object. One very nervous dog, with normal refraction, as demonstrated by the retinoscope, was allowed to smell a piece of meat. He became very much excited, pricked up his ears, arched his eyebrows and wagged his tail. The meat was then removed to a distance of twenty feet. The dog looked disappointed, but didn't lose interest. While he was watching the meat it was dropped into a box. A worried look came into his eyes. He strained to see what had become of it, and the retinoscope showed that he had become myopic. This experiment, it should be added, would succeed only with an animal possessing two active oblique muscles. Animals in which one of these muscles is absent or rudimentary are unable to elongate the eyeball under any circumstances.

Primarily the strain to see is a strain of the mind, and, as in all cases in which there is a strain of the mind, there is a loss of mental control. Anatomically the results of straining to see at a distance may be the same as those of regarding an object at the near point without strain; but in one case the eye does what the mind desires ; and in the other it does not.

These facts appear sufficiently to explain why visual acuity declines as civilization advances. Under the conditions of civilized life men's minds are under a continual strain. They have more things to worry them than uncivilized man had, and they are not obliged to keep cool and collected in order that they may see and do other things upon which existence depends. If he allowed himself to get nervous, primitive man was promptly

Relation of Civilization to Vision

Fig. 39. A Family Group Strikingly Illustrating the Effect of the Mind Upon the Vision

No. 1.—Girl of four with normal eyes. No. 2.—The child's mother with myopia. No. 3—The same girl at nine with myopia. Note that her expression has completely changed, and is now exactly like her mother's. Nos. 4, 5 and 6.—The girl's brother at two, six and eight. His eyes are normal in all three pictures. The girl has either inherited her mother's disposition to take things hard, or has been injuriously effected by her personality of strain. The boy has escaped both influences. In view of the prevailing theories about the relation of heredity to myopia, this picture is particularly interesting.

eliminated; but civilized man survives and transmits his mental characteristics to posterity. The lower animals when subjected to civilized conditions respond to them in precisely the same way as do human creatures. I have examined many domestic and menagerie animals, and have found them, in many cases, myopic, although they neither read, nor write, nor sew, nor set type.

Fig. 39. A Family Group Strikingly Illustrating the Effect of the Mind Upon the Vision. No. 1. Girl of four with normal eyes. No. 2. The child's mother with myopia. No. 3 The same girl at nine with myopia. Note that her expression has completely changed, and is now exactly like her mother's. Nos. 4, 5 and 6. The girl's brother at two, six and eight. His eyes are normal in all three pictures. The girl has either inherited her mother's disposition to take things hard, or has been injuriously effected by her personality of strain. The boy has escaped both influences. In view of the prevailing theories about the relation of heredity to myopia, this picture is particularly interesting.

A decline in visual acuity at the distance, however, is no more a peculiarity of civilization than is a similar decline at the near-point. Myopes, although they see better at the near-point than they do at the distance, never see as well as does the eye with normal sight; and in hypermetropia, which is more common than myopia, the sight is worse at the near-point than at the distance.

Fig. 40. Myopes Who Never Went to School, or Read in the Subway. No. 1. Myopic elephant in the Central Park Zoo, New York, thirty-nine years old. Young elephants and other young animals were found to have normal vision. No. 2. Cape buffalo with myopia, Central Park Zoo. No. 3. Myopic monkey, also in the Central Park Zoo. No. 4. Pet dog with myopia which progressed from year to year.

Relaxation Cures

The remedy is not to avoid either near work or distant vision, but to get rid of the mental strain which underlies the imperfect functioning of the eye at both points; and it has been demonstrated in thousands of cases that this can always be done.

Fortunately, all persons are able to relax under certain conditions at will. In all uncomplicated errors of refraction the strain to see can be relieved, temporarily, by having the patient look at a blank wall without trying to see. To secure permanent relaxation sometimes requires considerable time and much ingenuity. The same method cannot be used with everyone. The ways in which people strain to see are infinite, and the methods used to relieve the strain must be almost equally varied. Whatever the method that brings most relief, however, the end is always the same, namely relaxation. By constant repetition and frequent demonstration and by all means possible, the fact must be impressed upon the patient that perfect sight can be obtained only by relaxation. Nothing else matters.

Most people, when told that rest, or relaxation, will cure their eye troubles, ask why sleep does not do so. The answer to this question was given in Chapter VII. The eyes are rarely, if ever, completely relaxed in sleep, and if they are under a strain when the subject is awake, that strain will certainly be continued during sleep, to a greater or less degree, just as a strain of other parts of the body is continued.

 The idea that it rests the eyes not to use them is also erroneous. The eyes were made to see with, and if when they are open they do not see, it is because they are under such a strain and have such a great error of refraction that they cannot see. Near vision, although accomplished by a muscular act, is no more a strain on them than is distant vision, although accomplished without the intervention of the muscles. The use of the muscles does not necessarily produce fatigue. Some men can run for hours without becoming tired. Many birds support themselves upon one foot during sleep, the toes tightly clasping the swaying bough and the muscles remaining unfatigued by the apparent strain. Fabre tells of an insect which hung back downward for ten months from the roof of its wire cage, and in that position performed all the functions of life, even to mating and laying its eggs. Those who fear the effect of civilization, with its numerous demands for near vision, upon the eye may take courage from the example of this marvelous little animal which, in a state of nature, hangs by its feet only at intervals, but in captivity can do it for ten months on end, the whole of its life's span, apparently without inconvenience or fatigue. [1]

The fact is that when the mind is at rest nothing can tire the eyes, and when the mind is under a strain nothing can rest them. Anything that rests the mind will benefit the eyes. Almost everyone has observed that the eyes tire less quickly when reading an interesting book than when perusing something tiresome or difficult to comprehend. A schoolboy can sit up all night reading a novel without even thinking of his eyes, but if he tried to sit up all night studying his lessons he would soon find them getting very tired. A child whose vision was

[1] The Wonders of Instinct, English translation by de Mattos and Miall, 1918, pp. 36-38.

Time Required for a Cure

ordinarily so acute that she could see the moons of Jupiter with the naked eye became myopic when asked to do a sum in mental arithmetic, mathematics being a subject which was extremely distasteful to her. Sometimes the conditions which produce mental relaxation are very curious. One patient, for instance, was able to correct her error of refraction when she looked at the test card with her body bent over at an angle of about forty-five degrees, and the relaxation continued after she had assumed the upright position. Although the position was an unfavorable one, she had somehow got the idea that it improved her sight, and therefore it did so.

The time required to effect a permanent cure varies greatly with different individuals. In some cases five, ten, or fifteen minutes is sufficient, and I believe the time is coming when it will be possible to cure everyone quickly. It is only a question of accumulating more facts, and presenting these facts in such a way that the patient can grasp them quickly. At present, however, it is often necessary to continue the treatment for weeks and months, although the error of refraction may be no greater nor of longer duration than in those cases that are cured quickly. In most cases, too, the treatment must be continued for a few minutes every day to prevent relapse. Because a familiar object tends to relax the strain to see, the daily reading of the Snellen test card is usually sufficient for this purpose. It is also useful, particularly when the vision at the near point is imperfect, to read fine print every day as close to the eyes as it can be done. When a cure is complete it is always permanent; but complete cures, which mean the attainment, not of what is ordinarily called normal sight, but of a measure of telescopic and microscopic vision, are very rare. Even in these cases, too, the treatment can be continued with benefit; for it is impossible to place limits to the visual powers of man, and no matter how good the sight, it is always possible to improve it. Daily practice of the art of vision is also necessary to

Fig. 41. One of Many Thousands of Patients Cured of Errors of Refraction by the Methods Presented in This Book. No. 1. - Man of thirty-six, 1902, wearing glasses for myopia. Note the appearance of effort in his eyes. He was relieved in 1904 by means of exercises in distant vision and obtained normal sight without glasses.
No. 2. - The same man five years later. No relapse.

Fig. 41.—One of Many Thousands of Patients Cured of Errors of Refraction by the Methods Presented in This Book

No. 1.—Man of thirty-six, 1902, wearing glasses for myopia. Note the appearance of effort in his eyes. He was relieved in 1904 by means of exercises in distant vision and obtained normal sight without glasses.

No. 2.—The same man five years later. No relapse.

prevent those visual lapses to which every eye is liable, no matter how good its sight may ordinarily be. It is true that no system of training will provide an absolute safeguard against such lapses in all circumstances; but the daily reading of small distant, familiar letters will do much to lessen the tendency to strain when disturbing circumstances arise, and all persons upon whose eyesight the safety of others depends should be required to do this.

Cures at All Ages

Generally persons who have never worn glasses are more easily cured than those who have, and glasses should be discarded at the beginning of the treatment. When this cannot be done without too great discomfort, or when the patient has to continue his work during the treatment and cannot do so without glasses, their use must be permitted for a time ; but this always delays the cure. Persons of all ages have been benefited by this treatment of errors of refraction by relaxation; but children usually, though not invariably, respond much more quickly than adults. If they are under twelve years of age, or even under sixteen, and have never worn glasses, they are usually cured in a few days, weeks, or months, and always within a year, simply by reading the Snellen test card every day.

CHAPTER X

STRAIN

TEMPORARY conditions may contribute to the strain to see which results in the production of errors of refraction; but its foundation lies in wrong habits of thought. In attempting to relieve it the physician has continually to struggle against the idea that to do anything well requires effort. This idea is drilled into us from our cradles. The whole educational system is based upon it; and in spite of the wonderful results attained by Montessori through the total elimination of every species of compulsion in the educational process, educators who call themselves modern still cling to the club, under various disguises, as a necessary auxiliary to the process of imparting knowledge.

It is as natural for the eye to see as it is for the mind to acquire knowledge, and any effort in either case is not only useless, but defeats the end in view. You may force a few facts into a child's mind by various kinds of compulsion, but you cannot make it learn anything. The facts remain, if they remain at all, as dead lumber in the brain. They contribute nothing to the vital processes of thought; and because they were not acquired naturally and not assimilated, they destroy the natural impulse of the mind toward the acquisition of knowledge, and by the time the child leaves school or college, as the case may be, it not only knows nothing but is, in the majority of cases, no longer capable of learning.

In the same way you may temporarily improve the sight by effort, but you cannot improve it to normal, and

When the Eye Tries to See

if the effort is allowed to become continuous, the sight will steadily deteriorate and may eventually be destroyed. Very seldom is the impairment or destruction of vision due to any fault in the construction of the eye. Of two equally good pairs of eyes one will retain perfect sight to the end of life, and the other will lose it in the kindergarten, simply because one looks at things without effort and the other does not.

<u>The eye with normal sight never tries to see. If for any reason, such as the dimness of the light, or the distance of the object, it cannot see a particular point, it shifts to another. It never tries to bring out the point by staring at it, as the eye with imperfect sight is constantly doing.</u>

Whenever the eye tries to see, it at once ceases to have normal vision. A person may look at the stars with normal vision; but if he tries to count the stars in any particular constellation, he will probably become myopic, because the attempt to do these things usually results in an effort to see. A patient was able to look at the letter K on the Snellen test card with normal vision, but when asked to count its twenty-seven corners he lost it completely.

It obviously requires a strain to fail to see at the distance, because the eye at rest is adjusted for distant vision. If one does anything when one wants to see at the distance, one must do the wrong thing. The shape of the eyeball cannot be altered during distant vision without strain. It is equally a strain to fail to see at the near-point, because when the muscles respond to the mind's desire they do it without strain. Only by an effort can one prevent the eye from elongating at the near-point.

The eye possesses perfect vision only when it is absolutely at rest. Any movement, either in the organ or the object of vision, produces an error of refraction. With the retinoscope it can be demonstrated that even the necessary movements of the eyeball produce a slight error of refraction, and the moving pictures have given us a practical demonstration of the fact that it is impossible to see a moving object perfectly. When the movement of the object of vision is sufficiently slow, the resulting impairment of vision is so slight as to be inappreciable, just as the errors of refraction produced by slight movements of the eyeball are inappreciable; but when objects move very rapidly they can be seen only as a blur. For this reason it has been found necessary to arrange the machinery for exhibiting moving pictures in such a way that each picture is halted for a twenty-fourth of a second, and screened while it is moving into place. Moving pictures, accordingly, are never seen in motion.

The act of seeing is passive. Things are seen, just as they are felt, or heard, or tasted, without effort or volition on the part of the subject. When sight is perfect the letters on the test card are waiting, perfectly black and perfectly distinct, to be recognized. They do not have to be sought; they are there. In imperfect sight they are sought and chased. The eye goes after them. An effort is made to see them.

The muscles of the body are supposed never to be at rest. The blood-vessels, with their muscular coats, are never at rest. Even in sleep thought does not cease. But the normal condition of the nerves of sense - of hearing, sight, taste, smell and touch - is one of rest. They can be acted upon; they cannot act. The optic nerve, the

Mental Strain Reflected in the Eye

retina and the visual centers of the brain are as passive as the finger-nail. They have nothing whatever in their structure that makes it possible for them to do anything, and when they are the subject of effort from outside sources their efficiency is always impaired.

The mind is the source of all such efforts from outside sources brought to bear upon the eye. Every thought of effort in the mind, of whatever sort, transmits a motor impulse to the eye ; and every such impulse causes a deviation from the normal in the shape of the eyeball and lessens the sensitiveness of the center of sight. <u>If one wants to have perfect sight, therefore, one must have no thought of effort in the mind. Mental strain of any kind always produces a conscious or unconscious</u>

Demonstrate

1. That an effort to see always lowers the vision. Look at the Snellen test card at a distance of twenty feet. It may be possible for you to see the large letters and read them without any apparent effort, while the smaller letters produce a strain which you can feel. If you consciously increase the effort to see the smaller letters, your vision becomes more imperfect. It is not easy for you to realize that effort is always present when the vision is lowered. Knowing the cause of your imperfect sight is a great help in selecting the remedy.

2. That a stare always lowers the vision. It is a truth that the normal eye blinks very frequently. In order to have normal sight, the eyes must blink. One can demonstrate that, when the patient looks at one letter at the distance with normal sight, or looks at one letter at a near point where it is seen clearly, keeping the eyes continuously open without blinking for a minute or longer, always lowers the vision for the distance or for the near point. This should convince the patient that blinking is absolutely necessary in order to obtain good vision.

3. That palming, when done correctly, improves the vision. When the closed eyes are covered with one or both hands, and all light is excluded, the patient should see nothing at all, or a perfect black. This is a rest to the eyes and always improves the sight at least temporarily. Palming can be done wrong. When it is practiced incorrectly, the field imagined by the patient contains streaks of red, white, blue, or other colors. The eyes are under a strain, and the vision is not materially improved by the wrong method of palming. It can be demonstrated that palming for half an hour or longer is a greater benefit than palming for only a few minutes.

BETTER EYESIGHT
A MONTHLY MAGAZINE DEVOTED TO THE PREVENTION AND CURE OF IMPERFECT SIGHT WITHOUT GLASSES

Copyright, 1925, by the Central Fixation Publishing Company
Editor, W. H. BATES, M. D.
Publisher, CENTRAL FIXATION PUBLISHING COMPANY

Vol. X.   FEBRUARY, 1926   No. 8

Memory
By W. H. BATES, M.D.

When the sight is normal, the memory is perfect. The color and background of the letters or other objects seen, are remembered perfectly, instantaneously, and continuously.

ONE of the quickest cures of imperfect sight has been gained through the use of the memory. When the memory is perfect, the eyes at once become normal with normal vision. A perfect memory changes the elongated eyeball of myopia into the shorter length of the normal eye. No matter how high a degree of myopia one may have, when he has a perfect memory of some one thing, he is no longer myopic, but has normal eyes with normal vision.

An imperfect memory or an imperfect imagination may produce organic changes in the eyeball. The organic changes, which are present in many diseases of the eye, have been relieved with the aid of a perfect memory. In some cases the vision has been reduced to perception of light from scars on the front part of the eyeball. Perfect memory brings about the absorption of such opacities. A perfect memory has cured these obstinate cases.

Conical cornea is a very serious disease. Neither operation nor the use of drugs relieves or cures it. A perfect memory gives instant relief, the curvature of the cornea becomes normal, and the patient obtains normal vision.

eyestrain and if the strain takes the form of an effort to see, an error of refraction is always produced. A schoolboy was able to read the bottom line of the Snellen test card at ten feet, but when the teacher told him to mind what he was about he could not see the big C.1 Many children can see perfectly so long as their mothers are around ; but if the mother goes out of the room, they may at once become myopic, because of the strain produced by fear. Unfamiliar objects produce eyestrain and a consequent error of refraction, because they first produce mental strain. A person may have good vision when he is telling the truth ; but if he states what is not true, even with no intent to deceive, or if he imagines what is not true, an error of refraction will be produced, because it is impossible to state or imagine what is not true without an effort.

I may claim to have discovered that telling lies is bad

[1] In this case and others to be mentioned later, the large letter at the top of the card read by the eye with normal vision at two hundred feet, was a "C."

for the eyes, and whatever bearing this circumstance may have upon the universality of defects of vision, the fact can easily be demonstrated. If a patient can read all the small letters on the bottom line of the test card, and either deliberately or carelessly miscalls any of them, the retinoscope will indicate an error of refraction. In numerous cases patients have been asked to state their ages incorrectly, or to try to imagine that they were a year older or a year younger than they actually were, and in every case when they did this the retinoscope indicated an error of refraction. A patient twenty-five years old had no error of refraction when he looked at a blank wall without trying to see ; but if he said he was twenty-six or if someone else said he was twenty-six, or if he tried to imagine that he was twenty-six, he became myopic. The same thing happened when he stated or tried to imagine that he was twenty-four. When he stated or remembered the truth his vision was normal, but when he stated or imagined an error he had an error of refraction.

Two little girl patients arrived one after the other one day, and the first accused the second of having stopped at Huyler's for an ice cream soda, which she had been instructed not to do, being somewhat too much addicted to sweets. The second denied the charge, and the first, who had used the retinoscope and knew what it did to people who told lies, said :
"Do take the retinoscope and find out."
I followed the suggestion, and having thrown the light into the second child's eyes, I asked:
"Did you go to Huyler's?"
"Yes," was the response, and the retinoscope indicated no error of refraction.

Different Kinds of Strain

"Did you have an ice-cream soda?"

"No," said the child ; but the telltale shadow moved in a direction opposite to that of the mirror, showing that she had become myopic and was not telling the truth.

The child blushed when I told her this and acknowledged that the retinoscope was right; for she had heard of the ways of the uncanny instrument before and did not know what else it might do to her if she said anything more that was not true.

So sensitive is this test that if the subject, whether his vision is ordinarily normal or not, pronounces the initials of his name correctly while looking at a blank surface without trying to see, there will be no error of refraction; but if he miscalls one initial, even without any consciousness of effort, and with full knowledge that he is deceiving no one, myopia will be produced.

Mental strain may produce many different kinds of eyestrain. According to the statement of most authorities there is only one kind of eyestrain,' an indefinite thing resulting from so-called over-use of the eyes, or an effort to overcome a wrong shape of the eyeball. It can be demonstrated, however, that there is not only a different strain for each different error of refraction, but a different strain for most abnormal conditions of the eye. The strain that produces an error of refraction is not the same as the strain that produces a squint, or a cataract, [1] or glaucoma, [2] or amblyopia, [3] or inflammation of the conjunctiva [4] or of the margin of the lids, or disease of the optic nerve or retina. All these conditions may exist

1. An opacity of the lens. 2 A condition in which the eyeball becomes abnormally hard. 3 A condition in which there is a decline of vision without apparent cause. 4 A membrane covering the inner surface of the eyelid and the visible part of the white of the eye.

with only a slight error of refraction, and while the relief of one strain usually means the relief of any others that may coexist with it, it sometimes happens that the strain associated with such conditions as cataract and glaucoma is relieved without the complete relief of the strain that causes the error of refraction. Even the pain that so often accompanies errors of refraction is never caused by the same strain that causes these errors. Some myopes cannot read without pain or discomfort, but most of them suffer no inconvenience. When the hypermetrope regards an object at the distance the hypermetropia is lessened, but pain and discomfort may be increased. While there are many strains, however, there is only one cure for all of them, namely, relaxation.

The health of the eye depends upon the blood, and circulation is very largely influenced by thought. When thought is normal-that is, not attended by any excitement or strain-the circulation in the brain is normal, the supply of blood to the optic nerve and the visual centers is normal, and the vision is perfect. When thought is abnormal the circulation is disturbed, the supply of blood to the optic nerve and visual centers is altered, and the vision lowered. We can consciously think thoughts which disturb the circulation and lower the visual power ; we can also consciously think thoughts that will restore normal circulation, and thereby cure, not only all errors of refraction, but many other abnormal conditions of the eyes. We cannot by any amount of effort make ourselves see, but by learning to control our thoughts we can accomplish that end indirectly.

You can teach people how to produce any error of refraction, how to produce a squint, how to see two images of an object, one above another, or side by side,

As Quick as Thought

or at any desired angle from one another, simply by teaching them how to think in a particular way. When the disturbing thought is replaced by one that relaxes, the squint disappears, the double vision and the errors of refraction are corrected; and this is as true of abnormalties of long standing as of those produced voluntarily. No matter what their degree or their duration their cure is accomplished just as soon as the patient is able to secure mental control. The cause of any error of refraction, of a squint, or of any other functional disturbance of the eye, is simply a thought - a wrong thought - and the cure is as quick as the thought that relaxes. In a fraction of a second the highest degrees of refractive error may be corrected, a squint may disappear, or the blindness of amblyopia may be relieved. If the relaxation is only momentary, the correction is momentary. When it becomes permanent, the correction is permanent.

This relaxation cannot, however, be obtained by any sort of effort. It is fundamental that patients should understand this; for so long as they think, consciously or unconsciously, that relief from strain may be obtained by another strain their cure will be delayed.

CHAPTER XI

CENTRAL FIXATION

THE eye is a miniature camera, corresponding in many ways very exactly to the inanimate machine used in photography. In one respect, however, there is a great difference between the two instruments. The sensitive plate of the camera is equally sensitive in every part; but the retina has a point of maximum sensitiveness, and every other part is less sensitive in proportion as it is removed from that point. This point of maximum sensitiveness is called the "fovea centralis," literally the "central pit."

The retina, although it is an extremely delicate membrane, varying in thickness from one-eighth of an inch to less than half that amount, is highly complex. It is composed of nine layers, only one of which is supposed to be capable of receiving visual impressions. This layer is composed of minute rodlike and conical bodies which vary in form and are distributed very differently in its different parts. In the center of the retina is a small circular elevation known, from the yellow color which it assumes in death and sometimes also in life, as the "macula lutea," literally the "yellow spot." In the center of this spot is the fovea, a deep depression of darker color. In the center of this depression there are no rods, and the cones are elongated and pressed very closely together. The other layers, on the contrary, become here extremely thin, or disappear altogether, so that the cones are covered with barely perceptible traces of them. Beyond the center of the fovea the cones become thicker and fewer

Musculi oculi.—The muscles of the eyeball.

CENTRAL FIXATION - SEE CLEAR WITH THE CENTER OF THE VISUAL FIELD.
PLACE THE PART OF THE OBJECT THE EYES ARE LOOKING AT IN THE CENTER OF THE VISUAL FIELD.

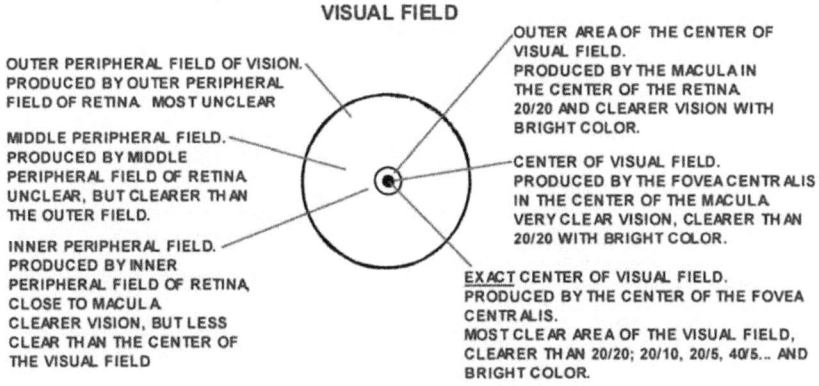

An Invariable Symptom of Imperfect Sight

and are interspersed with rods, the number of which increases toward the margin of the retina. The precise function of these rods and cones is not clear; but it is a fact that the center of the fovea, where all elements except the cones and their associated cells practically disappear, is the seat of the most acute vision. As we withdraw from this spot, the acuteness of the visual perceptions rapidly decreases. The eye with normal vision, therefore, sees one part of everything it looks at best, and everything else worse, in proportion as it is removed from the point of maximum vision ; and it is an invariable symptom of all abnormal conditions of the eyes, both functional and organic, that this central fixation is lost.

These conditions are due to the fact that when the sight is normal the sensitiveness of the fovea is normal, but when the sight is imperfect, from whatever cause, the sensitiveness of the fovea is lowered, so that the eye sees equally well, or even better, with other parts of the retina. Contrary to what is generally believed, the part seen best when the sight is normal is extremely small. The text-books say that at twenty feet an area having a diameter of half an inch can be seen with maximum vision, but anyone who tries at this distance to see every part of even the smallest letters of the Snellen test card - the diameter of which may be less than a quarter of an inch - equally well at one time will immediately become myopic. The fact is that the nearer the point of maximum vision approaches a mathematical point, which has no area, the better the sight.

The cause of this loss of function in the center of sight is mental strain; and as all abnormal conditions of the eyes, organic as well as functional, are accompanied by mental strain, all such conditions must necessarily be accompanied by loss of central fixation. When the mind is under a strain the eye usually goes more or less blind. The center of sight goes blind first, partially or completely, according to the degree of the strain, and if the strain is great enough the whole or the greater part of the retina may be involved. When the vision of the center of sight has been suppressed, partially or completely, the patient can no longer see the point which he is looking at best, but sees objects not regarded directly as well, or better, because the sensitiveness of the retina has now become approximately equal in every part, or is even better in the outer part than in the center. Therefore in all cases of defective vision the patient is unable to see best where he is looking.

This condition is sometimes so extreme that the patient may look as far away from an object as it is possible to see it, and yet see it just as well as when looking directly at it. In one case it had gone so far that the patient could see only with the edge of the retina on the nasal side. In other words, she could not see her fingers in front of her face, but could see them if held at the outer side of her eye. She had only a slight error of refraction, showing that while every error of refraction is accompanied by eccentric fixation, the strain which causes the one condition is different from that which produces the other. The patient had been examined by specialists in this country and Europe, who attributed her blindness to disease of the optic nerve or brain; but the fact that vision was restored by relaxation demonstrated that the condition had been due simply to mental strain.

Eccentric fixation, even in its lesser degrees, is so unnatural that great discomfort, or even pain, can be produced in a few seconds by trying to see every part of an

When the Eye Possesses Central Fixation

area three or four inches in extent at twenty feet, or even less, or an area of an inch or less at the near-point, equally well at one time, while at the same time the retinoscope will demonstrate that an error of refraction has been produced. This strain, when it is habitual, leads to all sorts of abnormal conditions and is, in fact, at the bottom of most eye troubles, both functional and organic. The discomfort and pain may be absent, however, in the chronic condition, and it is an encouraging symptom when the patient begins to experience them.

When the eye possesses central fixation it not only possesses perfect sight, but it is perfectly at rest and can be used indefinitely without fatigue. It is open and quiet; no nervous movements are observable; and when it regards a point at the distance the visual axes are parallel. In other words, there are no muscular insufficiencies. This fact is not generally known. The textbooks state that muscular insufficiencies occur in eyes having normal sight, but I have never seen such a case. The muscles of the face and of the whole body are also at rest, and when the condition is habitual there are no wrinkles or dark circles around the eyes.

In most cases of eccentric fixation, on the contrary, the eye quickly tires, and its appearance, with that of the face, is expressive of effort or strain. The ophthalmoscope 1 reveals that the eyeball moves at irregular intervals, from side to side, vertically or in other directions. These movements are often so extensive as to be manifest by ordinary inspection, and are sometimes sufficiently marked to resemble nystagmus.2 Nervous move-

1 A shorter movement can be noted when the observer watches the optic nerve with the ophthalmoscope than when he views merely the exterior of the eye. 2 A condition in which there is a conspicuous and more or less rhythmic movement of the eyeball from side to side.

ments of the eyelids may also be noted, either by ordinary inspection, or by lightly touching the lid of one eye while the other regards an object either at the near-point or the distance. The visual axes are never parallel, and the deviation from the normal may become so marked as to constitute the condition of squint. Redness of the conjunctiva and of the margins of the lids, wrinkles around the eyes, dark circles beneath them and tearing are other symptoms of eccentric fixation.

Eccentric fixation is a symptom of strain, and is relieved by any method that relieves strain; but in some cases the patient is cured just as soon as he is able to demonstrate the facts of central fixation. When he comes to realize, through actual demonstration of the fact, that he does not see best where he is looking, and that when he looks a sufficient distance away from a point he can see it worse than when he looks directly at it, he becomes able, in some way, to reduce the distance to which he has to look in order to see worse, until he can look directly at the top of a small letter and see the bottom worse, or look at the bottom and see the top worse. The smaller the letter regarded in this way, or the shorter the distance the patient has to look away from a letter in order to see the opposite part indistinctly, the greater the relaxation and the better the sight. When it becomes possible to look at the bottom of a letter and see the top worse, or to look at the top and see the bottom worse, it becomes possible to see the letter perfectly black and distinct. At first such vision may come only in flashes. The letter will come out distinctly for a moment and then disappear. But gradually, if the practice is continued, central fixation will become habitual.

Most patients can readily look at the bottom of the

The Use of Strong Lights

big C and see the top worse; but in some cases it is not only impossible for them to do this, but impossible for them to let go of the large letters at any distance at which they can be seen. In these extreme cases it sometimes requires considerable ingenuity, first to demonstrate to the patient that he does not see best where he is looking, and then to help him to see an object worse when he looks away from it than when he looks directly at it. The use of a strong light as one of the points of fixation, or of two lights five or ten feet apart, has been found helpful, the patient when he looks away from the light being able to see it less bright more readily than he can see a black letter worse when he looks away from it. It then becomes easier for him to see the letter worse when he looks away from it. This method was successful in the following case :

A patient with vision of 3/200, when she looked at a point a few feet away from the big C, said she saw the letter better than when she looked directly at it. Her attention was called to the fact that her eyes soon became tired and that her vision soon failed when she saw things in this way. Then she was directed to look at a bright object about three feet away from the card, and this attracted her attention to such an extent that she became able to see the large letter on the test card worse, after which she was able to look back at it and see it better. It was demonstrated to her that she could do one of two things: look away and see the letter better than she did before, or look away and see it worse. She then became able to see it worse all the time when she looked three feet away from it. Next she became able to shorten the distance successively to two feet, one foot, and six inches, with a constant improvement in vision; and finally she became able to look at the bottom of the letter and see the top worse, or look at the top and see the bottom worse. With practice she became able to look at the smaller letters in the same way, and finally she became able to read the ten line at twenty feet. By the same method also she became able to read diamond type, first at twelve inches and then at three inches. By these simple measures alone she became able, in short, to see best where she was looking, and her cure was complete.

The highest degrees of eccentric fixation occur in the high degrees of myopia, and in these cases, since the sight is best at the near-point, the patient is benefited by practicing seeing worse at this point. The distance can then be gradually extended until it becomes possible to do the same thing at twenty feet. One patient with a high degree of myopia said that the farther she looked away from an electric light the better she saw it, but by alternately looking at the light at the near-point and looking away from it she became able, in a short time, to see it brighter when she looked directly at it than when she looked away from it. Later she became able to do the same thing at twenty feet, and then she experienced a wonderful feeling of relief. No words, she said, could adequately describe it. Every nerve seemed to be relaxed, and a feeling of comfort and rest permeated her whole body. Afterward her progress was rapid. She soon became able to look at one part of the smallest letters on the card and see the rest worse, and then she became able to read the letters at twenty feet.

On the principle that a burnt child dreads the fire, some patients are benefited by consciously making their sight worse. When they learn, by actual demonstration of the facts, just how their visual defects are produced, they unconsciously avoid the unconscious strain which

Possibilities Cannot Be Limited

causes them. When the degree of eccentric fixation is not too extreme to be increased, therefore, it is a benefit to patients to teach them how to increase it. When a patient has consciously lowered his vision and produced discomfort and even pain by trying to see the big C, or a whole line of letters, equally well at one time, he becomes better able to correct the unconscious effort of the eye to see all parts of a smaller area equally well at one time.
(See the part of the object the eyes are looking at best, <u>clearest</u> in the <u>center</u> of the visual field by using the fovea centralis, center of the eyes retina.)

In learning to see best where he is looking it is usually best for the patient to think of the point not directly regarded as being seen less distinctly than the point he is looking at, instead of thinking of the point fixed as being seen best, as the latter practice has a tendency, in most cases, to intensify the strain under which the eye is already laboring. One part of an object is seen best only when the mind is content to see the greater part of it indistinctly, and as the degree of relaxation increases the area of the part seen worse increases, until that seen best becomes merely a point.

The limits of vision depend upon the degree of central fixation. A person may be able to read a sign half a mile away when he sees the letters all alike, but when taught to see one letter best he will be able to read smaller letters that he didn't know were there. The remarkable vision of savages, who can see with the naked eye objects for which most civilized persons require a telescope, is a matter of central fixation. Some people can see the rings of Saturn, or the moons of Jupiter, with the naked eye. It is not because of any superiority in the structure of their eyes, but because they have attained a higher degree of central fixation than most civilized persons do.

Not only do all errors of refraction and all functional disturbances of the eye disappear when it sees by central fixation, but many organic conditions are relieved or cured. I am unable to set any limits to its possibilities. I would not have ventured to predict that <u>glaucoma, incipient cataract and syphilitic iritis could be cured by central fixation; but it is a fact that these conditions have disappeared when central fixation was attained</u>. Relief was often obtained in a few minutes, and, in rare cases, this relief was permanent. Usually, however, a permanent cure required more prolonged treatment. Inflammatory conditions of all kinds, including inflammation of the cornea, iris, conjunctiva, the various coats of the eyeball and even the optic nerve itself, have been benefited by central fixation after other methods had failed. Infections, as well as diseases caused by protein poisoning and the poisons of typhoid fever, influenza, syphilis and gonorrhoea, have also been benefited by it. Even with a foreign body in the eye there is no redness and no pain so long as central fixation is retained.

Since central fixation is impossible without mental control, central fixation of the eye means central fixation of the mind. It means, therefore, health in all parts of the body, for all the operations of the physical mechanism depend upon the mind. Not only the sight, but all the other senses - touch, taste, hearing and smell - are benefited by central fixation. All the vital processes - digestion, assimilation, elimination, etc. - are improved by it. The symptoms of functional and organic diseases are relieved. The efficiency of the mind is enormously increased. The benefits of central fixation already observed are, in short, so great that the subject merits further investigation.

CHAPTER XII
PALMING

ALL the methods used in the cure of errors of refraction are simply different ways of obtaining relaxation, and most patients, though by no means all, find it easiest to relax with their eyes shut. This usually lessens the strain to see, and in such cases is followed by a temporary or more lasting improvement in vision.

Most patients are benefited merely by closing the eyes ; and by alternately resting them for a few minutes or longer in this way and then opening them and looking at the Snellen test card for a second or less, flashes of improved vision are, as a rule, very quickly obtained. Some temporarily obtain almost normal vision by this means; and in rare cases a complete cure has been effected, sometimes in less than an hour.

But since some light comes through the closed eyelids, a still greater degree of relaxation can be obtained, in all but a few exceptional cases, by excluding it. This is done by covering the closed eyes with the palms of the hands (the fingers being crossed upon the forehead) in such a way as to avoid pressure on the eyeballs. So efficacious is this practice, which I have called "palming," as a means of relieving strain, that we all instinctively resort to it at times, and from it most patients are able to get a considerable degree of relaxation.

But even with the eyes closed and covered in such a way as to exclude all the light, the visual centers of the brain may still be disturbed, the eye may still strain to see; and instead of seeing a field so black that it is impossible to remember, imagine, or see anything blacker, as one ought normally to do when the optic nerve is not subject to the stimulation of light, the patients will see illusions of lights and colors ranging all the way from an imperfect black to kaleidoscopic appearances so vivid that they seem to be actually seen with the eyes. The worse the condition of the eyesight, as a rule, the more numerous, vivid and persistent these appearances are. Yet some persons with very imperfect sight are able to palm almost perfectly from the beginning, and are, therefore, very quickly cured. Any disturbance of mind or body, such as fatigue, hunger, anger, worry or depression, also makes it difficult for patients to see black when they palm, persons who can see it perfectly under ordinary conditions being often unable to do so without assistance when they are ill or in pain.

It is impossible to see a perfect black unless the eyesight is perfect, because only when the eyesight is perfect is the mind at rest; but some patients can without difficulty approximate such a black nearly enough to improve their eyesight, and as the eyesight improves the deepness of the black increases. Patients who fail to see even an approximate black when they palm state that instead of black they see streaks or floating clouds of gray, flashes of light, patches of red, blue, green, yellow, etc. Sometimes instead of an immovable black, clouds of black will be seen moving across the field. In other cases the black will be seen for a few seconds and then some other color will take its place. The different ways in which patients can fail to see black when their eyes are closed and covered are, in fact, very numerous and often very peculiar.

(Modern Teachers state it is not mandatory to imagine and see black. Just relax and think pleasant thoughts, let the mind drift from one happy thought to another.)

Vivid Colors Seen When Palming

Some patients have been so impressed with the vividness of the colors which they imagined they saw that no amount of argument could, or did, convince them that they did not actually see them with their eyes. If

Fig. 42. Palming
This is one of the most effective methods of obtaining relaxation of all the sensory nerves.

Fig. 42. Palming. This is one of the most effective methods of obtaining relaxation of all the sensory nerves.

Palm and remember, shift on a favorite object: flower, colorful stone, jewelry, tree, land, old house... Improving the memory, imagination of clear mental pictures relaxes the mind, body, eyes and improves the vision.

other people saw bright lights or colors, with their eyes closed and covered, they admitted that these things would be illusions; but what they themselves saw under the same conditions was reality. They would not believe, until they had themselves demonstrated the truth, that their illusions were due to an imagination beyond their control.

Successful palming in these more difficult cases usually involves the practice of all the methods for improving the

Palm and imagine drifting down a river. See objects in color, clear, motion. Movement of the boat, water, wind, birds flying, sun shining, sparkling on the river, animals walking on the shore, colorful dragonflies... Imagine all the senses; touch, warmth of sun, feel the breeze, hear the water, birds, wind, taste your favorite drink...

sight described in succeeding chapters. For reasons which will be explained in the following chapter, the majority of such patients may be greatly helped by the memory of a black object. They are directed to look at such an object at the distance at which the color can be seen best, close the eyes and remember the color, and repeat until the memory appears to be equal to the sight. Then they are instructed, while still holding the memory of the black, to cover the closed eyes with the palms of the hands in the manner just described. If the memory of the black is perfect, the whole background will be black. If it is not, or if it does not become so in the course of a few seconds, the eyes are opened and the black object regarded again.

Palm and remember, imagine a pleasant object, scenery and shift throughout the scene; from object to object, part to part on objects. See objects in motion, action like a real life movie in the mind, in color, clear.

Many patients become able by this method to see black almost perfectly for a short time ; but most of them, even those whose eyes are not very bad, have great difficulty in seeing it continuously. Being unable to remember black for more than from three to five seconds, they cannot see black for a longer time than this. Such patients are helped by central fixation. When they have become able to see one part of a black object darker than the whole, they are able to remember the smaller area for a longer time than they could the larger one, and thus become able to see black for a longer period when they palm. They are also benefited by mental shifting (see Chapter XV) from one black object to another, or from one part of a black object to another. It is impossible to see, remember, or imagine anything, even for as much as

Mental Shifting

a second, without shifting from one part to another, or to some other object and back again; and the attempt to do so always produces strain. Those who think they are remembering a black object continuously are unconsciously comparing it with something not so black, or

Fig. 43 Patient with atrophy of the optic nerve gets flashes of improved vision after palming.

else its color and its position are constantly changing. It is impossible to remember even such a simple thing as a period perfectly black and stationary for more than a fraction of a second. When shifting is not done unconsciously patients must be encouraged to do it consciously. They may be directed, for instance, to remember successively a black hat, a black shoe, a black velvet dress, a black plush curtain, or a fold in the black dress or the black curtain, holding each one not more than a fraction of a second. Many persons have been benefited by remembering all the letters of the alphabet in turn perfectly black. Others prefer to shift from one small black object, such as a period or a small letter, to another, or to swing such an object in a manner to be described later (see Chapter XV).

In some cases the following method has proved successful: When the patient sees what he thinks is a perfect black, let him remember a piece of starch on this background, and on the starch the letter F as black as the background. Then let him let go of the starch and remember only the F, one part best, on the black background. In a short time the whole field may become as black as the blacker part of the F. The process can be repeated many times with a constant increase of blackness in the field.

In one case a patient who saw grey so vividly when she palmed that she was positive she saw it with her eyes, instead of merely imagining it, was able to obliterate nearly all of it by first imagining a black C on the grey field, then two black C's, and finally a multitude of overlapping C's.

It is impossible to remember black perfectly when it is not seen perfectly. If one sees it imperfectly, the best one can do is to remember it imperfectly. All persons, without exception, who can see or read diamond type at the near-point, no matter how great their myopia may be, or how much the interior of the eye may be diseased, become able, as a rule, to see black with their eyes closed and covered more readily than patients with hypermetropia or astigmatism; because, while myopes cannot see anything perfectly, even at the near-point, they see

Imperfect Memory Useful

better at that point than persons with hypermetropia or astigmatism do at any distance. Persons with high degrees of myopia, however, often find palming very difficult, since they not only see black very imperfectly, but, because of the effort they are making to see, cannot remember it more than one or two seconds. Any other condition of the eye which prevents the patient from seeing black perfectly also makes palming difficult. In some cases black is never seen as black, appearing to be grey, yellow, brown, or even bright red. In such cases it is usually best for the patient to improve his sight by other methods before trying to palm. Blind persons usually have more trouble in seeing black than those who can see, but may be helped by the memory of a black object familiar to them before they lost their sight. A blind painter who saw grey continually when he first tried to palm became able at last to see black by the aid of the memory of black paint. He had no perception of light whatever and was in terrible pain ; but when he succeeded in seeing black the pain vanished, and when he opened his eyes he saw light.

Even the imperfect memory of black is useful, for by its aid a still blacker black can be both remembered and seen; and this brings still further improvement. For instance, let the patient regard a letter on the Snellen test card at the distance at which the color is seen best, then close his eyes and remember it. If the palming produces relaxation, it will be possible to imagine a deeper shade of black than was seen, and by remembering this black when again regarding the letter it can be seen blacker than it was at first. A still deeper black can then be imagined, and this deeper black can, in turn, be transferred to the letter on the test card. By continuing this process a perfect perception of black, and hence perfect sight, are sometimes very quickly obtained. The deeper the shade of black obtained with the eyes closed, the more easily it can be remembered when regarding the letters on the test card.

The longer some people palm the greater the relaxation they obtain and the darker the shade of black they are able both to remember and see. Others are able to palm successfully for short periods, but begin to strain if they keep it up too long.

It is impossible to succeed by effort, or by attempting to "concentrate" on the black. As popularly understood, concentration means to do or think one thing only; but this is impossible, and an attempt to do the impossible is a strain which defeats its own end. The human mind is not capable of thinking of one thing only. It can think of one thing best, and is only at rest when it does so ; but it cannot think of one thing only. A patient who tried to see black only and to ignore the kaleidoscopic colors which intruded themselves upon her field of vision, becoming worse and worse the more they were ignored, actually went into convulsions from the strain, and was attended every day for a month by her family physician before she was able to resume the treatment. This patient was advised to stop palming, and, with her eyes open, to recall as many colors as possible, remembering each one as perfectly as possible. By thus taking the bull by the horns and consciously making the mind wander more than it did unconsciously, she became able, in some way, to palm for short periods.

Some particular kinds of black objects may be found to be more easily remembered than others. Black plush of a high grade for instance, proved to be an optimum

Optimum Blacks

(see Chapter XVIII) with many persons as compared with black velvet, silk, broadcloth, ink and the letters on the Snellen test card, although no blacker than these other blacks. A familiar black object can often be remembered more easily by the patient than those that

Fig. 44

No. 1.—Owing to paralysis of the seventh nerve on the right side, resulting from a mastoid operation on the right ear, the patient is unable to close her lips.

No. 2.—After palming and remembering a perfectly black period she became able not only to close the lips, but to whistle. The cure was permanent.

Fig. 44 No. 1. Owing to paralysis of the seventh nerve on the right side, resulting from a mastoid operation on the right ear, the patient is unable to close her lips. No. 2. After palming and remembering a perfectly black period she became able not only to close the lips, but to whistle. The cure was permanent.

are less so. A dressmaker, for instance, was able to remember a thread of black silk when she could not remember any other black object.

When a black letter is regarded before palming the patient will usually remember not only the blackness of the letter, but the white background as well. If the memory of the black is held for a few seconds, however, the background usually fades away and the whole field becomes black.

Patients often say that they remember black perfectly when they do not. One can usually tell whether or not this is the case by noting the effect of palming upon the vision. If there is no improvement in the sight when the eyes are opened, it can be demonstrated, by bringing the black closer to the patient, that it has not been remembered perfectly.

Although black is, as a rule, the easiest color to remember, for reasons explained in the next chapter, the following method sometimes succeeds when the memory of black fails: Remember a variety of colors - bright red, yellow, green, blue, purple, white especially - all in the most intense shade possible. Do not attempt to hold any of them more than a second. Keep this up for five or ten minutes. Then remember a piece of starch about half an inch in diameter as white as possible. Note the color of the background. Usually it will be a shade of black. If it is, note whether it is possible to remember anything blacker, or to see anything blacker with the eyes open. In all cases when the white starch is remembered perfectly the background will be so black that it will be impossible to remember anything blacker with the eyes closed, or to see anything blacker with them open.

When palming is successful it is one of the best methods I know of for securing relaxation of all the sensory nerves, including those of sight. When perfect relaxation is gained in this way, as indicated by the ability to see a perfect black, it is completely retained when the eyes are opened, and the patient is permanently cured.

When Palming Is Successful

At the same time pain in the eyes and head, and even in other parts of the body, is permanently relieved. Such cases are very rare, but they do occur. With a lesser

Fig 45. Fig. 1. Patient with absolute glaucoma of the right eye. He had suffered agonizing pain for six months and had no perception of light. He was photographed when testing the tension of his eyeball, which he found to be perfectly hard.
Fig. 2. The patient is palming and remembering a perfectly black period. After half an hour the eyeball became soft, the pain ceased, and the patient became able to see the light. After three years there was no return of the glaucoma.

degree of relaxation much of it is lost when the eyes are opened, and what is retained is not held permanently. In other words, the greater the degree of the relaxation produced by palming the more of it is retained when the eyes are opened and the longer it lasts. If you palm perfectly, you retain, when you open your eyes, all of the relaxation that you gain, and you do not lose it again. If you palm imperfectly, you retain only part of what you gain and retain it only temporarily - it may be only for a few moments. Even the smallest degree of relaxation is useful, however, for by means of it a still greater degree may be obtained.

Patients who succeed with palming from the beginning are to be congratulated, for they are always cured very quickly. A very remarkable case of this kind was that of a man nearly seventy years of age with compound hypermetropic astigmatism and presbyopia, complicated by incipient cataract. For more than forty years he had worn glasses to improve his distant vision, and for twenty years he had worn them for reading and desk work. Because of the cloudiness of the lens, he had now become unable to see well enough to do his work, even with glasses ; and the other physicians whom he had consulted had given him no hope of relief except by operation when the cataract was ripe. When he found palming helped him, he asked:

"Can I do that too much?"

"No," he was told. "Palming is simply a means of resting your eyes, and you cannot rest them too much."

A few days later he returned and said: "

Doctor, it was tedious, very tedious ; but I did it."

"What was tedious?" I asked.

"Palming," he replied. "I did it continuously for twenty hours."

"But you couldn't have kept it up for twenty hours continuously," I said incredulously. "You must have stopped to eat."

Tedious But Worth While

And then he related that from four o'clock in the morning until twelve at night he had eaten nothing, only drinking large quantities of water, and had devoted practically all of the time to palming. It must have been tedious, as he said, but it was also worth while. When he looked at the test card, without glasses, he read the bottom line at twenty feet. He also read fine print at six inches and at twenty. The cloudiness of the lens had become much less, and in the center had entirely disappeared. Two years later there had been no relapse.

Although the majority of patients are helped by palming, a minority are unable to see black, and only increase their strain by trying to get relaxation in this way. In most cases it is possible, by using some or all of the various methods outlined in this chapter, to enable the patient to palm successfully ; but if much difficulty is experienced, it is usually better and more expeditious to drop the method until the sight has been improved by other means. The patient may then become able to see black when he palms, but some never succeed in doing it until they are cured.

(It is not necessary to imagine and see black. Just relax and let the mind drift from one pleasant thought to another.)

CHAPTER XIII
MEMORY AS AN AID TO VISION

WHEN the mind is able to remember perfectly any phenomenon of the senses, it is always perfectly relaxed. The sight is normal, if the eyes are open; and when they are closed and covered so as to exclude all the light, one sees a perfectly black field - that is nothing at all. If you can remember the ticking of a watch, or an odor or a taste perfectly, your mind is perfectly at rest, and you will see a perfect black when your eyes are closed and covered. If your memory of a sensation of touch could be equal to the reality, you would see nothing but black when the light was excluded from your eyes. If you were to remember a bar of music perfectly when your eyes were closed and covered, you would see nothing but black. But in the case of any of these phenomena it is not easy to test the correctness of the memory, and the same is true of colors other than black. All other colors, including white, are altered by the amount of light to which they are exposed, and are seldom seen as perfectly as it is possible for the normal eye to see them. But when the sight is normal, black is just as black in a dim light as in a bright one. It is also just as black at the distance as at the near-point, while a small area is just as black as a large one, and, in fact, appears blacker. Black is, moreover, more readily

Memory a Measure of Relaxation

available than any other color. There is nothing blacker than printer's ink, and that is practically ubiquitous. By means of the memory of black, therefore, it is possible to measure accurately one's own relaxation. If the color is remembered perfectly, one is perfectly relaxed. If it is remembered almost perfectly, one's relaxation is almost perfect. If it cannot be remembered at all, one has very little or no relaxation.

By means of simultaneous retinoscopy, these facts can be readily demonstrated. An absolutely perfect memory is very rare, so much so that it need hardly be taken into consideration ; but a practically perfect memory, or what might be called normal, is attainable by every one under certain conditions. With such a memory of black, the retinoscope shows that all errors of refraction are corrected. If the memory is less than normal, the contrary will be the case. If it fluctuates, the shadow of the retinoscope will fluctuate. The testimony of the retinoscope is, in fact, more reliable than the statements of the patient. Patients often believe and state that they remember black perfectly, or normally, when the retinoscope indicates an error of refraction ; but in such cases it can usually be demonstrated by bringing the test card to the point at which the black letters can be seen best, that the memory is not equal to the sight. That the color cannot be remembered perfectly when the eyes and mind are under a strain, the reader can easily demonstrate by trying to remember it when making a conscious effort to see - by staring, partly closing the eyes, frowning, etc. - or while trying to see all the letters of a line equally well at one time. It will be found that it either cannot be remembered at all under these conditions, or that it is remembered very imperfectly.

When the two eyes of a patient are different, it has been found that the difference can be exactly measured by the length of time a black period can be remembered, while looking at the Snellen test card, with both eyes open, and with the better eye closed. A patient with normal vision in the right eye and half-normal vision in the left could, when looking at the test card with both eyes open, remember a period for twenty seconds continuously; but with the better eye closed, it could be remembered only ten seconds. A patient with half-normal vision in the right eye and one-quarter normal in the left could remember a period twelve seconds with both eyes open, and only six seconds with the better eye closed. A third patient, with normal sight in the right eye and vision of one-tenth in the left, could remember a period twenty seconds with both eyes open, and only two seconds when the better eye was closed. In other words, if the right eye is better than the left, the memory is better when the right eye is open than when only the left eye is open, the difference being in exact proportion to the difference in the vision of the two eyes.

In the treatment of functional eye troubles this relationship between relaxation and memory is of great practical importance. The sensations of the eye and of the mind supply very little information as to the strain to which both are being subjected, those who strain most often suffering the least discomfort; but by means of his ability to remember black the patient can always know whether he is straining or not, and is able, therefore, to avoid the conditions that produce strain. Whatever method of improving his sight the patient is using, he is advised to carry with him constantly the memory of a small area of black, such as a period, so that

Not Attainable by Effort

he may recognize and avoid the conditions that produce strain, and in some cases patients have obtained a complete cure in a very short time by this means alone. One advantage of the method is that it does not require a test card, for at any hour of the day or night, whatever the patient may be doing, he can always place himself in the conditions favorable to the perfect memory of a period.

The condition of mind in which a black period can be remembered cannot be attained by any sort of effort. The memory is not the cause of the relaxation, but must be preceded by it. It is obtained only during moments of relaxation, and retained only as long as the causes of strain are avoided; but how this is accomplished cannot be fully explained, just as many other psychological phenomena cannot be explained. We only know that under certain conditions that might be called favorable a degree of relaxation sufficient for the memory of a black period is possible, and that, by persistently seeking these conditions, the patient becomes able to increase the degree of the relaxation and prolong its duration, and finally becomes able to retain it under unfavorable conditions.

For most patients palming provides the most favorable conditions for the memory of black. When the strain to see is lessened by the exclusion of the light, the patient usually becomes able to remember a black object for a few seconds or longer, and this period of relaxation can be prolonged in one of two ways. Either the patient can open his eyes and look at a black object by central fixation at the distance at which it can be seen best, and at which the eyes are, therefore, most relaxed, or he can shift mentally from one black object to another, or from one part of a black object to another. By these means, and perhaps also through other influences that are not clearly understood, most patients become able, sooner or later, to remember black for an indefinite length of time with their eyes closed and covered.

With the eyes open and looking at a blank surface without trying consciously to see, the unconscious strain is lessened so that the patient becomes able to remember a black period, and all errors of refraction, as demonstrated by the retinoscope, are corrected. This result has been found to be invariable, and so long as the surface remains blank and the patient does not begin to remember or imagine things seen imperfectly, the memory and the vision may be retained. But if, with the improved vision, details upon the surface begin to come out, or if the patient begins to think of the test card, which he has seen imperfectly, the strain to see will return and the period will be lost.

When looking at a surface on which there is nothing particular to see, distance makes no difference to the memory, because the patient can always look at such a surface, no matter where it is, without straining to see it. When looking at letters, or other details, however, the memory is best at the point at which the patient's sight is best, because at that point the eyes and mind are more relaxed than when the same letters or objects are regarded at distances at which the vision is not so good. By practicing central fixation at the most favorable distance, therefore, and using any other means of improving the vision which are found effectual, the memory of the period may be improved, in some cases, very rapidly.

Improved Sight a Disturbing Influence

If the relaxation gained under these favorable conditions is perfect, the patient will be able to retain it when the mind is conscious of the impressions of sight at unfavorable distances. Such cases are, however, very rare. Usually the degree of relaxation gained is markedly imperfect, and is, therefore, lost to a greater or less degree when the conditions are unfavorable, as when letters or objects are being regarded at unfavorable distances. So disturbing are the impressions of sight under these circumstances, that just as soon as details begin to come out at distances at which they have not previously been seen, the patient usually loses his relaxation, and with it the memory of the period. In fact, the strain to see may even return before he has had time to become conscious of the image on his retina, as the following case strikingly illustrates:

A woman of fifty-five who had myopia of fifteen diopters, complicated with other conditions which made it impossible for her to see the big C at more than one foot, or to go about, either in her house or on the street, without an attendant, became able, when she looked at a green wall without trying to see it, to remember a perfectly black period and to see a small area of the wall-paper at the distance as well as she could at the near-point. When she had come close to the wall, she was asked to put her hand on the door-knob, which she did without hesitation. "But I don't see the knob," she hastened to explain. As a matter of fact she had seen it long enough to put her hand on it; but as soon as the idea of seeing it was suggested to her she lost the memory of the period, and with it her improved vision, and when she again tried to find the knob she could not do so.

When a period is remembered perfectly while a letter on the Snellen test card is being regarded, the letter improves, with or without the consciousness of the patient; because it is impossible to strain and relax at the same time, and if one relaxes sufficiently to remember the period, one must also relax sufficiently to see the letter, consciously or unconsciously. Letters on either side of the one regarded, or on the lines above and below it, also improve. When the patient is conscious of seeing the letters, this is very distracting, and usually causes him, at first, to forget the period ; while with some patients, as already noted, the strain may return even before the letters are consciously recognized.

Thus patients find themselves on the horns of a dilemma. The relaxation indicated by the memory of a period improves their sight, and the things they see with this improved vision cause them to lose their relaxation and their memory. It is very remarkable to me how the difficulty is ever overcome, but some patients are able to do it in five minutes or half an hour. With others the process is long and tedious.

There are various ways of helping patients to deal with this situation. One is to direct them to remember the period while looking a little to one side of the test card, say a foot or more; then to look a little nearer to it, and finally to look between the lines. In this way they may become able to see the letters in the eccentric field without losing the period; and when they can do this they may become able to go a step farther, and look directly at a letter without losing control of their memory. If they cannot do it, they are told to look at only one part of a letter - usually the bottom - or to see or imagine the period as part of the letter, while noting that the rest of the letter is less black and less distinct than the part

Dodging Improved Sight

directly regarded. When they can do this they become able to remember the period better than when the letter is seen all alike. If the letter is seen all alike, the perfect memory of the period is always lost. The next step is to ask the patient to note whether the bottom of the letter is straight, curved, or open, without losing the period on the bottom. When he can do this, he is asked to do the same with the sides and top of the letter, still holding the period on the bottom. Usually when the parts can be observed separately in this way, the whole letter can be seen without losing the memory of the period; but it occasionally happens that this is not the case, and further practice is needed before the patient can become conscious of all sides of the letter at once without losing the period. This may require moments, hours, days, or months. In one case the following method succeeded :

(Imagine the black letter is composed of many small black periods and look at one at a time, shifting from period to period or: shift 'move' one period with the eyes, visual attention to each part of the letter, one part at a time; shifting part to part to see the letter clear.)

The patient, a man with fifteen diopters of myopia, was so much disturbed by what he saw when his vision had been improved by the memory of a period that he was directed to look away from the Snellen test card, or whatever object he was regarding, when he found the letters or other details coming out; and for about a week he went around persistently dodging his improved sight. As his memory improved, it became more and more difficult for him to do this, and at the end of the week it was impossible. When he looked at the bottom line at a distance of twenty feet he remembered the period perfectly, and when asked if he could see the letters, he replied :

"I cannot help but see them."

Some patients retard their recovery by decorating the scenery with periods as they go about during the day, instead of simply remembering a period in their minds. This does them no good, but is, on the contrary, a cause of strain. The period can be imagined perfectly and with benefit as forming part of a black letter on the test card, because this merely means imagining that one sees one part of the black letter best; but it cannot be imagined perfectly on any surface which is not black, and to attempt to imagine it on such surfaces defeats the end in view.

The smaller the area of black which the patient is able to remember, the greater is the degree of relaxation indicated; but some patients find it easier, at first, to remember a somewhat larger area, such as one of the letters on the Snellen test card with one part blacker than the rest. They may begin with the big C, then proceed to the smaller letters, and finally get to a period. It is then found that this small area is remembered more easily than the larger ones, and that its black is more intense. Instead of a period, some patients find it easier to remember a colon, with one period blacker than the other, or a collection of periods, with one blacker than all the others, or the dot over an i or j. Others, again, prefer a comma to a period. In the beginning most patients find it helpful to shift consciously from one of these black areas to another, or from one part of such an area to another, and to realize the swing, or pulsation, produced by such shifting (see Chapter XV) ; but when the memory becomes perfect, one object may be held continuously, without conscious shifting, while the swing is realized only when attention is directed to the matter.

Although black is, as a rule, the best color to remember, some patients are bored or depressed by it, and prefer to remember white or some other color. A

A Help to Other Mental Processes

familiar object, or one with pleasant associations, is often easier to remember than one which has no particular interest. One patient was cured by the memory of a yellow buttercup, and another was able to remember the opal of her ring when she could not remember a period. Whatever the patient finds easiest to remember is the best to remember, because the memory can never be perfect unless it is easy.

When the memory of the period becomes habitual, it is not only not a burden, but is a great help to other mental processes. Then the mind, when it remembers one thing better than all other things, possesses central fixation, and its efficiency is thereby increased, just as the efficiency of the eye is increased by central fixation. In other words, the mind attains its greatest efficiency when it is at rest, and it is never at rest unless one thing is remembered better than all other things. When the mind is in such a condition that a period is remembered perfectly, the memory for other things is improved.

A high-school girl reports that when she was unable to remember the answer to a question in an examination, she remembered the period, and the answer came to her. When I cannot remember the name of a patient, I remember a period - and, behold, I have it! A musician who had perfect sight and could remember a period perfectly, had a perfect memory for music; but a musician with imperfect sight who could not remember a period could play nothing without his notes, only gaining that power when his sight and visual memory had become normal. In some exceptional cases, the strain to see letters on the Snellen test card has been so terrific that patients have said that they not only could not remember a period while they were looking at them, but could not remember even their own names.

Patients may measure the accuracy of their memory of the period, not only by comparing it with the sight, but by the following tests :

When the memory of the period is perfect it is instantaneous. If a few seconds or longer are necessary to obtain the memory, it is never perfect.

A perfect memory is not only instantaneous, but continuous.

When the period is remembered perfectly perfect sight comes instantaneously. If good vision is obtained only after a second or two, it can always be demonstrated that the memory of the period is imperfect and the sight also.

The memory of a period is a test of relaxation. It is the evidence by which the patient knows that his eyes and mind are at rest. It may be compared to the steamgauge of an engine, which has nothing to do with the machinery, but is of great importance in giving information as to the ability of the mechanism to do its work. When the period is black one knows that the engine of the eye is in good working order. When the period fades, or is lost, one knows that it is out of order, until a cure is effected. Then one does not need a period, or any other aid to vision, just as the engineer does not need a steam-gauge when the engine is going properly. One patient who had gained telescopic and microscopic vision by the methods presented in this book said, in answer to an inquiry from some one interested in investigating the treatment of errors of refraction without glasses, that he had not only done nothing to prevent a relapse, but had even forgotten how he was cured.

The Period no Longer Needed

The reply was unsatisfactory to the inquirer, but is quoted to illustrate the fact that when a patient is cured he does not need to do anything consciously in order to stay cured, although the treatment can always be continued with benefit, since even supernormal vision can be improved.

CHAPTER XIV

IMAGINATION AS AN AID TO VISION

WE see very largely with the mind, and only partly with the eyes. The phenomena of vision depend upon the mind's interpretation of the impression upon the retina. What we see is not that impression, but our own interpretation of it. Our impressions of size, color, form and location can be demonstrated to depend upon the interpretation by the mind of the retinal picture. The moon looks smaller at the zenith than it does at the horizon, though the optical angle is the same and the impression on the retina may be the same, because at the horizon the mind unconsciously compares the picture with the pictures of surrounding objects, while at the zenith there is nothing to compare it with. The figure of a man on a high building, or on the topmast of a vessel, looks small to the landsman; but to the sailor it appears to be of ordinary size, because he is accustomed to seeing the human figure in such positions.

Persons with normal vision use their memory, or imagination, as an aid to sight; and when the sight is imperfect it can be demonstrated, not only that the eye itself is at fault, but that the memory and imagination are impaired, so that the mind adds imperfections to the imperfect retinal image. No two persons with normal sight will get the same visual impressions from the same object; for their interpretations of the retinal picture will differ as much as their individualities differ, and

The Mind Out of Focus

when the sight is imperfect the interpretation is far more variable. It reflects, in fact, the loss of mental control which is responsible for the error of refraction. When the eye is out of focus, in short, the mind is also out of focus.

According to the accepted view most of the abnormalities of vision produced when there is an error of refraction in the eye are sufficiently accounted for by the existence of that error. Some are supposed to be due to diseases of the brain or retina. Multiple images are attributed to astigmatism, though only two can be legitimately accounted for in this way, while some patients state that they see half a dozen or more, and many persons with astigmatism do not see any. It can easily be demonstrated, however, that the inaccuracy of the focus accounts for only a small part of these results; and since they can all be corrected in a few seconds through the correction, by relaxation, of the error of refraction, it is evident that they cannot be due to any organic disease.

If we compare the picture on the glass screen of the camera when the camera is out of focus with the visual impressions of the mind when the eye is out of focus, there will be found to be a great difference between them. When the camera is out of focus it turns black into grey, and blurs the outlines of the picture; but it produces these results uniformly and constantly. On the screen of the camera an imperfect picture of a black letter would be equally imperfect in all parts, and the same adjustment of the focus would always produce the same picture. But when the eye is out of focus the imperfect picture which the patient imagines that he sees is always changing, whether the focus changes or not. There will be more grey on one part than on another, and both the shade and the position of the grey may vary within wide limits in a very short space of time. One part of the letter may appear grey and the rest black. Certain outlines may be seen better than others, the vertical lines, perhaps, appearing black and the diagonal grey, and vice versa. Again, the black may be changed into brown, yellow, green, or even red, transmutations impossible to the camera. Or there may be spots of color, or of black, on the grey, or on the white openings. There may also be spots of white, or of color, on the black.

When the camera is out of focus the picture which it produces of any object is always slightly larger than the image produced when the focus is correct; but when the eye is out of focus the picture which the mind sees may be either larger or smaller than it normally would be. To one patient the big C at ten feet appeared smaller than at either twenty feet or four inches. To some it appears larger than it actually is at twenty feet, and to others it seems smaller.

When the human eye is out of focus the form of the objects regarded by the patient frequently appears to be distorted, while their location may also appear to change. The image may be doubled, tripled, or still further multiplied, and while one object, or part of an object may be multiplied other objects or parts of objects in the field of vision may remain single. The location of these multiple images is sometimes constant and at others subject to continual change. Nothing like this could happen when the camera is out of focus.

How Imagination Cures

If two cameras are out of focus to the same degree, they will take two imperfect pictures exactly alike. If two eyes are out of focus to the same degree, similar impressions will be made upon the retina of each; but the impressions made upon the mind may be totally unlike, whether the eyes belong to the same person or to different persons. If the normal eye looks at an object through glasses that change its refraction, the greyness and blurring produced are uniform and constant; but when the eye has an error of refraction equivalent to that produced by the glasses, these phenomena are non-uniform and variable.

It is fundamental that the patient should understand that these aberrations of vision - which are treated more fully in a later chapter - are illusions, and not due to a fault of the eyes. When he knows that a thing is an illusion he is less likely to see it again. When he becomes convinced that what he sees is imaginary it helps to bring the imagination under control; and since a perfect imagination is impossible without perfect relaxation, a perfect imagination not only corrects the false interpretation of the retinal image, but corrects the error of refraction.

Imagination is closely allied to memory, although distinct from it. Imagination depends upon the memory, because a thing can be imagined only as well as it can be remembered. You cannot imagine a sunset unless you have seen one; and if you attempt to imagine a blue sun, which you have never seen, you will become myopic, as indicated by simultaneous retinoscopy. Neither imagination nor memory can be perfect unless the mind is perfectly relaxed. Therefore when the imagination and memory are perfect, the sight is perfect. Imagination, memory and sight are, in fact, coincident. When one is perfect, all are perfect, and when one is imperfect, all are imperfect. If you imagine a letter perfectly, you will see the letter and other letters in its neighborhood will come out more distinctly, because it is impossible for you to relax and imagine you see a perfect letter and at the same time strain and actually see an imperfect one. If you imagine a perfect period on the bottom of a letter, you will see the letter perfectly, because you cannot take the mental picture of a perfect period and put it on an imperfect letter. It is possible, however, as pointed out in the preceding chapter, for sight to be unconscious. In some cases patients may imagine the period perfectly, as demonstrated by the retinoscope, without being conscious of seeing the letter; and it is often some time before they are able to be conscious of it without losing the period.

When one treats patients who are willing to believe that the letters can be imagined, and who are content to imagine without trying to see, or compare what they see with what they imagine, which always brings back the strain, very remarkable results are sometimes obtained by the aid of the imagination. Some patients at once become able to read all the letters on the bottom line of the test card after they become able to imagine that they see one letter perfectly black and distinct. The majority, however, are so distracted by what they see when their vision has been improved by their imagination that they lose the latter. It is one thing to be able to imagine perfect sight of a letter, and another to be able to see the letter and other letters without losing control of the imagination.

In myopia the following method is often successful : First look at a letter at the point at which it is seen best. Then close the eyes and remember it. Repeat

Patients Who Succeed

until the memory is almost as good as the sight at the near-point. With the test card at a distance of twenty feet, look at a blank surface a foot or more to one side of it, and again remember the letter. Do the same at six inches and at three inches. At the last point note the appearance of the letters on the card - that is, in the eccentric field. If the memory is still perfect, they will appear to be a dim black, not grey, and those nearest the point of fixation will appear blacker than those more distant. Gradually reduce the distance between the point of fixation and the letter until able to look straight at it and imagine that it is seen as well as it is remembered. Occasionally it is well during the practice to close and cover the eyes and remember the letter, or a period, perfectly black. The rest and mental control gained in this way are a help in gaining control when one looks at the test card.

Patients who succeed with this method are not conscious while imagining a perfect letter, of seeing, at the same time, an imperfect one, and are not distracted when their vision is improved by their imagination. Many patients can remember perfectly with their eyes closed, or when they are looking at a place where they cannot see the letter; but just as soon as they look at it they begin to strain and lose control of their memory. Therefore, as the imagination depends upon the memory, they cannot imagine that they see the letter. In such cases it has been my custom to proceed somewhat in the manner described in the preceding chapter. I begin by saying to the patient:

"Can you imagine a black period on the bottom of this letter, and at the same time, while imagining the period perfectly, are you able to imagine that you see the letter?

Sometimes they are able to do this, but usually they are not. In that case they are asked to imagine part of the letter, usually the bottom. When they have become able to imagine this part straight, curved, or open, as the case may be, they become able to imagine the sides and top, while still holding the period on the bottom. But even after they have done this, they may still not be able to imagine the whole letter without losing the period. One may have to coax them along by bringing the card up a little closer, then moving it farther away; for when looking at a surface where there is anything to see, the imagination improves in proportion as one approaches the point where the sight is best, because at that point the eyes are most relaxed. When there is nothing particular to see, the distance makes no difference, because no effort is being made to see.

To encourage patients to imagine they see the letter it seems helpful to keep saying to them over and over again:

"Of course you do not see the letter. I am not asking you to see it. I am just asking you to imagine that you see it perfectly black and perfectly distinct."

When patients become able to see a known letter by the aid of their imagination, they become able to apply the same method to an unknown letter ; for just as soon as any part of a letter, such as an area equal to a period, can be imagined to be perfectly black, the whole letter is seen to be black, although the visual perception of this fact may not, at first, last long enough for the patient to become conscious of it.

In trying to distinguish unknown letters, the patient discovers that it is impossible to imagine perfectly unless one imagines the truth; for if a letter, or any part

One Way of Imagining Perfectly

of a letter, is imagined to be other than it is, the mental picture is foggy and inconstant, just like a letter which is seen imperfectly.

The ways in which the imagination can be interfered with are very numerous. There is one way of imagining perfectly and an infinite number of ways of imagining imperfectly. The right way is easy. The mental picture of the thing imagined comes as quick as thought, and can be held more or less continuously. The wrong way is difficult. The picture comes slowly, and is both variable and discontinuous. This can be demonstrated to the patient by asking him first to imagine or remember a black letter as perfectly as possible with the eyes closed, and then to imagine the same letter imperfectly. The first he can usually do easily; but it will be found very difficult to imagine a black letter with clear outlines to be grey, with fuzzy edges and clouded openings, and impossible to form a mental picture of it that will remain constant for an appreciable length of time. The letter will vary in color, shape and location in the visual field, precisely as a letter does when it is seen imperfectly; and just as the strain of imperfect sight produces discomfort and pain, the effort to imagine imperfectly will sometimes produce pain. The more nearly perfect the mental picture of the letter, on the contrary, the more easily and quickly it comes and the more constant it is.

Some very dramatic cures have been effected by means of the imagination. One patient, a physician, who had worn glasses for forty years and who could not without them see the big C at twenty feet, was cured in fifteen minutes simply by imagining that he saw the letters black. When asked to describe the big C with unaided vision he said it looked grey to him, and that the opening was obscured by a grey cloud to such an extent that he had to guess that it had an opening. He was told that the letter was black, perfectly black, and that the opening was perfectly white, with no grey cloud; and the card was brought close to him so that he could see that this was so. When he again regarded the letter at the distance, he remembered its blackness so vividly that he was able to imagine that he saw it just as black as he had seen it at the near-point, with the opening perfectly white; and therefore he saw the letter on the card perfectly black and distinct. In the same way he became able to read the seventy line; and so he went down the card, until in about five minutes he became able to read at twenty feet the line which the normal eye is supposed to read at ten feet. Next diamond type was given to him to read. The letters appeared grey to him, and he could not read them. His attention was called to the fact that the letters were really black, and immediately he imagined that he saw them black and became able to read them at ten inches.

The explanation of this remarkable occurrence is simply relaxation. All the nerves of the patient's body were relaxed when he imagined that he saw the letters black, and when he became conscious of seeing the letters on the card, he still retained control of his imagination. Therefore he did not begin to strain again, and actually saw the letters as black as he imagined them.

The patient not only had no relapse, but continued to improve. About a year later I visited him in his office and asked him how he was getting on. He replied that his sight was perfect, both for distance and the near-point. He could see the motor cars on the

Too Good To Be True

other side of the Hudson River and the people in them, and he could read the names of boats on the river which other people could make out only with a telescope. At the same time he had no difficulty in reading the newspapers, and to prove the latter part of this statement, he picked up a newspaper and read a few sentences aloud. I was astonished, and asked him how he did it.

"I did what you told me to do," he said.

"What did I tell you to do?" I asked.

"You told me to read the Snellen test card every day, which I have done, and to read fine print every day in a dim light, which I have also done."

Another patient, who had a high degree of myopia complicated with atrophy of the optic nerve, and who had been discouraged by many physicians, was benefited so wonderfully and rapidly by the aid of his imagination that one day while in the office he lost control of himself completely, and raising a test card which he held in his hand, he threw it across the room.

"It is too good to be true," he exclaimed; "I cannot believe it. The possibility of being cured and the fear of disappointment are more than I can stand."

He was calmed down with some difficulty and encouraged to continue. Later he became able to read the small letters on the test card with normal vision. He was then given fine print to read. When he looked at the diamond type, he at once said that it was impossible for him to read it. However, he was told to follow the same procedure that had benefited his distance sight. That is, he was to <u>imagine a period on one part of the small letters while holding the type at six inches.</u> After testing his memory of the period a number of times, he became able to imagine he saw a period perfectly black on one of the small letters. Then he lost control of his nerves again, and on being asked, "What is the trouble?" he said:

"I am beginning to read the fine print, and I am so overwhelmed that I lose my self-control."

In another case, that of a woman with high myopia complicated with incipient cataract, the vision improved in a few days from 3/200 to 20/50. Instead of going gradually down the card, a jump was made from the fifty line to the ten line. The card was brought up close to her, and she was asked to look at the letter O at three inches, the distance at which she saw it best, to imagine that she saw a period on the bottom of it and that the bottom was the blackest part. When she was able to do this at the near-point, the distance was gradually increased until she became able to see the O at three feet.

Then I placed the card at ten feet and she exclaimed:

"Oh, doctor, it is impossible! The letter is too small. It is too great a thing for me to do. Let me try a larger letter first."

Nevertheless she became able in fifteen minutes to read the small O on the ten line at twenty-feet.

(Close Vision Cure; Shift point to point on a period in a fine print letter and remember, imagine it dark black and clear.)

CHAPTER XV
SHIFTING AND SWINGING

WHEN the eye with normal vision regards a letter either at the near-point or at the distance, the letter may appear to pulsate, or to move in various directions, from side to side, up and down, or obliquely. When it looks from one letter to another on the Snellen test card, or from one side of a letter to another, not only the letter, but the whole line of letters and the whole card, may appear to move from side to side. This apparent movement is due to the shifting of the eye, and is always in a direction contrary to its movement. If one looks at the top of a letter, the letter is below the line of vision, and, therefore, appears to move downward. If one looks at the bottom, the letter is above the line of vision and appears to move upward. If one looks to the left of the letter, it is to the right of the line of vision and appears to move to the right. If one looks to the right, it is to the left of the line of vision and appears to move to the left.

Persons with normal vision are rarely conscious of this illusion, and may have difficulty in demonstrating it ; but in every case that has come under my observation they have always become able, in a longer or shorter time, to do so. When the sight is imperfect the letters may remain stationary, or even move in the same direction as the eye.

It is impossible for the eye to fix a point longer than a fraction of a second. If it tries to do so, it begins to strain and the vision is lowered. This can readily be demonstrated by trying to hold one part of a letter for an appreciable length of time. No matter how good the sight, it will begin to blur, or even disappear, very quickly, and sometimes the effort to hold it will produce pain. In the case of a few exceptional people a point may appear to be held for a considerable length of time; the subjects themselves may think that they are holding it ; but this is only because the eye shifts unconsciously, the movements being so rapid that objects seem to be seen all alike simultaneously.

The shifting of the eye with normal vision is usually not conspicuous, but by direct examination with the ophthalmoscope it can always be demonstrated. If one eye is examined with this instrument while the other is regarding a small area straight ahead, the eye being examined, which follows the movements of the other, is seen to move in various directions, from side to side, up and down in an orbit which is usually variable. If the vision is normal these movements are extremely rapid and unaccompanied by any appearance of effort. The shifting of the eye with imperfect sight, on the contrary, is slower, its excursions are wider, and the movements are jerky and made with apparent effort.

It can also be demonstrated that the eye is capable of shifting with a rapidity which the ophthalmoscope cannot measure. The normal eye can read fourteen letters on the bottom line of a Snellen test card, at a distance of ten or fifteen feet, in a dim light, so rapidly that they seem to be seen all at once. Yet it can be demonstrated that in order to recognize the letters under these conditions it is necessary to make about four shifts to each letter. At the near-point, even though one part of the

Rapidity of Eye's Motion

letter is seen best, the rest may be seen well enough to be recognized; but at the distance it is impossible to recognize the letters unless one shifts from the top to the bottom and from side to side. One must also shift from one letter to another, making about seventy shifts in a fraction of a second.

A line of small letters on the Snellen test card may be less than a foot long by a quarter of an inch in height; and if it requires seventy shifts to a fraction of a second to see it apparently all at once, it must require many thousands to see an area of the size of the screen of a moving picture, with all its detail of people, animals, houses, or trees, while to see sixteen such areas to a second, as is done in viewing moving pictures, must require a rapidity of shifting that can scarcely be realized. Yet it is admitted that the present rate of taking and projecting moving pictures is too slow. The results would be more satisfactory, authorities say, if the rate were raised to twenty, twenty-two, or twenty-four a second.

The human eye and mind are not only capable of this rapidity of action, and that without effort or strain, but it is only when the eye is able to shift thus rapidly that eye and mind are at rest, and the efficiency of both at their maximum. It is true that every motion of the eye produces an error of refraction ; but when the movement is short, this is very slight, and usually the shifts are so rapid that the error does not last long enough to be detected by the retinoscope, its existence being demonstrable only by reducing the rapidity of the movements to less than four or five a second. The period during which the eye is at rest is much longer than that during which an error of refraction is produced. Hence, when the eye shifts normally no error of refraction is manifest. The more rapid the unconscious shifting of the eye, the better the vision; but if one tries to be conscious of a too rapid shift, a strain will be produced.

Perfect sight is impossible without continual shifting, and such shifting is a striking illustration of the mental control necessary for normal vision. It requires perfect mental control to think of thousands of things in a fraction of a second; and each point of fixation has to be thought of separately, because it is impossible to think of two things, or of two parts of one thing, perfectly at the same time. The eye with imperfect sight tries to accomplish the impossible by looking fixedly at one point for an appreciable length of time; that is, by staring. When it looks at a strange letter and does not see it, it keeps on looking at it in an effort to see it better. Such efforts always fail, and are an important factor in the production of imperfect sight.

One of the best methods of improving the sight, therefore, is to imitate consciously the unconscious shifting of normal vision and to realize the apparent motion produced by such shifting. Whether one has imperfect or normal sight, conscious shifting and swinging are a great help and advantage to the eye; for not only may imperfect sight be improved in this way, but normal sight may be improved also. When the sight is imperfect, shifting, if done properly, rests the eye as much as palming, and always lessens or corrects the error of refraction.

The eye with normal sight never attempts to hold a point more than a fraction of a second, and when it shifts, as explained in the chapter on "Central Fixation," it always sees the previous point of fixation worse. When it ceases to shift rapidly and to see the point

The Shift That Rests

shifted from worse, the sight ceases to be normal, the swing being either prevented or lengthened, or (occasionally) reversed. These facts are the keynote of the treatment by shifting.

In order to see the previous point of fixation worse, the eye with imperfect sight has to look farther away from it than does the eye with normal sight. If it shifts only a quarter of an inch, for instance, it may see the previous point of fixation as well as or better than before; and instead of being rested by such a shift, its strain will be increased, there will be no swing, and the vision will be lowered. At a couple of inches it may be able to let go of the first point; and if neither point is held more than a fraction of a second, it will be rested by such a shift and the illusion of swinging may be produced. The shorter the shift the greater the benefit; but even a very long shift - as much as three feet or more - is a help to those who cannot accomplish a shorter one. When the patient is capable of a short shift, on the contrary, the long shift lowers the vision. The swing is an evidence that the shifting is being done properly, and when it occurs the vision is always improved. It is possible to shift without improvement; but it is impossible to produce the illusion of a swing without improvement, and when this can be done with a long shift, the movement can gradually be shortened until the patient can shift from the top to the bottom of the smallest letter, on the Snellen test card or elsewhere, and maintain the swing. Later he may become able to be conscious of the swinging of the letters without conscious shifting. (The Swing: Natural illusion of movement of the object, in the opposite direction the eyes, visual attention move to, upon the object; Oppositional Movement.)

No matter how imperfect the sight, it is always possible to shift and produce a swing, so long as the previous point of fixation is seen worse. Even diplopia and polyopia 1 do not prevent swinging with some improvement of vision. Usually the eye with imperfect vision is able to shift from one side of the card to the other, or from a point above the card to a point below it, and observe that in the first case the card appears to move from side to side, while in the second it appears to move up and down.

When patients are suffering from high degrees of eccentric fixation, it may be necessary, in order to help them to see worse when they shift, to use some of the methods described in the chapter on "Central Fixation." Usually, however, patients who cannot see worse when they shift at the distance can do it readily at the near-point, as the sight is best at that point, not only in myopia, but often in hypermetropia as well. When the swing can be produced at the near point, the distance can be gradually increased until the same thing can be done at twenty feet.

After resting the eyes by closing or palming, shifting and swinging are often more successful. By this method of alternately resting the eyes and then shifting, persons with very imperfect sight have sometimes obtained a temporary or permanent cure in a few weeks.

Shifting may be done slowly or rapidly, according to the state of the vision. At the beginning the patient will be likely to strain if he shifts too rapidly ; and then the point shifted from will not be seen worse, and there will be no swing. As improvement is made, the speed can be increased. It is usually impossible, however, to realize the swing if the shifting is more rapid than two or three times a second.

1 Double and multiple vision.

Imagination Helps

A mental picture of a letter can, as a rule, be made to swing precisely as can a letter on the test card. Occasionally one meets a patient with whom the reverse is true ; but for most patients the mental swing is easier at first than visual swinging; and when they become able to swing in this way, it becomes easier for them to swing the letters on the test card. By alternating mental with visual swinging and shifting, rapid progress is sometimes made. As relaxation becomes more perfect, the mental swing can be shortened, until it becomes possible to conceive and swing a letter the size of a period in a newspaper. This is easier, when it can be done, than swinging a larger letter, and many patients have derived great benefit from it.

All persons, no matter how great their error of refraction, when they shift and swing successfully, correct it partially or completely, as demonstrated by the retinoscope, for at least a fraction of a second. This time may be so short that the patient is not conscious of improved vision; but it is possible for him to imagine it, and then it becomes easier to maintain the relaxation long enough to be conscious of the improved sight. For instance, the patient, after looking away from the card, may look back to the big C, and for a fraction of a second the error of refraction may be lessened or corrected, as demonstrated by the retinoscope. Yet he may not be conscious of improved vision. By imagining that the C is seen better, however, the moment of relaxation may be sufficiently prolonged to be realized.

When swinging, either mental or visual, is successful, the patient may become conscious of a feeling of relaxation which is manifested as a sensation of universal swinging. This sensation communicates itself to any object of which the patient is conscious. The motion may be imagined in any part of the body to which the attention is directed. It may be communicated to the chair in which the patient is sitting, or to any object in the room, or elsewhere, which is remembered. The building, the city, the whole world, in fact, may appear to be swinging. When the patient becomes conscious of this universal swinging, he loses the memory of the object with which it started; but so long as he is able to maintain the movement in a direction contrary to the original movement of the eyes, or the movement imagined by the mind, relaxation is maintained. If the direction is changed, however, strain results. To imagine the universal swing with the eyes closed is easy, and some patients soon become able to do it with the eyes open. Later the feeling of relaxation which accompanies the swing may be realized without consciousness of the latter; but the swing can always be produced when the patient thinks of it.

There is but one cause of failure to produce a swing, and that is strain. Some people try to make the letters swing by effort. Such efforts always fail. The eyes and mind do not swing the letters; they swing of themselves. The eye can shift voluntarily. This is a muscular act resulting from a motor impulse. But the Swing comes of its own accord when the shifting is normal. It does not produce relaxation, but is an evidence of it; and while of no value in itself is, like the period, very valuable as an indication that relaxation is being maintained.

The following methods of shifting have been found useful in various cases :

One Cause of Failure

No. 1
(a) Regard a letter.
(b) Shift to a letter on the same line far enough away so that the first is seen worse.
(c) Look back at No. 1 and see No. 2 worse.
(d) Look at the letters alternately for a few seconds, seeing worse the one not regarded.

When successful, both letters improve and appear to move from side to side in a direction opposite to the movement of the eye.

No. 2
(a) Look at a large letter.
(b) Look at a smaller one a long distance away from it. The large one is then seen worse.
(c) Look back and see it better.
(d) Repeat half a dozen times.

When successful, both letters improve, and the card appears to move up and down.

No. 3
Shifting by the above methods enables the patient to see one letter on a line better than the other letters, and, usually, to distinguish it in flashes. In order to see the letter continuously it is necessary to become able to shift from the top to the bottom, or from the bottom to the top, seeing worse the part not directly regarded, and producing the illusion of a vertical swing.
(a) Look at a point far enough above the top of the letter to see the bottom, or the whole letter worse.
(b) Look at a point far enough below the bottom to see the top, or the whole letter, worse.
(c) Repeat half a dozen times.

If successful, the letter will appear to move up and down, and the vision will improve. The shift can then be shortened until it becomes possible to shift between the top and the bottom of the letter and maintain the swing. The letter is now seen continuously. If the method fails, rest the eyes, palm, and try again.

One may also practice by shifting from one side of the letter to a point beyond the other side, or from one corner to a point beyond the other corner.

No. 4
(a) Regard a letter at the distance at which it is seen best. In myopia this will be at the near-point, a foot or less from the face. Shift from the top to the bottom until able to see each worse alternately, when the letter will appear blacker than before, `and an illusion of swinging will be produced.
(b) Now close the eyes, and shift from the top to the bottom of the letter mentally.
(c) Regard a blank wall with the eyes open, and do the same. Compare the ability to shift and swing mentally with the ability to do the same visually at the near-point.
(d) Then regard the letter at the distance, and shift from the top to the bottom. If successful, the letter will improve, and an illusion of swinging will be produced.

No. 5
Some patients, particularly children, are able to see better when one points to the letters. In other cases

Pointing to the Letters

 this is a distraction. When the method is found successful one can proceed as follows :
(a) Place the tip of the finger three or four inches below the letter. Let the patient regard the letter, and shift to the tip of the finger, seeing the letter worse.
(b) Reduce the distance between the finger and the letter, first to two or three inches, then to one or two, and finally to half an inch, proceeding each time as in (a).

If successful, the patient will become able to look from the top to the bottom of the letter, seeing each worse alternately, and producing the illusion of swinging. It will then be possible to see the letter continuously.

No. 6
When the vision is imperfect it often happens that, when the patient looks at a small letter, some of the larger letters on the upper lines, or the big C at the top, look blacker than the letter regarded. This makes it impossible to see the smaller letters perfectly. To correct this eccentric fixation regard the letter which is seen best, and shift to the smaller letter. If successful, the small letter, after a few movements, will appear blacker than the larger one. If not successful after a few trials, rest the eyes by closing and palming, and try again. One may also shift from the large letter to a point some distance below the small letter, gradually approaching the latter as the vision improves.

No. 7
Shifting from a card at three or five feet to one at ten or twenty feet often proves helpful, as the unconscious memory of the letter seen at the near-point helps to bring out the one at the distance.

Different people will find these various methods of shifting more or less satisfactory. If any method does not succeed, it should be abandoned after one or two trials and something else tried. It is a mistake to continue the practice of any method which does not yield prompt results. The cause of the failure is strain, and it does no good to continue the strain.

When it is not possible to practice with the Snellen test card, other objects may be utilized. One can shift, for instance, from one window of a distant building to another, or from one part of a window to another part of the same window, from one auto to another, or from one part of an auto to another part, producing, in each case, the illusion that the objects are moving in a direction contrary to the movement of the eye. When talking to people, one can shift from one person to another, or from one part of the face to another part. When reading a book, or newspaper, one can shift consciously from one word or letter to another, or from one part of a letter to another.

Shifting and swinging, as they give the patient something definite to do, are often more successful than other methods of obtaining relaxation, and in some cases remarkable results have been obtained simply by demonstrating to the patient that staring lowers the vision and shifting improves it. One patient, a girl of sixteen with progressive myopia, obtained very prompt relief by shifting. She came to the office wearing a pair of glasses tinted a pale yellow, with shades at the sides; and in spite of this protection she was so annoyed by the light that her eyes were almost closed, and she had great

Cured by Shifting

difficulty in finding her way about the room. Her vision without glasses was 3/200. All reading had been forbidden, playing the piano from the notes was not allowed, and she had been obliged to give up the idea of going to college. The sensitiveness to light was relieved in a few minutes by focussing the light of the sun upon the upper part of the eyeball when she looked far down, by means of a burning glass (see Chapter XVII). The patient was then seated before a Snellen test card and directed to look away from it, rest her eyes, and then look at the big C. For a fraction of a second her vision was improved, and by frequent demonstrations she was made to realize that any effort to see the letters always lowered the vision. By alternately looking away, and then looking back at the letters for a fraction of a second, her vision improved so rapidly that in the course of half an hour it was almost normal for the distance. Then diamond type was given her to read. The attempt to read it at once brought on a severe pain. She was directed to proceed as she had in reading the Snellen test card; and in a few minutes, by alternately looking away and then looking at the first letter of each word in turn, she became able to read without fatigue, discomfort, or pain. She left the office without her glasses, and was able to see her way without difficulty. Other patients have been benefited as promptly by this simple method.

CHAPTER XVI

THE ILLUSIONS OF IMPERFECT AND OF NORMAL EYESIGHT

PERSONS with imperfect sight always have illusions of vision; so do persons with normal sight. But while the illusions of normal sight are an evidence of relaxation, the illusions of imperfect sight are an evidence of strain. Some persons with errors of refraction have few illusions, others have many; because the strain which causes the error of refraction is not the same strain that is responsible for the illusions.

The illusions of imperfect sight may relate to the color, size, location and form of the objects regarded. They may include appearances of things that have no existence at all, and various other curious and interesting manifestations.

ILLUSIONS OF COLOR

When a patient regards a black letter and believes it to be grey, yellow, brown, blue, or green, he is suffering from an illusion of color. This phenomenon differs from color-blindness. The color-blind person is unable to differentiate between different colors, usually blue and green, and his inability to do so is constant. The person suffering from an illusion of color does not see the false colors constantly or uniformly. When he looks at the Snellen test card the black letters may appear to him at one time to be grey; but at another moment they may appear to be a shade of yellow, blue, or brown. Some

Vagaries of Color and Size

patients always see the black letters red; to others, they appear red only occasionally. Although the letters are all of the same color, some may see the large letters black and the small ones yellow or blue. Usually the large letters are seen darker than the small ones, whatever color they appear to be. Often different colors appear in the same letter, part of it seeming to be black, perhaps, and the rest grey or some other color. Spots of black, or of color, may appear on the white; and spots of white, or of color, on the black.

ILLUSIONS OF SIZE

Large letters may appear small, or small letters large. One letter may appear to be of normal size, while another of the same size and at the same distance may appear larger or smaller than normal. Or a letter may appear to be of normal size at the near-point and at the distance, and only half that size at the middle distance. When a person can judge the size of a letter correctly at all distances up to twenty feet his vision is normal. If the size appears different to him at different distances, he is suffering from an illusion of size. At great distances the judgment of size is always imperfect, because the sight at such distances is imperfect, even though perfect at ordinary distances. The stars appear to be dots, because the eye does not possess perfect vision for objects at such distances. A candle seen half a mile away appears smaller than at the near-point; but seen through a telescope giving perfect vision at that distance it will be the same as at the near-point. With improved vision the ability to judge size improves.

The correction of an error of refraction by glasses seldom enables the patient to judge size as correctly as the normal eye does, and the ability to do this may differ very greatly in persons having the same error of refraction. A person with ten diopters of myopia corrected by glasses may (rarely) be able to judge the sizes of objects correctly. Another person, with the same degree of myopia and the same glasses, may see them only one-half or one-third their normal size. This indicates that errors of refraction have very little to do with incorrect perceptions of size.

ILLUSIONS OF FORM

Round letters may appear square or triangular ; straight letters may appear curved; letters of regular form may appear very irregular ; a round letter may appear to have a checker-board or a cross in the center. In short, an infinite variety of changing forms may be seen. Illumination, distance and environment are all factors in this form of imperfect sight. Many persons can see the form of a letter correctly when other letters are covered, but when the other letters are visible they cannot see it. The indication of the position of a letter by a pointer helps some people to see it. Others are so disturbed by the pointer that they cannot see the letter so well.

ILLUSIONS OF NUMBER

Multiple images are frequently seen by persons with imperfect sight, either with both eyes together, with each eye separately, or with only one eye. The manner in which these multiple images make their appearance is sometimes very curious. For instance, a patient with presbyopia read the word HAS normally with both eyes. The word PHONES he read correctly with the left eye;

Strange Tricks of the Mind

but when he read it with the right eye he saw the letter P double, the imaginary image being a little distance to the left of the real one. The left eye, while it had normal vision for the word PHONES, multiplied the shaft of a pin when this object was in a vertical position (the head remaining single), and multiplied the head when the position was changed to the horizontal (the shaft then remaining single). When the point of the pin was placed below a very small letter, the point was sometimes doubled while the letter remained single. No error of refraction can account for these phenomena. They are tricks of the mind only. The ways in which multiple images are arranged are endless. They are sometimes placed vertically, sometimes horizontally or obliquely, and sometimes in circles, triangles and other geometrical forms. Their number, too, may vary from two to three, four, or more. They may be stationary, or may change their position more or less rapidly. They also show an infinite variety of color, including a white even whiter than that of the background.

ILLUSIONS OF LOCATION

A period following a letter on the same horizontal level as the bottom of the letter may appear to change its position in a great variety of curious ways. Its distance from the letter may vary. It may even appear on the other side of the letter. It may also appear above or below the line. Some persons see letters arranged in irregular order. In the case of the word AND, for instance, the D may occupy the place of the N, or the first letter may change places with the last. All these things are mental illusions. The letters sometimes appear to be farther off than they really are. The small letters, twenty feet distant, may appear to be a mile away. Patients troubled by illusions of distance sometimes ask if the position of the card has not been changed.

ILLUSIONS OF NON-EXISTENT OBJECTS

When the eye has imperfect sight the mind not only distorts what the eye sees, but it imagines that it sees things that do not exist. Among illusions of this sort are the floating specks which so often appear before the eyes when the sight is imperfect, and even when it is ordinarily very good. These specks are known scientifically as "muscae volitantes," or "flying flies," and although they are of no real importance, being symptoms of nothing except mental strain, they have attracted so much attention, and usually cause so much alarm to the patient, that they will be discussed at length in another chapter.

ILLUSIONS OF COMPLEMENTARY COLORS

When the sight is imperfect, the subject, on looking away from a black, white, or brightly colored object, and closing the eyes, often imagines for a few seconds that he sees the object in a complementary, or approximately complementary, color. If the object is black upon a white background, a white object upon a black background will be seen. If the object is red, it may be seen as blue ; and if it is blue, it may appear to be red. These illusions, which are known as "after-images," may also be seen, though less commonly, with the eyes open, upon any background at which the subject happens to look, and are often so vivid that they appear to be real.

The Color of the Sun
ILLUSIONS OF THE COLOR OF THE SUN

Persons with normal sight see the sun white, the whitest white there is; but when the sight is imperfect it may appear to be any color in the spectrum - red, blue, green, purple, yellow, etc. In fact, it has even been described by persons with imperfect vision as totally black. The setting sun commonly appears to be red, because of atmospheric conditions; but in many cases these conditions are not such as to change the color, and while this still appears to be red to persons with imperfect vision, to persons with normal vision it appears to be white. When the redness of a red sun is an illusion, and not due to atmosphere conditions, its image on the ground glass of a camera will be white, not red, and the rays focussed with a burning glass will also be white. The same is true of a red moon.

BLIND SPOTS AFTER LOOKING AT THE SUN

After looking at the sun, most people see black or colored spots which may last from a few minutes to a year or longer, but are never permanent. These spots are also illusions, and are not due, as is commonly supposed, to any organic change in the eye. Even the total blindness which sometimes results, temporarily, from looking at the sun, is only an illusion.

(Modern Natural Eyesight Improvement Teachers state to CLOSE THE EYES when facing the sun (Sunning) and to move the eyes, had side to side, up, down...)

ILLUSIONS OF TWINKLING STARS

The idea that the stars should twinkle has been embodied in song and story, and is generally accepted as part of the natural order of things ; but it can be demonstrated that this appearance is simply an illusion of the mind.

CAUSE OF THE ILLUSIONS OF IMPERFECT SIGHT

All the illusions of imperfect sight are the result of a strain of the mind, and when the mind is disturbed for any reason, illusions of all kinds are very likely to occur. This strain is not only different from the strain that produces the error of refraction, but it can be demonstrated that for each and every one of these illusions there is a different kind of strain. Alterations of color do not necessarily affect the size or form of objects, or produce any other illusion, and it is possible to see the color of a letter, or of a part of a letter, perfectly, without recognizing the letter. To change black letters into blue, or yellow, or another color, requires a subconscious strain to remember or imagine the colors concerned, while to alter the form requires a subconscious strain to see the form in question. With a little practice anyone can learn to produce illusions of form and color by straining consciously in the same way that one strains unconsciously; and whenever illusions are produced in this way it will be found that eccentric fixation and an error of refraction have also been produced.

The strain which produces polyopia is different again from the strain which produces illusions of color, size and form. After a few attempts most patients easily learn to produce polyopia at will. Staring or squinting, if the strain is great enough, will usually make one see double. By looking above a light, or a letter, and then trying to see it as well as when directly regarded, one can produce an illusion of several lights, or letters, arranged vertically. If the strain is great enough, there

Conscious Production of Illusions

may be as many as a dozen of them. By looking to the side of the light or letter, or looking away obliquely at any angle, the images can be made to arrange themselves horizontally, or obliquely at any angle.

To see objects in the wrong location, as when the first letter of a word occupies the place of the last, requires an ingenuity of eccentric fixation and an education of the imagination which is unusual.

The black or colored spots seen after looking at the sun, and the strange colors which the sun sometimes seems to assume, are also the result of the mental strain. When one becomes able to look at the orb of day without strain, these phenomena immediately disappear.

After-images have been attributed to fatigue of the retina, which is supposed to have been so overstimulated by a certain color that it can no longer perceive it, and therefore seeks relief in the hue which is complementary to this color. If it gets tired looking at the black C on the Snellen test card, for instance, it is supposed to seek relief by seeing the C white. This explanation of the phenomenon is very ingenious but scarcely plausible. The eyes cannot see when they are closed; and if they appear to see under these conditions, it is obvious that the subject is suffering from a mental illusion with which the retina has nothing to do. Neither can they see what does not exist; and if they appear to see a white C on a green wall where there is no such object, it is obvious again that the subject is suffering from a mental illusion. The after-image indicates, in fact, simply a loss of mental control, and occurs when there is an error of refraction, because this condition also is due to a loss of mental control. Anyone can produce an after-image at will by trying to see the big C all alike - that is, under a strain ; but one can look at it indefinitely by central fixation without any such result.

While persons with imperfect sight usually see the stars twinkle, they do not necessarily do so. Therefore it is evident that the strain which causes the twinkling is different from that which causes the error of refraction. If one can look at a star without trying to see it, it does not twinkle; and when the illusion of twinkling has been produced, one can usually stop it by "swinging" the star. On the other hand, one can start the planets, or even the moon, to twinkling, if one strains sufficiently to see them.

ILLUSIONS OF NORMAL SIGHT

The illusions of normal sight include all the phenomena of central fixation. When the eye with normal sight looks at a letter on the Snellen test card, it sees the point fixed best, and everything else in the field of vision appears less distinct. As a matter of fact, the whole letter and all the letters may be perfectly black and distinct, and the impression that one letter is blacker than the others, or that one part of a letter is blacker than the rest, is an illusion. The normal eye, however, may shift so rapidly that it appears to see a whole line of small letters all alike simultaneously. As a matter of fact there is, of course, no such picture on the retina. Each letter has not only been seen separately, but it has been demonstrated in the chapter on "Shifting and Swinging" that if the letters are seen at a distance of fifteen or twenty feet, they could not be recognized unless about four shifts were made on each letter. To produce the impression of a simultaneous picture of fourteen letters,

All Vision an Illusion

therefore, some sixty or seventy pictures, each with some one point more distinct than the rest, must have been produced upon the retina. The idea that the letters are seen all alike simultaneously is therefore, an illusion. Here we have two different kinds of illusions. In the first case the impression made upon the brain is in accordance with the picture on the retina, but not in accordance with the fact. In the second the mental impression is in accordance with the fact, but not with the pictures upon the retina.

The normal eye usually sees the background of a letter whiter than it really is. In looking at the letters on the Snellen test card it sees white streaks at the margins of the letters, and in reading fine print it sees between the lines and the letters, and in the openings of the letters, a white more intense than the reality. Persons who cannot read fine print may see this illusion, but less clearly. The more clearly it is seen, the better the vision; and if it can be imagined consciously - it is imagined unconsciously when the sight is normal - the vision improves. If the lines of fine type are covered, the streaks between them disappear. When the letters are regarded through a magnifying glass by the eye with normal sight, the illusion is not destroyed, but the intensity of the white and black are lessened. With imperfect sight it may be increased to some extent by this means, but will remain less intense than the white and black seen by the normal eye. The facts demonstrate that perfect sight cannot be obtained with glasses.

The illusions of movement produced by the shifting of the eye and described in detail in the chapter on "Shifting and Swinging" must also be numbered among the illusions of normal sight, and so must the perception of objects in an upright position. This last is the most curious illusion of all. No matter what the position of the head, and regardless of the fact that the image on the retina is inverted, we always see things right side up.

CHAPTER XVII

VISION UNDER ADVERSE CONDITIONS A BENEFIT TO THE EYES

ACCORDING to accepted ideas of ocular hygiene, it is important to protect the eyes from a great variety of influences which are often very difficult to avoid, and to which most people resign themselves with the uneasy sense that they are thereby "ruining their eyesight." Bright lights, artificial lights, dim lights, sudden fluctuations of light, fine print, reading in moving vehicles, reading lying down, etc., have long been considered "bad for the eyes," and libraries of literature have been produced about their supposedly direful effects. These ideas are diametrically opposed to the truth. When the eyes are properly used, vision under adverse conditions not only does not injure them, but is an actual benefit, because a greater degree of relaxation is required to see under such conditions than under more favorable ones. It is true that the conditions in question may at first cause discomfort, even to persons with normal vision ; but a careful study of the facts has demonstrated that only persons with imperfect sight suffer seriously from them, and that such persons, if they practice central fixation, quickly become accustomed to them and derive great benefit from them.

(Fluorescent lights do impair health, function of the eyes and clarity of vision. It is best to use other light sources for artificial light, full spectrum. Natural sunlight through open windows or outside is best.)

Although the eyes were made to react to the light, a very general fear of the effect of this element upon the organs of vision is entertained both by the medical profession and by the laity. Extraordinary precautions are taken in our homes, offices and schools to temper the light, whether natural or artificial, and to insure that it shall not shine directly into the eyes ; smoked and amber glasses, eye-shades, broad-brimmed hats and parasols are commonly used to protect the organs of vision from what is considered an excess of light; and when actual disease is present, it is no uncommon thing for patients to be kept for weeks, months and years in dark rooms, or with bandages over their eyes.

The evidence on which this universal fear of the light has been based is of the slightest. In the voluminous literature of the subject one finds such a lack of information that in 1910 Dr. J. Herbert Parsons of the Royal Ophthalmic Hospital of London, addressing a meeting of the Ophthalmological Section of the American Medical Association, felt justified in saying that ophthalmologists, if they were honest with themselves, "must confess to a lamentable ignorance of the conditions which render bright light deleterious to the eyes." 1 Since then, Verhoeff and Bell have reported 2 an exhaustive series of experiments carried on at the Pathological Laboratory of the Massachusetts Charitable Eye and Ear Infirmary, which indicate that the danger of injury to the eye from light radiation as such has been "very greatly exaggerated." That brilliant sources of light sometimes produce unpleasant temporary symptoms cannot, of course, be denied; but as regards definite pathological effects, or permanent impairment of vision from exposure to light alone, Drs. Verhoeff and Bell were unable to find, either clinically or experimentally, anything of a positive nature.

1 Jour. Am. Med. Assn., Dec. 10, 1910, p. 2028.
2 Proc. Am. Acad. Arts and Sciences. 1916, Vol. 51, No. 13.

A Danger Greatly Exaggerated

As for danger from the heat effects of light, they consider this to be "ruled out of consideration by the immediate discomfort produced by excessive heat." They conclude, in short, that "the eye in the process of evolution has acquired the ability to take care of itself under extreme conditions of illumination to a degree hitherto deemed highly improbable." In their experiments, the eyes of rabbits, monkeys and human beings were flooded for an hour or more with light of extreme intensity, without any sign of permanent injury, the resulting scotomata[1] disappearing within a few hours. Commercial illuminants were found to be entirely free of danger under any ordinary conditions of their use. It was even found impossible to damage the retina with any artificial illuminant, except by exposures and intensities enormously greater than any likely to occur outside the laboratory. In one case an animal succumbed to heat after an exposure of an hour and a half to a 750-watt nitrogen lamp at twenty centimeters - about eight inches; but in a second experiment, in which it was well protected from the heat, there was no damage to the eye whatever after an exposure of two hours. As for the ultra-violet part of the spectrum, to which exaggerated importance has been attached by many recent writers, the situation was found to be much the same as with respect to the rest of the spectrum ; that is, "while under conceivable or realizable conditions of over-exposure, injury may be done to the external eye, yet under all practicable conditions found in actual use of artificial sources of light for illumination, the ultra-violet part of the spectrum may be left out as a possible source of injury."

1 Blind areas.

The results of these experiments are in complete accord with my own observations as to the effect of strong light upon the eyes. In my experience such light has never been permanently injurious. Persons with normal sight have been able to look at the sun for an indefinite length of time, even an hour or longer, without any discomfort or loss of vision. Immediately afterward they were able to read the Snellen test card with improved vision, their sight having become better than what is ordinarily considered normal. Some persons with normal sight do suffer discomfort and loss of vision when they look at the sun ; but in such cases the retinoscope always indicates an error of refraction, showing that this condition is due, not to the light, but to strain. In exceptional cases, persons with defective sight have been able to look at the sun, or have thought that they have looked at it, without discomfort and without loss of vision; but, as a rule, the strain in such eyes is enormously increased and the vision decidedly lowered by sun-gazing, as manifested by inability to read the Snellen test card. Blind areas (scotomata) may develop in various parts of the field - two or three or more. The sun, instead of appearing perfectly white, may appear to be slate-colored, yellow, red, blue, or even totally black. After looking away from the sun, patches of color of various kinds and sizes may be seen, continuing a variable length of time, from a few seconds to a few minutes, hours, or even months. In fact, one patient was troubled in this way for a year or more after looking at the sun for a few seconds. Even total blindness lasting a few hours has been produced. Organic changes may also be produced. Inflammation, redness of the conjunctiva, cloudiness of the lens and of the aqueous and vitreous humors, congestion and cloudiness of the retina, optic nerve and choroid, have all re

Ill Effects of Sun-Gazing Temporary

sulted from sun-gazing. These effects, however, are always temporary. The scotomata, the strange colors, even the total blindness, as explained in the preceding chapter, are only mental illusions. No matter how much the sight may have been impaired by sun-gazing, or how long the impairment may have lasted, a return to normal

Fig. 46.—Woman With Normal Vision Looking Directly at the Sun. Note That the Eyes are Wide Open and That There Is No Sign of Discomfort. Picture is Emily A. Bates (C. Lierman)

Fig. 46. Woman With Normal Vision Looking Directly at the Sun. Note That the Eyes are Wide Open and That There Is No Sign of Discomfort.
(MODERN NATURAL VISION IMPROVEMENT TEACHERS STATE: TO FACE THE SUN ONLY WITH THE EYES CLOSED and to MOVE THE EYES, HEAD/FACE SIDE TO SIDE... Looking at the bright sky away from the sun with eyes open is beneficial.) There are people, cultures that continue to Sun-Gaze with eyes open a specific way, but this is not allowed by some Modern Bates Teachers.

has always occurred ; while prompt relief of all the symptoms mentioned has always followed the relief of eyestrain, showing that the conditions are the result, not of the light, but of the strain. Some persons who have believed their eyes to have been permanently injured by the sun have been promptly cured by central fixation, indicating that their blindness had been simply functional.

By persistence in looking at the sun, a person with normal sight soon becomes able to do so without any loss of vision; but persons with imperfect sight usually find it impossible to accustom themselves to such a strong light until their vision has been improved by other means. One has to be very careful in recommending sun-gazing to persons with imperfect sight; because although no permanent harm can result from it, great temporary discomfort may be produced, with no permanent benefit. In some rare cases, however, complete cures have been effected by this means alone.

In one of these cases, the sensitiveness of the patient, even to ordinary daylight, was so great that an eminent specialist had felt justified in putting a black bandage over one eye and covering the other with a smoked glass so dark as to be nearly opaque. She was kept in this condition of almost total blindness for two years without any improvement. Other treatment extending over some months also failed to produce satisfactory results. She was then advised to look directly at the sun. The immediate result was total blindness, which lasted several hours; but next day the vision was not only restored to its former condition, but was improved. The sun-gazing was repeated, and each time the blindness lasted for a shorter period. At the end of a week the patient was able to look directly at the sun without discomfort, and her vision, which had been 20/200 without glasses and 20/70 with them, had improved to 20/10, twice the accepted standard for normal vision.

Patients of this class have also been greatly benefited by focussing the rays of the sun directly upon their eyes, marked relief being often obtained in a few minutes.

Like the sun, a strong electric light may also lower the vision temporarily, but never does any permanent harm.

Artificial Light May Be Beneficial

In those exceptional cases in which the patient can become accustomed to the light, it is beneficial. After looking at a strong electric light some patients have been able to read the Snellen test card better.

Fig. 47. Woman Aged 37, Child Aged 4, Both Looking Directly at Sun Without Discomfort
Picture; Emily C. Lierman, A. Bates

Fig. 47. Woman Aged 37, Child Aged 4, Both Looking Directly at Sun Without Discomfort

(MODERN TEACHERS STATE; SUNNING, SUN-GAZING IS DONE WITH CLOSED EYES ONLY and to MOVE, SHIFT THE EYES AND HEAD/FACE WITH THE EYES SIDE TO SIDE AND IN VARIOUS DIRECTIONS.) Sun-Gazing, Sunning is still practiced by some cultures with the eyes open & a specific way, with eye movement... Due to depletion of the ozone layer it must be done <u>CAREFULLY</u>!

It is not light but darkness that is dangerous to the eye. Prolonged exclusion from the light always lowers the vision, and may produce serious inflammatory conditions. Among young children living in tenements this is a somewhat frequent cause of ulcers upon the cornea, which ultimately destroy the sight. The children, finding their eyes sensitive to light, bury them in the pillows and thus shut out the light entirely. The universal fear of reading or doing fine work in a dim light is, however, unfounded. So long as the light is sufficient so that one can see without discomfort, this practice is not only harmless, but may be beneficial.

Sudden contrasts of light are supposed to be particularly harmful to the eye. The theory on which this idea is based is summed up as follows by Fletcher B. Dresslar, specialist in school hygiene and sanitation of the United States Bureau of Education:

"The muscles of the iris are automatic in their movements, but rather slow. Sudden contrasts of strong light and weak illumination are painful and likewise harmful to the retina. For example, if the eye, adjusted to a dim light, is suddenly turned toward a brilliantly lighted object, the retina will receive too much light and will be shocked before the muscles controlling the iris can react to shut out the superabundance of light. If contrasts are not strong, but frequently made, that is, if the eye is called upon to function where frequent adjustments in this way are necessary, the muscles controlling the iris become fatigued, respond more slowly and less perfectly. As a result, eyestrain in the ciliary muscles is produced and the retina is over-stimulated. This is one cause of headaches and tired eyes."1

There is no evidence whatever to support these statements. Sudden fluctuations of light undoubtedly cause discomfort to many persons, but, far from being injurious, I have found them, in all cases observed, to be actually beneficial. The pupil of the normal eye, when it has normal sight, does not change appreciably under

Fig. 48. Focussing the Rays of the Sun Upon the Eye of a Patient by Means of a Burning Glass.
(To be done by a Bates Method Ophthalmologist only! And only in extreme cases of vision impairment if necessary. Done wrong: it can burn, injure the eye. Done correct: it activates, brings to life the cells, nerves, cones, rods in the eyes, retina. Plain sunning, daily sunlight without eyeglasses is often all that is needed.)

1 School Hygiene, Brief Course Series in Education, edited by Monroe. 1916, p. 240.

the influence of changes of illumination ; and persons with normal vision are not inconvenienced by such changes. I have seen a patient look directly at the sun after coming from an imperfectly lighted room, and then, returning to the room, immediately pick up a newspaper and read it. When the eye has imperfect sight, the pupil usually contracts in the light and expands in the dark, but it has been observed to contract to the size of a pinhole in the dark. Whether the contraction takes place under the influence of light or of darkness, the cause is the same, namely, strain. Persons with imperfect sight suffer great inconvenience, resulting in lowered vision, from changes in the intensity of the light; but the lowered vision is always temporary, and if the eye is persistently exposed to these conditions, the sight is benefited. Such practices as reading alternately in a bright and a dim light, or going from a dark room to a well-lighted one, and vice versa, are to be recommended. Even such rapid and violent fluctuations of light as those involved in the production of the moving picture are, in the long run, beneficial to all eyes. I always advise patients under treatment for the cure of defective vision to go to the movies frequently and practice central fixation. They soon become accustomed to the flickering light, and afterward other light and reflections cause less annoyance.

(Practice alternating: Palming, Sunning, Palming, Sunning... to improve light tolerance and adjustment of the eyes to light and dark.)

Reading is supposed to be one of the necessary evils of civilization; but it is believed that by avoiding fine print, and taking care to read only under certain favorable conditions, its deleterious influences can be minimized. Extensive investigations as to the effect of various styles of print on the eyesight of school children have been made, and detailed rules have been laid down as to the size of the print, its shading, the distance of

Supposed Dangers of Reading

the letters from each other, the spaces between the lines, the length of the lines, etc. As regards the effects of different sorts of type on the human eye in general and those of children in particular, Dr. A. G. Young, in his much quoted report 1 to the Maine State Board of Health makes the following interesting observations: (These print size examples are not exact.)

Pearl, as the printers call it, is unfit for any eyes, yet the piles of Bibles and Testaments annually printed in it tempt many eyes to self-destruction.

Agate is the type in which a boy, to the writer's knowledge, undertook to read the Bible through. His outraged eyes broke down with asthenopia before he went far and could be used but little for school work the next two years.

Nonpareil is used in some papers and magazines for children, but, to spare the eyes, all such should, and do, go on the list of forbidden reading matter in those homes where the danger of such print is understood.

Minion is read by the healthy, normal young eye without appreciable difficulty, but even to the sound eye the danger of strain is so great that all books and magazines for children printed from it should be banished from the home and school.

Brevier is much used in newspapers, but is too small for magazines or books for young folks.

Bourgeois is much used in magazines, but should be used in only those school books to which a brief reference is made.

Long Primer is suitable for school readers for the higher and intermediate grades, and for text books generally.

Small Pica is still a more luxurious type, used in the North American Review and the Forum.

Pica is a good type for books for small children.

Great Primer should be used for the first reading book.

1 Seventh Annual Report to the Maine State Board of Health, by the secretary, Dr. A. G. Young, 1891. p. 193.

All this is directly contrary to my own experience. Children might be bored by books in excessively small print; but I have never seen any reason for supposing that their eyes or any other eyes, would be harmed by such type. On the contrary, <u>the reading of fine print, when it can be done without discomfort, has invariably proved to be beneficial, and the dimmer the light in which it can be read, and the closer to the eyes it can be held, the greater the benefit. By this means severe pain in the eyes has been relieved in a few minutes or even instantly.</u> The reason is that fine print cannot be read in a dim light and close to the eyes unless the eyes are relaxed, whereas large print can be read in a good light and at ordinary reading distance although the eyes may be under a strain. When fine print can be read under adverse conditions, the reading of ordinary print under ordinary conditions is vastly improved. <u>In myopia it may be a benefit to strain to see fine print, because myopia is always lessened when there is a strain to see near objects, and this has sometimes counteracted the tendency to strain in looking at distant objects, which is always associated with the production of myopia. Even straining to see print so fine that it cannot be read is a benefit to some myopes.</u>

Persons who wish to preserve their eyesight are frequently warned not to read in moving vehicles ; but since under modern conditions of life many persons have to spend a large part of their time in moving vehicles, and many of them have no other time to read, it is useless to expect that they will ever discontinue the practice. Fortunately the theory of its injuriousness is not borne out by the facts. When the object regarded is moved more or less rapidly, strain and lowered vision are, at

Seven Truths of Normal Sight

1. Normal Sight can always be demonstrated in the normal eye, but only under favorable conditions.
2. Central Fixation: The letter or part of the letter regarded is always seen best.
3. Shifting: The point regarded changes rapidly and continuously.
4. Swinging: When the shifting is slow, the letters appear to move from side to side, or in other directions with a pendulum-like motion.
5. Memory is perfect. The color and background of the letters or other objects seen, are remembered perfectly, instantaneously and continuously.
6. Imagination is good. One may even see the white part of letters whiter than it really is, while the black is not altered by distance, illumination, size, or form, of the letters.
7. Rest or relaxation of the eye and mind is perfect and can always be demonstrated. When one of these seven fundamentals is perfect, all are perfect.

Fig. 49. Specimen of Diamond Type. Many patients have been greatly benefited by reading type of this size.

Fig. 50. Photographic Type Reduction. Patients who can read photographic type reductions are instantly relieved of pain and discomfort when they do so, and those who cannot read such type may be benefited simply by looking at it.

first, always produced; but this is always temporary, and ultimately the vision is improved by the practice.

There is probably no visual habit against which we have been more persistently warned than that of reading in a recumbent posture. Many plausible reasons have been adduced for its supposed injuriousness; but so delightful is the practice that few, probably, have ever been deterred from it by fear of the consequences. It is gratifying to be able to state, therefore, that I have found these consequences to be beneficial rather than injurious. As in the case of the use of the eyes under other difficult conditions, it is a good thing to be able to read lying down, and the ability to do it improves with practice. In an upright position, with a good light coming over the left shoulder, one can read with the eyes under a considerable degree of strain; but in a recumbent posture, with the light and the angle of the page to the eye unfavorable, one cannot read unless one relaxes. Anyone who can read lying down without discomfort is not likely to have any difficulty in reading under ordinary conditions.

The fact is that vision under difficult conditions is good mental training. The mind may be disturbed at first by the unfavorable environment; but after it has become accustomed to such environments, the mental control, and, consequently, the eyesight are improved. To advise against using the eyes under unfavorable conditions is like telling a person who has been in bed for a few weeks and finds it difficult to walk to refrain from such exercise. Of course, discretion must be used in both cases. The convalescent must not at once try to run a Marathon, nor must the person with defective vision attempt, without some preparation, to outstare the

Discretion Must Be Used

sun at noonday. But just as the invalid may gradually increase his strength until the Marathon has no terrors for him, so may the eye with defective sight be educated until all the rules with which we have so long allowed ourselves to be harassed in the name of "eye hygiene" may be disregarded, not only with safety but with benefit.

CHAPTER XVIII
OPTIMUMS AND PESSIMUMS

IN nearly all cases of imperfect sight due to errors of refraction there is some object, or objects, which can be regarded with normal vision. Such objects I have called "optimums." On the other hand, there are some objects which persons with normal eyes and ordinarily normal sight always see imperfectly, an error of refraction being produced when they are regarded, as demonstrated by the retinoscope. Such objects I have called "pessimums." An object becomes an optimum, or a pessimum, according to the effect it produces upon the mind, and in some cases this effect is easily accounted for.

For many children their mother's face is an optimum, and the face of a stranger a pessimum. A dressmaker was always able to thread a No. 10 needle with a fine thread of silk without glasses, although she had to put on glasses to sew on buttons, because she could not see the holes. She was a teacher of dressmaking, and thought the children stupid because they could not tell the difference between two different shades of black. She could match colors without comparing the samples. Yet she could not see a black line in a photographic copy of the Bible which was no finer than a thread of silk, and she could not remember a black period. An employee in a cooperage factory, who had been engaged for years in picking out defective barrels as they went rapidly past him on an inclined plane, was able to continue his work

Idiosyncrasies of the Mind

after his sight for most other objects had become very defective, while persons with much better sight for the Snellen test card were unable to detect the defective barrels. The familiarity of these various objects made it possible for the subjects to look at them without strain - that is, without trying to see them. Therefore the barrels were to the cooper optimums ; while the needle's eye and the colors of silk and fabrics were optimums to the dressmaker. Unfamiliar objects, on the contrary, are always pessimums, as pointed out in the chapter on "The Variability of the Refraction of the Eye."

In other cases there is no accounting for the idiosyncrasy of the mind which makes one object a pessimum and another an optimum. It is also impossible to account for the fact that an object may be an optimum for one eye and not for the other, or an optimum at one time and at one distance and not at others. Among these unaccountable optimums one often finds a particular letter on the Snellen test card. One patient, for instance, was able to see the letter K on the forty, fifteen and ten lines, but could see none of the other letters on these lines, although most patients would see some of them, on account of the simplicity of their outlines, better than they would such a letter as K.

Pessimums may be as curious and unaccountable as optimums. The letter V is so simple in its outlines that many people can see it when they cannot see others on the same line. Yet some people are unable to distinguish it at any distance, although able to read other letters in the same word, or on the same line of the Snellen test card. Some people again will not only be unable to recognize the letter V in a word, but also to read any word that contains it, the pessimum lowering their sight not only for itself but for other objects. Some letters, or objects, become pessimums only in particular situations. A letter, for instance, may be a pessimum when located at the end or at the beginning of a line or sentence, and not in other places. When the attention of the patient is called to the fact that a letter seen in one location ought logically to be seen equally well in others, the letter often ceases to be a pessimum in any situation.

A pessimum, like an optimum, may be lost and later become manifest. It may vary according to the light and distance. An object which is a pessimum in a moderate light may not be so when the light is increased or diminished. A pessimum at twenty feet may not be one at two feet, or thirty feet, and an object which is a pessimum when directly regarded may be seen with normal vision in the eccentric field.

For most people the Snellen test card is a pessimum. If you can see the Snellen test card with normal vision, you can see almost anything else in the world. Patients who cannot see the letters on the Snellen test card can often see other objects of the same size and at the same distance with normal sight. When letters which are seen imperfectly, or even letters which cannot be seen at all, or which the patient is not conscious of seeing are regarded, the error of refraction is increased. The patient may regard a blank white card without any error of refraction ; but if he regards the lower part of a Snellen test card, which appears to him to be just as blank as the blank card, an error of refraction can always be demonstrated, and if the visible letters of the card are covered, the result is the same. The pessimum may, in short, be letters or objects which the patient is not conscious of seeing. This phenomenon is very common. When the

How Pessimums Become Optimums

card is seen in the eccentric field it may have the effect of lowering the vision for the point directly regarded. For instance, a patient may regard an area of green wallpaper at the distance, and see the color as well as at the near-point; but if a Snellen test card on which the letters are either seen imperfectly, or not seen at all, is placed in the neighborhood of the area being regarded, the retinoscope may indicate an error of refraction. When the vision improves, the number of letters on the card which are pessimums diminishes and the number of optimums increases, until the whole card becomes an optimum.

A pessimum, like an optimum, is a manifestation of the mind. It is something associated with a strain to see, just as an optimum is something which has no such association. It is not caused by the error of refraction, but always produces an error of refraction; and when the strain has been relieved it ceases to be a pessimum and becomes an optimum.

CHAPTER XIX

THE RELIEF OF PAIN AND OTHER SYMPTOMS BY THE AID OF THE MEMORY

MANY years ago patients who had been cured of imperfect sight by treatment without glasses quite often told me that after their vision had become perfect they were always relieved of pain, not only in the eyes and head, but in other parts of the body, even when the pain was apparently caused by some organic disease, or by an injury. The relief in many cases was so striking that I investigated some thousands of cases and found it to be a fact that persons with perfect sight, or the memory of perfect sight - that is, of something perfectly seen - do not suffer pain in any part of the body, while by a strain or effort to see I have produced pain in various parts of the body.

By perfect sight is not meant, necessarily, the perfect visual perception of words, letters, or objects, of a more or less complicated form. To see perfectly the color alone is sufficient, and the easiest color to see perfectly is black. But perfect sight is never continuous, careful scientific tests having shown that it is seldom maintained for more than a few minutes and usually not so long. For practical purposes in the relief of pain, therefore, the memory is more satisfactory than sight.

When black is remembered perfectly a temporary, if not a permanent, relief of pain always results. The skin may be pricked with a sharp instrument without causing discomfort. The lobe of the ear may be pinched be-

Pain of Operation Prevented

tween the nails of the thumb and first finger, and no pain will be felt. At the same time the sense of touch becomes more acute. The senses of taste, smell and hearing are also improved, while the efficiency of the mind is increased. The ability to distinguish different temperatures is increased, but one does not suffer from heat or cold. Organic conditions may not be changed; but all of the functional symptoms, such as fever, weakness, and shock, which these conditions cause, are relieved. Patients who have learned to remember black under all circumstances no longer dread to visit the dentist. When they remember a period the drill causes them no pain, and they are not annoyed even by the extraction of teeth. It is possible to perform surgical operations without anaesthetics when the patient is able to remember black perfectly. The following are only a few of many equally striking cases which might be given of the relief or prevention of pain by this means :

A patient suffered from ulceration of the eyeball, occurring at different times and resulting in the formation of holes through which the fluids in the interior escaped. These openings had to be closed by surgical operations. At first these operations were performed under the influence of cocaine ; but the progressive disease of the eye caused so much congestion that complete anaesthesia was no longer attainable by the use of this drug, and ether and chloroform were employed. As so many operations were needed, it became desirable to get along, if possible, without anaesthetics, and the patient's success in relieving pain by the memory of black suggested that she might also be able to prevent the pain of operations in the same way. Her ability to do this was tested by touching her eyeball lightly with a blunt probe. At first she forgot the black as soon as the probe touched her eye, but later she became able to remember it. The operation was then successfully performed ; the patient not only felt no pain,

Fig. 51. Operating Without Anaesthetics. The patient suffered from ulceration of the eyeball resulting in the formation of holes through which the fluids of the interior escaped. These holes had to be closed by surgical operations, and fourteen of these operations were performed without anaesthetics, because the patient was able to prevent pain by the memory of a black period.

but her self-control was better than when cocaine had been used. Later fourteen more operations were performed under the same conditions, the patient not only

No Pain in Dentist's Chair

suffering no pain, but, what was more remarkable, feeling no pain or soreness afterward. The patient stated that if she had been operated upon by a stranger she would probably have been so nervous that she would not have been able to remember the black; but later she was treated by a strange dentist, who made two extractions and did some other work, all without causing her any discomfort, because she was able to remember the period perfectly.

A man who had been extremely nervous in the dentist's chair, and had had four extractions made under gas, surprised his dentist, after having learned the effect of the memory of a period in relieving pain, by having a tooth extracted without cocaine, gas, or chloroform. The dentist complimented him on his nerve and looked incredulous when the patient said he had felt no pain at all. In a second case, that of a woman, the dentist removed the nerve from three teeth without causing the patient any pain.

A boy of fourteen came to the eye clinic of the Harlem Hospital, New York, with a foreign body deeply embedded in his cornea. It caused him much pain, and his mother stated that a number of physicians had been unable to remove it, because the child was so nervous that he could not keep

still long enough, although cocaine had been used quite freely. The boy was told to look at a black object, close and cover his eyes, and think of the black object until he saw black. He was soon able to do this, and the pain in his eye was relieved. He was next taught to remember the black with his eyes open. The foreign body was then removed from the cornea. The operation was one of much difficulty and required considerable time, but the boy felt no pain. While it was in progress he was asked if he was still remembering black.
"You bet I am," he replied.

In the same hospital a surgeon from the accident ward visited the eye clinic with a friend suffering from pain in his eyes and head. The patient was benefited very quickly by relaxation methods. The surgeon said it was unusual, and spoke slightingly of my methods. I challenged him to bring me a patient with pain that I could not relieve in five minutes.
"All right," he said. "I want you to understand that I am from Missouri."

He returned soon with a woman who had been suffering from severe pains in her head for several years. She had been operated upon a number of times, and had been under the care of the hospital for many months.
"You cannot help the pain in this patient's head," said the surgeon, "because she has a brain tumor."
I doubted the existence of a brain tumor, but I said:
"Brain tumor or no brain tumor, my assistant will stop the pain in five minutes."

He took out his watch, opened it, looked at the time, and told my assistant to go ahead. The patient was directed to look at a large black letter, note its blackness, then to cover her closed eyes with the palms of her hands, shutting out all the light, and to remember the blackness of the letter until she saw everything black. In less than three minutes she said:

"I now see everything perfectly black. I feel no pain in my head. I am completely relieved, and I thank you very much."

The surgeon looked bewildered, and left the room without a word.

Fig. 52. Neuralgia Relieved by Palming and the Memory of Black
While the visitor was explaining to her sceptical hostess the method of relieving pain by palming and the memory of black, another member of the family, who was suffering from trigeminal neuralgia, came in, and having heard what was being said, immediately put it into practice and was cured. The hostess later developed severe pain in her head and eyes, and did not obtain any relief until she also practiced palming and the memory of black.

Fig. 52. Neuralgia Relieved by Palming and the Memory of Black. While the visitor was explaining to her sceptical hostess the method of relieving pain by palming and the memory of black, another member of the family, who was suffering from trigeminal neuralgia, came in, and having heard what was being said, immediately put it into practice and was cured. The hostess later developed severe pain in her head and eyes, and did not obtain any relief until she also practiced palming and the memory of black.

To prevent a relapse, the patient was advised to palm six times a day or oftener. The pain did not return, and she came to the clinic some weeks later to express her gratitude.

Not only does the memory of perfect sight relieve pain and the symptoms of disease, but in some cases it produces manifest relief of the causes of these symptoms. Coughs, colds, hay fever, rheumatism and glaucoma are among the conditions that have been relieved in this way.

A patient under treatment for imperfect sight from a high degree of mixed astigmatism one day came to the office with a severe cold. She coughed continually, and there was a profuse discharge from both eyes and nose. There was some fever, with a severe pain in the eyes and head, and the patient was unable to breathe through her nose because of the inflammatory swelling. Palming was successful in half an hour, when the pain and discharge ceased, the nose opened, and the breathing and temperature became normal. The benefit was permanent - a very unusual thing after one treatment.

A boy of four with whooping-cough was always relieved by covering his eyes and remembering black. The relapses became less frequent, and in a few weeks he had completely recovered.

A man who suffered every summer from attacks of hay fever, beginning in June and lasting throughout the season was completely relieved by palming for half an hour ; and after three years there had been no relapse.

A man of sixty-five who had been under treatment for rheumatism for six months without improvement obtained temporary relief by palming, and by the time his vision had become normal the relief of the rheumatism was complete.

The Power of Thought

In many cases of glaucoma not only the pain, but the tension which is often associated with the pain, has been completely relieved by palming. In some cases permanent relief of the tension has followed one treatment. In others many treatments have been required.

Why the memory of black should have this effect cannot be fully explained, just as the action of many drugs cannot be explained; but it is evident that the body must be less susceptible to disturbances of all kinds when the mind is under control, and only when the mind is under control can black be remembered perfectly. That pain can be produced in any part of the body by the action of the mind is not a new observation; and if the mind can produce pain, it is not surprising that it should also be able to relieve pain and the conditions which produce it. This, doubtless, is the explanation of some of the remarkable cures reported by Faith Curists and Christian Scientists. Whatever the explanation, however, the facts have been attested by numerous proofs, and are of the greatest practical value.

With a little training, anyone with good sight can be taught to remember black perfectly with the eyes closed and covered, and with a little more training anyone can learn to do it with the eyes open. When one is suffering extreme pain, however, the control of the memory may be difficult, and the assistance of someone who understands the method may be necessary. With such assistance it is seldom or never impossible.

CHAPTER XX

PRESBYOPIA: ITS CAUSE AND CURE

AMONG people living under civilized conditions the accommodative power of the eye gradually declines, in most cases, until at the age of sixty or seventy it appears to have been entirely lost, the subject being absolutely dependent upon his glasses for vision at the near-point. As to whether the same thing happens among primitive people or people living under primitive conditions, very little information is available. Donders[1] says that the power of accommodation diminishes little, if at all, more rapidly among people who use their eyes much at the near-point than among agriculturists, sailors and others who use them mainly for distant vision; and Roosa and others[2] say the contrary.

This is a fact however, that people who cannot read, no matter what their age, will manifest a failure of near vision if asked to look at printed characters, although their sight for familiar objects at the near-point may be perfect. The fact that such persons, at the age of forty-five or fifty, cannot differentiate between printed characters is no warrant, therefore, for the conclusion that their accommodative powers are declining. A young illiterate would do no better, and a young student who can read Roman characters at the near-point without difficulty always develops symptoms of imperfect sight when he attempts to read, for the first time, old English, Greek, or Chinese characters.

1 On the Anomalies of Accommodation and Refraction of the Eye, p. 223.
2 Roosa: A Clinical Manual of Diseases of the Eye, 1894, p. 537; Oliver: System of Diseases of the Eye, vol. iv, p. 431.

Generally Accepted as Normal

When the accommodative power has declined to the point at which reading and writing become difficult, the patient is said to have "presbyopia," or, more popularly, "old sight" ; and the condition is generally accepted, both by the popular and the scientific mind, as one of the unavoidable inconveniences of old age. "Presbyopia," says Donders, "is the normal quality of the normal, emmetropic eye in advanced age," 1 and similar statements might be multiplied endlessly. De Schweinitz calls the condition "a normal result of growing old" ; 2 according to Fuchs it is "a physiological process which every eye undergoes";3 while Roosa speaks of the change as one which "ultimately affects every eye." 4

The decline of accommodative power with advancing years is commonly attributed to the hardening of the lens, an influence which is believed to be augmented, in later years, by a flattening of this body and a lowering of its refractive index, together with weakness or atrophy of the ciliary muscle; and so regular is the decline, in most cases, that tables have been compiled showing the nearpoint to be expected at various ages. From these it is said one might almost fit glasses without testing the vision of the subject; or, conversely, one might, from a man's glasses, judge his age within a year or two. The following table is quoted from Jackson's chapter on "The Dioptrics of the Eye," in Norris and Oliver's "System of Diseases of the Eye,"5 and does not differ materially from the tables given by Fuchs, Donders and Duane. The first

1 On the Anomalies of Accommodation and Refraction of the Eye, p. 210. 2 Diseases of the Eye, p. 148. 3 Text-book of Ophthalmology, authorized translation from the twelfth German edition by Duane, 1919, p. 862. Ernst Fuchs (1851-). Professor of Ophthalmology at Vienna from 1885 to 1915. His Text-book of Ophthalmology has been translated into many languages. 4 A Clinical Manual of Diseases of the Eye, p. 535. VoL i, p. 504.

column indicates the age ; the second, diopters of accommodative power; the third, the near-point for an emmetropic 1 eye, in inches.

Age	Diopters	Inches
10	14	2.81
15	12	3.28
20	10	3.94
25	8.5	4.63
30	7	5.63
35	5.5	7.16
40	4.5	8.75
45	3.5	11.25
50	2.5	15.75
55	1.5	26.25
60	.75	52.49
65	.25	157.48
70	0	0

According to these depressing figures, one must expect at thirty to have lost no less than half of one's original accommodative power, while at forty two-thirds of it would be gone, and at sixty it would be practically nonexistent.

There are many people, however, who do not fit this schedule. Many persons at forty can read fine print at four inches, although they ought, according to the table, to have lost that power shortly after twenty. Worse still, there are people who refuse to become presbyopic at all. Oliver Wendell Holmes mentions one of these cases in "The Autocrat of the Breakfast Table."

1 An eye which, when it is at rest, focusses parallel rays upon the retina, is said to be emmetropic or normal.

The Dead Hand of German Science

"There is now living in New York State," he says, "an old gentleman who, perceiving his sight to fail, immediately took to exercising it on the finest print, and in this way fairly bullied Nature out of her foolish habit of taking liberties at five-and-forty, or thereabout. And now this old gentleman performs the most extraordinary feats with his pen, showing that his eyes must be a pair of microscopes. I should be afraid to say how much he writes in the compass of a half-dime whether the Psalms or the Gospels, or the Psalms and the Gospels, I won't be positive." 1

There are also people who regain their near vision after having lost it for ten, fifteen, or more years ; and there are people who, while presbyopic for some objects, have perfect sight for others. Many dressmakers, for instance, can thread a needle with the naked eye, and with the retinoscope it can be demonstrated that they accurately focus their eyes upon such objects; and yet they cannot read or write without glasses.

So far as I am aware no one but myself has ever observed the last mentioned class of cases, but the others are known to every ophthalmologist of any experience. One hears of them at the meetings of ophthalmological societies ; they are even reported in the medical journals ; but such is the force of authority that when it comes to writing books they are either ignored or explained away, and every new treatise that comes from the press repeats the old superstition that presbyopia is "a normal result of growing old." We have beaten Germany; but the dead hand of German science still oppresses our intellects and prevents us from crediting the plainest evidence of our senses. Some of us are so filled with repugnance for

1 Everyman's Library, 1908, pp. 166-167.

the Hun that we can no longer endure the music of Bach, or the language of Goethe and Schiller; but German ophthalmology is still sacred, and no facts are allowed to cast discredit upon it.

Fortunately for those who feel called upon to defend the old theories, myopia postpones the advent of presbyopia, and a decrease in the size of the pupil, which often takes place in old age, has some effects in facilitating vision at the near-point. Reported cases of persons reading without glasses when over fifty-or fifty-five years of age, therefore, can be easily disposed of by assuming that the subjects must be myopic, or that their pupils are unusually small. If the case comes under actual observation, the matter may not be so simple, because it may be found that the patient, so far from being myopic, is hypermetropic, or emmetropic, and that the pupil is of normal size. There is nothing to do with these cases but to ignore them. Abnormal changes in the form of the lens have also been held responsible for the retention of near vision beyond the prescribed age, or for its restoration after it has been lost, the swelling of the lens in incipient cataract affording a very convenient and plausible explanation for the latter class of cases. In cases of premature presbyopia "accelerated sclerosis"1 of the lens and weakness of the ciliary muscle have been assumed ; and if such cases as the dressmakers who can thread their needles when they can no longer read the newspapers had been observed, no doubt some explanation consistent with the German viewpoint would have been found for them.

The truth about presbyopia is that it is not "a normal result of growing old," being both preventable and cu-

1 Fuchs: Text-book of Ophthalmology, p. 905.

A Form of Hypermetropia

rable. It is not caused by hardening of the lens, but by a strain to see at the near-point. It has no necessary connection with age, since it occurs, in some cases, as early as ten years, while in others it never occurs at all, although the subject may live far into the so-called presbyopic age. It is true that the lens does harden with advancing years, just as the bones harden and the structure of the skin changes ; but since the lens is not a factor in accommodation, this fact is immaterial, and while in some cases the lens may become flatter, or lose some of its refractive power with advancing years, it has been observed to remain perfectly clear and unchanged in shape up to the age of ninety. Since the ciliary muscle is also not a factor in accommodation, its weakness or atrophy can contribute nothing to the decline of accommodative power. Presbyopia is, in fact, simply a form of hypermetropia in which the vision for the near-point is chiefly affected, although the vision for the distance, contrary to what is generally believed, is always lowered also. The difference between the two conditions is not always clear. A person with hypermetropia may or may not read fine print, and a person at the presbyopic age may read it without apparent inconvenience and yet have imperfect sight for the distance. In both conditions the sight at both points is lowered, although the patient may not be aware of it.

It has been shown that when the eyes strain to see at the near-point the focus is always pushed farther away than it was before, in one or all meridians ; and by means of simultaneous retinoscopy it can always be demonstrated that when a person with presbyopia tries to read fine print and fails, the focus is always pushed farther away than it was before the attempt was made, indicating that the failure was caused by strain. Even the thought of making such an effort will produce strain, so that the refraction may be changed, and pain, discomfort and fatigue produced, before the fine print is regarded. Furthermore, when a person with presbyopia rests the eyes by closing them, or palming, he always becomes able, for a few moments at least, to read fine print at six inches, again indicating that his previous failure was due, not to any fault of the eyes, but to a strain to see. When the strain is permanently relieved, the presbyopia is permanently cured, and this has happened, not in a few cases, but in many, and at all ages, up to sixty, seventy and eighty.

The first patient that I cured of presbyopia was myself. Having demonstrated by means of experiments on the eyes of animals that the lens is not a factor in accommodation, I knew that presbyopia must be curable, and I realized that I could not look for any very general acceptance of the revolutionary conclusions I had reached so long as I wore glasses myself for a condition supposed to be due to the loss of the accommodative power of the lens. I was then suffering from the maximum degree of presbyopia. I had no accommodative power whatever, and had to have quite an outfit of glasses, because with a glass, for instance, which enabled me to read fine print at thirteen inches, I could not read it either at twelve inches or at fourteen. The retinoscope showed that when I tried to see anything at the near-point without glasses, my eyes were focussed for the distance, and when I tried to see anything at the distance they were focussed for the near-point. My problem, then, was to find some way of reversing this condition and inducing my eyes to focus for the point I wished to see at the moment that I wished

Only One Man Who Could Cure Me

to see it. I consulted various eye specialists but my language was to them like that of St. Paul to the Greeks, namely, foolishness. "Your lens is as hard as a stone," they said. "No one can do anything for you." Then I went to a nerve specialist. He used the retinoscope on me, and confirmed my own observations as to the peculiar contrariness of my accommodation ; but he had no idea what I could do about it. He would consult some of his colleagues, he said, and asked me to come back in a month, which I did. Then he told me he had come to the conclusion that there was only one man who could cure me, and that was Dr. William H. Bates of New York.

"Why do you say that?" I asked.
"Because you are the only man who seems to know anything about it," he answered.

Thus thrown upon my own resources, I was fortunate enough to find a non-medical gentleman who was willing to do what he could to assist me, the Rev. R. B. B. Foote, of Brooklyn. He kindly used the retinoscope through many long and tedious hours while I studied my own case, and tried to find some way of accommodating when I wanted to read, instead of when I wanted to see something at the distance. One day, while looking at a picture of the Rock of Gibralter which hung on the wall, I noted some black spots on its face. I imagined that these spots were the openings of caves, and that there were people in these caves moving about. When I did this my eyes were focussed for the reading distance. Then I looked at the same picture at the reading distance, still imagining that the spots were caves with people in them. The retinoscope showed that I had accommodated, and I was able to read the lettering beside the picture. I had, in fact, been temporarily cured by the use of my imagination. Later I found that when I imagined the letters black I was able to see them black, and when I saw them black I was able to distinguish their form. My progress after this was not what could be called rapid. It was six months before I could read the newspapers with any kind of comfort, and a year before I obtained my present accommodative range of fourteen inches, from four inches to eighteen; but the experience was extremely valuable, for I had in pronounced form every symptom subsequently observed in other presbyopic patients.

Fortunately for the patients, it has seldom taken me as long to cure other people as it did to cure myself. In some cases a complete and permanent cure was effected in a few minutes. Why, I do not know. I will never be satisfied till I find out. A patient who had worn glasses for presbyopia for about twenty years was cured in less than fifteen minutes by the use of his imagination.

When asked to read diamond type, he said he could not do so, because the letters were grey and looked all alike. I reminded him that the type was printer's ink and that there was nothing blacker than printer's ink. I asked him if he had ever seen printer's ink. He replied that he had. Did he remember how black it was? Yes. Did he believe that these letters were as black as the ink he remembered? He did, and then he read the letters; and because the improvement in his vision was permanent, he said that I had hypnotized him.

In another case a presbyope of ten years' standing was cured just as quickly by the same method. When reminded that the letters which he could not read were black, he replied that he knew they were black, but that they looked grey.

Responsible for Much Defective Eyesight

"If you know they are black, and yet see them grey," I said, "you must imagine them grey. Suppose you imagine that they are black. Can you do that?"

"Yes," he said, "I can imagine that they are black"; and then he proceeded to read them.

These extremely quick cures are rare. In nine cases out of ten progress has been much slower, and it has been necessary to resort to all the methods of obtaining relaxation found useful in the treatment of other errors of refraction. In the more difficult cases of presbyopia the patients often suffer from the same illusions of color, size, form and number, when they try to read fine print, as do patients with hypermetropia, astigmatism, and myopia when they try to read the letters on the Snellen test card at the distance. They are unable to remember or imagine, when trying to see at the near-point, even such a simple thing as a small black spot, but can remember it perfectly when they do not try to see. Their sight for the distance is often very imperfect and always below normal, although they may have thought it perfect; and just as in the case of other errors of refraction, improvement of the distant vision improves the vision at the near-point. Regardless, however, of the difficulty of the case and the age of the patient, some improvement has always been obtained, and if the treatment was continued long enough, the patient has been cured.

The idea that presbyopia is "a normal result of growing old" is responsible for much defective eyesight. When people who have reached the presbyopic age experience difficulty in reading, they are very likely to resort at once to glasses, either with or without professional advice. In some cases such persons may be actually presbyopic ; in others the difficulty may be something temporary, which they would have thought little about if they had been younger, and which would have passed away if Nature had been left to herself. But once the glasses are adopted, in the great majority of cases, they produce the condition they were designed to relieve, or, if it already existed, they make it worse, sometimes very rapidly, as every ophthalmologist knows. In a couple of weeks, sometimes, the patient finds, as noted in the chapter on "What Glasses Do to Us," that the large print which he could read without difficulty before he got his glasses, can no longer be read without their aid. In from five to ten years the accommodative power of the eye is usually gone ; and if from this point the patient does not go on to cataract, glaucoma, or inflammation of the retina, he may consider himself fortunate. Only occasionally do the eyes refuse to submit to the artificial conditions imposed upon them; but in such cases they may keep up an astonishing struggle against them for long periods. A woman of seventy, who had worn glasses for twenty years, was still able to read diamond type and had good vision for the distance without them. She said the glasses tired her eyes and blurred her vision, but that she had persisted in wearing them, in spite of a continual temptation to throw them off, because she had been told that it was necessary for her to do so.

If persons who find themselves getting presbyopic, or who have arrived at the presbyopic age, would, instead of resorting to glasses, follow the example of the gentleman mentioned by Dr.

Holmes, and make a practice of reading the finest print they can find, the idea that the decline of accommodative power is "a normal result of growing old" would soon die a natural death.

CHAPTER XXI
SQUINT AND AMBLYOPIA: THEIR CAUSE
(Wandering, Crossed eyes)

SINCE we have two eyes, it is obvious that in the act of sight two pictures must be formed; and in order that these two pictures shall be fused into one by the mind, it is necessary that there shall be perfect harmony of action between the two organs of vision. In looking at a distant object the two visual axes must be parallel, and in looking at an object at a less distance than infinity, which for practical purposes is less than twenty feet, they must converge to exactly the same degree. The absence of this harmony of action is known as "squint," or "strabismus," and is one of the most distressing of eye defects, not only because of the lowering of vision involved, but because the want of symmetry in the most expressive feature of the face which results from it has a most unpleasant effect upon the personal appearance. The condition is one which has long baffled ophthalmological science. While the theories as to its cause advanced in the text-books seem to fit some cases, they leave others unexplained, and all methods of treatment are admitted to be very uncertain in their results.

The idea that a lack of harmony in the movements of the eye is due to a corresponding lack of harmony in the strength of the muscles that turn them in their sockets seem such a natural one that this theory was almost universally accepted at one time. Operations based upon it once had a great vogue; but to-day they are advised, by most authorities, only as a last resort. It is true that many persons have been benefited by them ; but, at best, the correction of the squint is only approximate, and in many cases the condition has been made worse, while a restoration of binocular vision - the power of fusing the two visual images into one - is scarcely even hoped for.1

The muscle theory fitted the facts so badly that when Donders advanced the idea that squint was a condition growing out of refractive errors - hypermetropia being held responsible for the production of convergent and myopia for divergent squint - it was universally accepted. This theory, too, proved unsatisfactory, and now medical opinion is divided between various theories. Hansen-Grut attributed the condition, in the great majority of cases, to a defect, not of the muscles, but of the nerve supply; and this idea has had many supporters. Worth and his disciples lay stress on the lack of a so-called fusion faculty, and have recommended the use of prisms, or other measures, to develop it. Stevens believes that the anomaly results from a wrong shape of the orbit, and as it is impossible to alter this condition, advocates operations for the purpose of neutralizing its influence.

In order to make any of these theories appear consistent it is necessary to explain away a great many troublesome facts. The uncertain result of operations upon the eye muscles is sufficient to cast suspicion on the theory that the condition is due to any abnormality of the muscles, and many cases of marked paralysis of one or more muscles have been observed in which there was no squint. Relief of paralysis, moreover, may not relieve the squint, nor the relief of the squint the paralysis. Worth found

1 The result obtained by the operation is, as a rule, simply cosmetic. The sight of the squinting eye is not influenced by the operation, and in only a few instances is even binocular vision restored. Fuchs:-Text-book of Ophthalmology, p. 795. The result of even the most successful squint operation, in long-standing strabismus, is merely cosmetic in the vast majority of cases.-Eversbusch: The Diseases of Children, edited by Pfaunder and Schlossman. English translation by Shaw and La Fetra, second edition, 1912-1914, vol. vii, p. 316.

State of Vision Not Important Factor

so many cases which were not benefited by training designed to improve the fusion faculty that he recommended operations on the muscles in such cases; while Donders, noting that the majority of hypermetropes did not squint, was obliged to assume that hypermetropia

Fig. 53
No. 1—Reading the Snellen test card with normal vision; visual axes parallel.
No. 2—The same patient making an effort to see the test card; myopia and convergent squint of the left eye have been produced.

Fig. 53 No. 1 Reading the Snellen test card with normal vision; visual axes parallel. No. 2 The same patient making an effort to see the test card; myopia and convergent squint of the left eye have been produced.

did not cause this condition without the aid of co-operating circumstances.

That the state of the vision is not an important factor in the production of squint is attested by a multitude of facts. It is true, as Donders observed, that squint is usually associated with errors of refraction; but some people squint with a very slight error of refraction. It is also true that many persons with convergent squint have hypermetropia ; but many others have not. Some persons with convergent squint have myopia. A person may also have convergent squint with one eye normal and one hypermetropic or myopic, or with one eye blind. Usually the vision of the eye that turns in is less than that of the eye which is straight; yet there are cases in which the eye with the poorer vision is straight and the eye with the better vision turned in. With two blind eyes, both eyes may be straight, or one may turn in. With one good eye and one blind eye, both eyes may be straight. The blinder the eye, as a rule, the more marked the squint ; but exceptions are frequent, and in rare cases an eye with nearly normal vision may turn in persistently. A squint may disappear and return again, while convergent squint will change into divergent squint and back again. With the same error of refraction, one person will have squint and the other not. A third will squint with a different eye. A fourth will squint first with one eye and then with the other. In a fifth the amount of the squint will vary. One will get well without glasses, or other treatment, and another with these things. These cures may be temporary, or permanent, and the relapses may occur either with or without glasses.

However slight the error of refraction, the vision of many squinting eyes is inferior to that of the straight eye, and for this condition, usually, no apparent or sufficient cause can be found in the constitution of the eye. There is a difference of opinion as to whether this curious defect of vision is the result of the squint, or the squint the result of the defect of vision ; but the predominating opinion that it is, at least, aggravated by the squint has been crystallized in the name given to the condition, namely, "amblyopia ex anopsia," literally "dim-sighted-

Facts Versus Theory

ness from non-use" - for in order to avoid the annoyance of double vision the mind is believed to suppress the image of the deviating eye. There are, however, many squinting eyes without amblyopia, while such a condition has been found in eyes that have never squinted.

The literature of the subject is full of the impossibility of curing amblyopia, and in popular writings persons having the care of children are urged to have cases of squint treated early, so that the vision of the squinting eye may not be lost. According to Worth, not much improvement can ordinarily be obtained in amblyopic eyes after the age of six, while Fuchs says, 1 "The function of the retina never again becomes perfectly normal, even if the cause of the visual disturbance is done away with." Yet it is well known, as the translator of Fuchs points out in an editorial comment upon the above statement,2 that if the sight of the good eye is lost at any period of life, the vision of the amblyopic eye will often become normal. Furthermore, an eye may be amblyopic at one time and not at another. When the good eye is covered, a squinting eye may be so amblyopic that it can scarcely distinguish daylight from darkness; but when both eyes are open, the vision of the squinting eye may be found to be as good as that of the straight eye, if not better. In many cases, too, the amblyopia will change from one eye to the other.

Double vision occurs very seldom in squint, and when it does, it often assumes very curious forms. When the eyes turn in the image seen by the right eye should, according to all the laws of optics, be to the right, and the image seen by the left eye to the left. When the

1 Text-book of Ophthalmology, p. 633. 2 Cases have been reported, some surely authentic, in which an amblyopic squinting eye has acquired good vision, either through correction of the refraction, or because loss of sight in the good eye has compelled the use of the amblyopic eye.-Ibid.

eyes turn out, the opposite should be the case. But often the position of the images is reversed, the image of the right eye in convergent squint being seen to the left and that of the left eye to the right, while in divergent squint the opposite is the case. This condition is known as "paradoxical diplopia." Furthermore, persons with almost normal vision and both eyes perfectly straight may have both kinds of double vision.

All the theories heretofore suggested fail to explain the foregoing facts; but it is a fact that in all cases of squint a strain can be demonstrated, and that the relief of the strain is in all cases followed by the cure of the squint, as well as of the amblyopia and the error of refraction. It is also a fact that all persons with normal eyes can produce squint by a strain to see. It is not a difficult thing to do, and many children derive much amusement from the practice, while it gives their elders unnecessary concern, for fear the temporary squint may become permanent. To produce convergent squint is comparatively easy. Children usually do it by straining to see the end of the nose. The production of divergent squint is more difficult, but with practice persons with normal eyes become able to turn out either eye, or both, at will. They also become able to turn either eye upward and inward, or upward and outward, at any desired angle. Any kind of squint can, in fact, be produced at will by the appropriate kind of strain. Some persons retain the power to produce voluntary squint more or less permanently. Others quickly lose it if they do not keep in practice. There is usually a lowering of the vision when voluntary squint is produced, and accepted methods of measuring the strength of the muscles seem to show deficiencies corresponding to the nature of the squint.

CHAPTER XXII

SQUINT AND AMBLYOPIA: THEIR CURE

THE evidence is conclusive that squint and amblyopia, like errors of refraction, are purely functional troubles; and since they are always relieved by the relief of the strain with which they are associated, it follows that any of the methods which promote relaxation and central fixation may be employed for their cure. As in the case of errors of refraction, the squint disappears and the amblyopia is corrected just as soon as the patient gains sufficient mental control to remember a perfectly black period. In this way both conditions can be temporarily relieved in a few seconds, their permanent cure being a mere matter of making this temporary state permanent.

Strabismus Cure

One of the best ways of gaining mental control in cases of squint is to learn how to increase the squint, or produce other kinds of squint, voluntarily. In the case illustrated, the patient had divergent vertical squint in both eyes. When the left eye was straight the right eye turned out and up, and when the right eye was straight the left eye turned down and out. Both eyes were amblyopic and there was double vision, with the images sometimes on the same side and sometimes on opposite sides. The patient suffered from headaches, and having obtained no relief from glasses, or other methods of treatment, she made up her mind to an operation and consulted Dr. Gudmund J. Gislason, of Grand Forks, N. D., with a view to having one performed. Dr. Gislason, puzzled to find so many muscles apparently at fault, asked my opinion as to which of them should be operated upon. I showed the patient how to make her squint worse, and recommended that Dr. Gislason treat her by eye education without an operation. He did so, and in less than a month the patient had learned to turn both eyes in voluntarily. At first she did this by looking at a pencil held over the bridge of the nose; but later she became able to do it without the pencil, and ultimately she became able to produce every kind of squint at will. The treatment was not pleasant for her, because the production of new kinds of squint, or the making worse of the existing condition, gave her pain; but it effected a complete and permanent cure both of the squint and of the amblyopia. The same method has proved successful with other patients.

Some patients do not know whether they are looking straight at an object or not. These may be helped by watching the deviating eye and directing them to look more nearly in the proper direction. When the deviating eye looks directly at an object, the strain to see is less, and the vision is consequently improved. Covering the good eye with an opaque screen, or with ground glass, encourages a more proper use of the squinting eye, especially if the vision of that eye is imperfect.

Children of six years, or younger, can usually be cured of squint by the use of atropine, a one per cent solution being instilled into one or both eyes twice a day, for many months, a year, or longer. The atropine makes it more difficult for the child to see, and makes the sunlight disagreeable. In order to overcome this handicap it has to relax, and the relaxation cures the squint.

(Dr. Bates and Modern Teachers use Relaxation Methods... without atropine.)

The improvement resulting from eye education in cases of squint and amblyopia is sometimes so rapid as to be almost incredible. The following are a few of many other examples that might be quoted :

Learning to See Worse

A girl of eleven had convergent vertical squint of the left eye. The vision of this eye at the distance was 3/200, while at the near-point it was so imperfect that she was unable to read. The vision of the right eye was normal both for the near-point and the distance. She was wearing glasses when she came to the office - convex 4.00 D. S. combined with convex 0.50 D. C., axis 90, for the right eye; and convex 5.50 D. S. for the left eye - but had obtained no benefit from them. When she looked three feet away from the big C with the left eye, she saw it better than when she looked directly at it; but when asked to count my fingers held three feet away from the card, they so attracted her attention that she was able to see the large letter worse. The fact was impressed upon her that she could see the card better when she looked away from it, or she could see it worse, at will; and she was also asked to note that when she saw it worse her vision improved, and when she saw it better her vision declined. After shifting from the card to a point three feet away from it, and seeing the former worse a few times, her vision improved to 10/200. The ability to shift and see worse improved by practice so rapidly that in less than ten days her vision was normal in both eyes, and in less than two weeks it had improved to 20/10, while diamond type was read with each eye at from three inches to twenty inches. In less than three weeks her vision for the distance was 20/5, by artificial light, and she read photographic type reductions at two inches, the tests being made with both eyes together and with each eye separately. She also read strange test cards as readily as the familiar ones. She

Fig. 54. Case of Divergent Vertical Squint Cured by Eye Education.
No. 1. The right eye turns out and up, the left being straight. No. 2. The patient learns to look down and out with the left eye while the right looks straight. No. 3. The patient learns to turn both eyes in by looking at a pencil held over the bridge of the nose. No. 4. The patient is permanently cured. All four pictures were taken within fifteen minutes of each other, the patient having learned to reproduce the conditions represented at will.

Cured in Three Weeks

was advised to continue the treatment at home to prevent a relapse, and at the end of three years none had occurred. During the treatment at the office and practice at home the good eye was covered with an opaque screen, but this was not worn at other times.

(Seeing the letter worse when looking away from it=the letter is then in the peripheral field of vision and it should be worse, less clear. When the letter is placed in the central field, eyes looking directly at it, the letter is seen best, clear due to central fixation, the center of the visual field is clearest.)

A very remarkable case was that of a girl of fourteen who had squinted from childhood. The internal rectus of the right eye had been cut when she was two years old, but still pulled the eye inward. The patient objected to wearing a ground glass over her good eye, because her friends teased her about it and she thought it made her more conspicuous than the squint. One day she lost her glasses in the snow; but her father, who was a man of strong character, immediately provided another pair. Then she announced that she was ill, and couldn't go to school. I told the father that his daughter was hysterical, and simply imagined she was ill to avoid treatment. He insisted that she continue, and as she did not consider herself well enough to come to see me, I called upon her. With the assistance of her father she was made to understand that she would have to continue the treatment until she was cured, and she at once went to work with such energy and intelligence that in half an hour the vision of the squinting and amblyopic eye had improved from 3/200 to 20/30. She also became able to read fine print at twelve inches. She went back to school wearing the ground glass over the good eye; but whenever she wanted to see she looked over the top of it. Her father followed her to school, and insisted that she use the poorer eye instead of the better one. She became convinced that the simplest way out of her troubles would be to follow my instructions, and in less than a week the squint was corrected and she had perfect vision in both eyes. At the beginning of the treatment she could not count her fingers at three feet with the poorer eye, and in three weeks, including all the time that she wasted, she had perfect sight. When told that she was cured her main concern seemed to be to know whether she would have to wear the ground glass any more. She was assured that she would not have to do so unless there was a relapse, but there never was any relapse. 1

1 Bates; L'education de l'oeil dans l'amblyopie ex anopsia, Clin. Opht., Dec.10, 1912.

Fig. 55
No. 1.—Convergent squint of the right eye.
No. 2.—The patient is temporarily cured by the memory of a black period.

Fig. 55 No. 1. Convergent squint of the right eye. No. 2. The patient is temporarily cured by the memory of a black period.

Cured in Two Weeks

A girl of eight had had amblyopia and squint since childhood. The vision of the right eye was 10/40, while that of the left was 20/30. Glasses did not improve either eye. The patient was seated twenty feet from a Snellen test card and the right, or poorer eye, was covered with an opaque screen. She was directed to look with her better eye at the large letter on the card and to note its clearness. Next she was told to look at a point three feet to one side of the card, and her attention was called to the fact that she did not then see the large letter so well. The point of fixation was brought closer and closer to the letter, until she appreciated the fact that her vision was lowered when she looked only a few inches to one side of it. When she looked at a small letter she readily recognized that an eccentric fixation of less than an inch lowered the vision.

After she had learned to increase the amblyopia of the better eye, this eye was covered while she was taught how to lower the vision of the other, or poorer eye, by increasing its eccentric fixation. This was accomplished in a few minutes. She was told that the cause of her defective sight was her habit of looking at objects with a part of the retina to one side of the true center of sight. She was advised to see by looking straight at the Snellen card. In less than half an hour the vision of the left eye became normal, while the right improved from 10/40 to 10/10. The cure was complete in two weeks.

The following case was unusually prolonged, because as soon as one eye had been cured, the defect for which it had been treated appeared in the other eye. The patient, a child of ten, had imperfect sight in both eyes, but worse in the right than in the left. The vision of the right eye was restored after some weeks by eye education, when the left eye turned in and became amblyopic. The right eye was then covered, and after a few weeks of eye education the left became normal. The right eye then turned in and the vision became defective. It was necessary to educate the eyes alternately, for about a year, before both became normal at the same time. This patient had congenital paralysis of the external rectus muscle in both eyes, a condition which was apparently not relieved when the squint and amblyopia were cured.

In the following case the patient had an attack of infantile paralysis after her cure, resulting in a relapse, with new and more serious developments, which were, however quickly cured. The patient, a girl of six, seen first on December 11, 1914, had had divergent squint of the left eye for three years, and had worn glasses for two years without benefit - convex 2.50 D. S. for the right eye, and convex 6.00 D. S. combined with convex 1.00 D. C., axis 90, for the left. The vision of the right eye with glasses was 12/15 and of the left 12/200. Atropine was prescribed for the right eye for the purpose of partially blinding it and thus encouraging a more nearly proper use of the squinting eye, and the usual methods of securing relaxation, such as shifting, palming, the exercise of the memory, etc., were used. On January 13, 1915, the vision without glasses had improved to 10/70 for the right eye, and 10/50 for the left. On February 6, the vision of the right eye was 10/40 and of the left 10/30. The eyes were apparently straight, and scientific tests showed that both were used at the same time (binocular single vision). On April 17, after about four months' treatment, the vision of the left eye was normal, and there was binocular single vision at six inches. On May 1 the vision of the left eye was still normal, and whereas at the beginning the patient had been unable to read with it at all, even with glasses, she now read diamond type without glasses at six inches.

Accommodation Unaffected by Atropine

On August 16, 1916, the patient had an attack of infantile paralysis which was then epidemic. The sight of both eyes failed, the muscles that turned the eyes in and out were paralyzed, the eyelids twitched, and there was double vision. Various muscles of the head, the left leg and the left arm were also paralzyed. When she left the hospital after five weeks the left eye was turned in, and the vision of both eyes was so poor that she was unable to recognize her mother. Later she developed alternate convergent squint. On November 2 the paralysis in the right eye subsided, and four weeks later that of the left eye began to improve. On November 9 she returned for treatment without any conspicuous squint, but still suffering from double vision, with the images sometimes on the same side and sometimes on opposite sides. On November 23 the eyes were straight and the vision normal.

On July 11, 1918, the eyes were still straight and the vision normal, and there was binocular single vision at six inches. Although atropine had been used in the right eye every day for more than a year, and intermittently for a much longer time, and the pupil was dilated to the maximum, it read fine print without difficulty at six inches, central fixation overcoming the paralyzing effect of the drug. According to the current theory the accommodation should have been completely paralyzed, making near vision quite impossible. The patient also read fine print with the left eye as well as, or better than, with the right eye.

CHAPTER XXIII

FLOATING SPECKS: THEIR CAUSE AND CURE

A VERY common phenomenon of imperfect sight is the one known to medical science as "muscae volitantes" or "flying flies." These floating specks are usually dark or black, but sometimes appear like white bubbles, and in rare cases may assume all the colors of the rainbow. They move somewhat rapidly, usually in curving lines, before the eyes, and always appear to be just beyond the point of fixation. If one tries to look at them directly, they seem to move a little farther away. Hence their name of "flying flies."

The literature of the subject is full of speculations as to the origin of these appearances. Some have attributed them to the presence of floating specks - dead cells or the debris of cells - in the vitreous humor, the transparent substance that fills four-fifths of the eyeball behind the crystalline lens. Similar specks on the surface of the cornea have also been held responsible for them. It has even been surmised that they might be caused by the passage of tears over the cornea. They are so common in myopia that they have been supposed to be one of the symptoms of this condition, although they occur also with other errors of refraction, as well as in eyes otherwise normal. They have been attributed to disturbances of the circulation, the digestion and the kidneys, and because so many insane people have them, have been thought to be an evidence of incipient insanity. The patent-medicine business has thrived upon them, and it would be difficult to estimate the amount of mental torture they have caused, as the following cases illustrate.

A Pitiable Case

A clergyman who was much annoyed by the continual appearance of floating specks before his eyes was told by his eye specialist that they were a symptom of kidney disease, and that in many cases of kidney trouble disease of the retina might be an early symptom. So at regular intervals he went to the specialist to have his eyes examined, and when at length the latter died, he looked around immediately for some one else to make the periodical examination. His family physician directed him to me. I was by no means so well known as his previous ophthalmological adviser, but it happened that I had taught the family physician how to use the ophthalmoscope after others had failed to do so. He thought, therefore, that I must know a lot about the use of the instrument, and what the clergyman particularly wanted was some one capable of making a thorough examination of the interior of his eyes and detecting at once any signs of kidney disease that might make their appearance. So he came to me, and at least four times a year for ten years he continued to come.

Each time I made a very careful examination of his eyes, taking as much time over it as possible, so that he would believe that it was careful ; and each time he went away happy because I could find nothing wrong. Once when I was out of town he got a cinder in his eye, and went to another oculist to get it out. When I came back late at night I found him sitting on my doorstep, on the chance that I might return. His story was a pitiable one. The strange doctor had examined his eyes with the ophthalmoscope, and had suggested the possibility of glaucoma, describing the disease as a very treacherous one which might cause him to go suddenly blind and would be agonizingly painful. He emphasized what the patient had previously been told about the danger of kidney disease, suggested that the liver and heart might also be involved, and advised him to have all of these organs carefully examined. I made another examination of his eyes in general and their tension in particular ; I had him feel his eyeballs and compare them with my own, so that he might see for himself that they were not becoming hard as a stone; and finally I succeeded in reassuring him. I have no doubt, however, that he went at once to his family physician for an examination of his internal organs.

A man returning from Europe was looking at some white clouds one day when floating specks appeared before his eyes. He consulted the ship's doctor, who told him that the symptom was very serious, and might be the forerunner of blindness. It might also indicate incipient insanity, as well as other nervous or organic diseases. He advised him to consult his family physician and an eye specialist as soon as he landed, which he did. This was twenty-five years ago, but I shall never forget the terrible state of nervousness and terror into which the patient had worked himself by the time he came to me. It was even worse than that of the clergyman, who was always ready to admit that his fears were unreasonable. I examined his eyes very carefully, and found them absolutely normal. The vision was perfect both for the near-point and the distance. The color perception, the fields and the tension were normal; and under a strong magnifying glass I could find no opacities in the vitreous. In short, there were absolutely no symptoms of any

A Common Symptom

disease. I told the patient there was nothing wrong with his eyes, and I also showed him an advertisement of a quack medicine in a newspaper which gave a great deal of space to describing the dreadful things likely to follow the appearance of floating specks before the eyes, unless you began betimes to take the medicine in question at one dollar a bottle. I pointed out that the advertisement, which was appearing in all the big newspapers of the city every day, and probably in other cities, must have cost a lot of money, and must, therefore, be bringing in a lot of money. Evidently there must be a great many people suffering from this symptom, and if it were as serious as was generally believed, there would be a great many more blind and insane people in the community than there were. The patient went away somewhat comforted, but at eleven o'clock - his first visit had been at nine - he was back again. He still saw the floating specks, and was still worried about them. I examined his eyes again as carefully as before, and again was able to assure him that there was nothing wrong with them. In the afternoon I was not in my office, but I was told that he was there at three and at five. At seven he came again, bringing with him his family physician, an old friend of mine. I said to the latter:

"Please make this patient stay at home. I have to charge him for his visits, because he is taking up so much of my time; but it is a shame to take his money when there is nothing wrong with him."

What my friend said to him I don't know, but he did not come back again.

I did not know as much about muscae volitantes then as I know now, or I might have saved both of these patients a great deal of uneasiness. I could tell them that their eyes were normal, but I did not know how to relieve them of the symptom, which is <u>simply an illusion resulting from mental strain.</u> The specks are associated to a considerable extent with markedly imperfect eyesight, because persons whose eyesight is imperfect always strain to see; but persons whose eyesight is ordinarily normal may see them at times, because no eye has normal sight all the time. Most people can see muscae volitantes when they look at the sun, or any uniformly bright surface, like a sheet of white paper upon which the sun is shining. This is because most people strain when they look at surfaces of this kind. The specks are never seen, in short, except when the eyes and mind are under a strain, and they always disappear when the strain is relieved. <u>If one can remember a small letter on the Snellen test card by central fixation, the specks will immediately disappear, or cease to move ; but if one tries to remember two or more letters equally well at one time, they will reappear and move.</u>

Usually the strain that causes muscae volitantes is very easily relieved. A school teacher who had been annoyed by these appearances for years came to me because the condition had grown recently much worse. I was able in half an hour to improve her sight, which had been slightly myopic, to normal, whereupon the specks disappeared. Next day they came back, but another visit to the office brought relief. After that the patient was able to carry out the treatment at home, and had no more trouble.

A physician who suffered constantly from headaches and muscae volitantes was able to read only 20/70 when he looked at the Snellen test card, while the retinoscope showed mixed astigmatism and he saw the specks.

Cured in a Few Days

When he looked at a blank wall, or a blank white card, the retinoscope still showed mixed astigmatism and he still saw the specks. When, however, he remembered a black spot as well as he could see it, when looking at these surfaces, there were no specks, and the retinoscope indicated no error of refraction. In a few days he obtained complete relief from the astigmatism, the muscae volitantes, and the headaches, as well as from chronic conjunctivitis. His eyes, which had been partly closed, opened wide, and the sclera became white and clear. He became able to read in moving trains with no inconvenience, and - what impressed him more than anything else - he also became able to sit up all night with patients without having any trouble with his eyes next day.

CHAPTER XXIV

HOME TREATMENT

IT is not always possible for patients to go to a competent physician for relief. As the method of treating eye defects presented in this book is new, it may be impossible to find a physician in the neighborhood who understands it; and the patient may not be able to afford the expense of a long journey, or to take the time for treatment away from home. To such persons I wish to say that it is possible for a large number of people to be cured of defective eyesight without the aid, either of a physician or of anyone else. They can cure themselves, and for this purpose it is not necessary that they should understand all that has been written in this book, or in any other book. All that is necessary is to follow a few simple directions.

Place a Snellen test card on the wall at a distance of ten, fourteen, or twenty feet, and devote half a minute a day, or longer, to reading the smallest letters you can see, with each eye separately, covering the other with the palm of the hand in such a way as to avoid touching the eyeball. Keep a record of the progress made, with the dates. The simplest way to do this is by the method used by oculists, who record the vision in the form of a fraction, <u>with the distance at which the letter is read as the numerator and the distance at which it ought to be read as the denominator</u>. The figures above, or to one side of, the lines of letters on the test card indicate the distance at which these letters should be read by persons with normal eyesight. Thus a vision of 10/200 would

Children Quickly Cured

mean that the big C, which ought to be read at 200 feet, cannot be seen at a greater distance than ten feet. A vision of 20/10 would mean that the ten line, which the normal eye is not ordinarily expected to read at a greater distance than ten feet, is seen at double that distance. This is a standard commonly attained by persons who have practiced my methods.

Another and even better way to test the sight is to compare the blackness of the letter at the near-point and at the distance, in a dim light and in a good one. With perfect sight, black is not altered by illumination or distance. It appears just as black at the distance as at the near-point, and just as black in a dim light as in a good one. If it does not appear equally black to you under all these conditions, therefore, you may know that your sight is imperfect.

Children under twelve years who have not worn glasses are usually cured of defective eyesight by the above method in three months, six months, or a year. Adults who have never worn glasses are benefited in a very short time - a week or two - and if the trouble is not very bad, may be cured in the course of from three to six months. Children or adults who have worn glasses, however, are more difficult to relieve, and will usually have to practice the method of gaining relaxation described in other chapters; they will also have to devote considerable time to the treatment.

It is absolutely necessary that the glasses be discarded. No half-way measures can be tolerated, if a cure is desired. Do not attempt to wear weaker glasses, and do not wear glasses for emergencies. Persons who are unable to do without glasses for all purposes are not likely to be able to cure themselves. (Later, Dr. Bates changed this statement and allowed eyeglasses as long as the lens strength is continually reduced and worn only if absolutely necessary for work, safety, until vision is clear enough to go without them. Modern Teachers allow <u>reduced, weaker,</u> usually 20/40-20-50 eyeglass lenses if needed, temporarily as the vision is improving.)

Children and adults who have worn glasses will have to devote an hour or longer every day to practice with the test card and the balance of their time to practice on other objects. It will be well for such patients to have two test cards, one to be used at the near-point, where it can be seen best, and the other at ten or twenty feet. The patient will find it a great help to shift from the near card to the distant one, as the unconscious memory of the letters seen at the near-point helps to bring out those seen at the distance.

Make Your Own Eyechart

If you cannot obtain a test card, you can make one for yourself by painting black letters of appropriate size on a white card, or on a piece of white paper. The approximate diameter of these letters, reading from the top of the card to the bottom, is: 3 1/2 in., 1 3/4 in., 1 1/4 in., 7/8 in., 11/16 in., 1/2 in., 3/8 in., 1/4 in., 3/16 in.

If the patient can secure the aid of some person with normal sight, it will be a great advantage. In fact, persons whose cases are obstinate will find it very difficult, if not impossible, to cure themselves without the aid of a teacher. The teacher, if he is to benefit the patient, must himself be able to derive benefit from the various methods recommended. If his vision is 10/10, he must be able to improve it to 20/10, or more. If he can read fine print at twelve inches, he must become able to read it at six, or at three inches. He must also have sufficient control over his visual memory to relieve and prevent pain. A person who has defective sight, either for the distance or the near-point, and who cannot remember black well enough to relieve and prevent pain, will be unable to be of any material assistance in obstinate cases ; and no one will be able to be of any assistance in the application of any method which he himself has not used successfully.

The Duty of Parents

Parents who wish to preserve and improve the eyesight of their children should encourage them to read the Snellen test card every day. There should, in fact, be a Snellen test card in every family; for when properly used it always prevents myopia and other errors of refraction, always improves the vision, even when this is already normal, and always benefits functional nervous troubles. Parents should improve their own eyesight to normal, so that their children may not imitate wrong methods of using the eyes and will not be subject to the influence of an atmosphere of strain. They should also learn the principles of central fixation sufficiently well to relieve and prevent pain, in order that they may teach their children to do the same. This practice not only makes it possible to avoid suffering, but is a great benefit to the general health.

CHAPTER XXV
CORRESPONDENCE TREATMENT

CORRESPONDENCE treatment is usually regarded as quackery, and it would be manifestly impossible to treat many diseases in this way. Pneumonia and typhoid, for instance, could not possibly be treated by correspondence, even if the physician had a sure cure for these conditions and the mails were not too slow for the purpose. In the case of most diseases, in fact, there are serious objections to correspondence treatment.

But myopia, hypermetropia and astigmatism are functional conditions, not organic, as the text-books teach and as I believed myself until I learned better. Their treatment by correspondence, therefore, has not the drawbacks that exist in the case of most physical derangements. One cannot, it is true, fit glasses by correspondence as well as when the patient is in the office, but even this can be done, as the following case illustrates.

An old colored woman in the wilds of Honduras, far removed from any physician or optician, was unable to read her Bible, and her son, a waiter in New York, asked me if I could not do something for her. The suggestion gave me a distinct shock which I will remember as long as I live. I had never dreamed of the possibility of prescribing glasses for anyone I had not seen, and I had, besides, some very disquieting recollections of colored women whom I had tried to fit with glasses at my clinic.

Glasses Fitted by Mail

If I had so much difficulty in prescribing the proper glasses under favorable conditions, how could I be expected to fit a patient whom I could not even see? The waiter was deferentially persistent, however. He had more faith in my genius than I had, and as his mother was nearing the end of her life, he was very anxious to gratify her last wishes. So, like the unjust judge of the parable, I yielded at last to his importunity, and wrote a prescription for convex 3.00 D. S. The young man ordered the glasses and mailed them to his mother, and by return mail came a very grateful letter stating that they were perfectly satisfactory.

A little later the patient wrote that she couldn't see objects at the distance that were perfectly plain to other people, and asked if some glasses couldn't be sent that would make her see at the distance as well as she did at the near-point. This seemed a more difficult proposition than the first one; but again the son was persistent, and I myself could not get the old lady out of my mind. So again I decided to do what I could. The waiter had told me that his mother had read her Bible long after the age of forty. Therefore I knew she could not have much hypermetropia, and was probably slightly myopic. I knew also that she could not have much astigmatism, for in that case her sight would always have been noticeably imperfect. Accordingly I told her son to ask her to measure very accurately the distance between her eyes and the point at which she could read her Bible best with her glasses, and to send me the figures. In due time I received, not figures, but a piece of string about a quarter of an inch in diameter and exactly ten inches long. If the patient's vision had been normal for the distance, I knew that she would have been able to read her Bible best with her glasses at thirteen inches. The string showed that at ten inches she had a refraction of four diopters. Subtracting from this the three diopters of her reading glasses, I got one diopter of myopia. I accordingly wrote a prescription for concave 1.00 D. S., and the glasses were ordered and mailed to Honduras. The acknowledgment was even more grateful than in the case of the first pair. The patient said that for the first time in her life she was able to read signs and see other objects at a distance as well as other people did, and that the whole world looked entirely different to her.

Would anyone venture to say that it was unethical for me to try to help this patient? Would it have been better to leave her in her isolation without even the consolation of Bible reading? I do not think so. What I did for her required only an ordinary knowledge of physiological optics, and if I had failed, I could not have done her much harm.

In the case of the treatment of imperfect sight without glasses there can be even less objection to the correspondence method. It is true that in most cases progress is more rapid and the results more certain when the patient can be seen personally; but often this is impossible, and I see no reason why patients who cannot have the benefit of personal treatment should be denied such aid as can be given them by correspondence. I have been treating patients in this way for years, and often with extraordinary success.

Some years ago an English gentleman wrote to me that his glasses were very unsatisfactory. They not only did not give him good sight, but they increased, instead of lessening, his discomfort. He asked if I could help

Was It Unethical?

him, and since relaxation always relieves discomfort and improves the vision, I did not believe that I was doing him an injury in telling him how to rest his eyes. He followed my directions with such good results that in a short time he obtained perfect sight for both the distance and the near-point without glasses, and was completely relieved of his pain. Five years later he wrote me that he had qualified as a sharpshooter in the army. Did I do wrong in treating him by correspondence? I do not think so.

After the United States entered the European war, an officer wrote to me from the deserts of Arizona that the use of his eyes at the near-point caused him great discomfort, which glasses did not relieve, and that the strain had produced granulation of the lids. As it was impossible for him to come to New York, I undertook to treat him by correspondence. He improved very rapidly. The inflammation of the lids was relieved almost immediately, and in about four months he wrote me that he had read one of my own reprints - by no means a short one - in a dim light, with no bad after effects; that the glare of the Arizona sun, with the Government thermometer registering 114, did not annoy him; and that he could read the ten line on the test card at fifteen feet almost perfectly, while even at twenty feet he was able to make out most of the letters.

A third case was that of a forester in the employ of the U. S. Government. He had myopic astigmatism, and suffered extreme discomfort, which was not relieved either by glasses or by long summers in the mountains, where he used his eyes but little for close work. He was unable to come to New York for treatment, and although I told him that correspondence treatment was somewhat uncertain, he said he was willing to risk it. It took three days for his letters to reach me and another three for my reply to reach him, and as letters were not always written promptly on either side, he often did not hear from me more than once in three weeks. Progress under these conditions was necessarily slow; but his discomfort was relieved very quickly, and in about ten months his sight had improved from 20/50 to 20/20.

In almost every case the treatment of patients coming from a distance is continued by correspondence after they return to their homes; and although they do not get on so well as when they are coming to the office, they usually continue to make progress until they are cured.

At the same time it is often very difficult to make patients understand what they should do when one has to communicate with them entirely by writing, and probably all would get on better if they could have some personal treatment. At the present time the number of doctors in different parts of the United States who understand the treatment of imperfect sight without glasses is altogether too few, and my efforts to interest them in the matter have not been very successful.

CHAPTER XXVI

THE PREVENTION OF MYOPIA IN SCHOOLS : METHODS THAT FAILED

NO phase of ophthalmology, not even the problem of accommodation, has been the subject of so much investigation and discussion as the cause and prevention of myopia. Since hypermetropia was supposed to be due to a congenital deformation of the eyeball, and astigmatism, until recently, was also supposed to be congenital in most cases, these conditions were not thought to call for any explanation, nor to admit of any prevention; but myopia appeared to be acquired. It therefore presented a problem of immense practical importance to which many eminent men devoted years of labor.

Voluminous statistics were collected regarding its occurrence, and are still being collected. The subject has produced libraries of literature. But very little light is to be gained from the perusal of this material, and for the most part it leaves the reader with an impression of hopeless confusion. It is impossible even to arrive at any conclusion as to the prevalence of the complaint; for not only has there been no uniformity of standards and methods, but none of the investigators has taken into account the fact that the refraction of the eye is not a constant condition, but one which continually varies. There is no doubt, however, that most children, when they begin school, are free from this defect, and that both the number of cases and the degree of the myopia steadily increase as the educational process progresses. Professor Hermann Cohn, of Breslau,

Prevention of Myopia

whose report of his study of the eyes of upwards of 10,000 children first called general attention to this subject, found scarcely one per cent of myopia in the village schools, twenty to forty per cent in the "Realschulen," thirty to thirty-five in the gymnasia, and fifty-three to sixty-four in the professional schools. His investigations were repeated in many cities of Europe and America, and his observations, with some difference in percentages, everywhere confirmed.

These conditions were unanimously attributed to the excessive use of the eyes for near work, though, according to the theory that the lens is the agent of accommodation, it was a little difficult to see just why near work should have this effect. On the supposition that accommodation was effected by an elongation of the eyeball, it would have been easy to understand why an excessive amount of accommodation should produce a permanent elongation. But why should an abnormal demand on the accommodative power of the lens produce a change, not in the shape of that body, but in that of the eyeball? Numerous answers to this question have been proposed, but no one has yet succeeded in finding a satisfactory one.1 In the case of children it has been assumed by many authorities that, since the coats of the eye are softer in youth than in later years, they are unable to withstand a supposed intraocular tension produced by near work. When other errors of refraction, such as hypermetropia and astigmatism, believed to be congenital, were present, it has been supposed that the accommodative struggle for distinct vision produced irritation and strain which encouraged the production of short-

1 A satisfactory explanation of the mechanism by which near work produces myopia has not yet been given.-Tscherning: Physiologic Optics, p. 86. It is not yet determined how near work changes the longitudinal structure of the eye.-Eversbusch : The Diseases of Children, vol. vi, p. 291.

Myopia and the Educational Process

sight. When the condition developed in adults, the explanations had to be modified to fit the case, and the fact that a considerable number of cases were observed among peasants and others who did not use their eyes for near work led some authorities to divide the anomaly into two classes, one caused by near work and one unrelated to it, the latter being conveniently attributed to hereditary tendencies.

As it was impossible to abandon the educational system, attempts were made to minimize the supposed evil effects of the reading, writing and other near work which it demanded. Careful and detailed rules were laid down by various authorities as to the sizes of type to be used in schoolbooks, the length of the lines, their distance apart, the distance at which the book should be held, the amount and arrangement of the light, the construction of the desks, the length of time the eyes might be used without a change of focus, etc. Face-rests were even devised to hold the eyes at the prescribed distance from the desk and to prevent stooping, which was supposed to cause congestion of the eyeball and thus to encourage elongation. The Germans, with characteristic thoroughness, actually used these instruments of torture, Cohn never allowing his own children to write without one, "even when sitting at the best possible desk."1

The results of these preventive measures were disappointing. Some observers reported a slight decrease in the percentage of myopia in schools in which the prescribed reforms had been made, but on the whole, as Risley has observed in his discussion of the subject in Norris and Oliver's "System of Diseases of the Eye," "the injurious results of the educational process were not notably arrested." 1

1 The Hygiene of the Eye in Schools, p. 127.

"It is a significant, though discouraging, fact," he continues, "that the increase, as found by Cohn, both in the percentage and in the degree of myopia, had taken place in those schools where he had especially exerted himself to secure the introduction of hygienic reforms; and the same is true of the observations of Just, who had examined the eyes of twelve hundred and twenty-nine of the pupils of the two high schools of Zittau, in both of which the hygienic conditions were all that could be desired. He found, nevertheless, that the excellent arrangements had not in any degree lessened the percentage of increase in myopia."1

Fig. 56. Face-Rest Designed by Kallmann, a German Optician. Cohn never allowed his children to write without it, even when sitting at the best possible desk.

1 School Hygiene, System of Diseases of the Eye, vol. ii, p. 361.

The Theory Breaks Down

Further study of the subject has only added to its difficulty, while at the same time it has tended to relieve the schools of much of the responsibility formerly attributed to them for the production of myopia. As the "American Encyclopedia of Ophthalmology" points out, "the theory that myopia is due to close work aggravated by town life and badly lighted rooms is gradually giving ground before statistics."1

In an investigation in London, for instance, in which the schools were carefully selected to reveal any differences that might arise from the various influences, hygienic, social and racial, to which the children were subjected, the proportion of myopia in the best lighted building of the group was actually found to be higher than in the one where the lighting conditions were worst, although the higher degrees of myopia were more numerous in the latter than in the former. It has also been found that there is just as much myopia in schools where little near work is done as in those in which the demand upon the accommodative power of the eye is greater. 2 It is only a minority of children, moreover, that become myopic ; yet all are subject to practically the same influences, and even in the same child one eye may become myopic while the other remains normal. On the theory that shortsight results from any external influence to which the eye is exposed, it is impossible to account for the fact that under the same conditions of life the eyes of different individuals and the two eyes of the same individual behave differently.

Owing to the difficulty of reconciling these facts on the basis of the earlier theories, there is now a growing

1 American Encyclopedia and Dictionary of Ophthalmology, edited by Wood, 1913-1919, vol. xi, p. 8271. 2 Lawson: Brit. Med. Jour., June 18, 1898.

disposition to attribute myopia to hereditary tendencies; 1 but no satisfactory evidence on this point has been brought forward, and the fact that primitive peoples who have always had good eyesight become myopic just as quickly as any others when subjected to the conditions of civilized life, like the Indian pupils at Carlisle, 2 seems to be conclusive evidence against it.

In spite of the repeated failure of preventive measures based upon the limitation of near work and the regulation of lighting, desks, types, etc., the use of the eyes at the near-point under unfavorable conditions is still admitted by most exponents of the heredity theory as probably, if not certainly, a secondary cause of myopia. Sidler-Huguenin, however, whose startling conclusions as to the hopelessness of controlling shortsight were quoted earlier, has observed so little benefit from such precautions that he believes a myope may become an engineer just as well as a farmer, or a forester ; and as a result of his experiences with anisometropes, persons with an inequality of refraction between the two organs of vision, he even suggests that the use of myopic eyes may possibly be more favorable to their well-being than their non-use. In 150 cases in which, owing to this inequality and other conditions, the subjects practically used but one eye, the weaker organ, he reports, became gradually more and more myopic, sometimes excessively so, in open defiance of all the accepted theories relating to the matter.

The prevalence of myopia, the unsatisfactoriness of

1 It seems to have been amply demonstrated, by the studies of Motais, Steiger, Miss Barrington, and Karl Pearson, that errors of refraction are inherited. And while the use of the eyes for near work is probably a secondary cause, determining largely the development of the defect, it is not the primary cause. Cyclopedia of Education, edited by Monroe, 1911-1913, vol. iv, p. 361. 2 Fox (quoted by Risley) : System of Diseases of the Eye, vol. ii, p. 357.

Why Preventive Measures Have Failed

all explanations of its origin, and the futility of all methods of prevention, have led some writers of repute to the conclusion that the elongated eyeball is a natural physiological adaptation to the needs of civilization. Against this view two unanswerable arguments can be brought. One is that the myopic eye does not see so well even at the near-point as the normal eye, and the other that the defect tends to progression with very serious results, often ending in blindness. If Nature has attempted to adapt the eye to civilized conditions by an elongation of the globe, she has done it in a very clumsy manner. It is true that many authorities assume the existence of two kinds of myopia, one physiological, or at least harmless, and the other pathological; but since it is impossible to say with certainty whether a given case is going to progress or not, this distinction, even if it were correct, would be more important theoretically than practically.

Into such a slough of despair and contradiction have the misdirected labors of a hundred years led us! But in the light of truth the problem turns out to be a very simple one. In view of the facts given in Chapters V and IX, it is easy to understand why all previous attempts to prevent myopia have failed. All these attempts have aimed at lessening the strain of near work upon the eye, leaving the strain to see distant objects unaffected, and totally ignoring the mental strain which underlies the optical one. There are many differences between the conditions to which the children of primitive man were subjected, and those under which the offspring of civilized races spend their developing years, besides the mere fact that the latter learn things out of books and write things on paper, and the former did not. In the process of education, civilized children are shut up for hours every day within four walls, in the charge of teachers who are too often nervous and irritable. They are even compelled to remain for long periods in the same position. The things they are required to learn may be presented in such a way as to be excessively uninteresting; and they are under a continual compulsion to think of the gaining of marks and prizes rather than the acquisition of knowledge for its own sake. Some children endure these unnatural conditions better than others. Many cannot stand the strain, and thus the schools become the hotbed, not only of myopia, but of all other errors of refraction.

CHAPTER XXVII

THE PREVENTION AND CURE OF MYOPIA AND OTHER ERRORS OF REFRACTION IN SCHOOLS : A METHOD THAT SUCCEEDED

YOU cannot see anything with perfect sight unless you have seen it before. When the eye looks at an unfamiliar object it always strains more or less to see that object, and an error of refraction is always produced. When children look at unfamiliar writing or figures on the blackboard, distant maps, diagrams, or pictures, the retinoscope always shows that they are myopic, though their vision may be under other circumstances absolutely normal. The same thing happens when adults look at unfamiliar distant objects. When the eye regards a familiar object, however, the effect is quite otherwise. Not only can it be regarded without strain, but the strain of looking later at unfamiliar objects is lessened.

This fact furnishes us with a means of overcoming the mental strain to which children are subjected by the modern educational system. It is impossible to see anything perfectly when the mind is under a strain, and if children become able to relax when looking at familiar objects, they become able, sometimes in an incredibly brief space of time, to maintain their relaxation when looking at unfamiliar objects.

I discovered this fact while examining the eyes of 1,500 school children at Grand Forks, N. D., in 1903.[1] In

[1] Bates: The Prevention of Myopia in School Children, N. Y. Med. Jour.. July 29, 1911.

many cases, children who could not read all of the letters on the Snellen test card at the first test read them at the second or third test. After a class had been examined the children who had failed would sometimes ask for a second or third test. After a class had been examined, read the whole card with perfect vision. So frequent were these occurrences that there was no escaping the conclusion that in some way the vision was improved by reading the Snellen test card. In one class I found a boy who at first appeared to be very myopic, but who, after a little encouragement, read all the letters on the test card. The teacher asked me about this boy's vision, because she had found him to be very "nearsighted." When I said that his vision was normal she was incredulous, and suggested that he might have learned the letters by heart, or been prompted by another pupil. He was unable to read the writing or figures on the blackboard, she said, or to see the maps, charts and diagrams on the walls, and did not recognize people across the street. She asked me to test his sight again, which I did, very carefully, under her supervision, the sources of error which she had suggested being eliminated. Again the boy read all the letters on the card. Then the teacher tested his sight. She wrote some words and figures on the blackboard, and asked him to read them. He did so correctly. Then she wrote additional words and figures, which he read equally well. Finally she asked him to tell the hour by the clock, twenty-five feet distant, which he did correctly. It was a dramatic situation, both the teacher and the children being intensely interested. Three other cases in the class were similar, their vision, which had previously been very defective for distant objects, becoming normal in the few moments devoted

No More Defective Eyesight

to testing their eyes. It is not surprising that after such a demonstration the teacher asked to have a Snellen test card placed permanently in the room. The children were directed to read the smallest letters they could see from their seats at least once every day, with both eyes together and with each eye separately, the other being covered with the palm of the hand in such a way as to avoid pressure on the eyeball. Those whose vision was defective were encouraged to read it more frequently, and, in fact, needed no encouragement to do so after they found that the practice helped them to see the blackboard, and stopped the headaches, or other discomfort, previously resulting from the use of their eyes.

In another class of forty children, between six and eight, thirty of the pupils gained normal vision while their eyes were being tested. The remainder were cured later under the supervision of the teacher by exercises in distant vision with the Snellen card. This teacher had noted every year for fifteen years that at the opening of the school in the fall all the children could see the writing on the blackboard from their seats, but before school closed the following spring all of them without exception complained that they could not see it at a distance of more than ten feet. After learning of the benefits to be derived from the daily practice of distant vision with familiar objects as the points of fixation, this teacher kept a Snellen test card continually in her classroom and directed the children to read it every day. The result was that for eight years no more of the children under her care acquired defective eyesight.

This teacher had attributed the invariable deterioration in the eyesight of her charges during the school year to the fact that her classroom was in the basement and the light poor. But teachers with well-lighted classrooms had the same experience, and after the Snellen test card was introduced into both the well-lighted and the poorly lighted rooms, and the children read it every day, the deterioration of their eyesight not only ceased, but the vision of all improved. Vision which had been below normal improved, in most cases, to normal, while children who already had normal sight, usually reckoned at 20/20, became able to read 20/15, or 20/10. And not only was myopia cured, but the vision for near objects was improved.

At the request of the superintendent of the schools of Grand Forks, Mr. J. Nelson Kelly, the system was introduced into all the schools of the city and was used continuously for eight years, during which time it reduced myopia among the children, which I found at the beginning to be about six per cent, to less than one per cent.

In 1911 and 1912 the same system was introduced into some of the schools of New York City, 1 with an attendance of about ten thousand children. Many of the teachers neglected to use the cards, being unable to believe that such a simple method, and one so entirely at variance with previous teaching on the subject, could accomplish the desired results. Others kept the cards in a closet except when they were needed for the daily eye drill, lest the children should memorize them. Thus they not only put an unnecessary burden upon themselves, but did what they could to defeat the purpose of the system, which is to give the children daily exercise in distant vision with a familiar object as the point of fixation. A considerable number, however, used the system intelligently and persistently, and in less than a year were

1 Bates: Myopia Prevention by Teachers, N. Y. Med. Jour., Aug. 30, 1913.

Eyesight and Mentality Improved

able to present reports showing that of three thousand children with imperfect sight, over one thousand had obtained normal vision by its means. Some of these children, as in the case of the children of Grand Forks, were cured in a few minutes. Many of the teachers were also cured, some of them very quickly. In some cases the results of the system were so astonishing as to be scarcely credible.

In a class of mental defectives, where the teacher had kept records of the eyesight of the children for several years, it had been invariably found that their vision grew steadily worse as the term advanced. As soon as the Snellen test card had been introduced, however, they began to improve. Then came a doctor from the Board of Health who tested the eyes of the children and put glasses on all of them, even those whose sight was fairly good. The use of the card was then discontinued, as the teacher did not consider it proper to interfere while the children were wearing glasses prescribed by a physician. Very soon, however, the children began to lose, break, or discard their glasses. Some said that the spectacles gave them headaches, or that they felt better without them. In the course of a month or so most of the aids to vision which the Board of Health had supplied had disappeared. The teacher then felt herself at liberty to resume the use of the Snellen test card. Its benefits were immediate. The eyesight and the mentality of the children improved simultaneously, and soon they were all drafted into the regular classes, because it was found that they were making the same progress in their studies as the other children were.

Another teacher reported an equally interesting experience. She had a class of children who did not fit into the other grades. Many of them were backward in their studies. Some were persistent truants. All of them had defective eyesight. A Snellen test card was hung in the classroom where all the children could see it, and the teacher carried out my instructions literally. At the end of six months all but two had been cured, and these had improved very much, while the worst incorrigible and the worst truant had become good students. The incorrigible, who had previously refused to study, because, he said, it gave him a headache to look at a book, or at the blackboard, found out that the test card, in some way, did him a lot of good ; and although the teacher had asked him to read it but once a day, he read it whenever he felt uncomfortable. The result was that in a few weeks his vision had become normal and his objection to study had disappeared. The truant had been in the habit of remaining away from school two or three days every week, and neither his parents nor the truant officer had been able to do anything about it. To the great surprise of his teacher he never missed a day after having begun to read the Snellen test card. When she asked for an explanation, he told her that what had driven him away from school was the pain that came in his eyes whenever he tried to study, or to read the writing on the blackboard. After reading the Snellen test card, he said, his eyes and head were rested and he was able to read without any discomfort.

To remove any doubts that might arise as to the cause of the improvement noted in the eyesight of the children, comparative tests were made with and without cards. In one case six pupils with defective sight were examined daily for one week without the use of the test card. No improvement took place. The card was then restored to its place, and the group was instructed to read it every

Must Have Prevented Myopia

day. At the end of a week all had improved and five were cured. In the case of another group of defectives the results were similar. During the week that the card was not used, no improvement was noted ; but after a week of exercises in distant vision with the card all showed marked improvement, and at the end of a month all were cured. In order that there might be no question as to the reliability of the records of the teachers, some of the principals asked the Board of Health to send an inspector to test the vision of the pupils, and whenever this was done the records were found to be correct.

One day I visited the city of Rochester, and while there I called on the Superintendent of Public Schools and told him about my method of preventing myopia. He was very much interested and invited me to introduce it in one of his schools. I did so, and at the end of three months a report was sent to me showing that the vision of all the children had improved, while quite a number of them had obtained normal vision in both eyes.

The method has been used in a number of other cities and always with the same result. The vision of all the children improved, and many of them obtained normal vision in the course of a few minutes, days, weeks, or months.

It is difficult to prove a negative proposition, but since this system improved the vision of all the children who used it, it follows that none could have grown worse. It is therefore obvious that it must have prevented myopia. This cannot be said of any method of preventing myopia in schools which had previously been tried. All other methods are based on the idea that it is the excessive use of the eyes for near work that causes myopia, and all of them have admittedly failed.

It is also obvious that the method must have prevented other errors of refraction, a problem which previously had not even been seriously considered, because hypermetropia is supposed to be congenital, and astigmatism was until recently supposed also to be congenital in the great majority of cases. Anyone who knows how to use a retinoscope may, however, demonstrate in a few minutes that both of these conditions are acquired; for no matter how astigmatic or hypermetropic an eye may be, its vision always becomes normal when it looks at a blank surface without trying to see. It may also be demonstrated that when children are learning to read, write, draw, sew, or to do anything else that necessitates their looking at unfamiliar objects at the near-point, hypermetropia, or hypermetropic astigmatism, is always produced. The same is true of adults. These facts have not been reported before, so far as I am aware, and they strongly suggest that children need, first of all, eye education. They must be able to look at strange letters or objects at the near-point without strain before they can make much progress in their studies, and in every case in which the method has been tried it has been proven that this end is attained by daily exercise in distant vision with the Snellen test card. When their distant vision has been improved by this means, children invariably become able to use their eyes without strain at the near-point.

The method succeeded best when the teacher did not wear glasses. In fact, the effect upon the children of a teacher who wears glasses is so detrimental that no such person should be allowed to be a teacher, and since errors of refraction are curable, such a ruling would work no hardship on anyone. Not only do children imitate the visual habits of a teacher who wears glasses, but the

Why Should Our Children Suffer?

nervous strain of which the defective sight is an expression produces in them a similar condition. In classes of the same grade, with the same lighting, the sight of children whose teachers did not wear glasses has always been found to be better than the sight of children whose teachers did wear them. In one case I tested the sight of children whose teacher wore glasses, and found it very imperfect. The teacher went out of the room on an errand, and after she had gone I tested them again. The results were very much better. When the teacher returned she asked about the sight of a particular boy, a very nervous child, and as I was proceeding to test him she stood before him and said, "Now, when the doctor tells you to read the card, do it." The boy couldn't see anything. Then she went behind him, and the effect was the same as if she had left the room. The boy read the whole card.

Still better results would be obtained if we could reorganize the educational system on a rational basis. Then we might expect a general return of that primitive acuity of vision which we marvel at so greatly when we read about it in the memoirs of travelers. But even under existing conditions it has proven beyond the shadow of a doubt that errors of refraction are no necessary part of the price we must pay for education.

There are at least ten million children in the schools of the United States who have defective sight. This condition prevents them from taking full advantage of the educational opportunities which the State provides. It undermines their health and wastes the taxpayers' money. If allowed to continue, it will be an expense and a handicap to them throughout their lives. In many cases it will be a source of continual misery and suffering. And yet practically all of these cases could be cured and the development of new ones prevented by the daily reading of the Snellen test card.

Why should our children be compelled to suffer and wear glasses for want of this simple measure of relief? It costs practically nothing. In fact, it would not be necessary, in some cases, as in the schools of New York City, even to purchase the Snellen test cards, as they are already being used to test the eyes of the children. Not only does it place practically no additional burden upon the teachers, but, by improving the eyesight, health, disposition and mentality of their pupils, it greatly lightens their labors. No one would venture to suggest, further, that it could possibly do any harm. Why, then, should there be any delay about introducing it into the schools? If there is still thought to be need for further investigation and discussion, we can investigate and discuss just as well after the children get the cards as before, and by adopting that course we shall not run the risk of needlessly condemning another generation to that curse which heretofore has always dogged the footsteps of civilization, namely, defective eyesight. I appeal to all who read these lines to use whatever influence they possess toward the attainment of this end.

DIRECTIONS - FOR USING THE SNELLEN TEST CARD FOR THE PREVENTION AND CURE OF IMPERFECT SIGHT IN SCHOOLS

The Snellen Test Card is placed permanently upon the wall of the classroom, and every day the children silently read the smallest letters they can see from their seats with each eye separately, the other being covered

How to Use the Card

with the palm of the hand in such a way as to avoid pressure on the eyeball. This takes no appreciable amount of time and is sufficient to improve the sight of all children in one week and to cure all errors of refraction after some months, a year, or longer.

Children with markedly defective vision should be encouraged to read the card more frequently. Children wearing glasses should not be interfered with, as they are supposed to be under the care of a physician, and the practice will do them little or no good while the glasses are worn.

While not essential, it is a great advantage to have records made of the vision of each pupil at the time when the method is introduced, and thereafter at convenient intervals annually or more frequently. This may be done by the teacher.

The records should include the name and age of the pupils, the vision of each eye tested at twenty feet, and the date. For example:

John Smith, 10, Sept. 15, 1919
R. V. (vision of the right eye) 20/40
L. V. (vision of the left eye) 20/20
John Smith, 11, January 1, 1920
R. V. 20/30
L. V. 20/15

A certain amount of supervision is absolutely necessary. At least once a year some one who understands the method should visit each classroom for the purpose of answering questions, encouraging the teachers to continue the use of the method, and making some kind of a report to the proper authorities. It is not necessary that either the supervisor, the teachers, or the children should understand anything about the physiology of the eye.

CHAPTER XXVIII

THE STORY OF EMILY

THE efficacy of the method of treating imperfect sight without glasses presented in this book has been demonstrated in thousand of cases, not only in my own practice but in that of many persons of whom I may not even have heard; for almost all patients, when they are cured, proceed to cure others. At a social gathering one evening a lady told me that she had met a number of my patients; but when she mentioned their names I found that I did not remember any of them and said so.

"That is because you cured them by proxy," she said. "You didn't directly cure Mrs. Jones or Mrs. Brown, but you cured Mrs. Smith, and Mrs. Smith cured the other ladies. You didn't treat Mr. and Mrs. Simpkins, or Mr. Simpkins' mother and brother, but you may remember that you cured Mr. Simpkins' boy of a squint, and he cured the rest of the family."

In schools where the Snellen test card was used to prevent and cure imperfect sight, the children, after they were cured themselves, often took to the practice of ophthalmology with the greatest enthusiasm and success, curing their fellow students, their parents and their friends. They made a kind of game of the treatment, and the progress of each school case was watched with the most intense interest by all the children. On a bright day, when the patients saw well, there was great rejoicing, and on a dark day there was corresponding depression. One girl cured twenty-six children in six months; another cured twelve in three months; a third

Apparent Blindness Cured

developed quite a varied ophthalmological practice, and did things of which older and more experienced practitioners might well have been proud. Going to the school which she attended one day, I asked this girl about her sight, which had been very imperfect. She replied that it was now very good and that her headaches were quite gone. I tested her sight and found it normal. Then another child whose sight had also been very poor spoke up.
"I can see all right, too," she said. "Emily" - indicating girl No. 1 - "cured me."
"Indeed!" I replied. "How did she do that?"

The second girl explained that Emily had had her read the card, which she could not see at all from the back of the room, at a distance of a few feet. The next day she had moved it a little farther away, and so on, until the patient was able to read it from the back of the room, just as the other children did. Emily now told her to cover the right eye and read the card with her left, and both girls were considerably upset to find that the uncovered eye was apparently blind. The school doctor was consulted and said that nothing could be done. The eye had been blind from birth and no treatment would do any good.

Nothing daunted, however, Emily undertook the treatment. She told the patient to cover her good eye and go up close to the card, and at a distance of a foot or less it was found that she could read even the small letters. The little practitioner then proceeded confidently as with the other eye, and after many months of practice the patient became the happy possessor of normal vision in both eyes. The case had, in fact, been simply one of high myopia, and the school doctor, not being a specialist, had not detected the difference between this condition and blindness.

In the same classroom there had been a little girl with congenital cataract, but on the occasion of my visit the defect had disappeared. This, too, it appeared, was Emily's doing. The school doctor had said that there was no help for this eye except through operation, and as the sight of the other eye was pretty good, he fortunately did not think it necessary to urge such a course. Emily accordingly took the matter in hand. She had the patient stand close to the card, where, with the good eye covered, she was unable to see even the big C. Emily now held the card between the patient and the light, and moved it back and forth. At a distance of three or four feet this movement could be observed indistinctly by the patient. The card was then moved farther away, until the patient became able to see it move at ten feet and to see some of the larger letters indistinctly at a less distance. Finally, after six months, she became able to read the card with the bad eye as well as with the good one. After testing her sight and finding it normal in both eyes, I said to Emily:
"You are a splendid doctor. You beat them all. Have you done anything else?"
The child blushed, and turning to another of her classmates, said :
"Mamie, come here."
Mamie stepped forward and I looked at her eyes. There appeared to be nothing wrong with them.
"I cured her," said Emily.
"What of?" I inquired.
"Cross eyes," replied Emily.
"How?" I asked, with growing astonishment.
Emily described a procedure very similar to that adopted in the other cases. Finding that the sight of the crossed eye was very poor, so much so, indeed, that poor

An Astonishing Record

Mamie could see practically nothing with it, the obvious course of action seemed to her to be the restoration of its sight; and, never having read any medical literature, she did not know that this was impossible. So she went to it. She had Mamie cover her good eye and practice with the bad one at home and at school, until at last the sight became normal and the eye straight. The school doctor had wanted to have the eye operated upon, I was told, but, fortunately, Mamie was "scared" and would not consent. And here she was with two perfectly good, straight eyes.

"Anything else?" I inquired, when Mamie's case had been disposed of. Emily blushed again, and said: "Here's Rose. Her eyes used to hurt her all the time, and she couldn't see anything on the blackboard. Her headaches used to be so bad that she had to stay away from school every once in a while. The doctor gave her glasses, but they didn't help her and she wouldn't wear them. When you told us the card would help our eyes I got busy with her. I had her read the card close up, and then I moved it farther away, and now she can see all right and her head doesn't ache any more. She comes to school every day, and we all thank you very much."

This was a case of compound hypermetropic astigmatism.

Such stories might be multiplied indefinitely. Emily's astonishing record might not possibly be duplicated, but lesser cures by cured patients have been very numerous, and serve to show that the benefits of the method of preventing and curing defects of vision in the schools which is presented in the foregoing chapter would be far-reaching. Not only errors of refraction would be cured, but many more serious defects; and not only the children would be helped, but their families and friends also.

CHAPTER XXIX
MIND AND VISION

POOR sight is admitted to be one of the most fruitful causes of retardation in the schools. It is estimated[1] that it may reasonably be held responsible for a quarter of the habitually "left-backs," and it is commonly assumed that all this might be prevented by suitable glasses.

There is much more involved in defective vision, however, than mere inability to see the blackboard or to use the eyes without pain or discomfort. Defective vision is the result of an abnormal condition of the mind, and when the mind is in an abnormal condition it is obvious that none of the processes of education can be conducted with advantage. By putting glasses upon a child we may, in some cases, neutralize the effect of this condition upon the eyes, and by making the patient more comfortable may improve his mental faculties to some extent; but we do not alter fundamentally the condition of the mind, and by confirming it in a bad habit we may make it worse.

It can easily be demonstrated that among the faculties of the mind which are impaired when the vision is impaired is the memory; and as a large part of the educational process consists of storing the mind with facts, and all the other mental processes depend upon one's

[1] School Health News, published by the Department of Health of New York City, February, 1919.

Memory in Relation to Vision

knowledge of facts, it is easy to see how little is accomplished by merely putting glasses on a child that has "trouble with its eyes." The extraordinary memory of primitive people has been attributed to the fact that owing to the absence of any convenient means of making written records they had to depend upon their memories, which were strengthened accordingly; but in view of the known facts about the relation of memory to eyesight it is more reasonable to suppose that the retentive memory of primitive man was due to the same cause as his keen vision, namely, a mind at rest.

The primitive memory, as well as primitive keenness of vision, has been found among civilized people; and if the necessary tests had been made it would doubtless have been found that they always occur together, as they did in a case which recently came under my observation. The subject was a child of ten with such marvelous eyesight that she could see the moons of Jupiter with the naked eye a fact which was demonstrated by her drawing a diagram of these satellites which exactly corresponded to the diagrams made by persons who had used a telescope. Her memory was equally remarkable. She could recite the whole content of a book after reading it, as Lord Macaulay is said to have done, and she learned more Latin in a few days without a teacher than her sister, who had six diopters of myopia, had been able to do in several years. She remembered five years afterward what she ate at a restaurant, she called the name of the waiter, the number of the building and the street in which it stood. She also remembered what she wore on this occasion and what every one else in the party wore. The same was true of every other event which had awakened her interest in any way, and it was a favorite amusement in her family to ask her what the menu had been and what people had worn on particular occasions.

When the sight of two persons is different it has been found that their memories differ in exactly the same degree. Two sisters, one of whom had only ordinary good vision, indicated by the formula 20/20, while the other had 20/10, found that the time it took them to learn eight verses of a poem varied in almost exactly the same ratio as their sight. The one whose vision was 20/10 learned eight verses of the poem in fifteen minutes, while the one whose vision was only 20/20 required thirty-one minutes to do the same thing. After palming, the one with ordinary vision learned eight more verses in twenty-one minutes, while the one with 20/10 was able to reduce her time by only two minutes, a variation clearly within the limits of error. In other words, the mind of the latter being already in a normal or nearly normal condition, she could not improve it appreciably by palming, while the former, whose mind was under a strain, was able to gain relaxation, and hence improve her memory, by this means.

Even when the difference in sight is between the two eyes of the same person, it can be demonstrated, as was pointed out in the chapter on "Memory as an Aid to Vision," that there is a corresponding difference in the memory, according to whether both eyes are open, or the better eye closed.

Under the present educational system there is a constant effort to compel the children to remember. These efforts always fail. They spoil both the memory and the sight. The memory cannot be forced any more than the vision can be forced. We remember without effort,

Interest Necessary to Good Vision

just as we see without effort, and the harder we try to remember or see the less we are able to do so.

The sort of things we remember are the things that interest us, and the reason children have difficulty in learning their lessons is because they are bored by them. For the same reason, among others, their eyesight becomes impaired, boredom being a condition of mental strain in which it is impossible for the eye to function normally.

Some of the various kinds of compulsion now employed in the educational process may have the effect of awakening interest. Betty Smith's interest in winning a prize, for instance, or in merely getting ahead of Johnny Jones, may have the effect of rousing her interest in lessons that have hitherto bored her, and this interest may develop into a genuine interest in the acquisition of knowledge ; but this cannot be said of the various fear incentives still so largely employed by teachers. These, on the contrary, have the effect, usually, of completely paralyzing minds already benumbed by lack of interest, and the effect upon the vision is equally disastrous.

The fundamental reason, both for poor memory and poor eyesight in school children, in short, is our irrational and unnatural educational system. Montessori has taught us that it is only when children are interested that they can learn. It is equally true that it is only when they are interested that they can see. This fact was strikingly illustrated in the case of one of the two pairs of sisters mentioned above. Phebe, of the keen eyes, who could recite whole books if she happened to be interested in them, disliked mathematics and anatomy extremely, and not only could not learn them but became myopic when they were presented to her mind. She could read letters a quarter of an inch high at twenty feet in a poor light, but when asked to read figures one to two inches high in a good light at ten feet she miscalled half of them. When asked to tell how much 2 and 3 made she said "4," before finally deciding on "5;" and all the time she was occupied with this disagreeable subject the retinoscope showed that she was myopic. When I asked her to look into my eye with the ophthalmoscope, she could see nothing, although a much lower degree of visual acuity is required to note the details of the interior of the eye than to see the moons of Jupiter.

Shortsighted Isabel, on the contrary, had a passion for mathematics and anatomy and excelled in those subjects. She learned to use the ophthalmoscope as easily as Phebe had learned Latin. Almost immediately she saw the optic nerve, and noted that the center was whiter than the periphery. She saw the light-colored lines, the arteries; and the darker ones, the veins; and she saw the light streaks on the blood-vessels. Some specialists never become able to do this, and no one could do it without normal vision. Isabel's vision, therefore, must have been temporarily normal when she did it. Her vision for figures, although not normal, was better than for letters.

In both these cases the ability to learn and the ability to see went hand in hand with interest. Phebe could read a photographic reduction of the Bible and recite what she had read verbatum, she could see the moons of Jupiter and draw a diagram of them afterwards, because she was interested in these things ; but she could not see the interior of the eye, nor see figures even half as well as she saw letters, because these things bored her. When, however, it was suggested to her that it would be a good

Central Fixation of the Mind

joke to surprise her teachers, who were always reproaching her for her backwardness in mathematics, by taking a high mark in a coming examination, her interest in the subject awakened and she contrived to learn enough to get seventy-eight per cent. In Isabel's case letters were antagonistic. She was not interested in most of the subjects with which they dealt, and therefore she was backward in those subjects and had become habitually myopic. But when asked to look at objects which aroused an intense interest her vision became normal.

When one is not interested, in short, one's mind is not under control, and without mental control one can neither learn nor see. Not only the memory but all other mental faculties are improved when the eyesight becomes normal. It is a common experience with patients cured of defective sight to find that their ability to do their work has improved.

The teacher whose letter is quoted in a later chapter testified that after gaining perfect eyesight she "knew better how to get at the minds of the pupils," was "more direct, more definite, less diffused, less vague," possessed, in fact, "central fixation of the mind." In another letter she said: "The better my eyesight becomes, the greater is my ambition. On the days when my sight is best I have the greatest anxiety to do things."

Another teacher reported that one of her pupils used to sit doing nothing all day long and apparently was not interested in anything. After the test card was introduced into the classroom and his sight improved, he became anxious to learn, and speedily developed into one of the best students in the class. In other words, his eyes and his mind became normal together.

A bookkeeper nearly seventy years of age who had worn glasses for forty years found after he had gained perfect sight without glasses that he could work more rapidly and accurately and with less fatigue than ever in his life before. During busy seasons, or when short of help, he has worked for some weeks at a time from 7 a. m. until 11 p. m., and he insisted that he felt less tired at night after he was through than he did in the morning when he started. Previously, although he had done more work than any other man in the office, it always tired him very much. He also noticed an improvement in his temper. Having been so long in the office, and knowing so much more about the business than his fellow employees, he was frequently appealed to for advice. These interruptions, before his sight became normal, were very annoying to him and often caused him to lose his temper. Afterward, however, they caused him no irritation whatever.

In another case, symptoms of insanity were relieved when the vision became normal. The patient was a physician who had been seen by many nerve and eye specialists before he came to me, and who consulted me at last, not because he had any faith in my methods, but because nothing else seemed to be left for him to do. He brought with him quite a collection of glasses prescribed by different men, no two of them being alike. He had worn glasses, he told me, for many months at a time without benefit, and then he had left them off and had been apparently no worse. Outdoor life had also failed to help him. On the advice of some prominent neurologists he had even given up his practice for a couple of years to spend the time upon a ranch, but the vacation had done him no good.

I examined his eyes and found no organic defects and no error of refraction.

Under Terrific Strain

Yet his vision with each eye was only three-fourths of the normal and he suffered from double vision and all sorts of unpleasant symptoms. He used to see people standing on their heads and little devils dancing on the tops of the high buildings. He also had other illusions too numerous to be mentioned here. At night his sight was so bad that he had difficulty in finding his way about, and when walking along a country road he believed that he saw better when he turned his eyes far to one side and viewed the road with the side of the retina instead of with the center. At variable intervals, without warning and without loss of consciousness, he had attacks of blindness. These caused him great uneasiness, for he was a surgeon with a large and lucrative practice and he feared that he might have an attack while operating.

His memory was very poor. He could not remember the color of the eyes of any member of his family, although he had seen them all daily for years. Neither could he recall the color of his house, the number of rooms on the different floors or other details. The faces and names of patients and friends he recalled with difficulty or not at all.

His treatment proved to be very difficult, chiefly because he had an infinite number of erroneous ideas about physiological optics in general and his own case in particular, and insisted that all these should be discussed; while these discussions were going on he received no benefit. Every day for hours at a time over a long period he talked and argued. His logic was wonderful, apparently unanswerable, and yet utterly wrong.

His eccentric fixation was of such high degree that when he looked at a point forty-five degrees to one side of the big C on the Snellen test card he saw the letter just as black as when he looked directly at it. The strain to do this was terrific and produced much astigmatism; but the patient was unconscious of it and could not be convinced that there was anything abnormal in the symptom. If he saw the letter at all, he argued, he must see it as black at it really was, because he was not colorblind. Finally he became able to look away from one of the smaller letters on the card and see it worse than when he looked directly at it. It took eight or nine months to accomplish this, but when it had been done the patient said that it seemed as if a great burden had been lifted from his mind. He experienced a wonderful feeling of rest and relaxation throughout his whole body.

When asked to remember black with his eyes closed and covered he said he could not do so, and he saw every color but the black which one ought normally to see when the optic nerve is not subject to the stimulus of light. He had, however, been an enthusiastic football player at college, and he found at last that he could remember a black football. I asked him to imagine that this football had been thrown into the sea and that it was being carried outward by the tide, becoming constantly smaller but no less black. This he was able to do, and the strain floated with the football, until, by the time the latter had been reduced to the size of a period in a newspaper, it was entirely gone. The relief continued as long as he remembered the black spot, but as he could not remember it all the time, I suggested another method of gaining permanent relief. This was to make his sight voluntarily worse, a plan against which he protested with considerable emphasis.

"Good heavens!" he said. "Isn't my sight bad enough without making it worse?"

A Problem Not To Be Solved By Glasses

After a week of argument, however, he consented to try the method and the result was extremely satisfactory. After he had learned to see two or more lights where there was only one, by straining to see a point above the light while still trying to see the light as well as when looking directly at it, he became able to avoid the unconscious strain that had produced his double and multiple vision and was not troubled by these superfluous images any more. In a similar manner other illusions were prevented.

One of the last illusions to disappear was his belief that an effort was required to remember black. His logic on this point was overwhelming, but after many demonstrations he was convinced that no effort was required to let go, and when he realized this, both his vision and his mental condition immediately improved.

He finally became able to read 20/10 or more, and although more than fifty-five years of age, he also read diamond type at from six to twenty-four inches. His night blindness was relieved, his attacks of day blindness ceased, and he told me the color of the eyes of his wife and children. One day he said to me :

"Doctor, I thank you for what you have done for my sight, but no words can express the gratiude I feel for what you have done for my mind."

Some years later he called with his heart full of gratitude, because there had been no relapse.

From all these facts it will be seen that the problems of vision are far more intimately associated with the problems of education than we had supposed, and that they can by no means be solved by putting concave, or convex, or astigmatic lenses before the eyes of the children.

CHAPTER XXX
NORMAL SIGHT AND THE RELIEF OF PAIN FOR SOLDIERS AND SAILORS

THE Great War is over and among the millions of brave men who laid down their lives in the cruel conflict there were some who thought that they were doing so that wars might be no more. But the earth is still filled with wars and rumors of war, and in the countries of the victorious Allies the spirit of militarism is rampant. In the United States we are being urged to increase naval and military expenditure, and there is a strong demand for universal military training. Whether it is necessary for us to join in the competition of armaments which resulted in the terrific convulsion through which we have just passed is a question which need not be entered into here ; but if we are going to do so, we may as well have soldiers and sailors with normal sight; and if we attain this end we shall not have borne the burdens of militarism and navalism altogether in vain.

After the United States entered the recent war I had the privilege of making it possible for many young men who had been unable to meet the visual requirements for admission to the army and navy, or to favorite branches of these services, to gain normal vision; and seeing no reason why such benefits should be confined to the few, I supplied the Surgeon General of the Army with a plan whereby, with far less trouble and expense than was involved by the optical service upon which

A Leading Cause of Rejection

we were then depending to make the worst of the enlisted eye-defectives available for service at the front, normal vision without glasses might have been insured to all soldiers and sailors. This plan was not acted upon, and I now present it, with some modifications, to the public, in the hope that enough people will see its military value to secure its adoption.

If we are to have universal military training, we shall find, as the nations of Europe have found, that it will be necessary to take measures to provide suitable material for such training. In Europe this necessity has resulted in extensive systems of child care, but in this book we are concerned only with the question of eyesight. In the first draft for the recent war, defective eyesight was the greatest single cause for rejection, while in later drafts it became one of three leading causes only because of an enormous lowering of an already low standard. Yet there is no impediment to the raising of an army which might be more easily removed. If we want our children to grow big enough to be soldiers, without losing most of their teeth and developing flat feet and crooked spines before they reach the military age, we shall have to make some arrangements, as every one of the advanced countries of Europe has done, for providing material as well as intellectual food in the schools. We shall have to employ school physicians on full time, and pay them enough to compensate men of eminence for the loss of private practice. We shall also have to see that the children are not sacrificed to the ignorance or poverty of their parents before they reach school age. But to preserve their eyesight it is only necessary to place Snellen test cards in every school classroom and see that the children read them every day. With this simple system of eye education beginning in the kindergarten and extending through the whole educational process up to the university and the professional school, it would soon be found that the young men of the country, on arrival at the military age, were practically free from eye defects.

But some years must elapse before this happy result can be achieved; and all eyes, moreover, no matter how good their vision, are benefited by the daily practice of the art of seeing, while by such practice those visual lapses to which every eye is subject, and which are particularly dangerous in military and naval operations, are either prevented or minimized. Therefore a system of eye education for training camps and the front should also be provided. For this purpose the method used in the schools could be modified.

Under conditions of actual warfare, or on the parade grounds of training camps, a Snellen test card might be impracticable, but there are other letters, or small objects, on the uniforms, on the guns, on the wagons, or elsewhere, which would serve the purpose equally well.

Letters or objects which require a vision of 20/20 should be selected by some one who has been taught what 20/20 means, and the men should be required to regard these letters or objects twice a day. After reading the letters they should be directed to cover their closed eyes with the palms of their hands to shut out all the light, and remember some color, preferably black, as well as they are able to see it, for half a minute. Then they should read the letters again and note any improvement in vision. The whole procedure would not take more than a minute. It should be made part of the regular drill, night and morning, and men with imperfect sight

No Soldier Should Wear Glasses

should be encouraged to repeat it as many times a day as convenient. They will need no urging: for imperfect vision is a bar to advancement and excludes from the favorite branch of the service, namely, aviation.

In each regiment every ten men should be under the supervision of one man who understands the method, and who must possess normal vision without glasses. He should carry a pocket test card, consisting of a few of the smaller letters, and should test the vision of the men at the beginning of the training, and thereafter at intervals of three months, reporting the results to the medical officer in charge.

Since errors of refraction are curable, no soldier should be allowed to wear glasses; but if the use of these aids to vision is permitted, the men wearing them should not be required to take part in the eye drills, as the method will do them no good under these conditions. When they see the benefits of eye education, however, they may wish to share them and will, no doubt, be willing to submit to the inconvenience resulting, temporarily, from going without their glasses.

In military colleges the same method could be used as in the schools; but a daily eye drill should also form part of the maneuvers on the parade ground, so that the students may be prepared to use it later in training camps or at the front.

To aviators, whether engaged in military or civilian operations, or whether they are flying merely for pleasure, eye education is of particular importance. Accidents to aviators, otherwise unaccountable, are easily explained when one understands how dependent the aviator is upon his eyesight, and how easily perfect vision may be lost amid the unaccustomed surroundings, the dangers and hardships of the upper air. It was formerly supposed that aviators maintained their equilibrium in the air by the aid of the internal ear; but it is now becoming evident from the testimony of aviators who have found themselves emerging from a cloud with one wing down, or even with their machines turned completely upside down, that equilibrium is maintained almost entirely, if not altogether, by the sense of sight. 1 If the aviator loses his sight, therefore, he is lost, and we have one of those "unaccountable" accidents which, during the war, were so unhappily common in the air service. All aviators, therefore, should make a daily practice of reading small, familiar letters, or observing other small, familiar objects, at a distance of ten feet or more. In addition, they should have a few small letters, or a single letter, on their machines, at a distance of five, ten, or more feet from their eyes, arrangements being made to illuminate them for night flying and fogs, and should read them frequently while in the air. This would greatly lessen the danger of visual lapses with their accompanying loss of equilibrium and judgment.

As has already been pointed out, eye education not only improves the sight, but affords a means by which pain, fatigue, the symptoms of disease and other discomforts can be relieved. For this latter purpose it is of the greatest value to soldiers and sailors; and if, during the recent war, they had only understood the simple and always available method of relieving pain by the aid of the memory, not only much suffering, but many deaths from the destructive effects of pain upon the body might have been prevented. A soldier in a flooded trench, if he can remember black perfectly, will know the temperature of

1 Anderson: Lancet, March 16, 1918, p. 398: Hucks: Scientific American, October 6,1917, 0. 263

Palming Instead of Morphine

the water, but will not suffer from cold. Under the same conditions he may succumb from weakness on the march, but will not feel fatigue. He may die of hemorrhage, but he will die painlessly. It will not be necessary to give him morphine to relieve his pain; and thus to the dangers of the battlefields will not be added the danger of returning to civil life under the handicap of a lifelong morphine habit.

This danger, there is reason to believe, assumed enormous proportions during the war. The Germans used a bullet which broke when it struck the bone and caused intense pain. The men often died of this pain before help arrived. Whey they were rescued the surgeons at once gave them morphine. A few hours later the injection was probably repeated. Then the drug was given less frequently, but in many cases it was not discontinued entirely while the man was in the hospital. A Red Cross surgeon at a meeting of the New York County Medical Society stated that he had been responsible for producing the morphine habit in thousands of soldiers, and that every physician at the front had done the same. By such a simple method as palming all this might have been prevented.

If we are going to have universal military and naval training, an essential part of that training should be the instruction of the prospective soldiers and sailors in the art of relieving their own pain; and in the event of war every one who goes to the front, in whatever capacity, from the generals and admirals down to the ambulance drivers, should understand palming. Everyone in the war zone, no matter how far behind the lines, may need this knowledge to relieve his own pain, and everyone may need it to relieve the pain of others.

CHAPTER XXXI

LETTERS FROM PATIENTS

The following letters have been selected almost at random from the author's mail-bag, and are only specimens of many more that are equally interesting. They are published because it was felt that the personal stories of patients, told in their own language, might be more interesting and helpful to many readers than the more formal presentation of the facts in the preceding chapters.

ARMY OFFICER CURES HIMSELF

AS noted in the chapter on "What Glasses Do to Us," the sight always improves when glasses are discarded, though this improvement may be so slight as not to be noticed. In a few unusual cases, the patients when freed from the handicap of a condition which compels them to keep their eyes continually under a strain, find out, in some way, how to avoid strain, and thus regain a greater or less degree of their normal visual power. The writer of the following letter was able, without any help from anyone, to discover and put into practice the main principles presented in this book, and thus became able to read without his glasses. He is an engineer, and at the time the letter was written was fifty-one years of age. He had worn glasses since 1896, first for astigmatism, getting stronger ones every couple of years, and then for astigmatism and presbyopia. At one time he asked his oculist and several opticians if the eyes could not be strengthened by exercises, so as to

Glasses at the Front

make glasses unnecessary, but they said: "No. Once started on glasses you must keep to them." When the war broke out he was very nearly disqualified for service in the Expeditionary Forces by his eyes, but managed to pass the required tests, after which he was ordered abroad as an officer in the Gas Service. While there he saw in the "Literary Digest" of May 2, 1918, a reference to my method of curing defective eyesight without glasses, and on May 11 he wrote to me in part as follows:

"At the front I found glasses a horrible nuisance, and they could not be worn with gas masks. After I had been about six months abroad I asked an officer of the Medical Corps about going without glasses. He said I was right in my ideas and told me to try it. The first week was awful, but I persisted and only wore glasses for reading and writing. I stopped smoking at the same time to make it easier on my nerves.

"I brought to France two pairs of bow spectacles and two extra lenses for repairs. I have just removed the extra piece for near vision from these extra lenses and had them mounted as pince-nez, with shur-on mounts, to use for reading and writing, so that the only glasses I now use are for astigmatism, the age lens being off. Three months ago I could not read ordinary head-line type in newspapers without glasses. To-day, with a good light, I can read ordinary book type, held at a distance of eighteen inches from my eyes. Since the first week in February, when I discarded my glasses, I have had no headaches, stomach trouble, or dizziness, and am in good health generally. My eyes are coming back, and I believe it is due to sticking it out. I ride considerably in automobiles and trams, and somehow the idea has crept into my mind that after every trip my eyes are stronger. This, I think, is due to the rapid changing of focus in viewing scenery going by so fast. Other men have tried this plan on my advice, but gave it up after two or three days. Yet, from what they say, I believe they were not so uncomfortable as I was for a week or ten days. I believe most people wear glasses because they 'coddle' their eyes."

The patient was right in thinking that the motor and tram rides improved his sight. The rapid motion compelled rapid shifting.

A TEACHER'S EXPERIENCES

It has frequently been pointed out in this book that imperfect vision is always associated with an abnormal state of the mind, and that when the vision improves the mental faculties improve also, to a greater or lesser degree. The following letter is a striking illustration of this fact. The writer, a teacher forty years of age, was first treated on March 28, 1919. She was wearing the following glasses: right eye, convex 0.75D.S. with convex 4.00D.C., 105 deg.; left eye, convex 0.75D.S. with convex 3.50D.C., 105 deg. On June 9, 1919, she wrote:

"I will tell you about my eyes, but first let me tell you other things. You were the first to unfold your theories to me, and I found them good immediately - that is, I was favorably impressed from the start. I did not take up the cure because other people recommended it, but because I was convinced : first, that you believed in your discovery yourself ; second, that your theory of the cause of eye trouble was true. I don't know how I knew these two things, but I did. After a little conversation with you, you and your discovery both seemed to me to bear

Enjoys Her Sight

the ear-marks of the genuine article. As to the success of the method with myself I had a little doubt. You might cure others, but you might not be able to cure me. However, I took the plunge, and it has made a great change in me and my life.

"To begin with, I enjoy my sight. I love to look at things, to examine them in a leisurely, thorough way, much as a child examines things. I never realized it at the time, but it was irksome for me to look at things when I was wearing glasses, and I did as little of it as possible. The other day, going down on the Sandy Hook boat, I enjoyed a most wonderful sky without that hateful barrier of misted glasses, and I am positive I distinguished delicate shades of color that I never would have been able to see, even with clear glasses. Things seem to me now to have more form, more reality, than when I wore glasses. Looking into the mirror you see a solid representation on a flat surface, and the flat glass can't show you anything really solid. My eyeglasses, of course, never gave me this impression, but one curiously like it. I can see so clearly without them that it is like looking around corners without changing the position. I feel that I can almost do it.

"I very seldom have occasion to palm. Once in a great while I feel the necessity of it. The same with remembering a period. Nothing else is ever necessary. I seldom think of my eyes, but at times it is borne in upon me how much I do use and enjoy using them.

"My nerves are much better. I am more equable, have more poise, I am less shy. I never used to show that I was shy, or lacked confidence. I used to go ahead and do what was required, if not without hesitation; but it was hard. Now I find it easy. Glasses, or poor sight rather, made me self-conscious. It certainly is a great defect, and one people are sensitive to without realizing it. I mean the poor sight and the necessity for wearing glasses. I put on a pair of glasses the other day just for an experiment, and I found that they magnified things. My skin looked as if under a magnifying glass. Things seemed too near. The articles on my chiffonier looked so close I felt like pushing them away from me. The glasses I especially wanted to push away. They brought irritation at once. I took them off and felt peaceful. Things looked normal.

"From the beginning of the treatment I could use my eyes pretty well, but they used to tire. I remember making a large Liberty Loan poster two weeks after I took off my glasses, and I was amazed to find I could make the whole layout almost perfectly without a ruler, just as well as with my glasses. When I came to true it up with the ruler I found only the last row of letters a bit out of line at the very end. I couldn't have done better with glasses. However, this wasn't fine work. About the same time I sewed a hem at night in a black dress, using a fine needle. I suffered a little for this, but not much. I used to practice my exercises at that time, and palm faithfully. Now I don't have to practice, or palm; I feel no discomfort, and I am absolutely unsparing in my use of my eyes. I do everything I want to with them. I shirk nothing, pass up no opportunity of using them. From the first I did all my school work, read every notice, wrote all that was necessary, neglected nothing.

"Now to sum up the school end of it: I used to get headaches at the end of the month from adding columns of figures necessary to reports, etc. Now I do not get them. I used to get flustered when people came into my room.

Central Fixation of the Mind

Now I do not ; I welcome them. It is a pleasant change to feel this way. And - I suppose this is most important really, though I think of it last - I teach better. I know how to get at the mind and how to make the children see things in perspective. I gave a lesson on the horizontal cylinder recently, which, you know, is not a thrillingly interesting subject, and it was a remarkable lesson in its results and in the grip it got on every girl in the room, stupid or bright. What you have taught me makes me use the memory and imagination more, especially the latter, in teaching.

"To sum up the effect of being cured upon my own mind : I am more direct, more definite, less diffused, less vague. In short, I am conscious of being better centered. It is central fixation of the mind. I saw this in your latest paper, but I realized it long ago and knew what to call it."

A MENTAL TRANSITION

A man of forty-four who had worn glasses since the age of twenty was first seen on October 8, 1917, when he was suffering, not only from very imperfect sight, but from headache and discomfort. He was wearing for the right eye concave 5.00D.S. with concave 0.50D.C., 180 degrees, and for the left concave 2.50D.S. with concave 1.50D.C., 180 degrees. As his visits were not very frequent and he often went back to his glasses, his progress was slow. But his pain and discomfort were relieved very quickly, and almost from the beginning he had flashes of greatly improved and even of normal vision. This encouraged him to continue, and his progress, though slow, was steady. He has now gone without his glasses entirely for some months, and his nervous condition has improved as much as his sight. His wife was particularly impressed with the latter effect, and in December, 1919, she wrote:

"I have become very much interested in the thought of renewing my youth by becoming like a little child. The idea of the mental transition is not unfamiliar, but that this mental, or I should say spiritual, transition should produce a physical effect, which would lead to seeing clearly, is a sort of miracle very possible indeed, I should suppose, to those who have faith.

"In my husband's case, certainly some such miracle was wrought; for not only was he able to lay aside his spectacles after many years' constant use, and to see to read in almost any light, but I particularly noticed his serenity of mind after treatments. In this serenity he seemed able to do a great deal of work efficiently, and not under the high nervous pressure whose after-effect is the devastating scattering of forces.

"It did not occur to me for a long time that perhaps your treatment was quieting his nerves. But I think now that the quiet periods of relaxation, two or three times a day, during which he practiced with the letter card, must have had a very beneficial effect. He is so enthusiastic by nature, and his nerves are so easily stimulated, that for years he used to overdo periodically. Of course, his greatly improved eyesight and the relief from the former strain must have been a large factor in this improvement. But I am inclined to think that the intervals of quiet and peace were wonderfully beneficial, and why shouldn't they be? We are living on stimulants, physical stimulants, mental stimulants of all kinds. The minute these stop we feel we are merely existing, and yet, if we retain any of the normality of our youth, do you not think that we respond very happily to natural simple things?"

Relaxation Versus Glasses
RELIEF AFTER TWENTY-FIVE YEARS

While many persons are benefited by the accepted methods of treating defects of vision, there is a minority of cases, known to every eye specialist, which gets little or no help from them. These patients sometimes give up the search for relief in despair, and sometimes continue it with surprising pertinacity, never being able to abandon the belief, in spite of the testimony of experience, that somewhere in the world there must be some one with sufficient skill to fit them with the right glasses. The rapidity with which these patients respond to treatment by relaxation is often very dramatic, and affords a startling illustration of the superiority of this method to treatment by glasses and muscle-cutting. In the following case relaxation did in twenty-four hours what the old methods, as practiced by a succession of eminent specialists, could not do in twenty-five years.

The patient was a man of forty-nine, and his imperfect sight was accompanied by continual pain and misery, culminating twenty years before I saw him, in a complete nervous breakdown. As he was a writer, dependent upon his pen for a living, his condition was a serious economic handicap, and he consulted many specialists in the vain hope of obtaining relief. Glasses did little either to improve his sight, or to relieve his discomfort, and the eye specialists talked vaguely about disease of the optic nerve and brain as a possible cause of his troubles. The nerve specialists, however, were unable to do anything to relieve him. One specialist diagnosed his case as muscular, and gave him prisms, which helped him a little. Later, the same specialist, finding that all of the apparent muscular trouble was not corrected by glasses, cut the external muscles of both eyes. This also brought some relief, but not much. At the age of twenty-nine the patient suffered the nervous breakdown already mentioned. For this he was treated unsuccessfully by various specialists, and for nine years he was compelled to live out of doors. This life, although it benefited him, failed to restore his health, and when he came to me on September 13, 1919, he was still suffering from neurasthenia. His distant vision was less than 20/40, and could not be improved by glasses. He was able to read with glasses, but could not do so without discomfort. I could find no symptom of disease of the brain or of the interior of the eye. When he tried to palm he saw grey and yellow instead of black ; but he was able to rest his eyes simply by closing them, and by this means alone he became able, in twenty-four hours, to read diamond type and to make out most of the letters on the twenty line of the test card at twenty feet. At the same time his discomfort was materially relieved. He was under treatment for about six weeks, and on October 25 he wrote as follows :

"I saw you last on October 6, and at the end of the week, the 11th, I started off on a ten-day motor trip as one of the officials of the Cavalry Endurance Test for horses. The last touch of eyestrain which affected me nervously at all I experienced on the 8th and 9th. On the trip, though I averaged but five hours' sleep, rode all day in an open motor without goggles and wrote reports at night by bad lights, I had no trouble. After the third day the universal slow swing seemed to establish itself, and I have never had a moment's discomfort since. I stood fatigue and excitement better than I have ever

Out of the Woods

done, and went with less sleep. My practicing on the trip was necessarily somewhat curtailed, yet there was noticeable improvement in my vision. Since returning I have spent a couple of hours a day in practice, and have at the same time done a lot of writing.

"Yesterday, the 24th, I made a test with diamond type, and found that after twenty minutes' practice I could get the lines distinct, and make out the capital letters and bits of the text at a scant three inches. At seven I could read it readily, though I could not see it perfectly. This was by an average daylight - no sun. In a good daylight I can read the newspaper almost perfectly at a normal reading distance, say fifteen inches.

"I feel now that I am really out of the woods. I have done night work without suffering for it, a thing I have not done in twenty-five years, and I have worked steadily for more hours than I have been able to work at a time since my breakdown in 1899, all without sense of strain or nervous fatigue. You can imagine my gratitude to you. Not only for my own sake, but for yours, I shall leave no stone unturned to make the cure complete and get back the child eyes which seem perfectly possible in the light of the progress I have made in eight weeks."

SEEKING A MYOPIA CURE

In spite of the emphasis with which the medical profession denies the possibility of curing errors of refraction, there are many lay persons who refuse to believe that they are incurable. The author of the following statement represents a considerable class, and was remarkable only in the persistency with which he searched for relief. He was first seen on June 27, 1919, at which time he was thirty-two years of age. He was wearing concave 2.50D.S. for each eye, and his vision in each eye was 20/100. After he had obtained almost normal vision he wrote the following account of his experiences for "Better Eyesight":

"When the 'Lusitania' was sunk I knew that the United States was going to get into trouble, and I wanted to be in a position to join the Army. But I was suffering from a high degree of myopia, and I knew they wouldn't take me with glasses. Later on they took almost anyone who wasn't blind, but at that time I couldn't possibly have measured up to the standard. So I began to look about for a cure. I tried osteopathy, but didn't go very far with it. I asked the optician who had been fitting me with glasses for advice, but he said that myopia was incurable. I dismissed the matter for a time, but I didn't stop thinking about it. I am a farmer, and I knew from the experience of outdoor life that health is the normal condition of living beings. I knew that when health is lost it can often be regained. I knew that when I first tried to lift a barrel of apples onto a wagon I could not do so, but that after a little practice I became able to do it easily, and I did not see why, if one part of the body could be strengthened by exercise, others could not be strengthened also. I could remember a time when I was not myopic, and it seemed to me that if a normal eye could become myopic, it ought to be possible for a myopic eye to regain normality. After a while I went back to the optician and told him that I was convinced that there must be some cure for my condition. He replied that this was quite impossible, as everyone knew that myopia was incurable. The assurance with which he made this statement had an effect upon me quite the opposite of what he intended, for when he said that the cure of

It Ought To Be Possible

myopia was impossible I knew that it was not, and I resolved never to give up the search for a cure until I found it. Shortly after I had the good fortune to hear of Dr. Bates, and lost no time in going to see him. At the first visit I was able, just by closing and resting my eyes, to improve my sight considerably for the Snellen test card, and after a few months of intermittent treatment I became able to read 20/10 - in flashes. I am still improving, and when I can see a little better I mean to go back to that optician and tell him what I think of his ophthalmological learning."

FACTS VERSUS THEORIES

Reading fine print is commonly supposed to be an extremely dangerous practice, and reading print of any kind upon a moving vehicle is thought to be even worse. Looking away to the distance, however, and not seeing anything in particular is believed to be very beneficial to the eyes. In the light of these superstitions, the facts contained in the following letter are particularly interesting :

"On reaching home Monday morning I was surprised and pleased at the comments of my family regarding the appearance of my eyes. They all thought they looked so much brighter and rested, and that after two days of railroading. I didn't spare my eyes in the least on the way home. I read magazines and newspapers, looked at the scenery; in fact, used my eyes all the time. My sight for the near-point is splendid. Can read for hours without tiring my eyes. ... I went downtown today and my eyes were very tired when I got home. The fine print on the card [diamond type] helps me so... I would like to have your little Bible [a photographic reduction of the Bible with type much smaller than diamond]. I'm sure the very fine print has a soothing effect on one's eyes, regardless of what my previous ideas on the subject were."

It will be observed that the eyes of this patient were not tired by her two days' railroad journey, during which she read constantly; they were not tired by hours of reading after her return ; they were rested by reading extremely fine print; but they were very much tired by a trip downtown during which they were not called upon to focus upon small objects. Later a leaf from the Bible was sent to her, and she wrote:

"The effect even of the first effort to read it was wonderful. If you will believe it, I haven't been troubled having my eyes feel 'crossed' since, and while my actual vision does not seem to be any better, my eyes feel a great deal better."

CURED WITHOUT PERSONAL ASSISTANCE

I am constantly hearing of patients who have been able to improve their sight by the aid of information contained in my publications, without personal assistance. The writer of the following letter, a physician, is a remarkable example of these cases, as he was able not only to cure himself, but to relieve some very serious cases of defective vision among his patients.

"I first tried central fixation on myself and had marvelous results. I threw away my glasses and can now see better than I have ever done. I read very fine type (smaller than newspaper type) at a distance of six inches from the eyes, and can run it out at full arm's length and still read it without blurring the type.

Cataract Relieved

"I have instructed some of my patients in your methods, and all are getting results. One case who has a partial cataract of the left eye could not see anything on the Snellen test card at twenty feet, and could see the letters only faintly at ten feet. Now she can read 20/10 with both eyes together, and also with each eye separately; but the left eye seems, as she says, to be looking through a little fog. I could cite many other cases that have been benefited by central fixation, but this one is the most interesting to me."

CHAPTER XXXII
REASON AND AUTHORITY

SOME one - perhaps it was Bacon - has said: "You cannot by reasoning correct a man of ill opinion which by reasoning he never acquired." He might have gone a step further and stated that neither by reasoning, nor by actual demonstration of the facts, can you convince some people that an opinion which they have accepted on authority is wrong.

A man whose name I do not care to mention, a professor of ophthalmology, and a writer of books well known in this country and in Europe, saw me perform the experiment illustrated on Page 40, (Accommodation: Experiments on Animals) an experiment which, according to others who witnessed it, demonstrates beyond any possibility of error that the lens is not a factor in accommodation. At each step of the operation he testified to the facts; yet at the conclusion he preferred to discredit the evidence of his senses rather than accept the only conclusion that these facts admitted.

First he examined the eye of the animal to be experimented upon, with the retinoscope, and found it normal, and the fact was written down. Then the eye was stimulated with electricity, and he testified that it accommodated. This was also written down. I now divided the superior oblique muscle, and the eye was again stimulated with electricity. The doctor observed the eye with the retinoscope when this was being done and said: "You failed to produce accommodation." This fact, too, was written down. The doctor now used the electrode himself, but again failed to observe accommodation, and

Discredited His Own Observations

these facts were written down. I now sewed the cut ends of the muscle together, and once more stimulated the eye with electricity. The doctor said, "Now you have succeeded in producing accommodation," and this was written down. I now asked:

"Do you think that superior oblique had anything to do with producing accommodation?"
"Certainly not," he replied.
"Why?" I asked.
"Well," he said, "I have only the testimony of the retinoscope; I am getting on in years, and I don't feel that confidence in my ability to use the retinoscope that I once had. I would rather you wouldn't quote me on this."

While the operation was in progress, however, he gave no indication whatever of doubting his ability to use the retinoscope. He was very positive, in fact, that I had failed to produce accommodation after the cutting of the oblique muscle, and his tone suggested that he considered the failure ignominious. It was only after he found himself in a logical trap, with no way out except by discrediting his own observations, that he appeared to have any doubts as to their value.

Patients whom I have cured of various errors of refraction have frequently returned to specialists who had prescribed glasses for them, and, by reading fine print and the Snellen test card with normal vision, have demonstrated the fact that they were cured, without in any way shaking the faith of these practitioners in the doctrine that such cures are impossible.

The patient with progressive myopia whose case was mentioned in Chapter XV returned after her cure to the specialist who had prescribed her glasses, and who had said not only that there was no hope of improvement, but that the condition would probably progress until it ended in blindness, to tell him the good news which, as an old friend of her family, she felt he had a right to hear. But while he was unable to deny that her vision was, in fact, normal without glasses, he said it was impossible that she should have been cured of myopia, because myopia was incurable. How he reconciled this statement with his former patient's condition he was unable to make clear to her.

A lady with compound myopic astigmatism suffered from almost constant headaches which were very much worse when she took her glasses off. The theatre and the movies caused her so much discomfort that she feared to indulge in these recreations. She was told to take off her glasses and advised, among other things, to go to the movies ; to look first at the corner of the screen, then off to the dark, then back to the screen a little nearer to the center, and so forth. She did so, and soon became able to look directly at the pictures without discomfort. After that nothing troubled her. One day she called on her former ophthalmological adviser, in the company of a friend who wanted to have her glasses changed, and told him of her cure. The facts seemed to make no impression on him whatever. He only laughed and said, "I guess Dr. Bates is more popular with you than I am."

Sometimes patients themselves, after they are cured, allow themselves to be convinced that it was impossible that such a thing could have happened, and go back to their glasses. This happened in the case of a patient already mentioned in the chapter on "Presbyopia," who was cured in fifteen minutes by the aid of his imagination. He was very grateful for a time, and then he began to talk to eye specialists whom he knew and straightway grew skeptical as to the value of what I had done for him.

Discredited His Own Experience

One day I met him at the home of a mutual friend, and in the presence of a number of other people he accused me of having hypnotized him, adding that to hypnotize a patient without his knowledge or consent was to do him a grievous wrong. Some of the listeners protested that whether I had hypnotized him or not, I had not only done him no harm but had greatly benefited him, and he ought to forgive me. He was unable, however, to take this view of the matter. Later he called on a prominent eye specialist who told him that the presbyopia and astigmatism from which he had suffered were incurable, and that if he persisted in going without his glasses he might do himself great harm. The fact that his sight was perfect for the distance and the near-point without glasses had no effect upon the specialist, and the patient allowed himself to be frightened into disregarding it also. He went back to his glasses, and so far as I know has been wearing them ever since. The story obtained wide publicity, for the man had a large circle of friends and acquaintances; and if I had destroyed his sight I could scarcely have suffered more than I did for curing him.

Fifteen or twenty years ago the specialist mentioned in the foregoing story read a paper on cataract at a meeting of the ophthalmological section of the American Medical Association in Atlantic City, and asserted that anyone who said that cataract could be cured without the knife was a quack. At that time I was assistant surgeon at the New York Eye and Ear Infirmary, and it happened that I had been collecting statistics of the spontaneous cure of cataract at the request of the executive surgeon of this institution, Dr. Henry G. Noyes, Professor of Ophthalmology at the Bellevue Hospital Medical School. As a result of my inquiry, I had secured records of a large numher of cases which had recovered, not only without the knife, but without any treatment at all. I also had records of cases which I had sent to Dr. James E. Kelly of New York and which he had cured, largely by hygienic methods. Dr. Kelly is not a quack, and at that time was Professor of Anatomy in the New York Post Graduate Medical School and Hospital and attending surgeon to a large city hospital. In the five minutes allotted to those who wished to discuss the paper, I was able to tell the audience enough about these cases to make them want to hear more. My time was, therefore, extended, first to half an hour and then to an hour. Later both Dr. Kelly and myself received many letters from men in different parts of the country who had tried his treatment with success. The man who wrote the paper had blundered, but he did not lose any prestige because of my attack, with facts upon his theories. He is still a prominent and honored ophthalmologist, and in his latest book he gives no hint of having ever heard of any successful method of treating cataract other than by operation. He was not convinced by my record of spontaneous cures, nor by Dr. Kelly's record of cures by treatment; and while a few men were sufficiently impressed to try the treatment recommended, and while they obtained satisfactory results, the facts made no impression upon the profession as a whole, and did not modify the teaching of the schools. That spontaneous cures of cataract do sometimes occur cannot be denied; but they are supposed to be very rare, and any one who suggests that the condition can be cured by treatment still exposes himself to the suspicion of being a quack.

Between 1886 and 1891 I was a lecturer at the Post- Graduate Hospital and Medical School. The head of the institution was Dr. D. B. St. John Roosa. He was the

Man Not a Reasoning Being

author of many books, and was honored and respected by the whole medical profession. At the school they had got the habit of putting glasses on the nearsighted doctors, and I had got the habit of curing them without glasses. It was naturally annoying to a man who had put glasses on a student to have him appear at a lecture without them and say that Dr. Bates had cured him. Dr. Roosa found it particularly annoying, and the trouble reached a climax one evening at the annual banquet of the faculty when, in the presence of one hundred and fifty doctors, he suddenly poured out the vials of his wrath upon my head. He said that I was injuring the reputation of the Post Graduate by claiming to cure myopia. Every one knew that Donders said it was incurable, and I had no right to claim that I knew more than Donders. I reminded him that some of the men I had cured had been fitted with glasses by himself. He replied that if he had said they had myopia he had made a mistake. I suggested further investigation. "Fit some more doctors with glasses for myopia," I said, "and I will cure them. It is easy for you to examine them afterwards and see if the cure is genuine." This method did not appeal to him, however. He repeated that it was impossible to cure myopia, and to prove that it was impossible he expelled me from the Post Graduate, even the privilege of resignation being denied to me.

The fact is that, except in rare cases, man is not a reasoning being. He is dominated by authority, and when the facts are not in accord with the view imposed by authority, so much the worse for the facts. They may, and indeed must, win in the long run; but in the meantime the world gropes needlessly in darkness and endures much suffering that might have been avoided.

INDEX

Accommodation, 10, 26 (see also "Aphakia," "Myopia," "Presbyopia")
Arlt on, 29
Author on, 38, 54, 69
Brücke on, 29
Cohn on, 29
Cramer on, 25
Davis on, 33
Descartes on, 24
Donders on, 24, 29, 32, 38, 210, 211
Duane on, 211
Förster on, 32
Fuchs on, 211
von Graefe on, 32
Helmholtz on, 24, 26, 32
Hensen on, 29
Holmes on, 212
Huxley on, 29
Jackson on, 211
Kepler on, 23
Landolt on, 26
Langenbeck on, 24
Loring on, 33
Roosa on, 210
Sanson on, 29
Scheiner on, 24
Tscherning on, 27
de Schweinitz on, 36, 211
Völckers on, 29
Young on, 24, 30
Ainus, 16
Amblyopia, 111, 113 (see also "Squint")
Anisometropes, 256
Aphakia, 32, 47, 95, 96
Arlt, 29
  portrait, frontispiece

Armati, v, 81
Astigmatism, 12, 70, 149, 251
  prevention, 251, 265
  production, 12, 36, 39, 42, 43, 45, 89, 266, 282
  treatment, 229, 234, 273, 306 (see also "Refraction, errors of, treatment")
Atropine, 43, 48, 50, 69, 228, 234
Aviators, 287

Barrington, 256
Bell, 184
Brücke, 29

Camera, 13, 114, 149
Cataract, 89, 111, 214, 220
  treatment, 121, 134, 158, 272, 307
Central fixation, 114, 281
Christian Scientists, 209
Cohn, 29, 78, 251, 252, 253, 254
Colds, 208
Conjunctiva, 111, 118, 122
Cornea, 12, 36, 122 (see also "Images, on cornea")
Correspondence treatment, 246
Coughs, 208
Cramer, 25

Darkness, 189
Davis, 33
Descartes, 24
Donders, 23, 24, 25, 29, 32, 38, 210, 211, 222, 223
Dresslar, 190
Duane, 211, 225

Index

Myopia, 8, 10, 222 (see also "Accommodation")
Barrington on, 256
Cohn on, 251, 252, 253, 254
Donders on, 309
Eversbusch on, 252
Fox on, 256
Just on, 254
Lawson on, 255
Motais on, 256
Pearson on, 256
prevention, 8, 39, 251, 259
production, 2, 11, 14, 39, 63, 65, 75, 89, 109, 257
Risley on, 253
Roosa on, 308
Sidler-Huguenin on, 8, 82, 256
Steiger on, 256
  treatment, 8, 82, 120, 141, 157, 158, 170, 251, 259, 271, 299 (see also "Refraction, errors of, treatment")
Tscherning on, 252

Neuralgia, 207
Night blindness, 281, 283
Nystagmus, 117

Ophthalmology, 1, 214
Ophthalmometer, 34, 60, 66
Ophthalmoscope, 23, 117, 160
Optic nerve, 89, 108, 111, 112, 122, 127, 157
Optimums, 198

Pain, 133, 155, 202, 288
Palming, 123 (see also "Memory")
Paralysis, 131
Parsons, 184
Patagonians, 2
Pearson, 256
Pessimums, 198
Pigmies, 3
Polyopia, 112, 149, 174, 178, 179, 283
Presbyopia, 210

Pupil, 190, 214
Purkinje, 24, 25

Ray, 37
Reading, 192
Refraction, errors of (see also "Astigmatism," "Hypermetropia," "Myopia")
  cause, 1, 14, 89, 106 (see also "production")
  occurrence, 5, 75, 98, 251, 267, 285
  prevention, 1, 245, 285, 288
  production, 14, 38, 62, 75, 89, 106, 114
  treatment, 1, 101, 112, 118, 123, 136, 148, 159, 183, 242, 246, 259, 270, 274
Refraction, variability of, 10, 75, 85, 213, 215, 286, 287
Relaxation (see "Refraction, errors of, treatment")
Retina, 89, 109, 111, 114, 220
Retinoscope, 17, 110, 137
Rheumatism, 208
Risley, 253
Roosa, 210, 308
Rosenau, 4

Sanson, 29
Saturn, rings of, 121
Scheiner, 24
School-books, 192, 253
de Schweinitz, 36, 211
Sclera (see "Images, on sclera")
Scotomata, 177, 185, 186
Scott, 4
Sense, nerves of, 108
Shifting, 159
Sidler-Huguenin, 8, 82, 256
Snellen, 19
Snellen, jr., 69
Snellen test card, 19, 200, 242, 244, 268, 287
Soldiers and sailors, 5, 284
Squint, 112, 117, 118, 221, 227, 272
Steiger, 256
Stevens, 222

Index

Eccentric fixation (see "Central fixation")
Emmetropia, 11, 93
Eversbusch, 222, 252
Eye, 11, 13
  evolution of, 1
  muscles of, 38, 44
  retina of, 114
  unable to fix a point, 159

Fabre, 102
Face-rests, 253, 254
Faith Curists, 209
Förster, 32
Fovea, 114
Fox, 256
Fuchs, 211, 222, 225

Gislason, 227
Glasses, v, 8, 81, 181, 219
Glaucoma, 111
  treatment, 121, 133, 208
Gould, 4
von Graefe, 32

Hansen-Grut, 222
Hay fever, 208
Helmholtz, 24, 26, 32, 36, 38
  portrait, 31
Hensen, 29
Holmes, 212
Home treatment, 242
Huxley, 29
Hypermetropia, 10, 222, 251, 266
  prevention, 251, 266
  production, 14, 39, 42, 53, 63, 65, 66, 75, 89, 266
  treatment, 229, 234, 273 (see also "Refraction, errors of, treatment")

Illusions,
  of imperfect sight, 148, 172, 219, 280, 282
  of normal sight, 138, 172, 180

Images, 24, 54
  on cornea, 24, 54, 59, 60, 64, 66, 68
  on iris, 59, 63, 65
  on lens (back of), 24, 54, 62, 67
  on lens (front of), 24, 54
  on sclera, 59, 62, 63, 64
Imagination, 148, 165, 217
Indians, 2, 15, 256
Insanity, 280
Iritis, 121, 122

Jackson, 211
Johnson, 37
Jupiter, moons of, 103, 121, 275
Just, 254

Kelly, 308
Kepler, 23

Lancaster, 83
Landolt, 23, 26, 86
Langenbeck, 24
Lawson, 255
Lens (see "Accommodation," "Cataract," "Images," "Presbyopia")
Light, 78, 123, 183, 253, 261
Loring, 33

Macaulay, 275
Macula, 114
Memory, 126, 136, 151, 202, 274
Military training, 284
Mind, 89, 106, 115, 148, 196, 274, 295 (see also "Memory")
Montessori, 106
Moros, 6
Morphine, 289
Motais, 256
Moving pictures, 108, 161, 192
Muscae volitantes, 176, 236
Muscle, ciliary, 11, 29, 75, 85, 211, 215 (see also "Atropine")
Muscles, external, 32, 37, 38, 89

Index

Strain, 89, 106, 115, 172, 178, 192, 257
Swinging, 159

Truth, 74
Tscherning, 27, 30, 252

Verhoeff, 184
Vision, defects of, 4, 264 (see also "Refraction, errors of, occurrence;" "Refraction, variability of")
  limits of, 104, 121
  military standards of, 5

Vision, primitive, 1, 2, 3, 6, 15, 16, 121, 267, 275
  standard of normal, 19, 123
Visual centers, 108, 123
Völckers, 29

Webster, 35
Whooping cough, 208
Woinow, 33
Worth, 222, 223, 225

Young, Dr. A. G., 193
Young, Dr. Thomas, 24, 30
  portrait, 28

Index Page Numbers are for the Antique copy of this book. Free in PDF E-Book. Contact; mclearsight@aol.com - www.cleareyesight.info

Better Eyesight Magazine by William H. Bates, M. D.

Ophthalmologist - Eye, Ear, Nose & Throat

Central-Fixation Publishing Co.,
New York City, New York, USA

Original Antique Magazine Pages

Ophthalmologist William H. Bates

This E-book contains Photo-Copies of the <u>Original</u> printed pages of 'Better Eyesight Magazine' written and published by Ophthalmologist William H. Bates and his assistant/wife Emily C. A. Lierman/Bates. 11 Years - All 132 Monthly Magazine Issues; July 1919 to June 1930. A History Book, Antique Collection.

Dr. Bates discovered the natural principles, true function of the eyes (Visual System) and applied relaxation, natural methods to return the eyes, eye muscles, nerves, mind/brain, body to normal function with clear vision and healthy eyes. **The Bates Method**.

Emily C. Lierman, Bates

The Stories, articles in Better Eyesight Magazine describe how Dr. Bates, Emily Lierman Bates, other Doctors, School Teachers, Bates Method Students/Teachers, Children and Parents used Natural Treatments to prevent, remove many different eye problems without use of eyeglasses, surgery, drugs; unclear close and distant vision, astigmatism, cataracts, glaucoma, conical cornea, cornea scars, wandering and crossed eyes (Strabismus, Squint) and other conditions. Hundreds of Natural Treatments are listed. Dr. Bates used surgery only when necessary.

Better Eyesight Magazine consists of articles that are interesting, positive, fun to read. 'True Life Stories' of the doctors, patients, adults and children. Vision improvement based 'Fairy Stories' and other articles for children are included.

The magazines, books are the original source of Natural Eyesight (Vision) Improvement. The Original Better Eyesight Magazine collection is proof that Ophthalmologist William H. Bates discovered the Bates Method, Natural Eyesight Improvement and is the True Author of the Magazine.

Dr. Bates discovered Natural Eyesight Improvement over 100 years ago. The Optical and Medical Industry/Association and most Eye Doctors, Opticians have hidden Dr. Bates magazines, books, articles, Natural Eyesight Improvement from the public for over 100 years because: The writings are proof that Natural Eyesight Improvement works, produces clear vision, healthy eyes, it teaches people how to obtain clear vision '<u>on their own</u>' and prevents the need for purchasing eyeglasses, contact lenses, sunglasses, eye surgery and drugs.

Due to the truth about Natural Medicine becoming available to the modern public, Dr. Bates work has been recovered from individual owners and re-published. Many modern Ophthalmologists, Optometrists are now learning, teaching the Bates Method.

Cataract Number

Better Eyesight

A MONTHLY MAGAZINE DEVOTED TO THE PREVENTION AND CURE OF IMPERFECT SIGHT WITHOUT GLASSES

Vol. IV   JANUARY 1921   No. 1

The Treatment of Cataract
A Report of a Case

Cataract: Its Cause and Cure
By W. H. Bates, M.D.

Traumatic Cataract Disappears
By Margaret Downie

Incipient Cataract Relieved
By C. L. Steenson, M.D.

Cataract at the Clinic
By Emily C. Lierman

$2.00 per year   20 cents per copy

Published by the CENTRAL FIXATION PUBLISHING COMPANY
342 WEST 42nd STREET   NEW YORK, N. Y.

Original Antique Better Eyesight Magazine and a modern copy with 500 Pictures is free in color
PDF E-book download from the website and in paperback. Hard cover published in the future.

The 8 Correct Vision Habits, (natural, normal, relaxed eye, visual system function): Shifting, Central-fixation, Memory, Imagination, Switching Close and Far, Long Swing, Sunning, Palming and other activities described in this book are derived from Dr. Bates work, magazines.

Directions for the Original Better Eyesight Magazine

The Original Better Eyesight Magazine contains a few treatments that are no longer taught the old way to Natural Eyesight Improvement students. They have been changed, improved and new treatments, activities added. The E-Book 'Better Eyesight Magazine Illustrated with 500 Pictures' is attached free with this book. Read that modern text version of Better Eyesight Magazine to learn the new correct way a few of the old treatments in the original magazines are practiced.

Treatments, activities must be practiced correct to maintain healthy eyes, clear vision. Blue print and pictures in the text version describe the old, new, and improved treatments and the **correct new way to practice them**. The text version can also be used to check for correction of the old worn print in some copies of the original pages.

Fig. 8. The Usual Method of Using the Retinoscope
The observer is so near the subject that the latter is made nervous, and this changes the refraction.

Example of Older Methods That Have Been Changed;

<u>Open Eyes Sunning</u> is no longer practiced in this way. <u>Closed Eyes Sunning</u> only is practiced.
Some people still practice open eyed sunning but in a specific way: Eyes, head/face continually move, eyes blinking, eyes, head/face shifting to the sky near the left, right, top, bottom of the sun and across the sun quickly. The person faces the sun for a brief time. Other directions are applied for safety.
Modern Bates Teachers teach <u>Closed Eyes</u> Sunning only and with eye, head/face movement. Looking at the bright sky, clouds, trees... away from the sun is allowed.

<u>The Sunglass</u> is used only in special cases of near or complete blindness by an experienced Bates Method Ophthalmologist if other methods fail. It can burn the eye, like a magnifying glass when used incorrect, and, because it is a glass, it blocks full spectrum light resulting in partial spectrum, unbalanced light emitting through, from the glass. The light does not go into the eyes pupil and is not directed at the cornea. It is only directed at the sclera, white area of the eye, but it still must not be overused. Partial spectrum light is unhealthy. Pure full spectrum sunlight, not passing through glass is best, healthy for the eyes, brain, body, clarity of vision. The Sunglass is only a short, temporary treatment to <u>awaken, bring to life and action the cells in the eyes retina, lens</u>... to reverse extreme vision impairment, blindness. Done correct, by a Bates Method Eye Doctor, it is beneficial and will not harm the eye.

<u>Reading by 'first' looking at the white spaces between sentences</u> - Do not try to see-read the print clear while at the same time looking at the white spaces between sentences. Central-fixation must be used; look directly at the print to see, read it. In Better Eyesight Magazine, Dr. Bates explains in detail in his 'Questions and Answers Page' to; Use central-fixation when reading; Look directly at the object you want to see.
<u>First</u>: Look at, move the eyes (visual attention, <u>center of the visual field</u>) along the white spaces between the sentences to <u>relax the mind and eyes</u>. (Looking at the white spaces causes relaxation because there is nothing to see, there is no effort to see anything clear, so strain is avoided. This enables relaxation of the mind, eyes, eye muscles to occur. The relaxation produces clear vision, a 'Flash of Clarity'.) When the relaxation and clarity occur and the **print flashes dark black and clear**; then; look away from the spaces, look directly at the black print, <u>place the print in the center of the visual field</u> to read, see it clear. The relaxation and clear vision from looking at the white spaces continues when looking at the print. If it blurs, return to the spaces or Palm to regain relaxation. Then go back to the print. Use the memory and imagination when looking at the white spaces; Imagine painting the spaces pure, bright white with a white paint brush and pure white paint while imagining the white space is seen pure, bright, glowing white and clear. Relax, no effort. Move the paintbrush, eyes left and right along the spaces, blink, relax. Practice with the eyes open, then in the imagination with the eyes closed, then open again. Paint with an imaginary paint brush in the hand or use a white Nosefeather. Practice on Fine Print in the Sunlight. Jump back and forth from the white glowing-paper around the edges of the letters, to the letters, then glow, letters... The eyes and mind like the white & black, 'contrast'. When the print flashes clear; look at it and read. The fovea moves over the letters.

Some people misunderstood Dr. Bates in early times and would try to read the print while looking at the white spaces. Dr. Bates explained to; look at the space or the print; only one at a time, not both at the same time. Looking at, trying to see, think about 2 or more objects at the same time is the opposite of central-fixation: it is diffusion, eccentric fixation and causes tension, strain in the mind, (brain) eye muscles, eyes and unclear vision.

Look at one object at a time for clear vision. This is central-fixation: looking directly at the object of visual attention: first at the white spaces, then the black print, one object at a time, in the center of the visual field.

Palming and imagining, remembering, seeing perfect black on the closed eyes produces perfect relaxation and clear vision. Dr. Bates noticed that some patients used effort to imagine, see black and this prevented relaxation. Dr. Bates states that imagining, seeing black is not necessary to obtain perfect relaxation and clear vision. Remembering, imagining any pleasant thoughts, letting the mind drift from one happy thought, object to another while palming will produce the relaxation and clear vision. Then, black may also appear in front of the closed eyes. If black does not appear, it's alright, it will not make a difference in relaxation, clarity. See the palming chapter for examples.

Square, elliptical... swings - Some of the older swings are combined into the Infinity-Figure Eight Swing. The Long Swing, Sway (Rock)... remain as Dr. Bates created them and are also combined in the Figure Eight Swing. *For all swings and when shifting; move the head and body with the eyes - in the same direction.*

In later editions of Better Eyesight Magazine and books, Dr. Bates and Emily Lierman, Bates lists these changes. (The Sunglass and Open-Eyes Sunning remained in the 1930 final magazine and 1940 book.) Dr. Bates himself stated that the Bates Method is continually advancing, being improved. As he treated thousands of patients over the years the Bates Method was perfected. Bates Teachers state they learn much from their patients, students, each student being an individual and various treatments being successful for each condition, state of mind, body, eyes and personality.

A few original magazine pages that are old with unclear print have an additional new clear page attached, typed in present date print. A few misprints are corrected with additional print, leaving the original pages untouched.

Book printing settings for the original pages is best at: darkest black and highest quality. Not too dark or it will smear the print. The Original Antique Magazines are in Paperback on Amazon and other bookstores.

Distributing this book free to the public is encouraged. **Keep this page in the Original Better Eyesight Magazine E-book that states; The modern version is free with the original book and should also be read to insure correct application of some of the older original practices, treatments.** Corrections are in blue.

Thank-You, in Historical Order

+The University of California Library - http://www.lib.berkeley.edu/ and the Optometrist - Monroe J. Hirsch (name shown in old print, pictures in this book) and other Colleges, Libraries, Eye Doctors, Emily C. A. Lierman Bates, Bates Teachers, Individual Persons that preserved Ophthalmologist Bates Magazines, Books, hid them from the Optical Industry when these businesses, doctors were destroying Doctor Bates work. The law in Europe allowed preservation of Dr. Bates magazines, books.

+Thomas Quackenbush - http://www.naturalvisioncenter.com Bates Method, Natural Vision Improvement Teacher, Author of 'Relearning to See - Improve Your Eyesight Naturally' and 'Better Eyesight - The Complete Magazines of William H. Bates'. He is the first Natural Vision Improvement Teacher to re-publish and bring Dr. Bates work, treatments in Better Eyesight Magazine to the modern public.

+In 2005 people created the first public Internet PDF scan copy of the entire 132 issues of Dr. Bates Original Better Eyesight Magazine and Medical Articles. Every year, month, page in the original antique print! This proved that Dr. Bates discovered Natural Eyesight-Vision Improvement, he is the true source of the Bates Method.

In 2005-2012 people converted the PDFs and other photo-scan copies of the magazines, articles and Dr. Bates book into paper books. Small and fine microscopic print magazine, book versions were also created. Clark Night, Clearsight Publishing Co. placed Dr. Bates magazines, books on-line free in PDF after refining the quality. Four teachers, sellers tried to convince Clark to remove the free magazines or charge a high price for them. He kept the magazines, books free on-line for the public. Dr. Bates magazines, book are stored at the Library of Congress in microfilm along with other doctors and Dr. Bates trained Natural Eyesight teachers books. That magazine price is expensive. Buy it in person to be sure of the clarity and full content. There are a few extra things in that copy.

The following pages provide a sample of the 1919 Better Eyesight Magazine Issue Illustrated with 500 Pictures. Free in PDF form with this book.

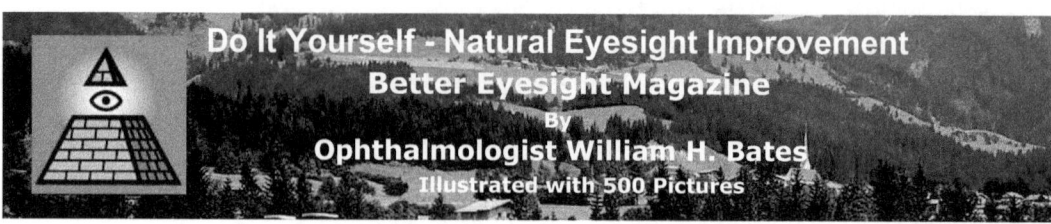

Better Eyesight Magazine by William H. Bates, M. D.
Ophthalmologist - Eye, Ear, Nose & Throat
Central-Fixation Publishing Co.
New York City, New York, USA

Ophthalmologist
William H. Bates

Do It Yourself - Natural Eyesight Improvement - Original and Modern Bates Method & Better Eyesight Magazine Illustrated with 500 Pictures by Ophthalmologist William H. Bates. Based on the Method, Treatments of Dr. Bates, the Eye Doctor that discovered The Bates Method of Natural Eyesight, (Vision) Improvement.

This Book contains Better Eyesight Magazine; a PDF text version of the magazines Illustrated with 500 pictures & additional Modern Natural Eyesight Improvement Training, Activities and a copy of the <u>Original Magazine Pages</u>. Better Eyesight Magazine contains all 132 Monthly Magazine Issues, 11 years-July, 1919 to June, 1930.

Emily C. Lierman, Bates

Stories From The Clinic included; 123 True Stories of Dr. Bates and Emily C.A. Lierman Bates patients varied treatments, eyesight improvement. Written and published by Ophthalmologist William Horatio Bates and his assistant, wife Emily C. A. Lierman, Bates. Eyecharts, Videos, Audio Lessons & 20 E-Books included by Dr. Bates and other Bates Teachers, Doctors. Learn the Modern Treatments and the Original Method, Treatments, Activities from Dr. Bates.

Introduction

Dr. Bates discovered the natural principles, true function of the eyes and applied relaxation, natural methods to return the eyes, eye muscles, nerves, mind/brain, thought patterns, body (entire visual system) to normal function with healthy eyes and clear vision. '<u>The Bates Method of Natural Eyesight Improvement</u>.'

Dr. Bates Better Eyesight Magazine stories, articles describe how Dr. Bates & Emily Lierman Bates, other Doctors, School Teachers, Bates Method Students/Teachers, Children and Parents used Natural Treatments to remove, correct, prevent many different eye problems without use of eyeglasses, surgery, drugs.

The natural treatments they applied removed/prevented; unclear close and distant vision, astigmatism, cataracts, glaucoma, conical cornea, cornea scars, wandering/crossed eyes (strabismus) and other conditions. Hundreds of Natural Treatments are listed.

Read more in Dr. Bates Dedication.

The 8 Correct, Relaxed, Vision Habits (natural, normal, <u>relaxed</u> eye, visual system function); Shifting, Central-fixation, Relaxation, Movement, Blinking, Abdominal Breathing, Switching Close and Far, Long Swing, Sway (Rock), Familiar Eyecharts, Memory and Imagination, Sunning, Palming, Reading Fine Print and other activities described on the Author's website www.cleareyesight.info and in this book are derived from Dr. Bates treatments, method and are listed in his Better Eyesight Magazine and books. The Natural Eyesight Improvement Student practices, imitates this normal eye function to gently coax, return the eyes (visual system) to normal, natural function and clear vision.

Dr. Bates Better Eyesight Magazines, books, Medical Articles are included in this E-Book to enable the Natural Eyesight Improvement student to learn directly from Ophthalmologist Bates, the original eye doctor that discovered Natural Eyesight Improvement, to provide the reader with access to Dr. Bates treatments, teaching method, true Natural Eyesight Improvement. The reader can avoid fraudulent teachers, harmful methods.

The Author, Clark Night is a Natural Eyesight Improvement Graduated Student and Self Trained Teacher that has maintained clear eyesight, freedom from eyeglasses for 37 years. Completed 5 different Natural Eyesight (Vision) Improvement Courses, Trained by Teachers in Person and Home School, studied many Bates and other Natural Vision Improvement books) Improved her close and distant vision to 20/20 and clearer at age 17. Age 59, can read fine print clear at 3 ft.+ and to 30 to 1 to 1/4 inches from the eyes. Teaches friends, family, public how to obtain clear vision without eyeglasses. http://www.cleareyesight.info

This Book Teaches a Variety of Natural Vision Improvement Treatments, Activities

Shifting; (Natural Eye movements), Central-fixation, Relaxation of the Mind/brain, body, eye muscles, eyes, Blinking, Memory and Imagination, Switching Close, Middle, Far for Perfect, Equally Clear Vision, Convergence, Accommodation, Divergence, Un-Accommodation in the Left and Right Eyes at all Distances, Left and Right Brain Hemisphere Activation and Integration, Color Treatment, Visualization, Alpha, Theta, Delta Brain Wave Frequency Deep Relaxation, Palming, Long Swing, Short Swing/Rock and Figure Eight Infinity Swings, Astigmatism Removal Swings, Positive Thinking, Constructive Thoughts, Emotions, Correct Posture, Neck, Shoulder Relaxation, Coordinated Body Movement Exercises, Physical Therapy, Abdominal Deep Breathing, Energy Circulation/Strengthening, Sunning, Saccadic Sunning, Reading, Seeing Fine Print and Eyecharts Clear, EFT, Acupressure, Headache Treatments, Nutrition Chapter-Eye, body Nutrition and other Activities for Clear Close, Distant, Day and Night Vision and Healthy Eyes. Treatments to reverse, remove, prevent: Myopia, Presbyopia (Unclear Distant & Close Vision), Astigmatism, Strabismus, Cataracts, Glaucoma and other eye/vision conditions.

Eyeglass Strength Reduction & Freedom From Glasses - Learn how to work with a Bates Method Behavioral Optometrist or Ophthalmologist for a complete eye exam and be prescribed <u>reduced</u>, weaker and weaker eyeglass lenses (if needed for driving, work safety...) temporarily as vision is improving. Gain complete freedom from eyeglasses.

Treatments are Derived from Dr. Bates Better Eyesight Magazines and Books

PAGE TWO

"PAGE TWO"

ON page two of this magazine are printed each month specific directions for improving the sight in various ways. Too many subscribers read the magazine once and then mislay it. We feel that at least page two should be kept for reference.

When the eyes are neglected the vision may fail. It is so easy to forget how to palm successfully. The long swing always helps but it has to be done right. One may under adverse conditions suffer a tension so great that the ability to remember or imagine perfectly is modified or lost and relaxation is not obtained. The long swing is always available and always brings sufficient relief to practice the short swing, central fixation, the perfect memory and imagination with perfect relief.

Be sure and review page two frequently; not only for your special benefit but also for the benefit of individuals you desire to help!

Persons with imperfect sight often have difficulty in obtaining relaxation by the various methods described in the book and in this magazine. It should be emphasized that persons with good vision are better able to help others than people who have imperfect sight or wear glasses. If you are trying to cure yourself avoid people who wear glasses or do not see well. Those individuals are always under a strain and the strain is manifested in their face, in their voices, in their walk, the way they sit, in short in everything that they do.

Strain is contagious. Teachers in Public Schools who wear glasses are a menace to their pupils' sight. Parents who wear glasses or who have imperfect sight lower the vision of their children. It is always well when treating children or adults to keep them away from people with imperfect sight.

This may be Dr. Bates signature.

Entire 132 PAGE TWO Training Articles from Dr. Bates' Better Eyesight Magazine, in the Original Antique Print. Free on the website; www.cleareyesight-batesmethod.info

RELAXATION FROM FINE PRINT

A BUSINESS card, 3" x 2" with fine print on one side is held in front of the eyes as near as possible, the upper part in contact with the eyebrows, the lower part resting lightly on the nose.

The patient looks directly at the fine print without trying to see. Being so close to the eyes most people realize that it is impossible to read the fine print and do not try, in this way they obtain a measure of relaxation which is sufficient to benefit the sight very much.

The patient moves the card from side to side a short distance slowly and sees the card moving provided the movement is not too short or too slow. The shorter the movement and the slower it is, the better.

Some patients, although the card is held very close, note that the white spaces between the lines become whiter and the black letters become blacker and clearer. In some cases one or more words of the fine print will be seen in flashes or even continuously as long as no effort is made to see or to read the fine print.

This movement of the card should be kept up to obtain the best results, for many hours every day. The hand which holds the card may soon become fatigued; one may then use the hands alternately. Some patients vary this by holding the card with both hands at the same time.

The amount of light is not important.

Comparisons

In practising with the Snellen test card, when the vision is imperfect, the blackness of the letters is modified and the white spaces inside the letters are also modified. By comparing the blackness of the large letters with the blackness of the smaller ones it can be demonstrated that the larger letters are imperfectly seen.

When one notes the whiteness in the center of a large letter, seen indistinctly, it is usually possible to compare the whiteness seen with the remembered whiteness of something else. By alternately comparing the whiteness in the center of a letter with the memory of a better white, as the snow on the top of a mountain, the whiteness of the letter usually improves. In the same way, comparing the shade of black of a letter with the memory of a darker shade of black of some other object may be also a benefit to the black.

Most persons with myopia are able to read fine print at a near point quite perfectly. They see the blackness and whiteness of the letters much better than they are able to see the blackness of the larger letters on the Snellen test card at 15 or 20 feet. Alternately reading the fine print and regarding the Snellen test card, comparing the black and white of the small letters with the black and white of the large letters, is often times very beneficial. Some cases of myopia have been cured very promptly by this method.

All persons with imperfect sight for reading are benefited by comparing the whiteness of the spaces between the lines with the memory of objects which are whiter. Many persons can remember white snow with the eyes closed whiter than the spaces between the lines. By alternately closing the eyes for a minute or longer, remembering white snow, white starch, white paint, a white cloud in the sky with the sun shining on it, and flashing the white spaces without trying to read, many persons have materially improved their sight and been cured.

Have You a Bible?

You all know fine print is beneficial.
Do you practice reading it?
Doctor Bates has proven that by reading a few lines of very fine print daily you are giving your eyes the relaxing "exercise" that will tend to prevent many common defects.

We publish a Bible that is printed in microscopic type, and measures one by one and a half inches and contains the new and old Testament.

Many patients past fifty have learned to read this with ease. Send for yours today.

Price $4.00

Snellen Test Cards

THERE should be a Snellen test card in every family and in every school classroom. When properly used it always improves the sight even when sight is already normal. Children or adults with errors of refraction, if they have never worn glasses, are cured simply by reading every day the smallest letters they can see at a distance of ten, fifteen, or twenty feet.

PAPER .... 50 CENTS
CARDBOARD (*folding*) 75 CENTS
DELIVERED

Back numbers Better Eyesight............$ .30
Bound vols., 1st, 2nd and 3rd years, each.. 4.25
Photographic reduction of the Bible......... 4.00
Ophthalmoscopes, with and without Battery,
   from ....10.00 to 50.00
Retinoscopes 4.00
Burning glasses 5.00
Reprints of articles by Dr. Bates in other medical journals: a limited number for sale. Send for list.

For Sale By
Central Fixation Publishing Company
383 Madison Avenue, New York City

Demonstrate

1. That a short, swaying movement improves the vision more than a long sway.

Place the test card at a distance where only the large letter at the top of the card can be distinguished. This may be ten feet, further or nearer. Stand with the feet about one foot apart and sway the body from side to side. When the body sways to the right, look to the right of the card. When the body sways to the left, look to the left of the card. Do not look at the Snellen test card. Sway the body from side to side and look to the right of the Snellen test card, and alternately to the left of it. Note that the test card appears to be moving. Increase the length of the sway and notice that the test card seems to move a longer distance from side to side. Observe the whiteness of the card and the blackness of the letters. Now shorten the sway, which, of course, shortens the movement of the card. The card appears whiter and the letters blacker when the movement of the card is short, than when the movement of the card is long.

2. Demonstrate that when the eyes are stationary, they are under a tremendous strain. Stand before the Snellen test card at a distance of fifteen or twenty feet. Look directly at one small area of a large letter, which can be seen clearly. Stare at that part of the letter without closing the eyes and without shifting the eyes to some other point. The vision becomes worse and the letter blurs. Stare continuously, and note that the longer you stare, the more difficult it is to keep the eyes focused on that one point or part of the letter. Not only does the stare become more difficult, but the eyes become tired; and by making a greater effort, the eyes pain, or a headache is produced. The stare can cause fatigue of the whole body when the effort is sufficiently strong and prolonged.

The Fundamental Principle

THE FLASHING CURE

Do you read imperfectly? Can you observe then that when you look at the first word, or the first letter, of a sentence you do not see best where you are looking; that you see other words, or other letters, just as well as or better than the ones you are looking at? Do you observe also that the harder you try to see the worse you see?

Now close your eyes and rest them, remembering some color, like black or white, that you can remember perfectly. Keep them closed until they feel rested, or until the feeling of strain has been completely relieved. Now open them and look at the first word or letter of a sentence for a fraction of a second. If you have been able to relax, partially or completely, you will have a flash of improved or clear vision, and the area seen best will be smaller.

After opening the eyes for this fraction of a second, close them again quickly, still remembering the color, and keep them closed until they again feel rested. Then again open them for a fraction of a second. Continue this alternate resting of the eyes and flashing of the letters for a time, and you may soon find that you can keep your eyes open longer than a fraction of a second without losing the improved vision.

If your trouble is with distant instead of near vision, use the same method with distant letters.

In this way you can demonstrate for yourself the fundamental principles of the cure of imperfect sight by treatment without glasses.

If you fail, ask someone with perfect sight to help you.

THE SWINGING CURE

If you see a letter perfectly, you may note that it appears to pulsate, or move slightly in various directions. If your sight is imperfect, the letter will appear to be stationary. The apparent movement is caused by the unconscious shifting of the eye. The lack of movement is due to the fact that the eye stares, or looks too long at one point. This is an invariable symptom of imperfect sight, and may often be relieved by the following method:

Close your eyes and cover them with the palms of the hands so as to exclude all the light, and shift mentally from one side of a black letter to the other. As you do this, the mental picture of the letter will appear to move back and forth in a direction contrary to the imagined movement of the eye. Just so long as you imagine that the letter is moving, or swinging, you will find that you are able to remember it, and the shorter and more regular the swing, the blacker and more distinct the letter will appear. If you are able to imagine the letter stationary, which may be difficult, you will find that your memory of it will be much less perfect.

Now open your eyes and look first at one side and then at the other of the real letter. If it appears to move in a direction opposite to the movement of the eye, you will find that your vision has improved. If you can imagine the swing of the letter as well with your eyes open as with your eyes closed, as short, as regular and as continuous, your vision will be normal.

PERFECT SIGHT

If you learn the fundamental principles of perfect sight and will consciously keep them in mind your defective vision will disappear. The following discoveries were made by Dr. Bates and his method is based on them. With it he has cured so-called incurable cases:

1. Many blind people are curable.

2. All errors of refraction are functional, therefore curable.

3. All defective vision is due to strain in some form.

4. Strain is relieved by relaxation.

You can demonstrate to your own satisfaction that strain lowers the vision. When you stare, you strain. Look fixedly at one object for five seconds or longer. What happens? The object blurs and finally disappears. Also, your eyes are made uncomfortable by this experiment. When you rest your eyes for a few moments the vision is improved and the discomfort relieved.

Have some one with perfect sight demonstrate the fundamental principles contained in Dr. Bates' book, "Perfect Sight Without Glasses." If the suggestions and instructions are carried out, and glasses discarded, it is possible to improve the vision without personally consulting a physician.

"Perfect Sight Without Glasses" will be sent C. O. D. on five days' approval. Price, $5.00.

Central Fixation Publishing Company
383 Madison Avenue, New York City

Practice Time

A large number of people have bought the book "Perfect Sight Without Glasses" but do not derive as much benefit from it as they should because they do not know how long they should practice.

Rest: The eyes are rested in various ways. One of the best methods is to close the eyes for half an hour after testing the sight. This usually improves the vision.

Palming: With the eyes closed and covered with the palms of both hands the vision is usually benefited. The patient should do this five minutes hourly.

Shifting: The patient looks from one side of the room to the other, alternately resting the eyes. This may be done three times daily for half an hour at a time. The head should move with the eyes and the patient should blink.

Swinging: When the shifting is slow, stationary objects appear to move from side to side. This should be observed whenever the head and eyes move.

Long Swing: Nearly all persons should practice the long swing one hundred times daily.

Memory: When the vision is perfect, it is impossible for the memory to be imperfect. One can improve the memory by alternately remembering a letter with the eyes open and closed. This should be practiced for half an hour twice daily.

Imagination: It has been frequently demonstrated and published in this magazine that the vision is only what we imagine it to be. Imagination should be practiced whenever the vision is tested. Imagine a known letter with the eyes open and with the eyes closed. This should be practiced for ten minutes twice daily.

Repetition: When one method is found which improves the vision more than any other method, it should be practiced until the vision is continuously improved.

SNELLEN TEST CARDS

There should be a Snellen test card in every family and in every school classroom. When properly used it always improves the sight even when it is already normal. Children or adults with errors of refraction, if they have never worn glasses, are cured simply by reading every day the smallest letters they can see at a distance of ten, fifteen, or twenty feet.

For Sale By

The Central Fixation Publishing Company

Paper .... 50 Cents
Cardboard (folding) .... 75 Cents
DELIVERED

Back numbers BETTER EYESIGHT.................$ .30
Bound vols., 1st and 2nd years, each............ 4.25
Photographic reductions of the Bible............ 4.00
Ophthalmoscopes (best quality) 4.00
Burning glasses 4.00

Reprints of articles by Dr. Bates in other medical journals, a limited number for sale. Send for list.

FOR SALE BY

Central Fixation Publishing Company
18 East 48th Street, New York

SNELLEN TEST CARDS

There should be a Snellen Test Card in every home and schoolroom. When properly used, it always improves the sight, even when this is already normal, and children and adults are often cured of errors of refraction simply by reading every day the smallest letters they can see at a distance of ten, fifteen, or twenty feet.

Cardboard (folding), 25 cents, postpaid.

Numeral Test Cards and other special styles, 50 cents and $1.00, postage prepaid.

Fundamental Cards, 10 cents each.

BETTER EYESIGHT

A magazine devoted to the prevention and cure of imperfect sight without glasses.

W. H. BATES, M.D., Editor

This monthly contains the latest discoveries of the editor, and gives simple instructions for self-treatment by the aid of which many persons have been able to cure themselves. $2.00 per year.

Back numbers: 30 cents a copy; bound volumes, twelve issues each, $3.00.

REPRINTS OF ARTICLES BY DR. BATES
from medical journals
in book form,

$0.50 Each.

TREATMENT. One patient, forty years of age, had been blind from birth. The corneas of both eyes were totally opaque, so that it was impossible to see the color of the iris. The patient was helpless on the street and required someone to lead him. Central fixation, the use of his memory and imagination, and other methods for the relief of eyestrain were practiced. The sun treatment was especially beneficial. The patient was taught to expose his closed eyelids to the sun for many hours daily.

At the end of a few months' treatment, he became able to recognize people on the street. He was taught the alphabet and the names of the figures. When his knowledge of the letters became perfect, he was able to read the Snellen test card, 20/20. He was also able to read fine print without glasses. After thirty-five years, his friends reported that his eyes were still normal.

Another case was that of a woman, aged seventy-five, who had to be led into the office. She had suffered from inflammation of the cornea of both eyes for many years, and had frequent attacks of ulcers. From time to time, these ulcers would heal, but they always left a scar.

When the patient was first seen, a scar tissue involved the whole cornea, so that one could not distinguish the colored part of the eye. I believe that eyestrain was the only cause of the trouble, because the sun treatment, palming and swinging, brought about an improvement so that the cornea became perfectly clear, and the vision of the patient for distant and near objects was normal.

The Blindness of Squint or Amblyopia Ex Anopsia

In cases of squint, the vision of the eye which turns either in or out is variable. In many cases, the squinting eye may have normal vision, but in the majority of cases, the vision may be very much lowered, and in rare cases, the squinting eye may be totally blind with no perception of light.

CAUSE. There have been many theories proposed to account for the blindness of squint. I have found, however, that the cause of the blindness is due to eyestrain.

TREATMENT. The vision of these cases is benefited by relaxation methods—palming, swinging, and the use of the memory or the imagination. A letter may be imagined perfectly or imperfectly. When imagined imperfectly, the vision is always lowered. When imagined perfectly, with the eyes open as well as with the eyes closed, the vision is always improved. By remembering or imagining a letter, with the eyes closed for half a minute or longer, one becomes able to imagine a letter quite perfectly with the eyes open for a few seconds. Repeat.

CASE HISTORY. In one case, a woman, about thirty years of age, was totally blind in the right eye which turned in, although the eye itself was apparently normal. That is to say, there were no opacities in any part of the eye, and the retina and optic nerve were normal.

With both eyes open, the vision was 15/20. By practice, with the aid of her memory and imagination, the vision, with both eyes, soon became normal without glasses, 15/10. Coincident with the improvement of the vision of both eyes together, which meant an improvement in the vision of the left eye, the patient gradually became able to distinguish light in the right or blind eye. In less than two weeks, after daily treatment, the vision of the right eye became normal and the eyes straight.

It seems curious that so many articles have been published on amblyopia (dim-sightedness) ex-anopsia (from lack of education or use of eye) without going further and studying the results of the opposite of ex-anopsia,—relaxation methods of treatment.

SAVED FROM BLINDNESS
By Patricia Palmer

It is very hard for an active young girl to suddenly learn that in a short time she may lose her eyesight. I had always felt a great deal of pity for blind people, but I never stopped to realize how many beautiful things they missed until I knew that I was going blind myself. I only wore glasses for three years, but in that short time I developed a very bad case of progressive myopia. In the summer of 1918 my sight became so poor that I had to stop reading altogether and even a moderately bright day hurt my eyes so much that I kept them bandaged a great part of the time. Finally I had to put on a dark Krux lens, and the goggle-like glasses that I wore shut out all light. In the fall I started school, but as I could not see to read I was working under great difficulties. Then, through an article published some months before in the *Scientific American,* we learned of Dr. Bates's work and it seemed the last possible hope. I declared that there was no use in taking the trip to New York, because I knew he could do nothing for me, but in the end I went.

The first time I looked at the test card I could not see the big "C" until I stood within four feet of it, but in two hours I was able to flash all the letters of the third line and part of the fourth at ten feet. In four weeks I had 10/10 vision and my hearing, which had been bad, was normal.

Some weeks after I returned home a friend, who was calling, complained of a bad headache. I persuaded him to take off his glasses and showed him how to palm and swing the letters on the chart. A short time later he discovered, to his surprise, that his headache was entirely gone.

This incident made me realize that if I showed others what Dr. Bates had shown me I could relieve, if not cure, their troubles. The next person that I worked with was a little girl with progressive myopia which had not become very serious. She worked very conscientiously, and about a month after we started, when she visited Dr. Bates, her sight was nearly perfect.

I have helped a number of people, some successfully, others not so successfully. One of my most interesting cases was a chauffeur who thought that he was unusually farsighted, but who could not see to read the paper. When I tested his eyes I found that he had only 10/20 vision. In a short time, however, he attained normal sight by palming and swinging the letters. I then told him to close his eyes and count ten, then open them for a fraction of a second. I held a book in front of him and in a short time, by closing his eyes and then glancing at it, he read parts of it. He practices on signboards, automobile licenses, or anything that he sees, and now he reads the entire paper every evening. He has noticed, too, that he is not blinded by bright lights at night as he used to be.

As to the value of swinging the little black period I am very decided. I find it my best friend, especially in a test. One time in a French examination, in the excitement of the moment, I could not think of a certain word which I knew well enough and which was very important to me. I closed my eyes and palmed for a second and remembered the period. In a flash my self-control returned to me and with it the word. I have tried this several times since, usually with success.

I often wonder now how I could possibly have managed without my eyes, even with glasses. It is such a joy to be able to read from morning to night if I want to.

MAKE YOUR SIGHT WORSE

Strange as it may seem there is no better way of improving the sight than by making it worse. To see things worse when one is already seeing them badly requires mental control of a degree greater than that required to improve the sight. The importance of these facts is very great. When patients become able to lower their vision by conscious staring, they become better able to avoid unconscious staring. When they demonstrate by increasing their eccentric fixation that trying to see objects not regarded lowers the vision, they may stop trying to do the same thing unconsciously.

What is true of the sight is also true of the imagination and memory. If one's memory and imagination are imperfect, they can be improved by consciously making them worse than they are. Persons with imperfect sight never remember or imagine the letters on the test card as perfectly black and distinct, but to imagine them as grey and cloudy is very difficult, or even impossible, and when a patient has done it, or tried to do it, he may become able to avoid the unconscious strain which has prevented him from forming mental pictures as black and distinct as the reality.

To make imperfect sight worse is always more difficult than to lower normal vision. In other words, to make a letter which already appears grey and indistinct noticeably more cloudy is harder than to blur a letter seen distinctly. To make an imperfect mental picture worse is harder than to blur a perfect one. Both practices require much effort, much hard disagreeable work; but they always, when successful, improve the memory, imagination and vision.

BETTER EYESIGHT

A MAGAZINE DEVOTED TO THE PREVENTION AND CURE OF IMPERFECT SIGHT WITHOUT GLASSES

Copyright, 1920, by the Central Fixation Publishing Company
Editor—W. H. BATES, M.D.
Publisher—CENTRAL FIXATION PUBLISHING CO.

Vol. III   SEPTEMBER, 1920   No. 3

EXPERIENCES WITH CENTRAL FIXATION
By M. H. STUART, M.D.
Moultrie, Ga.

We are greatly indebted to Dr. Stuart for sending us this remarkable story of his own cure and that of his patients, all of which was accomplished without personal assistance by means of the information presented in this magazine.

Some sixteen years ago, when working as a stenographer, I developed indigestion and became extremely nervous, one of my symptoms being a tension in the spinal cord between the shoulder blades which was extremely uncomfortable. In the late afternoon and evening I would become so nervous that I could scarcely sit still, and I have walked five miles into the country and back again to get relief. I tried dieting for the indigestion, but after two months failed to get any relief. A medical student then suggested that the trouble might be due to my eyes. I went to an oculist, who fitted me with glasses, and all my troubles ceased.

The glasses given to me were convex 0.25, axis 90. A few years later, when I was in New York doing post-graduate work at the Polyclinic, they were changed to concave 0.25, axis 180, my refraction having changed from hypermetropia to myopia. In succeeding years the myopic astigmatism increased to concave 0.75, axis 180, and finally, after I had worn glasses for some fourteen years, to concave 1.00, axis 180. The last correction I had worn for about two years when I discarded glasses for good.

Slight as my error of refraction was, I was not able to leave off my glasses for more than an hour or two without suffering from nervousness and the feeling of tenseness in the spinal cord alluded to above. At other times I was perfectly comfortable except for the last year or two, during which I had so much to do that I suffered at times from the old nervous trouble. I had no pain in my head or eyes, but the trouble in my back was so bad last fall that I had to have the services of a masseur in order to do my work.

Five years ago I first read about Dr. Bates' experiments upon the eye muscles of animals. While interested I was not prepared to abandon the accepted teachings on the subject, and I waited to hear more. Recently I read, in the May (1920) number of BETTER EYESIGHT, Dr. Arnau's story of how his headaches were cured, and I was so impressed by it that I determined to try the relaxation method upon myself. I palmed for five minutes and then read the card three times with each eye as far as I could without effort. I did this six times a day for five days, and at the end of this time I had gained a very decided degree of relaxation. I had, of course, discarded glasses, and, although this caused me a little discomfort at first, I was able, about a week later, to perform, without them, three tonsilectomies and one operation for cataract, and to remove two blind eyes. At the same time I went through my daily routine of treating ten to thirty patients, examining eyes, ears, noses and throats, much of which work requires extra good vision. At noon I lay down to rest as usual and read the Atlanta paper. At night I read the Moultrie daily paper and anything else that I wanted to.

After the first five days of systematic relaxation I have never done anything in a routine way for myself, but if I feel nervous, or my eyes feel drawn, I swing twenty times and palm. In this way I am always able to get relief. Another method of gaining relaxation that I have resorted to is to look at an imaginary period in any dark, distant object. In this pine-woods district there are thousands of stumps, many of which have been burned and blackened. The third day after I discarded my glasses I had to drive about twenty-eight miles, and whenever my eyes felt drawn I would look in an easy relaxed way at a small point on one of these stumps and always got relaxation.

Nearly every afternoon at half past four I go out for a game of golf, and often I palm before going, as I find it gives me better control of my nervous system, and enables me to play a more consistent game.

I was so pleased with the results of the new treatment in my own case that I have since taught central fixation to about forty of my patients, and in only about two did I fail to improve the vision at the first sitting.

The following are some of my more notable cases.

Mr. S, an automobile mechanic, had been mentally deranged for two weeks, following an atttack of flu, after which he gradually became rational, only to find that he saw double and his vision was imperfect in each eye. At the first examination he read with his right 20/120, and with the left 20/60. I suggested that he palm at least six times a day for five minutes, and on the second day he was greatly improved, reading with the right eye 20/80, left 20/40. On the third day he read with the right eye 20/40, left 20/30, an increase of vision in the right eye of 200 per cent, and in the left of 100 per cent. He is now at work, and when, occasionally, he has to lay off, it is not on account of any trouble with his eyes, but because of weakness in his knees.

A year ago a Mr. B consulted me about the sight of his right eye, the left having been blind for years. His vision was 10/40, and could not be improved by any lens. I advised him to have the left eye removed, since it was a menace to the other eye. He would not consent to this and I did not see him again until May 5, of this year, when he came to my office practically blind in his right eye from sympathetic opthalmia. At one foot he could only count fingers. I advised the immediate removal of the blind eye and of a few teeth that had pus about them; but I could not promise that his vision would be saved. That afternoon I removed the eye, and the following day I was gratified to find that he could count fingers at three feet. I sent him home with some large letters to use for the practice of central fixation, and by the fifteenth he was able to count fingers at five feet. I then told him how to practice the universal swing, and on the twenty-second he could count fingers at seven feet. On the twenty-ninth he could read the small type on the 20 line of the test card at four inches, whereas he had been entirely unable to see them previously. He states that he can now see the small chickens running about near his feet, and can see small cotton plants seven feet away. I am confident that in a year, or some such matter, he will have sufficient vision to attend to the necessary work of his farm.

I have treated three cases of squint, all of them with success. One of them, Delia S, aged twelve, came to me on May 15, with her right eye turned in to such a degree that the cornea was partly hidden. The sight of this eye was so imperfect that at three feet she could only count fingers. With her left eye she could read 20/30. She was told to palm, and when she returned on May 24 she was able, with the squinting eye, to count fingers at six feet, twice as far as at her first visit, and the eye was straighter. On June 5 she came again, and counted fingers at eight feet, an increase of vision since the beginning of 700 per cent. On July 3, while I was writing this report, she came in, and I found that her right eye had improved to 20/60, one third of normal, while her left had become entirely normal, 20/20. Her right eye was entirely straight at times, and I feel sure that in a few months this condition will have become permanent.

Another case of squint was that of a young girl of fourteen with rather large, pretty blue eyes, one of which, the right, was slightly crossed inwardly. Her sight was very imperfect—half normal in the right eye and one-third normal in the left—while, like most cross-eyed people, she was troubled with double vision. I asked her to palm at least six times a day, and she came back with her eyes straighter and able to read 20/30 with both. The next week showed normal vision, the eyes being at times perfectly straight.

I was particularly pleased to be able to relieve these little girls of a disfigurement which means so much more to them than it would mean to a boy, and I was much interested to note how much prettier their eyes were, apart from the disappearance of the squint, after a few treatments. They were wide open, softer-looking, in short, relaxed.

REST

All methods of curing errors of refraction are simply different ways of obtaining rest.

Different persons do this in different ways. Some patients are able to rest their eyes simply by closing them, and complete cures have been obtained by this means, the closing of the eyes for a longer or shorter period being alternated with looking at the test card for a moment. In other cases patients have strained more when their eyes were shut than when they were open. Some can rest their eyes when all light is excluded from them by covering with the palms of the hands; others cannot, and have to be helped by other means before they can palm. Some become able at once to remember or imagine that the letters they wish to see are perfectly black, and with the accompanying relaxation their vision immediately becomes normal. Others become able to do this only after a considerable time. Shifting is a very simple method of relieving strain, and most patients soon become able to shift from one letter to another, or from one side of a letter to another in such a way that these forms seem to move in a direction opposite to the movement of the eye. A few are unable to do this, but can do it with a mental picture of a letter, after which they become able to do it visually.

Patients who do not succeed with any particular method of obtaining rest for their eyes should abandon it and try something else. The cause of the failure is strain, and it does no good to go on straining.

BETTER EYESIGHT
A MAGAZINE DEVOTED TO THE PREVENTION AND CURE OF IMPERFECT SIGHT WITHOUT GLASSES

Copyright, 1920, by the Central Fixation Publishing Company
Editor—W. H. BATES, M.D.
Publisher—CENTRAL FIXATION PUBLISHING CO.

Vol. II   APRIL, 1920   No. 4

HOW I HELPED OTHERS

By Victoria Coolidge

When I had become able to read without glasses, and my headaches had become less and less frequent, and less severe each time, I was so enthusiastic over my experience that I was anxious to help others. My brother was my first patient. He was so much interested in what had been done for me that he wanted to try it himself; but I never dreamed of being able to help him, because his eyes were almost as bad as my own had been, his glasses being: right eye convex 3.25 D.S.; left eye, convex 3.75 D.S. combined with 0.50 D.C., 180 degrees. However, I knew the treatment could do no harm, so I decided that I would try to show him as nearly as I could what Dr. Bates had done for me. Imagine my surprise, then, when I found that he, too, by holding the fine print six inches from his eyes and looking alternately at the top and bottom of the letters, became able to read it just as I had become able to do so. He proved to be a model pupil as soon as he had demonstrated to his own satisfaction that he must leave off his glasses all the time if he wanted to make any appreciable progress. He has now done without them for about a year, and has made remarkable progress in that time, the secret of his success being a great desire to be cured, an intelligent grasp of the idea of central fixation, and perseverance in practicing central fixation at every possible opportunity.

The next person I was able to help was a friend who, while visiting me, happened to notice the Snellen test card hanging on the wall. She asked me what I was doing with it, and I explained, adding that she was very fortunate in having normal vision. "I thought I had," she said, "but I have had so many headaches that I consulted an eye specialist the other day and he gave me glasses." She was so displeased to think she had to wear them, and had found it so difficult to get used to seeing with them, that I asked her if she would like to try Dr. Bates' treatment without glasses. She said that she would jump at the chance. I told her to read the card every day at ten, fifteen, and twenty feet, and to palm whenever she had a headache. That was in August. On December 19 she telephoned that she had practiced reading the card every day, that she had no trouble with headaches, and that she was reading 20/10 easily with the better eye, and fairly well with the other. Shortly after she began the treatment herself, she was able to improve the vision of a child nine years old from 20/50 to 20/20.

It has been many times pointed out in this magazine that children under twelve years of age who have never worn glasses are easily cured; and so for the past month I have been trying to see what I could do for such children, and for some who were older—including two who had worn glasses, one some time previously and the other up to the time I began to treat her. I have worked with six and they have all improved. One girl, fifteen, who had worn glasses a few years ago for imperfect sight in one eye, but who had discarded them, improved in a half hour from 20/70 to 20/50, by alternating palming, or sometimes just closing her eyes, and then reading the Snellen test card. This improvement was permanent.

Another girl, sixteen, had worn glasses for a year, chiefly for headache, she said, although her vision in both eyes was but 20/200. As she could read without her glasses without much difficulty, she was only too glad to take them off, as most girls of that age are, but she was afraid of the headaches. I asked her to try it, and she has done so for about three weeks, during which time her vision improved to 20/70 and she had no headaches.

The following is the record of four little girls who have improved by reading the Snellen test card daily, and palming:

Name	Age	Vision Sept. 1919 Phys. Rec. Card	Dec. 11	Dec. 31
Catherine	10	R. 20/50	20/40	20/40
		L. 20/50	20/40	20/40
Blanche	10	R. 4/50	6/40	6/30
		L. 4/50	6/40	6/30
Vinnie	9	R. 20/50	20/40	
		L. 20/40	20/30	absent
Sylvia	10	R. 20/40	20/15	20/10
		L. 20/40	20/15	20/10

Catherine's vision afterwards (January 22) improved to 20/20. The case of Sylvia was so interesting that it will be treated in more detail next month.

Better Eyesight

A Monthly Magazine Devoted to the Prevention and Cure of Imperfect Sight without Glasses

Published by the Central Fixation Company, 300 Madison Ave., New York, as the official organ of the BETTER EYESIGHT LEAGUE, a national organization to relieve the sufferings and discomfort of those afflicted with imperfect eyesight, to disseminate the knowledge of the scientific cure and prevention of imperfect sight without the use of glasses, and to promote further research and investigation into the causes for imperfect eyesight and its improvement without the use of artificial lenses.

W. H. BATES, M. D., Editor

VOL. VII.   JULY, 1922   No. 1

THE STORY OF VIOLET
By W. H. BATES, M. D.

Just what, in simple words, is Central Fixation? If you will read this story of a ten-year-old girl who discovered it for herself you will know, not in terms of theory or in scientific phrases, but in practical simplicity.

SOME years ago a young girl, aged 10, was brought to me for the cure of imperfect sight and squint. She was wearing quite strong glasses for relief.

The right or squinting eye, even with her strong glasses, had very poor vision. The best she could see with this eye with or without glasses was counting fingers at about three feet. Looking straight ahead of her with this squinting eye, with the other eye covered, everything was visible and, she said, perfectly dark, and what she did see at any time with this eye was off to one side. She was unable to read with this eye with or without her glasses.

With her left eye her vision was improved by glasses so that she had about one-quarter of normal vision and could read large print with more or less difficulty for short periods of time. She usually had a headache every day and at times great pain in one or both eyes.

Reading or studying her lessons was a punishment. Unlike other children she had no pleasure in reading story books. The trouble with her eyes interfered with her play. She spent most of her time sitting alone with no desire to talk and kept her eyes closed a good deal of the time. Without her glasses she could not read at all ordinary print.

The case to me was very interesting because of the results obtained in a short time, three weeks. When the mother asked me how long it would take, I believed and told her that if the girl got any improvement in three months she would be very fortunate. In fact she was practically cured in a week but I was so fearful of a relapse I had her come a few weeks longer to be sure she retained what she had gained.

GLASSES OFF

The first thing I had her do was to discard her glasses altogether. With both eyes open her vision was 10/200. When she was able to see the large letter on the card clearly or well enough to tell what the letter was, I asked her if she saw it all alike. She said "No." She told me that she noticed that when she looked at the top of the letter she saw it best and the bottom worse. When she looked at the bottom of the letter she saw the bottom of the letter best and the top worse.

"But," I said, "The top is just as black as the bottom and one side is just as black as the other side. The letter is perfectly black in all parts."

"Yes," she said, "but I do not see it that way."

I told her to try it that way. She said at once the letter blurred so that she could not tell it. When I brought the letter up close, at three feet away she saw it more distinctly than at ten feet.

"Now," I said to her, "when you try to see the letter all alike what happens?"

She answered, "It blurs and if I try hard enough I cannot even tell what the letter is."

I said to her, "You know the letter is perfectly black and when you see one part best you are seeing something that is not so, aren't you?"

"Yes," she answered.

"Now when you see something that is not so you do not really see it— you only imagine it, don't you?"

She answered, "I do not see one part best, I only imagine it."

Then I pointed to the second line, first letter, "Can you imagine the top of this letter is blacker than the bottom? Make believe it is," I told her.

"Oh," she said, "I can make believe it is, I can imagine the top best."

"Can you imagine the bottom best if you want to?"

"Yes I can imagine the bottom best and the top worse."

"What letter is it?" she answered: "A letter R."

"Is the letter R as black as the big C?"

"No," she answered, "it is quite gray and all blurred on the edges."

"You know it isn't gray don't you?"

"Yes, I know it isn't gray but that is the way I see it."

"Isn't that an illusion?" when you see gray you are seeing something that isn't true, aren't you?"

"Yes, when I see it gray I am seeing something that isn't true."

"Now suppose you make believe that the letter R is just as black as the big C, which it really is. Can you do that?"

"I can make believe it is, I can imagine it is, but I have to imagine one part at a time."

"All right," I said, "I can forgive you for that. Keep on imagining one part is blacker than the rest," and then she screamed with delight.

"Oh goody, the whole card is getting better and I can see a thousand times more then I could before."

BETTER VISION QUICKLY

In her eagerness to prove that her sight was better, almost breathlessly, she read several lines.

I said to her, "Why do you stop?"

She answered, "They all turn gray."

"Oh," I said, "Nonsense, they didn't all turn gray. You only made believe they did. Suppose you make believe they are black all the time, not some times gray, and other times black, because they are not. You know those letters are continuously black."

"Yes I know it but I do not always imagine or make believe they are."

"Can you make believe they are?"

"Oh, yes I can and can read more of them," and this she did and apologized, saying that she could not read them or imagine them perfectly black unless she made believe she saw a part of the letter best.

I was very much impressed with the fact that this child had discovered for herself what I call Central Fixation or the ability to see a part of a letter better than the rest of it. She found, without any suggestion on my part, that she could not read any of the letters with maximum vision unless she did see one part best. When she came to the smaller letters she hesitated and failed to see them.

"What is the trouble?" I asked.

"Oh," she said, "They are so small it seems as though I ought at least to see a small letter all alike and tell what it is."

Then I called her attention to the fact that she could not tell any of those small letters when she tried to imagine the letters all alike. I brought the card closer and encouraged her to imagine one part best of the smaller letters. At a nearer point than ten feet she was able to imagine even the letters on the bottom line, one part best, and distinguish them. She was able to demonstrate that when she saw the small letters all alike that her sight was not so good. When she looked at the card at ten feet she became able, by alternating with looking at the card nearer, to see the small letters, one part best, as well as she could at a nearer point.

REAL PRACTICE

She practiced with the card at home and did what very few of my patients are able to do, she improved her sight practicing by herself. In a few days her vision with both eyes together became normal. Then I had her cover the good eye, the left, and practice in the same way with the squinting eye, which had such very poor sight. With her eyes closed she could imagine one part best of a large letter at ten feet continuously. By flashing the large letter with the squinting eye, alternately, her ability to see one part best improved, at first in flashes and later more continuously.

When she was at home her mother said the child was spending all her time with the card. She shortened the time of her meals in order to be busy with the Snellen Test Card for a longer time. She even brought the card to the table and practiced with it while she was eating. It was difficult to induce her to go to sleep because she wanted to practice more. She was up in the morning soon after daylight and practiced with her card while she was dressing.

She very soon had her reward, for in less than a week's time she had normal vision with each eye and the squint disappeared never to return.

It was very interesting how she improved her ability to read fine print at the near point. When I asked her, "Do you see those small letters of the diamond type one part best?" she answered "Yes."

"Do you see the period of the diamond type one part best?"

"Yes, but when I get started I can read it so fast that I do not have time to notice that I am seeing the letters one part best."

HIGHER MENTAL EFFICIENCY

This child accomplished what I have never seen anybody else do. She could read the diamond type with each eye by central fixation so close to her eyes that the page touched her eye lashes. She could read signs further off than any person I ever knew.

With the wonderful improvement in her sight came an increased mental efficiency. Her memory was unusual. She could read perfectly a page of history and because she saw it perfectly she was able to remember it perfectly. As a consequence her scholarship became very good indeed. Formerly she was at the foot of her class, afterwards she was at the head. She astonished her teacher with the quickness of her perceptions, her ability to understand. Formerly when her sight was poor she was a very unhappy, depressed person, later she was full of life and action and seemed to enjoy life to the utmost.

One day she met one of my patients on the street. "How are you getting along?" she asked. The patient answered gloomily, "Not as well as I would like. How are you?"

"Oh, I am all right, I am cured and I am very glad and happy over it. How much do you practice and how often do you go to see Doctor?"

"Oh, I practice once in a while, half an hour or so a day when I think of it and I call on the Doctor about once a week."

Then Violet exclaimed, "Oh how foolish, that isn't the way I did it. I wanted to get well and I wanted to get well quick and I did just exactly what the Doctor told me to do and the more I practiced the more I improved. I found it was a good thing to do what he said, so I did it. When he told me to remember a period all day long I did it. He told me to do a whole lot of other things and some of them seemed hard, difficult, but when I found I could do them they seemed easier to do and I am glad of it."

When the patient told me of the meeting with Violet he asked me why she improved so much more than he had improved.

I asked him, "Did you follow my instructions as enthusiastically as Violet did? Was there any reason, any real reason why you could not do it?"

"No," he answered, "There was no reason why I should not have practiced as faithfully as Violet but my eyes are so bad that it is difficult for me to do the right thing although you repeatedly had me demonstarate that to do the wrong thing was a strain, an effort and required hard work and made me uncomfortable. When I did the right thing it was easier and I felt more comfortable."

This patient after his meeting and talk with Violet came to the office more frequently, practiced more continuously and made surprising progress. In a few weeks he went back to his former state of mind, and did not do so well. I have always thought if he could have had Violet with him most of the time or could have seen her daily he would have done much better. Most of my patients always do better when they have someone with perfect sight to encourage them by their example or advice.

Better Eyesight Magazine by Ophthalmologist William H. Bates
July - December, Year 1919

Better Eyesight

A MONTHLY MAGAZINE DEVOTED TO THE PREVENTION AND CURE OF IMPERFECT SIGHT WITHOUT GLASSES

Vol. I   JULY, 1919   No. 1

THE LIBRARY
OF
THE UNIVERSITY
OF CALIFORNIA

Foreword

Fundamental Facts

Central Fixation

A Teacher's Experiences

Army Officer Cures Himself

GIVEN WITH LOVE TO THE
OPTOMETRY LIBRARY
BY
MONROE J. HIRSCH, O.D., Ph.D.

$2.00 per year   20 cents per copy
Published by the CENTRAL FIXATION PUBLISHING COMPANY
39-45 EAST 42nd STREET   NEW YORK, N. Y.

Ophthalmologist
William H. Bates

Emily C. Lierman, Bates

BETTER EYESIGHT

**A MONTHLY MAGAZINE DEVOTED TO THE PREVENTION AND
CURE OF IMPERFECT SIGHT WITHOUT GLASSES**

July, 1919 - June, 1930 - 132 Magazine Issues

Central Fixation Publishing Co.

New York, N. Y. USA

July, 1919

Do you read imperfectly? Can you observe then that when you look a tthe first word, or the first letter, of a sentence you do not see best where you are looking; that you see other words, or other letters, just as well as or better than the ones you are looking at? Do you observe also that the harder you try to see the worse you see?

Now close your eyes and rest them, remembering some color, like black or white, that you can remember perfectly. Keep them closed until they feel rested, or until the feeling of strain has been completely relieved. Now open them and look at the first word or letter of a sentence for a fraction of a second. If you have been able to relax, partially or completely, you will have a flash of improved or clear vision, and the area seen best will be smaller.

After opening the eyes for this fraction of a second, close them again quickly, still remembering the color, and keep them closed until they again feel rested. Then again open them for a fraction of a second. Continue this alternate resting of the eyes and flashing of the letters for a time, and you may soon find that you can keep your eyes open longer than a fraction of a second without losing the improved vision.

If your trouble is with distant instead of near vision, use the same method with distant letters.

In this way you can demonstrate for yourself the fundamental principles of the cure of imperfect sight by treatment without glasses. If you fail, ask someone with perfect sight to help you.

Do You Read Imperfectly? - This first article and others are placed on page 2 on the inside cover of each monthly Better Eyesight Magazine issue. The articles consist of a variety of the Best of Dr. Bates Original Natural Eyesight Improvement Treatments, Activities. The student can copy, paste these into a small fine print booklet to carry in a pocket and practice in your spare time.

FOREWORD

WHEN the United States entered the European war recruits for general military service were required to have a visual acuity of 20/40 in one eye and 20/100 in the other.1 This very low standard, although it is a matter of common knowledge that it was interpreted with great liberality, proved to be the greatest physical obstacle to the raising of an army. Under it 21.68 per cent of the registrants were rejected, 13 per cent more than for any other single cause.2

Later the standard was lowered3 so that men might be "unconditionally accepted for general military service" with a vision of 20/100 in each eye without glasses, provided one eye was correctible to 20/40. For special or limited service they might be accepted with only 20/200 in each eye without glasses, provided one was correctible to 20/40. At the same time a great many defects other than errors of refraction were admitted in both classes, such as squint not interfering with vision, slight nystagmus, and color blindness. Even total blindness in one eye was not a cause for rejection to the limited service class, provided it was not due to progressive or organic change, and the vision of the other eye was normal. Under this incredible standard eye defects still remained one of three leading causes of rejection.

Over ten per cent, (10.65) of the registrants were disqualified by them, while defects of the bones and joints and of the heart and blood-vessels ran respectively one and one and a half percent higher.4 Most of the revelations about the physical condition of the American people which resulted from the operation of the draft law had been anticipated by persons who had been giving their attention to such matters - and whose warnings had long fallen upon deaf ears - but it is doubtful if anyone had formed an adequate conception of the truth regarding the condition of the nation's eyesight. That it should be impossible to raise an army with even half normal vision in one eye, and that one man in every ten rejected for military service should have been unable, even by the aid of glasses, to attain this standard, is a situation so appalling that words fail to characterize it, so incredible that only the most unimpeachable evidence could compel belief in it. Under these circumstances it seems to me the plain duty of anyone who has found any means of controlling the evil in question to give the facts the widest possible publicity.

Most writers on ophthalmology today appear to believe that defective eyesight is part of the price we must pay for civilization. The human eye, they say, was not designed for the uses to which it is now put. Eons before there were any schools, or printing presses, electric lights, or moving pictures, its evolution was complete. In those days it served the needs of the human animal perfectly, but it is not to be expected, we are told, that it should respond without injury to the new demands. By care it is thought that this injury may be minimized, but to eliminate it wholly is considered to be too much to hope for. Such is the depressing conclusion to which the monumental labors of a hundred years and more have led us.

I have no hesitation in stating that this conclusion is unqualifiedly wrong. Nature did not blunder when she made the human eye, but has given us in this intricate and wonderful mechanism, upon which so much of the usefulness as well as the pleasure of life depends, an organ as fully equal to the needs of civilization as to those of the Stone Age. After thirty-three years of clinical and experimental work, I have demonstrated to my own satisfaction and that of others that the eye is capable of meeting the utmost demands of civilization; that the errors of refraction which have so long dogged the footsteps of progress, and which have made the raising of an army during the recent war so difficult, are both preventable and curable; and that many other forms of imperfect sight, long held to be incurable, may be either improved or completely relieved.

All these discoveries have been published in the medical press, but while their reliability has never been publicly disputed, the medical profession has so far failed to make use of them. Meantime the sight of our children is being destroyed daily in the schools, and our young men and women are entering life with a defect which, if uncorrected, must be a source of continual misery and expense to them, sometimes ending in blindness or economic ruin. Admitting for the sake of argument that I may be wrong in my conclusion that these things are unnecessary, it is time I was proven to be wrong. I should not be allowed to play on the forlorn hope of a suffering world. If I am right, as I know I am, a suffering world should no longer be deprived of the benefit of my discoveries.

To give publicity to these discoveries and arouse discussion regarding them is one of the objects for which this magazine has been started. At the same time its pages are open to everyone who has any light to throw upon the problem. It has too long been the custom of ophthalmologists to disregard every fact at variance with the accepted theories. Such facts, when observed, have usually not been published, and when published they have either been ignored or explained away in some more or less plausible manner. The management of this magazine wishes to make it a medium for the publication of such facts, which, it may safely be asserted, are known to every ophthalmologist of any experience, and which, if they had received proper consideration, would long ago have led us out of the blind alley in which we are now languishing.

While I think it may be truthfully said that many of my methods are new and original, other physicians, both in this country and in Europe, have cured themselves and others by treatment without glasses. Lay persons have done the same.

Fine Print – For Clear Close Vision

In *The Autocrat of the Breakfast Table*, Oliver Wendell Holmes published a very remarkable case of the cure of presbyopia.

"There is now living in New York State," he says, "an old gentleman who, perceiving his sight to fail, immediately took to exercising it on the finest print, and in this way fairly bullied Nature out of her foolish habit of taking liberties at five-and-forty, or thereabouts. And now this old gentleman performs the most extraordinary feats with his pen, showing that his eyes must be a pair of microscopes. I should be afraid to say how much he writes in the compass of a half-dime, whether the Psalms or the Gospels, or the Psalms and the Gospels, I won't be positive."5

An officer in the American Expeditionary Forces, whose letter is published elsewhere, wrote to me about a year ago that he has cured himself of presbyopia, and after half a lifetime of misery was entirely free from eye discomfort.
There must be many more of these cases, and we want to hear of them.

(Five and forty=fifties, forties... year of age.) Reading fine print maintains clear close and distant vision at all ages and keeps the eyes healthy, prevents development of eye diseases.

FUNDAMENTAL FACTS

For about seventy years it has been believed that the eye accommodates for vision at different distances by changing the curvature of the lens, and this theory has given birth to another, namely, that errors of refraction are due to a permanent organic change in the shape of the eyeball. On these two ideas the whole system of treating errors of refraction is based at the present time.

My experiments and clinical observations have demonstrated that both these theories are wrong.6 They have shown:

(1) That the lens is not a factor in accommodation;
(2) That the change of focus necessary for vision at different distances is brought about by the action of the superior and inferior obliques, which, by their contraction and relaxation, change the length of the eyeball as the length of the camera is changed by the shortening and lengthening of the bellows;
(3) That errors of refraction are due to the abnormal action of these muscles and of the recti, the obliques being responsible for myopia and the recti for hypermetropia, while both may combine in the production of astigmatism;
(4) That this abnormal action of the muscles on the outside of the eyeball is always due to mental strain of some kind.

This being the case it follows that all errors of refraction can be cured by relaxation. All methods of treatment, therefore, are simply different ways of obtaining relaxation. And because it is impossible to relax the eye muscles without relaxing the mind - and the relaxation of the mind means the relaxation of the whole body - it also follows that improvement in the eyesight is always accompanied by an improvement in health and mental efficiency.

The fact that all errors of refraction are functional can often be demonstrated within five minutes. When a person with myopia, hypermetropia, or astigmatism, looks at a blank wall without trying to see, the retinoscope, with a plane mirror, at six feet, indicates, in flashes or more continuously no error of refraction. The conditions should be favorable for relaxation and the doctor should be as much at his ease as the patient.

It can also be demonstrated with the retinoscope that persons with normal sight do not have it all the time.7 When the vision of such persons becomes imperfect at the distance it will be found that myopic refraction has been produced;8 when it becomes imperfect at the near point it will be found that hypermetropia has been produced.

CENTRAL FIXATION

An invariable symptom of all abnormal conditions of the eyes, whether functional or organic, is the loss of central fixation. When a person with perfect vision looks at a letter on the Snellen test card he can always observe that all the other letters in his field of vision are seen less distinctly. He can also observe that when he looks at the bottom of even the smallest letter on the card, the top appears less black and less distinct than the part directly regarded, while the same is true of a letter of diamond type, or of the smallest letters that are printed. When a person with imperfect sight looks at the card he can usually observe that when he can read a line of letters he is able to look at one letter of a line and see it better than the others, but the letters of a line he cannot read may look all alike, or those not directly regarded may even be seen better than the one fixed.

These conditions are due to the fact that when the sight is normal the sensitiveness of the fovea is normal, but when the sight is imperfect, from whatever cause, the sensitiveness of the fovea is lowered, so that the eye sees equally well, or even better, with other parts of the retina. Contrary to what is generally believed, the part seen best when the sight is normal is extremely small. **The text-books say that at twenty feet an area having a diameter of a quarter of an inch can be seen with maximum vision, but anyone who tries at this distance to see every part of one of the small letters of the Snellen test card - the diameter of which is about a quarter of an inch - equally well at one time will immediately become myopic. The fact is that the nearer the point of maximum vision approaches a mathematical point, which has no area, the better the sight.**

The cause of this loss of function in the center of sight is mental strain; and as all abnormal conditions of the eyes, organic as well as functional, are accompanied by mental strain, all such conditions must necessarily be accompanied by loss of central fixation. When the mind is under a strain the eye usually goes more or less blind. The center of sight goes blind first, partially or completely, according to the degree of the strain, and if the strain is great enough the whole or the greater part of the retina may be involved. When the vision of the center of sight has been suppressed, partially or completely, the patient can no longer see the point which he is looking at best, but sees objects not regarded directly as well, or better, because the sensitiveness of the retina has now become approximately equal in every part, or is even better in the outer part than in the center. Therefore in all cases of defective vision the patient is unable to see best where he is looking. When the person with imperfect vision sees the peripheral field clearest, it is not as clear as the central field is when the vision is normal.

This condition is sometimes so extreme that the patient may look as far away from an object as it is possible to see it and yet see it just as well as when looking directly at it. In one case it had gone so far that the patient could see only with the edge of the retina on the nasal side. In other words, she could not see her fingers in front of her face, but could see them if she held them at the outer side of her eye. She had no error of refraction, showing that while every error of refraction is accompanied by eccentric fixation, the strain which causes the one condition is different from that which produces the other. The patient had been examined by specialists in this country and Europe, who attributed her blindness to disease of the optic nerve, or brain; but the fact that vision was restored by relaxation demonstrated that the condition had been due simply to mental strain.

Eccentric fixation, even in its lesser degrees, is so unnatural that great discomfort, or even pain, can be produced in a few seconds by trying to see every part of an area three or four inches in extent at twenty feet, or even less, or an area of an inch or less at the near point, equally well at one time, while at the same time the retinoscope will demonstrate that an error of refraction has been produced. This strain, when it is habitual, leads to all sorts of abnormal conditions and is, in fact, at the bottom of most eye troubles, both functional and organic. The discomfort and pain may be absent, however, in the chronic condition, and it is an encouraging symptom when the patient begins to experience them.

Natural health improvement doctors state; When health or vision is impaired, pain and other symptoms occur. When health/vision impairment increases, sometimes the pain, other uncomfortable symptoms vanish, are not felt. New symptoms may take their place. When healing occurs and the health/vision is reversing back to normal, is being corrected/cured; the old pains, symptoms may temporarily re-appear as the health/vision is passing backwards through previous beginning stages of the health or vision problem. Then, as the health/vision improves to perfect health, clear vision; the pain, symptoms are completely removed. Complete recovery without passing through pain, uncomfortable symptoms can also occur.

The center of the retina, macula and fovea centralis with its many cones produce the clearest vision and brightest color in the center of the visual field. The peripheral field of the retina produces less clear vision and less color in the peripheral field of vision. When the vision is normal, clear; the center of the visual field is clearest and the peripheral field less clear. The exact center of the visual field is produced by the fovea centralis and is the size of the pointed end of a pin and produces very clear vision, much clearer than 20/20 and brightest color, fine detailed vision, ability to see very small parts of objects at close and far distances.

Central fixation – To look at/see one small part of a object clearest at a time in the center of the visual field. Shifting is combined with central fixation- The eyes, center of the visual field moves, shifts continually from part to part (point to point) on a object to see the object clear. The center of the visual field also moves with the eyes from object to object seeing one object at as time clearest.
Natural Eyesight Improvement returns perfect clear central vision and brings the peripheral to its maximum possible clarity.

Look at the dot on the top of the E.
The dot is in the center of the visual field and is clearest. The dot on the bottom is in the peripheral field and is less clear.
Shift dot to dot seeing one dot clearest at a time.

When the eye possesses central fixation it not only possesses perfect sight, but it is perfectly at rest and can be used indefinitely without fatigue. It is open and quiet; no nervous movements are observable; and when it regards a point at the distance the visual axes are parallel. In other words, there are no muscular insufficiencies. This fact is not generally known. The text-books state that muscular insufficiencies occur in eyes having normal sight, but I have never seen such a case. The muscles of the face and of the whole body are also at rest, and when the condition is habitual there are no wrinkles or dark circles around the eyes.

In most cases of eccentric fixation, on the contrary, the eye quickly tires, and its appearance, with that of the face, is expressive of effort or strain. The ophthalmoscope reveals that the eyeball moves at irregular intervals, from side to side, vertically or in other directions. These movements are often so extensive as to be manifest by ordinary inspection, and are sometimes sufficiently marked to resemble nystagmus. Nervous movements of the eyelids may also be noted, either by ordinary inspection, or by lightly touching the lid of one eye while the other regards an object either at the near point or the distance. The visual axes are never parallel, and the deviation from the normal may become so marked as to constitute the condition of **squint**. Strain, eccentric fixation, diffusion causes squint, crossed, wandering eyes, imperfect convergence, divergence. Redness of the conjuctiva and of the margins of the lids, wrinkles around the eyes, dark circles beneath them and tearing are other symptoms of eccentric fixation.

Eccentric fixation is a symptom of strain, and is relieved by any method that relieves strain; but in some cases the patient is cured just as soon as he is able to demonstrate the facts of central fixation. When he comes to realize, through actual demonstration of the fact, that (when experiencing blur, eccentric fixation, diffusion, not seeing with the center of the visual field) he does not see best where he is looking, and that when he looks a sufficient distance away from a point (when the eyes are working correct, relaxed, with central fixation) he can see it worse than when he looks directly at it, he becomes able, in some way, to reduce the distance to which he has to look in order to see worse, until he can look directly at the top of a small letter and see the bottom worse, or look at the bottom and see the top worse. The smaller the letter regarded in this way, or the shorter the distance the patient has to look away from a letter in order to see the opposite part indistinctly, the greater the relaxation and the better the sight. When it becomes possible to look at the bottom of a letter and see the top worse, or to look at the top and see the bottom worse, it becomes possible to see the letter perfectly black and distinct. At first such vision may come only in flashes. The letter will come out distinctly for a moment and then disappear. But gradually, if the practice is continued, central fixation will become habitual.

Most patients can readily look at the bottom of the big C and see the top worse; but in some cases it is not only impossible for them to do this, but impossible for them to let go of the large letters at any distance at which they can be seen. In these extreme cases it sometimes requires considerable ingenuity, first to demonstrate to the patient that he does not see best where he is looking, and then to help him to see an object worse when he looks away from it than when he looks directly at it. The use of a strong light as one of the points of fixation, or of two lights five or ten feet apart, has been found helpful, the patient when he looks away from the light being able to see it less bright more readily than he can see a black letter worse when he looks away from it. It then becomes easier for him to see the letter worse when he looks away from it. This method was successful in the following case:

A patient with vision of 3/200, when she looked at a point a few feet away from the big C, said she saw the letter better than when she looked directly at it. Her attention was called to the fact that her eyes soon became tired and that her vision soon failed when she saw things in this way. Then she was directed to look at a bright object about three feet away from the card, and this attracted her attention to such an extent that she became able to see the large letter on the test card worse, after which she was able to look back at it and see it better. It was demonstrated to her that she could do one of two things: look away and see the letter better than she did before, or look away and see it worse. She then became able to see it worse all the time when she looked three feet away from it. Next she became able to shorten the distance successively to two feet, one foot and six inches, with a constant improvement in vision; and finally she became able to look at the bottom of the letter and see the top worse, or look at the top and see the bottom worse. With practice she became able to look at the smaller letters in the same way, and finally she became able to read the ten line at twenty feet. By the same method also she became able to read diamond type, first at twelve inches and then at three inches. By these simple measures alone she became able, in short, to see best where she was looking, and her cure was complete.

The highest degrees of eccentric fixation occur in the high degrees of myopia, and in these cases, since the sight is best at the near point, the patient is benefited by practicing seeing worse at this point. The distance can then be gradually extended until it becomes possible to do the same thing at twenty feet. One patient with a high degree of myopia said that the farther she looked away from an electric light the better she saw it, but by alternately looking at the light at the near point and looking away from it she became able, in a short time, to see it brighter when she looked directly at it than when she looked away from it. Later she became able to do the same thing at twenty feet, and then she experienced a wonderful feeling of relief. No words, she said, could adequately describe it. Every nerve seemed to be relaxed, and a feeling of comfort and rest permeated her whole body. Afterward her progress was rapid. She soon became able to look at one part of the smallest letters on the card and see the rest worse, and then she became able to read the letters at twenty feet.

On the principle that a burnt child dreads the fire, some patients are benefited by consciously making their sight worse. When they learn, by actual demonstration of the facts, just how their visual defects are produced, they unconsciously avoid the unconscious strain which causes them. When the degree of eccentric fixation is not too extreme to be increased, therefore, it is a benefit to patients to teach them how to increase it. **When a patient has consciously lowered his vision and produced discomfort and even pain by trying to see the big C, or a whole line of letters, equally well at one time, he becomes better able to correct the unconscious effort of the eye to see all parts of a smaller area equally well at one time.** (experience strain=learn to avoid it.)

In learning to see best where he is looking it is usually best for the patient to think of the point not directly regarded as being seen less distinctly than the point he is looking at, instead of thinking of the point fixed as being seen best, as the latter practice has a tendency, in most cases, to intensify the strain under which the eye is already laboring. One part of an object is seen best only when the mind is content to see the greater part of it indistinctly, and as the degree of relaxation increases the area of the part seen worse increases until that seen best becomes merely a point. (Exact center of visual field, fovea centralis, clearer than 20/20)

The limits of vision depend upon the degree of central fixation. A person may be able to read a sign half a mile away when he sees the letters all alike, but when taught to see one letter best he will be able to read smaller letters that he didn't know were there.

The remarkable vision of savages, who can see with the naked eye objects for which most civilized persons require a telescope, is a matter of central fixation. Some people can see the rings of Saturn, or the moons of Jupiter, with the naked eye. It is not because of any superiority in the structure of their eyes, but because they have attained a higher degree of central fixation than most civilized persons do.

Not only do all errors of refraction and all functional disturbances of the eye disappear when it sees by central fixation, but many organic conditions are relieved or cured. I am unable to set any limits to its possibilities. I would not have ventured to predict that glaucoma, incipient cataract and syphilitic iritis could be cured by central fixation; but it is a fact that these conditions have disappeared when central fixation was attained. Relief was often obtained in a few minutes, and sometimes this relief was permanent. Usually, however, a permanent cure required more prolonged treatment. Inflammatory conditions of all kinds, including inflammation of the cornea, iris, conjunctiva, the various coats of the eyeball and even the optic nerve itself, have been benefited by central fixation after other methods had failed. Infections, as well as diseases caused by protein poisoning and the poisons of typhoid fever, influenza, syphilis and gonorrhoea, have also been benefited by it. Even with a foreign body in the eye there is no redness and no pain so long as central fixation is retained.

Since central fixation is impossible without mental control, central fixation of the eye means central fixation of the mind. It means, therefore, health in all parts of the body, for all the operations of the physical mechanism depend upon the mind. Not only the sight, but all the other senses - touch, taste, hearing and smell - are benefited by central fixation. All the vital processes - digestion, assimilation, elimination, etc. - are improved by it. The symptoms of functional and organic diseases are relieved. The efficiency of the mind is enormously increased. The benefits of central fixation already observed are, in short, so great that the subject merits further investigation.

Central fixation example:
Look at the top part of the letter C. Place it in the center of the visual field. Shift on it to avoid staring. While looking at that part, in the center of the visual field; that part is clearest. Other parts of the C away from the part the eyes are looking directly at are in the peripheral field are seen worse, less clear.
When the eyes move, shift to a new part, example; a part on the bottom of the C; this part is now in the center of the visual field, is clearest and the top of the C and other parts are in the peripheral field, away from the central field and are seen less clear.
Shift from part to part on the C and see one small part at a time clearest in the center of the visual field – Central Fixation.
Practice on large, then smaller letters, any objects, then on small objects, a fine print letter.
When the eyes can shift: small point to small point on a small object, small part of a object, fine print letter and use central fixation, vision is very clear.
Central fixation must be combined with shifting; shifting from point to point.
Central fixation does not mean to fix the eyes immobile on a point.

Look at/see clearest - one part (dot) of the C at a time, in the <u>center</u> of the visual field. The part (dot) in the peripheral field is less clear.

Eccentric fixation is – Diffusion – trying to see two or more objects or more than one part of a object at the same time, objects in the central and peripheral field equally clear at the same time. Not shifting from part to part, object to object. To space the visual attention out to cover the entire field without moving the eyes. Using the peripheral area of the retina and field of vision to see with, placing the object of visual attention in the peripheral field.

A TEACHER'S EXPERIENCES

A teacher forty years of age was first treated on March 28, 1919. She was wearing the following glasses: O. D. convex 0.75 D. S. with convex 4.00 D. C., 105 deg.; O. S. convex 0.75 D. S. with convex 3.50 D. C., 105 deg. On June 9, 1919, she wrote:

I will tell you about my eyes, but first let me tell you other things. You were the first to unfold your theories to me, and I found them good immediately - that is, I was favorably impressed from the start. I did not take up the cure because other people recommended it, but because I was convinced: first, that you believed in your discovery yourself; second, that your theory of the cause of eye trouble was true. I don't know how I knew these two things, but I did. After a little conversation with you, you and your discovery both seemed to me to bear the ear-marks of the genuine article. As to the success of the method with myself I had a little doubt. You might cure others, but you might not be able to cure me, However, I took the plunge, and it has made a great change in me and my life.

To begin with, I enjoy my sight. I love to look at things, to examine them in a leisurely, thorough way, much as a child examines things. I never realized it at the time, but it was irksome for me to look at things when I was wearing glasses, and I did as little of it as possible. The other day, going down on the Sandy Hook boat, I enjoyed a most wonderful sky without that hateful barrier, of misted glasses, and I am positive I distinguished delicate shades of color that I never would have been able to see, even with clear glasses. Things seem to me now to have more form, more reality than when I wore glasses. Looking into the mirror you see a solid representation on a flat surface, and the flat glass can't show you anything really solid. My eye-glasses, of course, never gave me this impression, but one curiously like it. I can see so clearly without them that it is like looking around corners without changing the position. I feel that I can almost do it.

I very seldom have occasion to **palm**.9 Once in a great while I feel the necessity of it. The same with **remembering a period**.10 Nothing else is ever necessary. I seldom think of my eyes, but at times it is borne in upon me how much I do use and enjoy using them.

My nerves are much better. I am more equable, have more poise, am less shy. I never used to show that I was shy, or lacked confidence. I used to go ahead and do what was required, if not without hesitation, but it was hard. Now I find it easy. Glasses, or poor sight rather, made me self-conscious. It certainly is a great defect and one people are sensitive to without realizing it. I mean the poor sight and the necessity for wearing glasses. I put on a pair of glasses the other day just for an experiment, and I found that they magnified things. My skin looked as if under a magnifying glass. Things seemed too near. The articles on my chiffonier looked so close I felt like pushing them away from me. The glasses I especially wanted to push away. They brought irritation at once. I took them off and felt peaceful. Things looked normal.

I see better in the street than I ever did with glasses. I can see what people look like across the street, can distinguish their features, etc., a thing I could not do with glasses, or before I wore them. I can see better across the river and further into people's houses across the street. Not that I indulge, but I noticed an increase of power while looking out of the window in school.

Speaking of school, I corrected an immense pile of examination papers the other day, five hours at a stretch, with an occasional look off the paper and an occasional turn about the room. I felt absolutely no discomfort after it. Two weeks previous to this feat I handled two hundred designs over and over again, looking at each one dozens and dozens of times to note changes and improvement in line and color. Occasionally, while this work was going on. I had to palm in the mornings on rising.

I use my eyes with as much success writing, though once in a while after a lot of steady writing they are a little bit tired. I can read at night without having to get close to a light. I mention this because last summer I had to sit immediately under the light, or I could not see.

From the beginning of the treatment I could use my eyes pretty well, but they used to tire. I remember making a large Liberty Loan poster two weeks after I took off my glasses, and I was amazed to find I could make the whole layout almost perfectly without a ruler, just as well as with my glasses. When I came to true it up with the ruler I found only the last row of letters a bit out of line at the very end. I couldn't have done better with glasses. However this wasn't fine work. About the same time I sewed a hem at night in a black dress, using a fine needle. I suffered a little for this, but not much. I used to practice my exercises at that time and palm faithfully. Now I don't have to practice, or palm; I feel no discomfort, and I am absolutely unsparing in my use of my eyes. I do everything I want to with them. I shirk nothing, pass up no opportunity of using them. From the first I did all my school work, read every notice, wrote all that was necessary, neglected nothing. Everything I was called upon to do I attempted. For instance, I had to read President Wilson's "Fourteen Points" in the assembly room without notice in a poor light-unusual wording, too,-and I read it unhesitatingly. I have yet to fail to make good.

Now to sum up the school end of it, I used to get headaches at the end of the month from adding columns of figures necessary to reports, etc. Now I do not get them. I used to get flustered when people came into my room. Now I do not; I welcome them. It is a peasant change to feel this way. And-I suppose this is most important really, though I think of it last-I teach better. I know how to get at the mind and how to make the children see things in perspective. I gave a lesson on the horizontal cylinder recently, which, you know, is not a thrillingly interesting subject, and it was a remarkable lesson in its results and in the grip it got on every girl in the room, stupid and bright. What you have taught me makes me use the memory and imagination more, especially the latter, in teaching.

Now, to sum up the effect of being cured upon my own mind. I am more direct, more definite, less diffused, less vague. In short, I am conscious of being better centered. It is central fixation of the mind. I saw this in your latest paper, but I realized it long ago and knew what to call it.

ARMY OFFICER CURES HIMSELF

An engineer, fifty-one years of age, had worn glasses since 1896, first for astigmatism, getting stronger ones every couple of years, and then for astigmatism and presbyopia. At one time he asked his oculist and several opticians if the eyes could not be strengthened by exercises, so as to make glasses unnecessary, but they said: "No. Once started on glasses you must keep to them." When the war broke out he was very nearly disqualified for service in the Expeditionary Forces by his eyes, but managed to pass the required tests, after which he was ordered abroad as an officer in the Gas Service. While there he saw in the Literary Digest of May 2, 1918, a reference to my method of curing defective eyesight without glasses, and on May 11 he wrote to me in part as follows:

At the front I found glasses a horrible nuisance, and they could not be worn with gas masks. After I had been about six months abroad I asked an officer of the Medical Corps about going without glasses. He said I was right in my ideas and told me to try it. The first week was awful, but I persisted and only wore glasses for reading and writing. I stopped smoking at the same time to make it easier on my nerves.

I brought to France two pairs of bow spectacles and two extra lenses for repairs. I have just removed the extra piece for near vision from these extra lenses and had them mounted as pince-nez, with shur-on mounts, to use for reading and writing, so that the only glasses I now use are for astigmatism, the age lens being off. Three months ago I could not read ordinary head-line type in newspapers without glasses. Today, with a good light, I can read ordinary book type (18 point), held at a distance of eighteen inches from my eyes. Since the first week in February, when I discarded my glasses, I have had no headaches, stomach trouble, or dizziness, and am in good health generally. My eyes are coming back, and I believe it is due to sticking it out. I ride considerably in automobiles and trams, and somehow the idea has crept into my mind that after every trip my eyes are stronger. This, I think, is due to the rapid changing of focus in viewing scenery going by so fast.

Other men have tried this plan on my advice, but gave it up after two or three days. Yet, from what they say, I believe they were not so uncomfortable as I was for a week or ten days.

I believe most people wear glasses because they "coddle" their eyes.

July, 1919 footnotes

1 - Harvard: Manual of Military Hygiene for the Military services of United States, third revised edition 1917, p. 195.
2 - Report of the Provost Marshal General to the Secretary of War on the First Draft under the Selective Service Act, 1917.
3 - Standards of Physical Examination for the Use of Local Boards, District Boards and Medical Advisory Boards under the Selective Service Act, Form 75, issued through office of the Provost Marshal General.
4 - Second Report of the Provost Marshal General to the Secretary of War on the Operations of the Selective Service System to December 20, 1918.
5 - Everyman's Library, 1908, pp. 166 and 167.
6 - Bates: The Cure of Defective Eyesight by Treatment Without Glasses. N. Y. Med. Jour., May 8, 1915. A Study of Images Reflected from the Cornea, Iris, Lens and Sclera. N. Y. Med. Jour., May 18, 1918.
7 - Bates: The Imperfect Sight of the Normal Eye. N. Y. Med. Jour., Sept 8, 1917.
8 – Bates: The Cause of Myopia. N. Y. Med. Jour., March 16, 1912.
9 - By palming is meant the covering of the closed eyes with the palms of the hands in such a way as to exclude all the light, while remembering some color, usually black.
10 - Bates: *Memory as an Aid to Vision.* N. Y. Med. Jour., May 24, 1919.

SCHOOL NUMBER
BETTER EYESIGHT
A MONTHLY MAGAZINE DEVOTED TO THE PREVENTION AND CURE OF IMPERFECT SIGHT WITHOUT GLASSES
August, 1919

How to Use the Snellen Test Card
FOR THE
Prevention and Cure of Imperfect Sight in Children

The Snellen Test Card is placed permanently upon the wall of the classroom, and every day the children silently read the smallest letters they can see from their seats with each eye separately, the other being covered with the palm of the hand in such a way as to avoid pressure on the eyeball. This takes no appreciable amount of time, and is sufficient to improve the sight of all children in one week and to cure all errors of refraction after some months, a year, or longer.

Children with markedly defective vision should be encouraged to read the card more frequently.

Records may be kept as follows:

John Smith, 10, Sept. 15, 1918.
   R. V. (vision of the right eye) 20/40.
   L. V. (vision of the left, eye) 20/20.

John Smith, 11, Jan. 1, 1919.
   R. V. 20/30.
   L. V. 20/15.

20/20
The numerator (top number) of the fraction indicates the distance of the test card from the pupil;
The denominator (bottom number) denotes the line read, as designated by the figures printed above the middle of each line of the Snellen Test Card.

A certain amount of supervision is absolutely necessary. At least once a year some one who understands the method should visit each classroom for the purpose of answering questions, encouraging the teachers to continue the use of the method, and making a report to the proper authorities.

It is not necessary that either the inspector, the teachers, or the children, should understand anything about the physiology of the eye.

SNELLEN TEST CARDS

There should be a Snellen test card in every family and in every school classroom. When properly used it always improves the sight even when it is already normal. Children or adults with errors of refraction, if they have never worn glasses, are cured simply by reading every day the smallest letters they can see at a distance of ten, fifteen, or twenty feet.

For Sale By
THE CENTRAL FIXATION PUBLISHING COMPANY

Paper ....50 Cents
Cardboard (folding) ....75 Cents
DELIVERED

A limited number of reprints of articles by Dr. Bates published in other medical journals also for sale. Send for list.

Dr. Hermann Von Helmholtz
Inventor of the Ophthalmoscope

Hermann Von Helmholtz (1821–1894) A German Physician, Physicist

Dr. Helmholtz studied and contributed to developments in mechanics, physics, science, mathematics, energy conservation, electrodynamics, fluid dynamics, thermodynamics, chemical thermodynamics, chemistry, electricity, magnetism, meteorology, philosophy, fine arts, physiology of the eye and the ear, hearing, acoustics, motion perception, physiological optics, mathematics of the eye, theories of vision, visual perception of space, color vision, color blindness, dioptrics (study of the refraction of light, especially by lenses) of the eye and many other areas of science.
He studied electrodynamics by Michael Faraday and James Clerk Maxwell, began the revolution in wireless communication, wrote the 'Handbook of Physiological Optics'.

He invented the Ophthalmoscope to examine/inspect the interior of the eye/retinal blood vessels, detect high blood pressure and arterial disease… He also invented the Ophthalmometer to measure the eyes accommodation/the eye's curvature.

Dr. Helmholtz created the 'Theory of Accommodation' – which states that the human eyes lens changes shape due to the action of the Ciliary Muscle to produce accommodation in the eye for clear vision when looking at close distances.

For years the Optical Industry, Eye Doctors stated Helmholtz's Theory as an absolute fact and stated that due to this fact, unclear vision cannot be cured, that only glasses, surgery, drugs can correct unclear vision and other eye problems.

Dr. William H. Bates, Ophthalmologist, eye, ear… doctor proved that the outer eye muscles (Oblique, Recti) can change the shape of the eye, produce accommodation and affect the clarity of vision. Relaxed, normally functioning outer eye muscles produced clear vision. Bates stated the lens does not produce accommodation. Dr. Bates proved as fact that unclear vision and a variety of other eye problems can be corrected, cured by natural methods of relaxing the mind, body, eye muscles, returning mind, body, eye muscles, eyes to normal function without eyeglasses, surgery, drugs. The Bates Method.

Modern day Ophthalmologists state that: with new technology, they have proven that the lens does change shape and can produce accommodation.

Some Scientists, Ophthalmologists state that Helmholtz and Bates were correct, that the eye and lens change shape, work together (and the lens might also move) to produce accommodation.

The Bates Method relaxes, improves function, health of the entire visual system, eyes, mind, body and relaxes, improves function of <u>all the eye muscles</u>; outer (Oblique, Recti & other outer muscles), inner (ciliary/lens, iris…) and continues to produce clear vision for over 100 years. Even before Bates time, the Bates Method was used naturally by the human eye.

A HOUSE BUILT ON SAND

That the results of the present method of treating defects of vision are far from satisfactory is something which no one would attempt to deny. It is well known that many patients wander from one specialist to another, seeking vainly for relief, while others give up in despair and either bear their visual ills as best they may without assistance, or else resort to Christian Science, mental science, osteopathy, physical culture, or some of the other healing cults to which the incompetence of orthodox medicine has given birth. The specialists themselves, having daily to handle each other's failures, are scarcely better satisfied. Privately they criticize each other with great asperity and freedom, and publicly they indulge in much speculation as to the underlying causes of this deplorable state of affairs.

At the recent meeting of the Ophthalmological Section of the American Medical Association, Dr. E. J. Gardiner, of Chicago, in a paper on *The Present Status of Refraction Work*,[1] finds that ignorance is responsible for the largest quota of failure to get satisfactory results from what he calls the "rich heritage" of ophthalmic science, but that a considerable percentage must be attributed to other causes. Among these causes he enumerates a too great dependence on measuring devices, the delegation of refraction work to assistants, and the tendency to eliminate cycloplegics, in deference to the prejudices of patients who have a natural objection to being incapacitated by "drops."

On the same occasion, Dr. Samuel Theobald, of Johns Hopkins University, noted a tendency to "minimize the importance of muscular anomalies" as an important cause of many failures to give relief to eye patients. Among cases that have come into his hands after glasses had been prescribed by other ophthalmologists he has often found that "though great pains had been taken to correct even minor faults of refraction, grave muscular errors had been entirely overlooked." From this fact and from the small number of latent muscular defects noted in the hospital reports which he has examined, the conclusion seems to him inevitable that such faults are in large measure ignored.

Dr. Walter Pyle, of Philadelphia, laid stress on "necessary but often neglected refinements in examination of ocular refraction." "Long practice, infinite care and attention to finer details," he said, "are imperative requisites, since a slight fault in the correction of a refractive error aggravates rather than relieves the accompanying asthenopic symptoms." This care, he says, must be exercised not only by the oculist but by the optician, and to the end that the latter may be inspired to do his part, he suggests that the oculist provide himself with the means for keeping tabs on him in the form of a mechanical lens measure, axis finder and centering machine.

Dr. Charles Emerson, of the Indiana University School of Medicine, suggested a closer co-operation between the ophthalmologist and the physician, as there were many patients who could not be helped by the ophthalmologist alone.

The fitting of glasses by opticians is usually condemned without qualification, but in the discussion which followed these papers, Dr. Dunbar Roy, of Atlanta, said that the optician, just because he does not use cycloplegics, frequently fits patients with comfortable glasses where the ophthalmologist has failed. When a patient needs glasses, said Dr. Roy, he needs them when his eyes are in their natural or normal condition and not when the muscle of accommodation is partially paralyzed. Even the heavy frames used in the adjustment of trial lenses were not forgotten in the search for possible causes of failure, Dr. Roy believing that the patient is often so annoyed by these contrivances that he does not know which is causing him the most discomfort, the frames or the glasses.

Nowhere in the whole discussion was there any suggestion that this great mass of acknowledged failure could possibly be due to any defect in fundamental principles. These are a "rich heritage," the usefulness of which is not to be questioned. If they do not produce satisfactory results, it must be due to their faulty application, and it is taken for granted that there are a select few who understand and are willing to take the trouble to use them properly.

The simple fact, however, is that the fitting of glasses can never be satisfactory. The refraction of the eye is continually changing.2 Myopia, hypermetropia and astigmatism come and go, diminish and increase, and the same adjustment of glasses cannot suit the affected eyes at all times. One may be able, in many cases, to make the patient comfortable, to improve his sight, or to relieve nervous symptoms; but there will always be a considerable number of persons who get little or no help from glasses, while practically everyone who wears them is more or less dissatisfied. The optician may succeed in making what is considered to be a satisfactory adjustment, and the most eminent ophthalmologist may fail. I personally know of one specialist, a man of international reputation, who fitted a patient sixty times with glasses without affording him the slightest relief.

And even when the glasses do what is expected of them they do very little. Considering the nature of the superstructure built on the foundation of Donders, and the excellent work being done by leading men, Dr. Gardiner thinks the present status of refraction work might be deemed eminently satisfactory if it were not for the great amount of bad and careless work being done; but I do not consider it satisfactory when all we can do for people with imperfect sight is to give them eye crutches that do not even check the progress of the trouble, when the only help we can offer to the millions of myopic and hypermetropic and astigmatic and squinting children in our schools is to put spectacles on them. If this is the best that ophthalmology can do after building for three-quarters of a century upon the foundation of Donders, is it not time that we began to examine that foundation of which Dr. Gardiner boasts that "not one stone has been removed"? Instead of seeking the cause of our failure to accomplish even the little we claim to be able to do in the ignorance and carelessness of the average practitioner, great as that ignorance and carelessness often are; in the neglect of cycloplegics and the refinements of lens adjustment: in the failure to detect latent muscular anomalies; in the absence of co-operation between specialist and general practitioner: would it not be wiser to examine the foundation of our superstructure and see whether it is of stone or of sand?

THE PREVENTION OF MYOPIA
Methods That Failed

The publication in 1867 by Professor Hermann Cohn of Breslau of a study of the eyes of ten thousand school children first called general attention to the fact that while myopia is seldom found in the pre-school age, the defect increases steadily both in percentage of cases and in degree during the educational period. Professor Cohn's investigations were repeated in all the advanced countries, and his observations, with some difference in percentages, were everywhere confirmed. The conditions were unanimously attributed to the excessive use of the eyes for near work, and as it was impossible to abandon the educational system, attempts were made to minimize the supposed evil effects of the reading, writing and other near work which it demanded. Careful and detailed rules were laid down by various authorities as to the size of type to be used in school books, the length of the lines, their distance apart, the distance at which the book should be held, the amount and arrangement of the light, the construction of the desks, the length of time the eyes might be used without a change of focus, etc. Face rests were even devised to hold the eyes at the prescribed distance from the desk and to prevent stooping, which was supposed to cause congestion of the eyeball and thus to encourage elongation. The Germans, with characteristic thoroughness, actually used these instruments of torture, Cohn never allowing his children to write without one, "even at the best possible desk."3

The results of these preventive measures were disappointing. Some observers reported a slight decrease in the percentage of myopia in schools in which the prescribed reforms had been made; but on the whole, as Risley has observed in his discussion of the subject in Norris and Oliver's *System of Diseases of the Eye*, "the injurious effects of the educational process were not noticeably arrested."

"It is a significant, though discouraging fact," he continues, "that the increase, as found by Cohn, both in the percentage and in the degree of myopia, had taken place in those schools where he had especially exerted himself to secure the introduction of hygienic forms, and the same is true of the observations of Just, who had examined the eyes of twelve hundred and twenty-nine of the pupils of the two High Schools of Zittau, in both of which the hygienic conditions were all that could be desired. He found, nevertheless, that the excellent arrangements had not in any degree lessened the percentage of increase in myopia. It became necessary, therefore, to look beyond faulty hygienic environments for the cause of the pathological states represented by Myopia."4

With the passage of time further evidence to the same effect has steadily accumulated. In an investigation in London, for instance, in which the schools were carefully selected to reveal any difference that might arise from the various influences, hygienic, social and racial, to which the children were subjected, the proportion of myopia in the best lighted and ventilated school of the group was actually found to be higher than in the one where these conditions were worst.5 It has also been found that there is just as much myopia in schools where little near work is done as in those in which the demands upon the accommodative power of the eye are greater, while in any case it is only a minority of the children in any school who become myopic, although all may be exposed to practically the same eye conditions. Dr. Adolf Steiger, in his recent hook on *Spherical Refraction*, bears witness, after a comprehensive survey of the whole question, to the "absolutely negative results of school hygiene,"6 and Dr. Sidler-Huguenin reports7 that in the thousands of cases that have come under his care he has observed no appreciable benefit from any method of treatment at his command.

Facts of this sort have led to a modification of the myopia theory, but have produced no change in methods of myopia prevention. An hereditary tendency toward the development of the defect is now assumed by most authorities; but although no one has ever been able to offer even a plausible explanation for its supposed injuriousness, and though its restriction has been proven over and over again to be useless, near work is still generally held to be a contributing cause and ophthalmologists still go on in the same old way, trying to limit the use of the eyes at the near-point and encourage vision at the distance. It is incomprehensible that men calling themselves scientific, and having had at least a scientific training, can be so foolish. One might excuse a layman for such irrational conduct, but how men of scientific repute who are supposed to write authoritative textbooks can go on year after year copying each other's mistakes and ignoring all facts which are in conflict with them is a thing which reasonable people can hardly be expected to understand.

In 1912,8 and a good many times since, I published the observation that myopia is always lessened when the subject strains to see at the near point, and always produced in the normal eye when the subject strains to see at the distance. These observations are

of the greatest practical importance, for if they are correct, they prove our present methods of preventing myopia to be a monumental blunder. Yet no one, so far as I have heard, has taken the trouble to test their accuracy. I challenged the medical profession to produce a single exception to the statements I made in the 1912 publication, and that challenge has stood for seven years, although every member of the Ophthalmological Section of the American Medical Association must have had an opportunity to see it, and anyone who knows how to use a retinoscope could have made the necessary tests in a few minutes. If any did this, they failed to publish the results of their observations, and are, therefore, responsible for the effects of their silence. If they found that I was right and neglected to say so, they are responsible for the fact that the benefits that must ultimately result from this discovery have been delayed. If they found that I was wrong, they are responsible for any harm that may have resulted from their indifference.

THE PREVENTION AND CURE OF MYOPIA AND OTHER ERRORS OF REFRACTION
A Method That Succeeded

You cannot see anything with perfect sight unless you have seen it before. When the eye looks at an unfamiliar object it always strains more or less to see that object, and an error of refraction is always produced. When children look at unfamiliar writing, or figures, on the blackboard, distant maps, diagrams, or pictures, the retinoscope always shows that they are myopic, though their vision may be under other circumstances absolutely normal. The same thing happens when adults look at unfamiliar distant objects. When the eye regards a familiar object, however, the affect is quite otherwise. Not only can it be regarded without strain, but the strain of looking later at unfamiliar objects is lessened.

This fact furnishes us with a means of overcoming the mental strain to which children are subjected by the modern educational system. It is impossible to see anything perfectly when the mind is under a strain, and if children become able to relax when looking at familiar objects, they become able, sometimes in an incredibly brief space of time, to maintain their relaxation when looking at unfamiliar objects.

I discovered this fact while examining the eyes of 1,500 school children at Grand Forks, N. D., in 1903.9 In many cases children who could not read all of the letters on the Snellen test card at the first test read them at the second or third test. After a class had been examined the children who had failed would sometimes ask for a second test, and then it often happened that they would read the whole card with perfect vision. So frequent were these occurrences that there was no escaping the conclusion that in some way the vision was improved by reading the Snellen test card. In one class I found a boy who at first appeared to be very myopic, but who, after a little encouragement, read all the letters on the test card. The teacher asked me about this boy's vision, because she had found him to be very "near-sighted." When I said that his vision was normal she was incredulous, and suggested that he might have learned the letters by heart, or been prompted by another pupil. He was unable to read the writing or figures on the blackboard, she said, or to see the maps, charts, and diagrams on the walls, and did not recognize people across the street. She asked me to test his sight again, which I did, very carefully, under her supervision, the sources of error which she had suggested being eliminated. Again the boy read all the letters on the card. Then the teacher tested his sight. She wrote some words and figures on the blackboard and asked him to read them. He did so correctly. Then she wrote additional words and figures, which he read equally well. Finally she asked him to tell the hour by the clock twenty-five feet distant, which he did correctly. It was a dramatic situation, both the teacher and the children being intensely interested. Three other cases in the class were similar, their vision, which had previously been very defective for distant objects, becoming normal in the few moments devoted to testing their eyes. It is not surprising that after such a demonstration the teacher asked to have a Snellen test card placed permanently in the room.

The children were directed to read the smallest letters they could see from their seats at least once every day, with both eyes together and with each eye separately, the other being covered with the palm of the hand in such a way as to avoid pressure on the eyeball. (Use of eye patch is best so the hand does not need to be held up – holding hand up to eye causes the muscles in hand, arm, shoulder, neck, then eyes to become tense.)

Practice shifting on a familiar object - letters on a test card daily with; Both eyes together, one eye at a time, both eyes together again.

Those whose vision was defective were encouraged to read it more frequently, and in fact needed no encouragement to do so after they found that the practice helped them to see the blackboard, and stopped the headaches, or other discomfort, previously resulting from the use of their eyes.

In another class of forty children, between six and eight, thirty of the pupils gained normal vision while their eyes were being tested. The remainder were cured later under the supervision of the teacher by exercises in distant vision with the Snellen card. This teacher had noted every year for fifteen years that at the opening of the school in the fall all the children could see the writing on the blackboard from their seats, but before school closed the following spring all of them without exception complained that they could not see it at a distance of more than ten feet. After learning of the benefits to be derived from the daily practice of distant vision with familiar objects as the points of fixation, this teacher kept a Snellen test card continually in her classroom and directed the children to read it every day. The result was that for eight years no more of the children under her care acquired defective eyesight.

This teacher had attributed the invariable deterioration in the eyesight of her charges during the school year to the fact that her classroom was in the basement and the light poor. But teachers with well-lighted classrooms had the same experience, and after the Snellen test card was introduced into both the well-lighted and the poorly lighted rooms, and the children read it every day, the deterioration of their eyesight not only ceased, but the vision of all improved. Vision which had been below normal improved, in most cases, to normal, while children who already had normal sight, usually reckoned at 20/20, became able to read 20/15 or 20/10. And not only was myopia cured, but the vision for near objects was improved.

At the request of the superintendent of the schools of Grand Forks, Mr. J. Nelson Kelly, the system was introduced into all the schools of the city and was used continuously for eight years, during which time it reduced myopia among the children, which I found at the beginning to be about six per cent, to less than one per cent.

In 1911 and 1912 the same system was introduced into some of the schools of New York City[10] with an attendance of about ten thousand children. Many of the teachers neglected to use the cards, being unable to believe that such a simple method, and one so entirely at variance with previous teaching on the subject, could accomplish the desired results. Others kept the cards in a closet except when they were needed for the daily eye drill, lest the children should memorize them. Thus they not only put an unnecessary burden upon themselves, but did what they could to defeat the purpose of the system, which is to give the children **daily exercise in distant vision with a familiar object as the point of fixation**. A considerable number, however, used the system intelligently and persistently, and in less than a year were able to present reports showing that of three thousand children with imperfect sight over one thousand had obtained normal vision by its means. Some of these children, as in the case of the children of Grand Forks, were cured in a few minutes. Many of the teachers were also cured, some of them very quickly. In some cases the results of the system were so astonishing as to be scarcely credible.

In a class of mental defectives, where the teacher had kept records of the eyesight of the children for several years, it had been invariably found that their vision grew steadily worse as the term advanced. As soon as the Snellen test card had been introduced, however, they began to improve. Then came a doctor from the Board of Health who tested the eyes of the children and put glasses on all of them, even those whose sight was fairly good. The use of the card was then discontinued, as the teacher did not consider it proper to interfere while the children were wearing glasses prescribed by a physician. Very soon, however, the children began to lose, break, or discard, their glasses. Some said that the spectacles gave them headaches, or that they felt better without them. In the course of a month or so most of the aids to vision which the Board of Health had supplied had disappeared. The teacher then felt herself at liberty to resume the use of the Snellen test card. Its benefits were immediate. The eyesight and the mentality of the children improved simultaneously, and soon they were all drafted into the regular classes, because it was found that they were making the same progress in their studies as the other children were.

Another teacher reported an equally interesting experience. She had a class of children who did not fit into the other grades. Many of them were backward in their studies. Some were persistent truants. All of them had defective eyesight. A Snellen test card was hung in the classroom where all the children could see it, and the teacher carried out my instructions literally. At the end of six months all but two had been cured and these had improved very much, while the worst incorrigible and the worst truant had become good students. The incorrigible, who had previously refused to study, because, he said, it gave him a headache to look at a book, or at the blackboard, found out that the test card, in some way, did him a lot of good; and although the teacher had asked him to read it but once a day, he read it whenever he felt uncomfortable. The result was that in a few weeks his vision had become normal and his objection to study had disappeared. The truant had been in the habit of remaining away from school two or three days every week, and neither his parents nor the truant officer had been able to do anything about it. To the great surprise of his teacher he never missed a day after having begun to read the Snellen test card. When she asked for an explanation he told her that what had driven him away from school was the pain that came in his eyes whenever he tried to study, or to read the writing on the blackboard. After reading the Snellen test card, he said, his eyes and head were rested and he was able to read without any discomfort.

To remove any doubts that might arise as to the cause of the improvement noted in the eyesight of the children comparative tests were made with and without cards. In one case six pupils with defective sight were examined daily for one week without the use of the test card. No improvement took place. The card was then restored to its place and the group was instructed to read it every day. At the end of a week all had improved and five were cured. In the case of another group of defectives the results were similar. During the week that the card was not used no improvement was noted, but after a week of exercises in distant vision with the card all showed marked improvement, and at the end of a month all were cured. In order that there might be no question as to the reliability of the records of the teachers some of the principals asked the Board of Health to send an inspector to test the vision of the pupils, and whenever this was done the records were found to be correct. Dr. Bates has the children read the eyechart with both eyes together, then one eye at a time, then both eyes together again. He also has the children look close and distant, shifting on exact letters on two identical eyecharts placed at close and far distances. Also done with both eyes together, then one eye at a time, then both eyes together again. If vision needs more improvement in one eye, extra time is spent practicing with that eye to bring the vision equally clear, perfect in both left and right eyes. Basic Behavioral Optometry.

One day I visited the city of Rochester, and while there I called on the Superintendent of Public Schools and told him about my method of preventing myopia. He was very much interested and invited me to introduce it in one of his schools. I did so, and at the end of three months a report was sent to me showing that the vision of all the children had improved, while quite a number of them had obtained perfect sight in both eyes.

The method has been used in a number of other cities and always with the same result. The vision of all the children improved, and many of them obtained perfect sight in the course of a few minutes, days, weeks or months.

It is difficult to prove a negative proposition, but since this system improved the vision of all the children who used it, it follows that none could have grown worse. It is therefore obvious that it must have prevented myopia. This cannot be said of any method of preventing myopia in schools which had previously been tried. All other methods are based on the idea that it is the excessive use of the eyes for near work that causes myopia, and all of them have admittedly failed.

It is also obvious that the method must have prevented other errors of refraction, a problem which previously had not even been seriously considered, because hypermetropia is supposed to be congenital, and astigmatism was until recently supposed also to be congenital in the great majority of cases. Anyone who knows how to use a retinoscope may, however, demonstrate in a few minutes that both of these conditions are acquired; for no matter how astigmatic or hypermetropic an eye may be, its vision always becomes normal when it looks at a blank surface without trying to see. It may also be demonstrated that when children are learning to read, write, draw, sew, or to do anything else that necessitates their looking at unfamiliar objects at the near-point, hypermetropia, or hypermetropic astigmatism, is always produced. The same is true of adults. These facts have not been reported before, so far as I am aware, and they strongly suggest that children need, first of all, eye education. They must be able to look at strange letters or objects at the near-point without strain before they can make much progress in their studies, and in every case in which the method has been tried it has proven that this end is attained by daily exercise in distant vision with the Snellen test card. When their distant vision has been improved by this means children invariably become able to use their eyes without strain at the near-point.

The method succeeded best when the teacher did not wear glasses. In fact, the effect upon the children of a teacher who wears glasses is so detrimental that no such person should be allowed to be a teacher, and since errors of refraction are curable, such a ruling would work no hardship on anyone. Not only do children imitate the visual habits of a teacher who wears glasses, but the nervous strain of which the defective sight is an expression produces in them a similar condition. In classes of the same grade, with the same lighting, the sight of children whose teachers did not wear glasses has always been found to be better than the sight of children whose teachers did wear them. In one case I tested the sight of children whose teacher wore glasses and found it very imperfect. The teacher went out of the room on an errand, and after she had gone I tested them again. The results were very much better. When the teacher returned she asked about the sight of a particular boy, a very nervous child, and as I was proceeding to test him she stood before him and said, "Now, when the doctor tells you to read the card, do it." The boy couldn't see anything. Then she went behind him, and the effect was the same as if she had left the room. The boy read the whole card.

Still better results would be obtained if we could reorganize the educational system on a rational basis. Then we might expect a general return of that **primitive acuity of vision** which we marvel at so greatly when we read about it in the memoirs of travelers. But even under existing conditions it has been proven beyond the shadow of a doubt that errors of refraction are no necessary part of the price we must pay for education.

There are at least ten million children in the schools of the United States who have defective sight. This condition prevents them from taking full advantage of the educational opportunities which the State provides. It undermines their health and wastes the taxpayers' money. If allowed to continue, it will be an expense and a handicap to them throughout their lives. In many cases it will be a source of continual misery and suffering. And yet practically all of these cases could be cured and the development of new ones prevented by the daily reading of the Snellen test card.

Why should our children be compelled to suffer and wear glasses for want of this simple measure of relief? It costs practically nothing. In fact, it would not be necessary, in some cases, as in the schools of New York City, even to purchase the Snellen test cards, as they are already being used to test the eyes of the children. Not only does it place practically no additional burden upon the teachers, but, by improving the eyesight, health, disposition and mentality of their pupils, it greatly lightens their labors. No one would venture to suggest, further, that it could possibly do any harm. Why, then, should there be any delay about introducing it into the schools? If there is still thought to be need for further investigation and discussion, we can investigate and discuss just as well after the children get the cards as before, and by adopting that course we will not run the risk of needlessly condemning another generation to that curse which heretofore has always dogged the footsteps of civilization, namely, defective eyesight. I appeal to all who read these lines to use whatever influence they possess toward the attainment of this end.

Native American Indians had perfect eyesight and health before they were forced into the white mans culture, schools, religion diet. Modern Indians are now reclaiming their heritage. An American Indian would be a great U.S. President.
This book is free for Native American Indians to read, distribute, sell.

THE STORY OF EMILY

**Children cured of defective eyesight by Dr. Bates, teach the Bates Method,
cure defective sight; blur, astigmatism, cataract, crossed eyes in other children.**

The efficacy of the method of treating imperfect sight without glasses has been demonstrated in thousands of cases, not only in my own practice but in that of many persons of whom I may not even have heard; for almost all patients when they are cured proceed to cure others. At a social gathering one evening a lady told me that she had met a number of my patients; but when she mentioned their names, I found that I did not remember any of them, and said so.

"That is because you cured them by proxy," she said. "You didn't directly cure Mrs. Jones or Mrs. Brown, but you cured Mrs. Smith and Mrs. Smith cured the other ladies. You didn't treat Mr. and Mrs. Simpkins or Mr. Simpkins' mother and brother, but you may remember that you cured Mr. Simpkins' boy of a squint, and he cured the rest of the family."

In schools where the Snellen test card was used to prevent and cure imperfect sight, the children, after they were cured themselves, often took to the practice of ophthalmology with the greatest enthusiasm and success, curing their fellow students, their parents and their friends. They made a kind of game of the treatment, and the progress of each school case was watched with the most intense interest by all the children. On a bright day, when the patients saw well, there was great rejoicing, and on a dark day there was corresponding depression. One girl cured twenty-six children in six months; another cured twelve in three months; a third developed quite a varied ophthalmological practice and did things of which older and more experienced practitioners might well have been proud. Going to the school which she attended one day, I asked this girl about her sight, which had been very imperfect. She replied that it was now very good, and that her headaches were quite gone. I tested her sight and found it normal. Then another child whose sight had also been very poor spoke up,

"I can see all right too," she said. "Emily"—indicating girl No. I—"cured me."

"Indeed"" I replied. "How did she do that?"

The second girl explained that Emily had had her read the card, which she could not see at all from the back of the room, at a distance of a few feet. The next day she had moved it a little further way, and so on, until the patient was able to read it from the back of the room, just as the other children did. Emily now told her to cover the right eye and read the card with her left, and both girls were considerably upset to find that the **uncovered eye was apparently blind.** The school doctor was consulted and said that nothing could be done. The eye had been blind from birth and no treatment would do any good.

Nothing daunted, however, Emily undertook the treatment. She told the patient to cover her good eye and go up close to the card, and at a distance of a foot or less it was found that she could read even the small letters. The little practitioner then proceeded confidently as with the other eye, and after many months of practice the patient became the happy possessor of normal vision in both eyes. The case had, in fact, been simply one of high myopia, and the school doctor, not being a specialist, had not detected the difference between this condition and blindness.

In the same classroom, there had been a little girl with congenital **cataract**, but on the occasion of my visit the defect had disappeared. This, too, it appeared, was Emily's doing. The school doctor had said that there was no help for this eye except through operation, and as the sight of the other eye was pretty good, he fortunately did not think it necessary to urge such a course. Emily accordingly took the matter in hand. She had the patient stand close to the card, and at that distance it was found that she could not see even the big C. Emily now held the card between the patient and the light and moved it back and forth. At a distance of three or four feet this movement could be observed indistinctly by the patient. The card was then moved farther away, until the patient became able to see it move at ten feet and to see some of the larger letters indistinctly at a less distance. Finally, after six months, she became able to read the card with the bad eye as well as with the good one. After testing her sight and finding it normal in both eyes, I said to Emily

"You are a splendid doctor. You beat them all. Have you done anything else?"

The child blushed, and turning to another of her classmates, said:

"Mamie, come here."

Mamie stepped forward and I looked at her eyes. There appeared to be nothing wrong with them.

"I cured her," said Emily.

"What of?" I inquired.

"Cross eyes," replied Emily.

"How," I asked, with growing astonishment.

Emily described a procedure very similar to that adopted in the other cases. Finding that the sight of the **crossed eye** was very poor, so much so, indeed, that poor Mamie could see practically nothing with it, the obvious course of action seemed to her to be the restoration of its sight; and, never having read any medical literature she did not know that this was impossible. So she went to it. She had Mamie cover her good eye and practice with the bad one at home and at school, until at last the sight became normal and the eye straight. The school doctor had wanted to have the eye operated upon, I was told, but fortunately Mamie was "scared" and would not consent. And here she was with two perfectly good, straight eyes.

"Anything else?" I inquired, when Mamie's case had been disposed of. Emily blushed again, and said:

"Here's Rose. Her eyes used to hurt her all the time, and she couldn't see anything on the blackboard. Her headaches used to be so bad that she had to stay away from school every once in a while. The doctor gave her glasses; but they didn't help her, and she wouldn't wear them. When you told us the card would help our eyes I got busy with her. I had her read the card close up, and then I moved it farther away, and now she can see all right, and her head doesn't ache any more. She comes to school every day, and we all thank you very much."

This was a case of compound hypermetropic astigmatism. Such stories might be multiplied indefinitely. Emily's astonishing record cannot, it is true, be duplicated, but lesser cures by cured patients have been very numerous and serve to show that the benefits of the method of preventing and curing defects of vision in the schools which is presented in this number of BETTER EYESIGHT would be far-reaching. Not only errors of refraction would be cured, but many more serious defects; and not only the children would be helped, but their families and friends also.

THE CURE OF IMPERFECT SIGHT

By Treatment Without Glasses

By W. H. BATES, M.D., New York

A RESUME of animal experiments and clinical observations which demonstrate that the lens is not a factor in accommodation and that all **errors of refraction are functional and therefore curable.**

METHODS OF TREATMENT whereby such **cures have been effected in thousands of cases.** These methods will enable not only physicians, but parents, teachers, and others who themselves possess normal vision to cure all children under twelve years of age who have never worn glasses, and many children and adults who have. Many persons with minor defects of vision are able to cure themselves.

Thoroughly scientific, the book is at the same time written in language which any intelligent layman can understand. It is profusely illustrated with original photographs and drawings, and will be published shortly at $3, post-paid. Orders may be placed now with the

Central Fixation Publishing Company, 39-45 East 42nd Street, New York.

August, 1919 -

1 - For reports of all the papers quoted, see Jour. Am. Med. Assoc. June 21, 1919.
2 - Bates: The Imperfect Sight of the Normal Eye, N. Y. Med. Jour., Sept. 8, 1917.
3 - The Hygiene of the Eye in Schools, English translation, edited by Turnbull, p. 127.
4 - System of Diseases of the Eye, 1897. Vol. II, p. 361.
5 - Brit. Med. Jour., June 18, 1898.
6 - Die Entstehung der sphärischen Refraktionen des menschlichen Auges, Berlin, 1913, p. 540.
7 - Archiv f. Augenhlk., Vol. LXXIX, 1915, translated in Archives of Ophthalmology, Vol. XLV, No. 6, November 1916.
8 - Bates: The Cause of Myopia, N. Y. Med. Jour., March 16, 1912.
9 - Bates: The Prevention of Myopia in School Children, N. Y. Med. Jour., July 29, 1911.
10 - Bates: Myopia Prevention by Teachers, N. Y. Med. Jour., Aug. 30, 1913.

BETTER EYESIGHT
A MONTHLY MAGAZINE DEVOTED TO THE PREVENTION AND CURE OF IMPERFECT SIGHT WITHOUT GLASSES
September, 1919
THE FLASHING CURE

Do you read imperfectly? Can you observe then that when you look at the first word, or the first letter, of a sentence you do not see best where you are looking; that you see other words, or other letters, just as well as or better than the ones you are looking at? Do you observe also that the harder you try to see the worse you see?

Now close your eyes and rest them, remembering some color, like black or white, that you can remember perfectly. Keep them closed until they feel rested, or until the feeling of strain has been completely relieved. Now open them and **look at the first word or letter of a sentence for a fraction of a second**. If you have been able to relax, partially or completely, you will have a **flash of improved or clear vision**, and the area seen best will be smaller.

After opening the eyes for this fraction of a second, close them again quickly, still remembering the color, and keep them closed until they again feel rested. Then again open them for a fraction of a second. Continue this alternate resting of the eyes and flashing of the letters for a time, and you may soon find that you can keep your eyes open longer than a fraction of a second without losing the improved vision.

If your trouble is with distant instead of near vision, use the same method with distant letters.

In this way you can demonstrate for yourself the fundamental principles of the cure of imperfect sight by treatment without glasses.

If you fail, ask someone with perfect sight to help you.

When looking at a letter: shift on it part to part. Blink. The letter remains clear.
Shift dot to dot (part to part) on the E.

VISION AND EDUCATION

Poor sight is admitted to be one of the most fruitful causes of retardation in the schools. It is estimated1 that it may reasonably be held responsible for a quarter of the habitually "left-backs," and it is commonly assumed that all this might be prevented by suitable glasses.

There is much more involved in defective vision, however, than mere inability to see the blackboard, or to use the eyes without pain or discomfort. Defective vision is the result of an abnormal condition of the mind, and when the mind is in an abnormal condition it is obvious that none of the processes of education can be conducted with advantage. By putting glasses upon a child we may, in some cases, neutralize the effect of this condition upon the eyes and by making the patient more comfortable may improve his mental faculties to some extent, but we do not alter fundamentally the condition of the mind and by confirming it in a bad habit we may make it worse.

It can easily be demonstrated that among the faculties of the mind which are impaired when the vision is impaired is the memory; and as a large part of the educational process consists of storing the mind with facts, and all the other mental processes depend upon one's knowledge of facts, it is easy to see how little is accomplished by merely putting glasses on a child that has "trouble with its eyes." The **extraordinary memory of primitive people** has been attributed to the fact that owing to the absence of any convenient means of making written records they had to depend upon their memories, which were strengthened accordingly; but in view of the known facts about the relation of memory to eyesight it is more reasonable to suppose that the retentive memory of primitive man was due to the same cause as his **keen vision**, namely, **a mind at rest**.

The primitive memory as well as primitive keenness of vision have been found among civilized people, and if the necessary tests had been made it would doubtless have been found that they always occur together, as they did in a case which recently came under my observation. The subject was a child of ten with such marvelous eyesight that **she could see the moons of Jupiter with the naked eye**, a fact which was demonstrated by her drawing a diagram of these satellites which exactly corresponded to the diagrams made by persons who had used a telescope. **Her memory was equally remarkable.** She could recite the whole content of a book after reading it, as Lord Macauley is said to have done, and she learned more Latin in a few days without a teacher than her sister who had six diopters of myopia had been able to do in several years. She remembered five years afterward what she ate at a restaurant, she recalled the name of the waiter, the number of the building and the street in which it stood. She also remembered what she wore on this occasion and what every one else in the party wore. The same was true of every other event which had awakened her interest in any way, and it was a favorite amusement in her family to ask her what the menu had been and what people had worn on particular occasions.

When the sight of two persons is different it has been found that their memories differ in exactly the same degree. Two sisters, one of whom had only ordinary good vision, indicated by the formula 20/20, while the other had 20/10, found that the time it took them to learn eight verses of a poem varied in almost exactly the same ratio as their sight. The one whose vision was 20/10 learned eight verses of the poem in fifteen minutes, while the one whose vision was only 20/20 required thirty-one minutes to do the same thing. After palming the one with ordinary vision learned eight more verses in twenty-one minutes, while the one with 20/10 was only able to reduce her time by two minutes, a variation clearly within the limits of error. In other words, the mind of the latter being already in a normal or nearly normal condition, she could not improve it appreciably by palming, while the former whose mind was under a strain was able to gain relaxation, and hence improve her memory, by this means.

When the two eyes of the same person are different a corresponding difference in the memory has been noted according to whether both eyes were open, or the better eye closed. A patient with normal vision in the right eye and half-normal vision in the left when looking at the Snellen test card with both eyes open could remember a period for twenty seconds continuously, but could remember it only ten seconds when the better eye was closed. A patient with half-normal vision in the right eye and one-quarter normal in the left could remember a period for twelve seconds with both eyes open and only six seconds with better eye closed. A third patient with normal sight in the right eye and vision of one-tenth in the left could remember a period twelve seconds with both eyes open and only two seconds when the better eye was closed. In other words if the right eye is better than the left the memory is better when the right eye is open than when only the left eye is open.

Under the present educational system there is a constant effort to compel the children to remember. These efforts always fail. They spoil both the memory and the sight. The memory cannot be forced any more than the vision can be forced. **We remember without effort, just as we see without effort, and the harder we try to remember or see the less we are able to do so.**

The sort of things we remember are the things that interest us, and the reason children have difficulty in learning their lessons is because they are bored by them. For the same reason, among others, their eyesight becomes impaired, boredom being a condition of mental strain in which it is impossible for the eye to function normally.

Some of the various kinds of compulsion now employed in the educational process may have the effect of awakening interest. Betty Smith's interest in winning a prize, for instance, or in merely getting ahead of Johnny Jones, may have the effect of rousing her interest in lessons that have hitherto bored her, and this interest may develop into a genuine interest in the acquisition of knowledge; but this cannot be said of the various fear incentives still so largely employed by teachers. These, on the contrary, have the effect, usually, of completely paralyzing minds already benumbed by lack of interest, and the effect upon the vision is equally disastrous.

The fundamental reason, both for poor memory and poor eyesight in school children, in short, is our irrational and unnatural educational system. **Montessori has taught us that it is only when children are interested that they can learn. It is equally true that it is only when they are interested that they can see.** This fact was strikingly illustrated in the case of one of the two pairs of sisters mentioned above. Phebe, of the keen eyes, who could recite whole books if she happened to be interested in them, disliked mathematics and anatomy extremely, and not only could not learn them but became myopic when they were presented to her mind. She could read letters a quarter of an inch high at twenty feet in a poor light, but when asked to read figures one to two inches high in a good light at ten feet she miscalled half of them. When asked to tell how much 2 and 3 made, she said "4," before finally deciding on "5"; and all the time she was occupied with this disagreeable subject the retinoscope showed that she was myopic. When I asked her to look into my eye with the ophthalmoscope she could see nothing, although a much lower degree of visual acuity is required to note the details of the interior of the eye than to see the moons of Jupiter.

Short-sighted Isabel, on the contrary, had a passion for mathematics and anatomy, and excelled in those subjects. She learned to use the ophthalmoscope as easily as Phebe had learned Latin. Almost immediately she saw the optic nerve, and noted that the center was whiter than the periphery. She saw the light-colored lines, the arteries; and the darker ones, the veins; and she saw the light streaks on the blood-vessels. Some specialists never become able to do this, and no one could do it without normal vision. Isabel's vision, therefore, must have been temporarily normal when she did it. Her vision for figures, although not normal, was better than for letters.

In both these cases the ability to learn and the ability to see went hand in hand with interest. Phebe could read a photographic reduction of the Bible and recite what she had read verbatim, she could see the moons of Jupiter and draw a diagram of them afterwards, because she was interested in these things; but she could not see the interior of the eye, nor see figures even half as well as she saw letters, because these things bored her. When, however, it was suggested to her that it would be a good joke to surprise her teachers, who were always reproaching her for her backwardness in mathematics, by taking a high mark in a coming examination, her interest in the subject awakened and she contrived to learn enough to get seventy-eight per cent. In Isabel's case letters were antagonistic. She was not interested in most of the subjects with which they dealt and, therefore, she was backward in those subjects and had become habitually myopic. But when asked to look at objects which aroused an intense interest her vision became normal.

When one is not interested, in short, one's mind is not under control, and without mental control one can neither learn nor see. Not only the memory but all other mental faculties are improved when the eyesight becomes normal. It is a common experience with patients cured of defective sight to find that their ability to do their work has improved.

The teacher whose letter was quoted in the first issue of BETTER EYESIGHT testified that after gaining perfect eyesight she "knew better how to get at the minds of the pupils, was "more direct, more definite, less diffused, less vague," possessed, in fact, "central fixation of the mind." In another letter she said, "The better my eyesight becomes the greater is my ambition. On the days when my sight is best I have the greatest anxiety to do things."

Another teacher reports that one of her pupils used to sit doing nothing all day long and apparently was not interested in anything. After the test card was introduced into the classroom and his sight improved, he became anxious to learn, and speedily developed into one of the best students in the class. In other words his eyes and his mind became normal together.

A bookkeeper nearly **seventy years of age** who had **worn glasses for forty years** found after he had **gained perfect sight without glasses** that he could work more rapidly and accurately and with less fatigue than ever in his life before. During busy seasons, or when short of help, he has worked for some weeks at a time from 7 a. m, until 11 p. m., and he reports that he felt less tired at night after he was through than he did in the morning when he started. Previously, although he had done more work than any other man in the office, it always tired him very much. He also noticed an improvement in his temper. Having been so long in the office and knowing so much more about the business than his fellow employees, he was frequently appealed to for advice. These interruptions, before his sight became normal, were very annoying to him and often caused him to lose his temper. Afterward, however, they caused him no irritation whatever. In the case of another patient whose story is given elsewhere symptoms of insanity were relieved when the vision became normal.

From all these facts it will be seen that the problems of vision are far more intimately associated with the problems of education than we had supposed, and that they can by no means be solved by putting concave, or convex, or astigmatic lenses before the eyes of the children.

THE DOCTOR'S STORY

One of the most striking cases of the relation of mind to vision that ever came to my attention was that of a physician whose mental troubles, at one time so serious that they suggested to him the idea that he might be going insane, were completely relieved when his sight became normal. He had been seen by many eye and nerve specialists before he came to me and consulted me at last, not because he had any faith in my methods, but because nothing else seemed to be left for him to do. He brought with him quite a collection of glasses prescribed by different men, no two of them being alike. He had worn glasses, he told me, for many months at a time without benefit and then he had left them off and had been apparently no worse. Outdoor life had also failed to help him. On the advice of some prominent neurologists he had even given up his practice for a couple of years to spend the time upon a ranch, but the vacation had done him no good.

I examined his eyes and found no organic defects and no error of refraction. Yet his vision with each eye was only three-fourths of the normal, and he suffered from **double vision and all sorts of unpleasant symptoms**. He used to see people standing on their heads, and little devils dancing on the tops of the high buildings. He also had other **illusions** too numerous to mention in a short paper. At night his sight was so bad that he had difficulty in finding his way about, and when walking along a country road he believed that he saw better when he turned his eyes far to one side and viewed the road with the side of the retina instead of with the center. At variable intervals, without warning and without loss of consciousness, **he had attacks of blindness**. These caused him great uneasiness, for he, was a surgeon with a large and lucrative practice, and he feared that he might have an attack while operating.

His memory was very poor. He could not remember the color of the eyes of any member of his family, although he had seen them all daily for years. Neither could he recall the color of his house, the number of rooms on the different floors, or other details. The faces and names of patients and friends he recalled with difficulty, or not at all.

His treatment proved to be very difficult, chiefly because he had an infinite number of erroneous ideas about physiological optics in general and his own case in particular and insisted that all these should be discussed; while these discussions were going on he received no benefit. Every day for hours at a time over a long period he talked and argued. Never have I met a person whose logic was so wonderful, so apparently unanswerable, and yet so utterly wrong.

His eccentric fixation was of such high degree that when he looked at a point forty-five degrees to one side of the big C on the Snellen test card, he saw the letter just as black as when he looked directly at it. The strain to do this was terrific, and produced much astigmatism; but the patient was unconscious of it, and could not be convinced that there was anything abnormal in the symptom. If he saw the letter at all, he argued, he must see it as black as it really was, because he was not color-blind. Finally he became able to look away from one of the smaller letters on the card and see it worse than when he looked directly at it. It took eight or nine months to accomplish this, but when it had been done the patient said that it seemed as if a great burden had been lifted from his mind. He experienced a wonderful feeling of rest and relaxation throughout his whole body.

When asked to remember black with his eyes closed and covered he said he could not do so, and he saw every color but the black which one ought normally to see when the optic nerve is not subject to the stimulus of light. He had, however, been an enthusiastic football player at college, and he found at last that he could remember a black football. I asked him to imagine that this football had been thrown into the sea and that it was being carried outward by the tide, becoming constantly smaller but no less black. This he was able to do, and the strain floated with the football, until, by the time the latter had been reduced to the size of a period in a newspaper, it was entirely gone. The relief continued as long as he remembered the black spot, but as he could not remember it all the time, I suggested another method of gaining permanent relief. This was to make his sight voluntarily worse, a plan against which he protested with considerable emphasis.

"Good heavens!" he said, "Is not my sight bad enough without making it worse."

After a week of argument, however, he consented to try the method, and the result was extremely satisfactory. After he had learned to see two or more lights where there was only one, by straining to see a point above the light while still trying to see the light as well as when looking directly at it, he became able to avoid the unconscious strain that had produced his double and multiple vision and was not troubled by these superfluous images any more. In a similar manner other illusions were prevented.

One of the last illusions to disappear was his belief that an effort was required to remember black. His logic on this point was overwhelming, but after many demonstrations he was convinced that no effort was required to let go, and when he realized this, both his vision and his mental condition immediately improved.

He finally became able to read 20/10 or more, and although more than fifty-five years of age, he also read diamond type at from six to twenty-four inches. His night blindness was relieved, his attacks of day blindness ceased, and he told me the color of the eyes of his wife and children. One day he said to me:

"Doctor, I thank you for what you have done for my sight; but no words can express the gratitude I feel for what you have done for my mind."

Some years later he called with his heart full of gratitude, because there had been no relapse.

LYING A CAUSE OF MYOPIA

I may claim to have discovered the fact that telling lies is bad for the eyes. Whatever bearing this circumstance may have upon the universality of defects of vision, it can easily be demonstrated that it is impossible to say what is not true, even with no intent to deceive, or even to imagine a falsehood, without producing an error of refraction.

If a patient can read all the small letters on the bottom line of the test card, and either deliberately or carelessly miscalls any of them, the retinoscope will indicate an error of refraction. In numerous cases patients have been asked to state their ages incorrectly, or to try to imagine that they were a year older, or a year younger, than they actually were, and in every case when they did this the retinoscope indicated an error of refraction. A patient twenty-five years old had no error of refraction when he looked at a blank wall without trying to see; but if he said he was twenty-six, or if someone else said he was twenty-six, or if he tried to imagine that he was twenty-six, he became myopic. The same thing happened when he stated or tried to imagine that he was twenty-four. When he stated or remembered the truth his vision was normal, but when he stated or imagined an error he had an error of refraction.

Two little girl patients arrived one after the other one day, and the first accused the second of having stopped at Huyler's for an ice-cream soda, which she had been instructed not to do, being somewhat too much addicted to sweets. The second denied the charge, and the first, who had used the retinoscope and knew what it did to people who told lies, said:

"Do take the retinoscope and find out."

"I followed the suggestion, and having thrown the light into the second child's eyes, I asked:

"Did you go to Huyler's?"

"Yes," was the response, and the retinoscope indicated no error of refraction.

"Did you have an ice-cream soda?"

"No," Said the child; but the tell-tale shadow moved in a direction opposite to that of the mirror, showing that she had become myopic and was not telling the truth.

The child blushed when I told her this and acknowledged that the retinoscope was right, for she had heard of the ways of the uncanny instrument before and did not know what else it might do to her if she said anything more that was not true.

The fact is that it requires an effort to state what is not true, and this effort always results in a deviation from the normal in the refraction of the eye. So sensitive is the test that if the subject, whether his vision is ordinarily normal, or not, pronounces the initials of his name correctly while looking at a blank surface without trying to see, there will be no error of refraction; but if he miscalls one initial, even without any consciousness of effort, and with full knowledge that he is deceiving no one, myopia will be produced.

CURED IN FIFTEEN MINUTES

Patients often ask how long it takes to be cured. The answer is that it takes only as long as it takes to relax. If this can be done in five minutes, the patient is cured in five minutes, no matter how great the degree of his error of refraction, or how long its duration. All persons with errors of refraction are able to relax in a few seconds under certain conditions, but to gain permanent relaxation usually requires considerable time. Some persons, however, are able to get it very quickly. These quick cures are very rare, except in the case of children under twelve; but they do occur, and I believe the time is coming when it will be possible to cure everyone quickly. It is only a question of accumulating more facts and presenting them in such a way that the patient can grasp them quickly.

A very remarkable case of a quick cure was that of a man of fifty-five who had worn glasses for thirty years for distant vision and ten years for reading, and whose distant vision at the time he consulted me was 20/200.

When he looked at the Snellen test card the letters appeared grey to him instead of black. He was told that they were black, and the fact was demonstrated by bringing the card close to him. His attention was also called to the fact that the small letters were just as black as the large ones. He was then directed to close and cover his eyes with the palms of his hands, shutting out all the light. When he did this he saw a perfect black, indicating that he had secured perfect relaxation and that the optic nerve and visual centers of the brain were not disturbed. While his eyes were still closed he was asked:

"Do you think that you can remember with your eyes open the perfect black that you now see?"

"Yes," he answered, "I know I can,"

When he opened his eyes, however, his memory of the black was imperfect, and though able to read the large letters, he could not read the small ones. A second time he was told to close and cover his eyes, and again he saw a perfect black. When he opened them he was able to retain complete control of his memory, and so was able to read the whole card. This was ten minutes after he entered the office.

Diamond type was now given him to read, but the letters looked grey to him, and he could not distinguish them. Neither could he remember black when he was looking at them, because in order to see them grey he had to strain, and in order to remember black he would have had to relax, and he could not do both at the same time. He was told that the letters were perfectly black, and when he looked away from them he was able to remember them black. When he looked back he still remembered them black, and was able to read them with normal vision at twelve inches. This took five minutes, making the whole time in the office fifteen minutes. The cure was permanent, the patient not only retaining what he had gained, but continuing to improve his sight, by daily reading of fine print and the Snellen test card, till it became almost **telescopic**.

September, 1919

1 -School Health News, published by the Department of Health of New York City, February, 1919.

BETTER EYESIGHT

A MONTHLY MAGAZINE DEVOTED TO THE PREVENTION AND CURE OF IMPERFECT SIGHT WITHOUT GLASSES

October, 1919

THE SWINGING CURE

If you see a letter perfectly, you may note that it appears to pulsate, or move slightly in various directions. If your sight is imperfect, the letter will appear to be stationary. The apparent movement is caused by the unconscious shifting of the eye. The lack of movement is due to the fact that the eye stares, or looks too long at one point. This is an invariable symptom of imperfect sight, and may often be relieved by the following method:

Close your eyes and cover them with the palms of the hands so as to exclude all the light, and shift mentally from one side of a black letter to the other. As you do this, the mental picture of the letter will appear to move back and forth in a direction contrary to the imagined movement of the eye. Just so long as you imagine that the letter is moving, or swinging, you will find that you are able to remember it, and the **shorter and more regular the swing, the blacker and more distinct the letter will appear**. If you are able to imagine the letter stationary, which may be difficult, you will find that your memory of it will be much less perfect.

Now open your eyes and look first at one side and then at the other of the real letter. If it appears to move in a direction opposite to the movement of the eye, you will find that your vision has improved. If you can imagine the swing of the letter as well with your eyes open as with your eyes closed, as **short**, as **regular** and as **continuous**, your vision will be normal.

SIMULTANEOUS RETINOSCOPY

Much of my information about the eye has been obtained by means of simultaneous retinoscopy.

The retinoscope is an instrument used to measure the refraction of the eye. It throws a beam of light into the pupil by reflection from a mirror, the light being either outside the instrument—above and behind the subject—or arranged within it by means of an electric battery. On looking through the sight-hole one sees a larger or smaller part of the pupil filled with light, which in normal human eyes is a reddish yellow, because this is the color of the retina, but which is green in a cat's eye, and might be white if the retina were diseased. Unless the eye is exactly focused at the point from which it is being observed one sees also a dark shadow at the edge of the pupil, and it is the behavior of this shadow when the mirror is moved in various directions which reveals the refractive condition of the eye. If the instrument is used at a distance of six feet or more, and the shadow moves in a direction opposite to the movement of the mirror, the eye is myopic. If it moves in the same direction as the mirror, the eye is either hypermetropic or normal; but in the case of hypermetropia the movement is more pronounced than in that of normality, and an expert can usually tell the difference between the two states merely by the nature of the movement. In astigmatism the movement is different in different meridians. To determine the degree of the error, or to distinguish accurately between hypermetropia and normality, or between the different kinds of astigmatism, it is usually necessary to place a glass before the eye of the subject.

This exceedingly useful instrument has possibilities which have not been generally realized by the medical profession. It is commonly employed only under certain artificial conditions in a dark room; but it is possible to use it under all sorts of normal and abnormal conditions on the eyes both of human beings and of the lower animals. I have used it in the daytime and at night; when the subjects were comfortable and when they were excited; when they were trying to see and when they were not; when they were lying and when they were telling the truth. I have also used it, under varying conditions, on the eyes of many cats, dogs, rabbits, birds, turtles, reptiles and fish.

Most ophthalmologists depend upon the Snellen test card, supplemented by trial lenses, to determine whether the vision is normal or not, and to determine the degree of any abnormality that may exist. This is a slow, awkward and unreliable method of testing the vision, and absolutely unavailable for the study of the refraction of the lower animals and that of human beings under the conditions of life. The test card can be used only under certain favorable conditions, but the retinoscope can be used anywhere. It is a little easier to use it in a dim light than in a bright one, but it may be used in any light, even with the strong light of the sun shining directly into the eye. It is available whether the subject is at rest or in motion, asleep or awake, or even under ether or chloroform. It is also available when the observer is in motion. It has been used successfully when the eyelids were partly closed, shutting off part of the area of the pupil; when the pupil was dilated; also when it was contracted to a pin-point; when the subject was reading fine print at six inches, or at a greater distance; and when the eye was oscillating from side to side, from above downward, or in other directions.

It takes a considerable time, varying from minutes to hours, to measure the refraction with the Snellen test card and trial lenses. With the retinoscope, however, the refraction can be determined in a fraction of a second. With the Snellen test card and trial lenses it would be impossible to get any information about the refraction of a baseball player at the moment he swings for the ball, at the moment he strikes it, and at the moment after he strikes it. With the retinoscope, however, it is quite easy to determine whether his vision is normal, or whether he is myopic, hypermetropic, or astigmatic, when he does these things; and if any errors of refraction are noted, one can guess their degree pretty accurately by the rapidity of the movement of the shadow.

With the Snellen test card and trial lenses conclusions must be drawn from the patient's statements as to what he sees; but the patient often becomes so worried and confused during the examination that he does not know what he sees, or whether different glasses make his sight better, or worse; and, moreover, visual acuity is not reliable evidence of the state of the refraction. One patient with two diopters of myopia may see twice as much as another with the same error of refraction. The evidence of the test card is, in fact, entirely subjective; that of the retinoscope is entirely objective, depending in no way upon the statements of the patient.

By means of simultaneous retinoscopy it has been demonstrated that the refraction of the eye is never constant; that all persons with errors of refraction have, at frequent intervals during the day and night, moments of normal vision when their myopia, hypermetropia, or astigmatism, disappears completely; and that all persons, no matter how good their sight may ordinarily be, have moments of imperfect sight when they become myopic, hypermetropic, or astigmatic. It has also been demonstrated that when the eye makes an effort to see, an error of refraction is always produced, and that when it looks at objects without effort, all errors of refraction disappear, no matter how great their degree, or how long their duration. It has been further demonstrated that when the eye strains to see distant objects myopia is always produced in one or all meridians, and when it strains to see near objects hypermetropia is always produced in one or all meridians.

The examination of the eyes of persons while asleep, or under the influence of ether or chloroform, has shown that the eye is rarely at rest during sleep, or while the subject is unconscious from any cause. Persons whose sight was normal while awake were found to have myopia, hypermetropia and astigmatism when asleep, and if these errors were present when they were awake, they were increased during sleep. This explains why so many people are unable to see as well in the morning as at other times, and why people waken with headaches and pain in the eyes. Under ether or chloroform, errors of refraction are also produced or increased, and when people are sleepy they have invariably been found to have errors of refraction.

Under conditions of mental or physical discomfort, such as pain, cough, fever, discomfort from heat or cold, depression, anger, or anxiety, errors of refraction are always produced in the normal eye, or increased in the eye in which they already exist. In a dim light, in a fog, or in the rain, the retinoscope may indicate no error of refraction in eyes which ordinarily have normal sight; but a pilot on a ship on a rainy night usually has an error of refraction, because he is straining to see, and it is rare to find persons in positions of responsibility under unfavorable conditions with normal vision.

In order to obtain reliable results with the retinoscope it must be used at a distance of six feet or more from the subject. When used at a distance of three feet or less, as it commonly is, the subject becomes nervous and unconsciously strains, thus altering his refraction.

FLOATING SPECKS

A very common phenomenon of imperfect sight is the one known to medical science as *muscae volitantes*, or *flying flies*. These floating specks are usually dark, or black; but sometimes appear like white bubbles, and in rare cases may assume all the colors of the rainbow. They move somewhat rapidly, usually in curving lines, before the eyes, and always appear to be just beyond the point of fixation. If one tries to look at them directly, they seem to move a little farther away. Hence their name of *flying flies*.

The literature of the subject is full of speculations as to the origin of these appearances. Some have attributed them to the presence of floating specks—dead cells or the debris of cells—in the vitreous humor, the transparent substance that fills four-fifths of the eyeball behind the crystalline lens. Similar specks on the surface of the cornea have also been held responsible for them. It has even been surmised that they might be caused by the passage of tears over the cornea. They are so common in myopia that they have been supposed to be one of the symptoms of this condition, although they occur also with other errors of refraction, as well as in eyes otherwise normal. They have been attributed to disturbances of the circulation, the digestion and the kidneys, and because so many insane people have them, have been thought to be an evidence of incipient insanity. The patent-medicine business has thrived upon them, and it would be difficult to estimate the amount of mental torture they have caused, as the following cases illustrate.

A clergyman who was much annoyed by the continual appearance of floating specks before his eyes was told by his eye specialist that they were a symptom of kidney disease, and that in many cases of kidney trouble, disease of the retina might be an early symptom. So at regular intervals he went to the specialist to have his eyes examined, and when at length the latter died, he looked around immediately for some one else to make the periodical examination. His family physician directed him to me. I was by no means so well known as his previous ophthalmological adviser, but it happened that I had taught the family physician how to use the ophthalmoscope after others had failed to do so. He thought, therefore, that I must know a lot about the use of the instrument, and what the clergyman particularly wanted was some one capable of making a thorough examination of the interior of his eyes, and detecting at once any signs of kidney disease that might make their appearance. So he came to me, and at least four times a year for ten years he continued to come.

Each time I made a very careful examination of his eyes, taking as much time over it as possible, so that he would believe that it was careful; and each time he went away happy because I could find nothing wrong. Once when I was out of town he got a cinder in his eye and went to another oculist to get it out. When I came back late at night I found him sitting on my doorstep, on the chance that I might return. His story was a pitiable one. The strange doctor had examined his eyes with the ophthalmoscope, and had suggested the possibility of glaucoma, describing the disease as a very treacherous one which might cause him to go suddenly blind and would be agonizingly painful. He emphasized what the patient had previously been told about the danger of kidney disease, suggested that the liver and heart might also be involved, and advised him to have all of these organs carefully examined. I made another examination of his eyes in general and their tension in particular; I had him feel his eyeballs and compare them with my own, so that he might see for himself that they were not becoming hard as a stone; and finally I succeeded in reassuring him. I have no doubt, however, that he went at once to his family physician for an examination of his internal organs.

A man returning from Europe was looking at some white clouds one day when floating specks appeared before his eyes. He consulted the ship's doctor, who told him that the symptom was very serious, and might be the forerunner of blindness. It might also indicate incipient insanity, as well as other nervous or organic diseases. He advised him to consult his family physician and an eye specialist as soon as he landed, which he did. This was twenty-five years ago, but I shall never forget the terrible state of nervousness and terror into which the patient had worked himself by the time he came to me. It was even worse than that of the clergyman, who was always ready to admit that his fears were unreasonable. I examined his eyes very carefully, and found them absolutely normal. The vision was perfect both for the near-point and the distance. The color perception, the fields and the tension were normal; and under a strong magnifying glass I could find no opacities in the vitreous. In short, there were absolutely no symptoms of any disease. I told the patient there was nothing wrong with his eyes, and I also showed him an advertisement of a quack medicine in a newspaper which gave a great deal of space to describing the dreadful things likely to follow the appearance of floating specks before the eyes, unless you began betimes (in good time, early) to take the medicine in question at one dollar a bottle. I pointed out that the advertisement, which was appearing in all the big newspapers of the city every day, and probably in other cities, must have cost a lot of money, and must, therefore, be bringing in a lot of money. Evidently there must be a great many people suffering from this symptom, and if it were as serious as was generally believed, there would be a great many more blind and insane people in the community than there were. The patient went away somewhat comforted, but at eleven o'clock—his first visit had been at nine—he was back again. He still saw the floating specks, and was still worried about them. I examined his eyes again as carefully as before, and again was able to assure him that there was nothing wrong with them. In the afternoon I was not in my office, but I was told that he was there at three and at five. At seven he came again, bringing with him his family physician, an old friend of mine. I said to the latter:

"Please make this patient stay at home. I have to charge him for his visits, because he is taking up so much of my time; but it is a shame to take his money when there is nothing wrong with him."

What my friend said to him I don't know, but he did not come back again.

I did not know as much about **muscae volitantes** then as I know now, or I might have saved both of these patients a great deal of uneasiness. I could tell them that their eyes were normal, but I did not know how to relieve them of the symptom, which is simply **an illusion resulting from mental strain**. The specks are associated to a considerable extent with markedly **imperfect eyesight**, because persons whose eyesight is imperfect always strain to see; but persons whose eyesight is ordinarily normal may see them at times, because no eye has normal sight all the time. Most people can see muscae volitantes when they look at the sun, or any uniformly bright surface, like a sheet of white paper upon which the sun is shining. This is because most people strain when they look at surfaces of this kind. The specks are never seen, in short, except when the eyes and mind are under a strain, and they always disappear when the strain is relieved. **If one can remember a small letter on the Snellen test card by central fixation, the specks will immediately disappear, or cease to move; but if one tries to remember two or more letters equally well at one time, they will reappear and move.**

Usually the strain that causes muscae volitantes is very easily relieved.   See; April, 1925
Floating specks may be debris in the eyeball. A cleansing diet, improved circulation of blood, fluid to/in the eye can break down floaters and enable them to flow out of the eye. Eyestrain, mental strain, staring, poor diet, sugar, can cause floaters. Shifting, central fixation, relaxation can stop the appearance of floaters.

CORRESPONDENCE TREATMENT

Correspondence treatment is usually regarded as quackery, and it would be manifestly impossible to treat many diseases in this way. Pneumonia and typhoid, for instance, could not possibly be treated by correspondence, even if the physician had a sure cure for these conditions and the mails were not too slow for the purpose. In the case of most diseases, in fact, there are serious objections to correspondence treatment.

But myopia, hypermetropia and astigmatism are functional conditions, not organic, as the text-books teach, and as I believed myself until I learned better. Their treatment by correspondence, therefore, has not the drawbacks that exist in the case of most physical derangements. One cannot, it is true, fit glasses by correspondence as well as when the patient is in the office, but even this can be done, as the following case illustrates.

An old colored woman in the wilds of Honduras, far removed from any physician or optician, was unable to read her Bible, and her son, a waiter in New York, asked me if I could not do something for her. The suggestion gave me a distinct shock which I will remember as long as I live. I had never dreamed of the possibility of prescribing glasses for anyone I had not seen, and I had, besides, some very disquieting recollections of colored women whom I had tried to fit with glasses at my clinic. If I had so much difficulty in prescribing the proper glasses under favorable conditions, how could I be expected to fit a patient whom I could not even see? The waiter was deferentially persistent, however. He had more faith in my genius than I had, and as his mother was nearing the end of her life, he was very anxious to gratify her last wishes. So, like the unjust judge of the parable, I yielded at last to his importunity, and wrote a prescription for convex 3.00 D. S. The young man ordered the glasses and mailed them to his mother, and by return mail came a very grateful letter stating that they were perfectly satisfactory.

A little later the patient wrote that she couldn't see objects at the distance that were perfectly plain to other people, and asked if some glasses couldn't be sent that would make her see at the distance as well as she did at the near-point. This seemed a more difficult proposition than the first one; but again the son was persistent, and I myself could not get the old lady out of my mind. So again I decided to do what I could. The waiter had told me that his mother had read her Bible long after the age of forty. Therefore I knew she could not have much hypermetropia, and was probably slightly myopic. I knew also that she could not have much astigmatism, for in that case her sight would always have been noticeably imperfect. Accordingly I told her son to ask her to measure very accurately the distance between her eyes and the point at which she could read her Bible best with her glasses, and to send me the figures. In due time I received, not figures, but a piece of string about a quarter of an inch in diameter and exactly ten inches long. If the patient's vision had been normal for the distance, I knew that she would have been able to read her Bible best with her glasses at thirteen inches. The string showed that at ten inches she had a refraction of four diopters. Subtracting from this the three diopters of her reading glasses, I got one diopter of myopia. I accordingly wrote a prescription for concave 1.00 D. S., and the glasses were ordered and mailed to Honduras. The acknowledgment was even more grateful than in the case of the first pair. The patient said that for the first time in her life she was able to read signs and see other objects at a distance as well as other people did, and that the whole world looked entirely different to her.

Would anyone venture to say that it was unethical for me to try to help this patient? Would it have been better to leave her in her isolation without even the consolation of Bible reading? I do not think so. What I did for her required only an ordinary knowledge of physiological optics, and if I had failed, I could not have done her much harm.

In the case of the treatment of imperfect sight without glasses there can be even less objection to the correspondence method. It is true that in most cases progress is more rapid and the results more certain when the patient can be seen personally; but often this is impossible, and I see no reason why patients who can not have the benefit of personal treatment should be denied such aid as can be given them by correspondence. I have been treating patients in this way for years, and often with extraordinary success.

Some years ago an English gentleman wrote to me that his glasses were very unsatisfactory. They not only did not give him good sight, but they increased instead of lessening his discomfort. He asked if I could help him, and since relaxation always relieves discomfort and improves the vision, I did not believe that I was doing him an injury in telling him how to rest his eyes. He followed my directions with such good results that in a short time he obtained perfect sight for both the distance and the near-point without glasses, and was completely relieved of his pain. Five years later he wrote me that he had qualified as a sharpshooter in the army. Did I do wrong in treating him by correspondence? I do not think so.

After the United States entered the European war, an officer wrote to me from the deserts of Arizona that the use of his eyes at the near-point caused him great discomfort, which glasses did not relieve, and that the strain had produced granulation of the lids. As it was impossible for him to come to New York, I undertook to treat him by correspondence. He improved very rapidly. The inflammation of the lids was relieved almost immediately, and in about four months he wrote me that he had read one of my own reprints-by no means a short one-in a dim light, with no bad after effects; that the glare of the Arizona sun, with the Government thermometer registering 114, did not annoy him, and that he could read the ten line on the test card at fifteen feet almost perfectly, while even at twenty feet he was able to make out most of the letters.

A third case was that of a forester in the employ of the U. S. Government. He had myopic astigmatism, and suffered extreme discomfort, which was not relieved either by glasses or by long summers in the mountains, where he used his eyes but little for close work. He was unable to come to New York for treatment, and although I told him that correspondence treatment was somewhat uncertain, he said he was willing to risk it. It took three days for his letters to reach me and another three for my reply to reach him, and as letters were not always written promptly on either side, he often did not hear from me more than once in three weeks. Progress under these conditions was necessarily slow; but his discomfort was relieved very quickly, and in about ten months his sight had improved from 20/50 to 20/20.

In almost every case the treatment of cases coming from a distance is continued by correspondence after they return to their homes; and although the patients do not get on so well as when they are coming to the office, they usually continue to make progress till they are cured.

At the same time it is often very difficult to make patients understand what they should do when one has to communicate with them entirely by writing, and probably all would get on better if they could have some personal treatment. At the present time the number of doctors in different parts of the United States who understand the treatment of imperfect sight without glasses is altogether too few, and my efforts to interest them in the matter have not been very successful. I would consider it a privilege to treat medical men without a fee, and when cured they will be able to assist me in the treatment of patients in their various localities.

BETTER EYESIGHT
A MONTHLY MAGAZINE DEVOTED TO THE PREVENTION AND CURE OF IMPERFECT SIGHT WITHOUT GLASSES
November, 1919
THE MEMORY CURE

When the sight is perfect, the memory is also perfect, because the mind is perfectly relaxed. Therefore the sight may be improved by any method that improves the memory. The easiest thing to remember is a small black spot of no particular size and form; but when the sight is imperfect it will be found impossible to remember it with the eyes open and looking at letters, or other objects with definite outlines. It may, however, be remembered for a few seconds or longer, when the eyes are closed and covered, or when looking at a blank surface where there is nothing particular to see. By cultivating the memory under these favorable conditions, it gradually becomes possible to retain it under unfavorable ones, that is, when the eyes are open and the mind conscious of the impressions of sight. By alternately remembering the period with the eyes closed and covered and then looking at the Snellen test card, or other letters or objects; or by remembering it when looking away from the card where there is nothing particular to see, and then looking back; the patient becomes able, in a longer or shorter time, to retain the memory when looking at the card, and thus becomes able to read the letters with normal vision. Many children have been cured very quickly by this method. Adults who have worn glasses have greater difficulty. Even under favorable conditions, the period cannot be remembered for more than a few seconds, unless one shifts from one part of it to another. One can also shift from one period, or other small black object, to another.

REASON AND AUTHORITY

This article describes how eye doctors fought against Dr. Bates, tried to hide the Bates Method from the public so they could continue selling eyeglasses, surgery, drugs.

Some one—perhaps it was Bacon—has said: "You cannot by reasoning correct a man of ill opinion which by reasoning, he never acquired." He might have gone a step farther and stated that neither by reasoning, nor by actual demonstration of the facts, can you convince some people that an opinion which they have accepted on authority is wrong. A man whose name I do not care to mention, a professor of ophthalmology, and a writer of books well known in this country and in Europe, saw me perform an experiment upon the eye of a rabbit which, according to others who had witnessed it, demonstrated beyond any possibility of error that the lens is not a factor in accommodation. At each step of the operation he testified to the facts; yet at the conclusion he preferred to discredit the evidence of his senses rather than accept the only conclusion that these facts admitted.

First he examined the eye of the animal to be experimented upon with the retinoscope and found it normal, and the fact was written down. Then the eye was stimulated with electricity, and he testified that it accommodated. This was also written down. I now divided the superior oblique muscle, and the eye was again stimulated with electricity. The doctor observed the eye with the retinoscope when this was being done and said, "You failed to produce accommodation." This fact, too, was written down. The doctor now used the electrode himself, but again failed to observe accommodation, and these facts were written down. I now sewed the cut ends of the muscle together, and once more stimulated the eye with electricity. The doctor said, "Now you have succeeded in producing accommodation," and this was written down. I now asked:

"Do you think that superior oblique had anything to do with producing accommodation?"

"Certainly not," he replied.

"Why?" I asked.

"Well," he said, "I have only the testimony of the retinoscope. I am getting on in years, and I don't feel that confidence in my ability to use the retinoscope that I once had. I would rather you wouldn't quote me on this."

While the operation was in progress, however, he gave no indication whatever of doubting his ability to use the retinoscope. He was very positive, in fact, that I had failed to produce accommodation after the cutting of the oblique muscle and his tone suggested that he considered the failure ignominious. It was only after he found himself in a logical trap, with no way out except by discrediting his own observations, that he appeared to have any doubts as to their value.

Patients whom I have cured of various errors of refraction have frequently returned to specialists who had prescribed glasses for them, and, by reading fine print and the Snellen test card with normal vision, have demonstrated the fact that they were cured, without in any way shaking the faith of these practitioners in the doctrine that such cures are impossible. A girl of sixteen who had progressive myopia of such high degree that she was not allowed to read, and was unable to go about on the streets without a guide, was assured by the specialist whom her family consulted that her condition was quite hopeless, and that it was likely to progress until it ended in blindness. She was cured in a very short time by means of the methods advocated in this magazine, becoming able to discard her glasses and resume all the ordinary activities of life. She then returned to the specialist who had condemned her to blindness to tell him the good news; but, while he was unable to deny the fact that her vision was normal without glasses, he said it was impossible that she would have been cured of myopia, because myopia was incurable. How he reconciled this statement with his former patient's condition he was unable to make clear to her.

A lady with compound myopic astigmatism1 suffered from almost constant headaches which were very much worse when she took her glasses off. Every week, no matter what she did, she was so prostrated by eyestrain that she had to spend a few days in bed; and if she went to a theatre, or to a social function, she had to stay there longer. She was told to take off her glasses and go to the movies: to look first at the corner of the screen, then off to the dark, then back to the screen a little nearer to the center, and so forth. She did so, and soon became able to look directly at the pictures without discomfort. After that nothing troubled her. One day she called on her former ophthalmological adviser, in the company of a friend who wanted to have her glasses changed, and told him of her cure. The facts seemed to make no impression on him whatever. He only laughed and said, "I guess Dr. Bates is more popular with you than I am."

In some cases patients themselves, after they are cured, allow themselves to be convinced that it was impossible that such a thing could have happened, and go back to their glasses. A clergyman and writer, aged forty-seven, who had worn glasses for years for distance and reading, had what I should have considered the good fortune to be very quickly cured. By the aid of his imagination he was able to relax in less than five minutes, and to stay relaxed. When he looked at fine print it appeared grey to him, and he could not read it. I asked him if he had ever seen printer's ink. He replied, of course, that he had. I then told him that the paragraph of printed matter which he held in his hand was printed in printer's ink, and that it was black and not grey. I asked him if he did not know and believe that it was black, or if he could not at least imagine that it was black. "Yes," he said, "I can do that"; and immediately he read the print. It took him only about a minute to do this, and he was not more than five minutes in the office. The cure was permanent, and he was very grateful-for a time. Then he began to talk to eye specialists whom he knew, and thereupon grew skeptical as to the value of what I had done for him. One day I met him at the home of a mutual friend, and in the presence of a number of other people he accused me of having hypnotized him, adding that to hypnotize a patient without his knowledge or consent was to do him a grievous wrong. Some of the listeners protested that whether I had hypnotized him or not, I had not only done him no harm, but had greatly benefited him, and he ought to forgive me. He was unable, however, to take this view of the matter. Later he called on a prominent eye specialist who told him that the presbyopia (old sight) and astigmatism from which he had suffered were incurable, and that if he persisted in going without his glasses he might do himself great harm. The fact that his sight was perfect for the distance and the near-point had no effect upon the specialist and the patient allowed himself to be frightened into disregarding it also. He went back to his glasses, and so far as I know has been wearing them ever since. The story obtained wide publicity, for the man had a large circle of friends and acquaintances; and if I had destroyed his sight I could scarcely have suffered more than I did for curing him.

Other Doctors try to hide Dr. Bates discoveries from the public. Doctors expel Dr. Bates from the Hospital he worked at after Dr. Bates cures patients without glasses, surgery, drugs and proves the facts of Natural Eyesight Improvement.

Fifteen or twenty years ago the specialist mentioned in the foregoing story read a paper on cataract at a meeting of the ophthalmological section of the American Medical Association in Atlantic City, and asserted that anyone who said that cataract could be cured without the knife was a quack. At that time I was assistant surgeon at the New York Eye and Ear Infirmary, and it happened that I had been collecting statistics of the spontaneous cure of cataract at the request of the executive surgeon of this institution, Dr. Henry G. Noyes, Professor of Ophthalmology at the Bellevue Hospital Medical School. As a result of my inquiry I had secured records of a large number of cases which had recovered, not only without the knife, but without any treatment at all. I also had records of cases which I had sent to Dr. James E. Kelly of New York and which he had cured, largely by hygienic methods. Dr. Kelly is not a quack, and at that time was Professor of Anatomy in the New York Post Graduate Medical School and Hospital and attending surgeon to a large city hospital. In the five minutes allotted to those who wished to discuss the paper, I was able to tell the audience enough about these cases to make them want to hear more. My time was, therefore, extended, first to half an hour and then to an hour. Later both Dr. Kelly and myself received many letters from men in different parts of the country who had tried his treatment with success. The man who wrote the paper had blundered, but he did not lose any prestige because of my attack with facts upon his theories. He is still a prominent and honored ophthalmologist and in his latest book he gives no hint of having ever heard of any successful method of treating cataract other than by operation. He was not convinced by my record of spontaneous cures, nor by Dr. Kelly's record of cures by treatment; and while a few men were sufficiently impressed to try the treatment recommended, and while they obtained satisfactory results, the facts made no impression upon the profession as a whole, and did not modify the teaching of the schools. That spontaneous cures of cataract do sometimes occur cannot be denied; but they are supposed to be very rare, and any one who suggests that the condition can be cured by treatment still exposes himself to the suspicion of being a quack.

Between 1886 and 1891 I was a lecturer at the Post Graduate Hospital and Medical School. The head of the institution was Dr. D. B. St. John Roosa. He was the author of many books, and was honored and respected by the whole medical profession. At the school they had got the habit of putting glasses on the nearsighted doctors, and I had got the habit of curing them without glasses. It was naturally annoying to a man who had put glasses on a student to have him appear at a lecture without them and say that Dr. Bates had cured him. Dr. Roosa found it particularly annoying, and the trouble reached a climax one evening at the annual banquet of the faculty when, in the presence of one hundred and fifty doctors, he suddenly poured out the vials of his wrath upon my head. He said that I was injuring the reputation of the Post Graduate by claiming to cure myopia. Every one knew that Donders said it was incurable, and I had no right to claim that I knew more than Donders. I reminded him that some of the men I had cured had been fitted with glasses by himself. He replied that if he had said they had myopia he had made a mistake. I suggested further investigation. "Fit some more doctors with glasses for myopia," I said, "and I will cure them. It is easy for you to examine them afterwards and see if the cure is genuine." This method did not appeal to him, however. He repeated that it was impossible to cure myopia, and to prove that it was impossible **he expelled me from the Post Graduate, even the privilege of resignation being denied to me.** The fact is that, except in rare cases, man is not a reasoning being. He is dominated by authority, and when the facts are not in accord with the view imposed by authority, so much the worse for the facts. They may and indeed must win in the long run; but in the meantime the world gropes needlessly in darkness and endures much suffering that might have been avoided.

THE EFFECT OF LIGHT UPON THE EYES

Although the eyes were made to react to the light, a very general fear of the effect of this element upon the organs of vision is entertained both by the medical profession and by the laity. Extraordinary precautions are taken in our homes, offices and schools to temper the light, whether natural or artificial, and to insure that it shall not shine directly into the eyes; smoked and amber glasses, eye-shades, broad-brimmed hats and parasols are commonly used to protect the organs of vision from what is considered an excess of light; and when actual disease is present, it is no uncommon thing for patients to be kept for weeks, months and years in dark rooms, or with bandages over their eyes.

The evidence on which this universal fear of the light has been based is of the slightest. In the voluminous literature of the subject one finds such a lack of information that, in 1910, Dr. J. Herbert Parsons of the Royal Ophthalmic Hospital of London, addressing a meeting of the Ophthalmological Section of the American Medical Association, felt justified in saying that ophthalmologists, if they were honest with themselves, "must confess to a lamentable ignorance of the conditions which render bright light injurious to the eyes."[2] Since then, Verhoeff and Bell have reported[3] an exhaustive series of experiments carried on at the Pathological Laboratory of the Massachusetts Charitable Eye and Ear Infirmary, which indicate that the danger of injury to the eye from light radiation as such has been "very greatly exaggerated." That brilliant sources of light sometimes produce unpleasant temporary symptoms cannot, of course, be denied; but as regards definite pathological effects, or permanent impairment of vision from exposure to light alone, Drs. Verhoeff and Bell were unable to find, either clinically or experimentally, anything of a positive nature.

The results of these experiments are in complete accord with my own observations as to the effect of strong light upon the eyes. In my experience such light has never been permanently injurious. Persons with normal sight have been able to look at the sun for an indefinite length of time, even an hour or longer, without any discomfort or loss of vision. Immediately afterward they were able to read the Snellen test card with improved vision, their sight having become better than what is ordinarily considered normal. Some persons with normal sight do suffer discomfort and loss of vision when they look at the sun; but in such cases the retinoscope always indicates an error of refraction, showing that this condition is due, not to the light, but to strain. In exceptional cases persons with defective sight have been able to look at the sun, or have thought that they have looked at it, without discomfort and without loss of vision; but, as a rule, the strain in such eyes is enormously increased and the vision decidedly lowered by sun-gazing, as manifested by inability to read the Snellen test card. **Blind areas (scotomata)** may develop in various parts of the field—two or three or more. The sun, instead of appearing perfectly white, may appear to be slate-colored, yellow, red, blue, or even totally black. After looking away from the sun, patches of color of various kinds and sizes may be seen, continuing a variable length of time, from a few seconds to a few minutes, hours, or even months. In fact, one patient was troubled in this way for a year or more after looking at the sun for a few seconds. Even total blindness lasting a few hours has been produced. Organic changes may also be produced. Inflammation, redness of the conjunctiva, cloudiness of the lens and of the aqueous and viterous humours, congestion and cloudiness of the retina, optic nerve and choroid, have all resulted from **sun-gazing**. These effects, however, are **always temporary**. The scotomata, the strange colors, even the total blindness, as explained in the preceding chapter, are only mental illusions. No matter how much the sight may have been impaired by **sun-gazing**, or how long the impairment may have lasted, a return to normal has always occurred; while prompt relief of all the symptoms mentioned has always followed the relief of eyestrain, showing that the conditions are the result, not of the light, but of the strain. **Some persons who have believed their eyes to have been permanently injured by the sun have been promptly cured by central fixation, indicating that their blindness had been simply functional.**

By persistence in looking at the sun, a person with normal sight soon becomes able to do so without any loss of vision; but persons with imperfect sight usually find it impossible to accustom themselves to such a strong light until their vision has been improved by other means. **One has to be very careful in recommending sun-gazing to persons with imperfect sight; because, although no permanent harm can result from it, great temporary discomfort may be produced, with no permanent benefit. In some rare cases, however, complete cures have been effected by this means alone.**
Diet must also be healthy. No prescription, non-prescription drugs, including sinus sprays, cough/cold medicines...

In one of these cases the sensitiveness of the patient, even to ordinary daylight, was so great that an eminent specialist had felt justified in putting a black bandage over one eye and covering the other with a smoked glass so dark as to be nearly opaque. She was kept in this condition of almost total blindness for two years without any improvement. Other treatment extending over some months also failed to produce satisfactory results. She was then advised to look directly at the sun. The immediate result was total blindness, which lasted several hours; but next day the vision was not only restored to its former condition, but was improved. The sun-gazing was repeated, and each time the blindness lasted for a shorter period. At the end of a week the patient was able to look directly at the sun without discomfort, and her vision, which had been 20/200 without glasses and 20/70 with them, had improved to 20/10, twice the accepted standard for normal vision.

Like the sun, a strong electric light may also lower the vision temporarily, but never does any permanent harm. In those exceptional cases in which the patient can become accustomed to the light, it is beneficial. After looking at a strong electric light some patients have been able to read the Snellen test card better.

It is not light but darkness that is dangerous to the eye. Prolonged exclusion from the light always lowers the vision, and may produce serious inflammatory conditions. Among young children living in tenements this is a somewhat frequent cause of ulcers upon the cornea, which ultimately destroy the sight. The children, finding their eyes sensitive to light, bury them in the pillows and thus shut out the light entirely. **The universal fear of reading or doing fine work in a dim light is, however, unfounded. So long as the light is sufficient so that one can see without discomfort, this practice is not only harmless, but may be beneficial.**

Sudden contrasts of light are supposed to be particularly harmful to the eye. The theory on which this idea is based is summed up as follows by Fletcher B. Dresslar, specialist in school-hygiene and sanitation of the United States Bureau of Education:

"The muscles of the iris are automatic in their movements, but rather slow. Sudden strong light and weak illumination are painful and likewise harmful to the retina. For example, if the eye adjusted to a dim light is suddenly turned toward a brilliantly lighted object, the retina will receive too much light, and will be shocked before the muscles controlling the iris can react to shut out the superabundance of light. If contrasts are not strong, but are frequently made, that is, if the eye is called upon to function where frequent adjustments in this way are necessary, the muscles controlling the iris become fatigued, respond more slowly and less perfectly. As a result, eyestrain in the ciliary muscles is produced and the retina is over stimulated. This is one cause of headaches and tired eyes."4   There is no evidence whatever to support these statements. Sudden fluctuations of light undoubtedly cause discomfort to many persons, but far from being injurious, I have found them, in all cases observed, to be actually beneficial. The pupil of the normal eye, when it has normal sight, does not change appreciably under the influence of changes of illumination; and persons with normal vision are not inconvenienced by such changes. I have seen a patient look directly at the sun after coming from an imperfectly lighted room, and then, returning to the room, immediately pick up a newspaper and read it. When the eye has imperfect sight, the pupil usually contracts in the light and expands in the dark, but it has been observed to contract to the size of a pinhole in the dark. Whether the contraction takes place under the influence of light or of darkness, the cause is the same, namely, strain. Persons with imperfect sight suffer great inconvenience, resulting in lowered vision, from changes in the intensity of the light; but the lowered vision is always temporary, and if the eye is persistently exposed to these conditions, the sight is benefited. Such practices as reading alternately in a bright and a dim light, or going from a dark room to a well-lighted one, and vice versa, are to be recommended. Even such rapid and violent fluctuations of light as those involved in the production of the moving picture are, in the long run, beneficial to all eyes. I always advise patients under treatment for the cure of defective vision to go to the movies frequently and practice central fixation. They soon become accustomed to the flickering light, and afterward other lights and reflections cause less annoyance.

In later years Dr. Bates advises <u>closed eyes sunning</u>.

TWO POINTS OF VIEW

Being anxious to know what my colleagues think of BETTER EYESIGHT, I lately sent notes to a number of them asking for their opinion. The following replies were so interesting that I think the readers of the magazine have a right to see them.

Dear Doctor:

As long as you ask for my opinion of your new magazine entitled BETTER EYESIGHT, permit me to give it to you in all frankness. It is what we call in the vernacular, "PUNK."

Meaning no personal offense, I am,
              Your colleague.

Dear Doctor

Your little note received this morning and am glad to have the opportunity to tell you what I think of BETTER EYESIGHT.

It is all that you claim for it, and I am always glad to receive it, as I know that I am going to get something beneficial for myself as well as something for the good of my patients.

If the medical bigots had BETTER EYESIGHT on their desks, and would put into practice what you give in each number, it would be a great blessing to the people who are putting eye crutches on their eyes. I first tried central fixation on myself and had marvelous results. I threw away my glasses and can now see better than I have ever done. I read very fine type (smaller than newspaper type) at a distance of six inches from the eyes, and can run it out at full arm's length and still read it without blurring the type.

I have instructed some of my patients in your methods, and all are getting results. One case who has a partial cataract of the left eye could not see anything on the Snellen test card at twenty feet, and could see the letters only faintly at ten feet. Now she can read 20/10 with both eyes together and also with each eye separately, but the left eye seems, as she says, to be looking through a little fog. I could cite many other cases that have been benefited by central fixation, but this one is the most interesting to me. Kindly send me more of the subscription slips, as I want to hand them out to my patients.
Yours very truly,

November, 1919

1 - A condition in which the eye is shortsighted in all meridians, but more so in one than in the others.
2 - Jour. Am. Med. Assn., Dec. 10, 1910, p. 2028.
3 - Proc. Am. Acad. Arts and Sciences, July, 1916, vol. 51, No. 13.
4 - School Hygiene, Brief Course Series in Education, edited by Paul Monroe, Ph.D., 1916, pp. 235-236.

BETTER EYESIGHT
A MONTHLY MAGAZINE DEVOTED TO THE PREVENTION AND CURE OF IMPERFECT SIGHT WITHOUT GLASSES
December, 1919
THE IMAGINATION CURE

When the imagination is perfect the mind is always perfectly relaxed, and as it is impossible to relax and imagine a letter perfectly, and at the same time strain and see it imperfectly, it follows that when one imagines that one sees a letter perfectly one actually does see it, as demonstrated by the retinoscope, no matter how great an error of refraction the eye may previously have had. The sight, therefore, may often be improved very quickly by the aid of the imagination. To use this method the patient may proceed as follows:

Look at a letter at the distance at which it is seen best. Close and cover the eyes so as to exclude all the light, and remember it. Do this alternately until the memory is nearly equal to the sight. Next, after remembering the letter with the eyes closed and covered, and while still holding the mental picture of it, look at a blank surface a foot or more to the side of it, at the distance at which you wish to see it. Again close and cover the eyes and remember the letter, and on opening them look a little nearer to t. Gradually reduce the distance between the point of fixation and the letter, until able to look directly at it and imagine it aswell as it is remembered with the eyes closed and covered. The letter will then be seen perfectly, and other letters in its neighborhood will come out. **If unable to remember the whole letter, you may be able to imagine a black period as forming part of it. If you can do this, the letter will also be seen perfectly.**
Imagine the letter is composed of many black periods and shift from period to period (part to part) on the letter.

THE MENACE OF LARGE PRINT

If you look at the big "C" on the Snellen test card (or any other large letter of the same size) at ten, fifteen, or twenty feet, and try to see it all alike, you may note a feeling of strain and the letter may not appear perfectly black and distinct. If you now look at only one part of the letter, and see the rest of it worse, you will note that the part seen best appears blacker than the whole letter when seen all alike, and you may also note a relief of strain. If you look at the small "c" on the bottom line of the test card, you may be able to note that it seems blacker than the big "C." If not, imagine it as forming part of the area of the big "C." If you are able to see this part blacker than the rest of the letter, the imagined letter will, of course, appear blacker also. If your sight is normal, you may now go a step further and note that when you look at one part of the small "c" this part looks blacker than the whole letter, and that it is easier to see the letter in this way than to see it all alike.

If you look at a line of the smaller letters that you can read readily, and try to see them all alike-all equally black and equally distinct in outline-you will probably find it to be impossible, and the effort will produce discomfort and, perhaps, pain. You may, however, succeed in seeing two or more of them alike. This, too, may cause much discomfort, and if continued long enough, will produce pain. If you now look at only the first letter of the line, seeing the adjoining ones worse, the strain will at once be relieved, and the letter will appear blacker and more distinct than when it was seen equally well with the others.

If your sight is normal at the near-point, you can repeat these experiments with a letter seen at this point, with the same results. A number of letters seen equally well at one time will appear less black and less distinct than a single letter seen best, and a large letter will seem less black and distinct than a small one; while in the case of both the large letter and the several letters seen all alike, a feeling of strain may be produced in the eye. You may also be able to note that the reading of very fine print, when t can be done perfectly, is markedly restful to the eye.

The smaller the point of maximum vision, in short, the better the sight, and the less the strain upon the eye. This fact can usually be demonstrated in a few minutes by any one whose sight is not markedly imperfect; and in view of some of our educational methods, is very interesting and instructive.

Probably every man who has written a book upon the eye for the last hundred years has issued a warning against fine print in school books, and recommended particularly large print for small children. This advice has been followed so assiduously that one could probably not find a lesson book for small children anywhere printed in ordinary reading type, while alphabets are often printed in characters one and two inches high. The British Association for the Advancement of Science does not wish to see children read books at all before they are seven years old, and would conduct their education previous to that age by means of large printed wall-sheets, blackboards, pictures, and oral teaching. If they must read, however, it wants them to have 24- and 30-point type, with capitals about a quarter of an inch in height. This is carefully graded down, a size smaller each year, until at the age of twelve the children are permitted to have the same kind of type as their elders. Bijou editions of Bible, prayer-book and hymnals are forbidden, however, to children of all ages.1

In the London myope classes, which have become the model for many others of the same kind, books are eliminated entirely, and only the older children are allowed to print their lessons in one- and two-inch types.2

Yet it has just been shown that large print is a strain upon the eyes, while the retinoscope demonstrates that a strain to see at the near-point always produces hypermetropia3 (commonly but erroneously called "farsight"). We should naturally expect, therefore, to find hypermetropia very common among small children, and it is. Of children eight and a half years old in the public schools of Philadelphia, Risley4 found that more than eighty-eight per cent were hypermetropic, and similar figures may be found in all statistics of the subject. The percentage declines as the children become older, but hypermetropia, or hypermetropic astigmatism, remains at all ages the most common of all errors of refraction. Hypermetropia is, in fact, a much more serious problem than myopia, or nearsight. Yet we have heard very little about it, for the specialists have concluded, from its prevalence and its tendency to pass away or become less pronounced with the growth of the body, that it is the normal state of the immature human eye and therefore beyond the reach of preventive measures. It is true that many young children are not hypermetropic, but this fact is easily disposed of by the theory that the ciliary muscle alters the shape of the lens in such cases sufficiently to compensate for the shortness of the eyeball.

The baselessness of this theory, as well as the relation of large print to the production of hypermetropia, may be demonstrated by the fact that the condition can be relieved, and has been relieved in numerous cases, by the reading of fine print, combined with rest of the eyes. A child of eight was cured in a few visits by this means. Yet according to the British Association she should not, at this age, have been allowed to read any type larger than 12-point, with capitals more than an eighth of an inch in height. Many grown people have been cured of hypermetropia in the same way, and in all forms of functional imperfect sight the reading of fine print, when it can be done with comfort, has been found to be a benefit to the eyes. Even straining to see fine print is sometimes a benefit in myopia.   Large letters are not a strain if central fixation, shifting are applied.   Avoid diffusion, eccentric fixation.

SHIFTING AND SWINGING
Correct Appearance of Oppositional Movement

When the eye with normal vision regards a letter either at the near-point or at the distance, the letter may appear to pulsate, or move in various directions, from side to side, up and down, or obliquely. When it looks from one letter to another on the Snellen test card, or from one side of a letter to another, not only the letters, but the whole line of letters and the whole card, may appear to move from side to side. This apparent movement is due to the shifting of the eye, and is always in a direction contrary to its movement. If one looks at the top of a letter, the letter is below the line of vision, and therefore appears to move downward. If one looks at the bottom, the letter is above the line of vision and appears to move upward. If one looks to the left of the letter, it is to the right of the line of vision and appears to move to the right. If one looks to the right, it is to the left of the line of vision and appears to move to the left.

Persons with normal vision are rarely conscious of this illusion, and may have difficulty in demonstrating it; but in every case that has come under my observation they have always become able, in a longer or shorter time, to do so. When the sight is imperfect the letters may remain stationary, or even move in the same direction as the eye.

It is impossible for the eye to fix a point longer than a fraction of a second. If it tries to do so, it begins to strain and the vision is lowered. This can readily be demonstrated by trying to hold one part of a letter for an appreciable length of time. No matter how good the sight, it will begin to blur, or even disappear, very quickly, and sometimes the effort to hold it will produce pain. In the case of a few exceptional people a point may appear to be held for a considerable length of time; the subjects themselves may think that they are holding it; but this is only because the eye shifts unconsciously, the movements being so rapid that objects seem to be seen all alike simultaneously.

The shifting of the eye with normal vision is usually not conspicuous, but by direct examination with the opthalmoscope5 it can always be demonstrated. If one eye is examined with this instrument while the other is regarding a small area straight ahead, the eye being examined, which follows the movements of the other, is seen to move in various directions, from side to side, up and down, in an orbit which is usually variable. If the vision is normal, these movements are extremely rapid and unaccompanied by any appearance of effort. The shifting of the eye with imperfect sight, on the contrary, is slower, its excursions are wider, and the movements are jerky and made with apparent effort.

It can also be demonstrated that the **eye is capable of shifting with a rapidity which the ophthalmoscope cannot measure.** (Saccadic movements) The normal eye can read fourteen letters on the bottom line of a Snellen test card, at a distance of ten or fifteen feet, in a dim light, so rapidly that they seem to be seen all at once. Yet it can be demonstrated that in order to recognize the letters under these conditions it is necessary to make about four shifts to each letter. At the near-point, even though one part of the letter is seen best, the rest may be seen well enough to be recognized; but at the distance it is impossible to recognize the letters unless one shifts from the top to the bottom and from side to side. One must also shift from one letter to another, making about **seventy shifts in a fraction of a second**.

A line of small letters on the Snellen test card may be less than a foot long by a quarter of an inch in height; and if it requires seventy shifts to a fraction of a second to see it apparently all at once, it must require many thousands to see an area of the size of the screen of a moving picture with all its detail of people, animals, houses, or trees, while to see sixteen such areas to a second, as is done in viewing moving pictures, must require a rapidity of shifting that can scarcely be realized. Yet it is admitted that the present rate of taking and projecting moving pictures is too slow. The results would be more satisfactory, authorities say, if the rate were raised to twenty, twenty-two or twenty-four a second. The human eye and mind are not only capable of this rapidity of action, and that without effort or strain, but it is only when the eye is able to shift thus rapidly that eye and mind are at rest, and the efficiency of both at their maximum. It is true that every motion of the eye produces an error of refraction; but when the movement is short, this is very slight, and usually the shifts are so rapid that the error does not last long enough to be detected by the retinoscope, its existence being demonstrable only by reducing the rapidity of the movements to less than four or five a second. The period during which the eye is at rest is much longer than that during which an error of refraction is produced. Hence, when the eye shifts normally no error of refraction is manifest. The more rapid the unconscious shifting of the eye, the better the vision; but if one tries to be conscious of a too rapid shift, a strain will be produced.

Perfect sight is impossible without continual shifting, and such shifting is a striking illustration of the mental control necessary for normal vision. It requires perfect mental control to think of thousands of things in a fraction of a second; and each point of fixation has to be thought of separately, because it is impossible to think of two things, or of two parts of one thing, perfectly at the same time. The eye with imperfect sight tries to accomplish the impossible by looking fixedly at one point for an appreciable length of time; that is, by staring. When it looks at a strange letter and does not see it, it keeps on looking at it in an effort to see it better. Such efforts always fail, and are an important factor in the production of imperfect sight.

+ One of the best methods of improving the sight, therefore, is to imitate consciously the unconscious shifting of normal vision, and to realize the apparent motion produced by such shifting. Whether one has imperfect or normal

sight, conscious shifting and swinging are a great help and advantage to the eye; for not only may imperfect sight be improved in this way, but normal sight may be improved also.

Detailed instructions for improving the sight by this method will be given in my forthcoming book, *The Cure of Imperfect Sight by Treatment without Glasses*.

Rapid and tiny shifts, the eyes ability to shift many times per fraction of a second are called Saccadic eye movements, vibrations. The eye produces many different movements, high frequency...

OPTIMUMS AND PESSIMUMS

In nearly all cases of imperfect sight due to errors of refraction there is some object, or objects, which can be regarded with normal vision. Such objects I have called *optimums*. On the other hand, there are some objects which persons with normal eyes and ordinarily normal sight always see imperfectly, an error of refraction being produced when they are regarded, as demonstrated by the retinoscope. Such objects I have called *pessimums*. An object becomes an optimum, or a pessimum, according to the effect it produces upon the mind, and in some cases this effect is easily accounted for.

For many children their mother's face is an optimum, and the face of a stranger a pessimum. A dressmaker was always able to thread a No. 10 needle with a fine thread of silk without glasses, although she had to put on glasses to sew on buttons, because she could not see the holes. She was a teacher of dressmaking, and thought the children stupid because they could not tell the difference between two different shades of black. She could match colors without comparing the samples. Yet she could not see a black line in a photographic copy of the Bible which was no finer than a thread of silk, and she could not remember a black period. An employee in a cooperage factory, who had been engaged for years in picking out defective barrels as they went rapidly past him on an inclined plane, was able to continue his work after his sight for most other objects had become very defective, while persons with much better sight for the Snellen test card were unable to detect the defective barrels. The familiarity of these various objects made it possible for the subjects to look at them without strain—that is, without trying to seem them. Therefore the barrels were to the cooper optimums; while the needle's eye and the colors of silk and fabrics were optimums to the dressmaker. Unfamiliar objects, on the contrary, are always pessimums.

In other cases there is no accounting for the idiosyncracy of the mind which makes one object a pessimum and another an optimum. It is also impossible to account for the fact that an object may be an optimum for one eye and not for the other, or an optimum at one time and at one distance and not at others. Among these unaccountable optimums one often finds a particular letter on the Snellen test card. One patient, for instance, was able to see the letter K on the forty, fifteen and ten lines, but could see none of the other letters on these lines, although most patients would see some of them, on account of the simplicity of their outlines, better than they would such a letter as K.

Pessimums may be as curious and unaccountable as optimums. The letter V is so simple in its outlines that many people can see it when they cannot see others on the same line. Yet some people are unable to distinguish it at any distance, although able to read other letters in the same word, or on the same line of the Snellen test card. Some people again will not only be unable to recognize the letter V in a word, but also to read any word that contains it, the pessimum lowering their sight not only for itself but for other objects. Some letters, or objects, become pessimums only in particular situations. A letter, for instance, may be a pessimum when located at the end, or at the beginning of a line, or sentence, and not in other places. When the attention of the patient is called to the fact that a letter seen in one location ought logically to be seen equally well in others, the letter often ceases to be a pessimum in any situation.

A pessimum, like an optimum, may be lost and later become manifest. It may vary according to the light and distance. An object which is a pessimum in a moderate light may not be so when the light is increased or diminished. A pessimum at twenty feet may not be one at two feet, or thirty feet, and an object which is a pessimum when directly regarded may be seen with normal vision in the eccentric field—that is, when not directly regarded.

For most people the Snellen test card is a pessimum. If you can see the Snellen test card with normal vision, you can see almost anything else in the world. Patients who cannot see the letters on the Snellen test card can often see other objects of the same size and at the same distance with normal sight. When letters which are seen imperfectly, or even letters which cannot be seen at all, or which the patient is not conscious of seeing, are regarded, the error of refraction is increased. The patient may regard a blank white card without any error of refraction; but if he regards the lower part of a Snellen test card, which appears to him to be just as blank as the blank card, an error of refraction can always be demonstrated, and if the visible letters of the card are covered the result is the same. The pessimum may, in short, be letters or objects which the patient is not conscious of seeing. This phenomenon is very common. When the card is seen in the eccentric field it may have the effect of lowering the vision for the point directly regarded. For instance, a patient may regard an area of green wall-paper at the distance, and see the color as well as at the near-point; but if a Snellen test card on which the letters are either seen imperfectly, or not seen at all, is placed in the neighborhood of the area being regarded, the retinoscope may indicate an error of refraction. When the vision improves, the number of letters on the card which are pessimums diminishes and the number of optimums increases, until the whole card becomes an optimum.

A pessimum, like an optimum, is a manifestation of the mind. It is something associated with a strain to see, just as an optimum is something which has no such association. It is not caused by the error of refraction, but always produces an error of refraction; and when the strain has been relieved it ceases to be a pessimum and becomes an optimum.

HOME TREATMENT

It is not always possible for patients to go to a competent physician for relief. As the method of treating eye defects presented in this magazine is new, it may be impossible to find a physician in the neighborhood who understands it; and the patient may not be able to afford the expense of a long journey, or to take the time for treatment away from home. To such persons I wish to say that it is possible for a large number of people to be cured of defective eyesight without the aid either of a physician or of anyone else.

They can cure themselves, and for this purpose it is not necessary that they should understand all that has been written in this magazine, or anywhere else. All that is necessary is to follow a few simple directions.

Place a Snellen test card on the wall at a distance of ten, fourteen, or twenty feet, and devote half a minute a day, or longer, to reading the smallest letters you can see, with each eye separately, covering the other with the palm of the hand in such a way as to avoid touching the eyeball.

Keep a record of the progress made, with the dates. The simplest way to do this is by the method used by oculists, who record the vision in the form of a fraction, with the distance at which the letter is read as the numerator and the distance at which it ought to be read as the denominator. As already explained, the figures above the lines of letters on the test card indicate the distance at which these letters should be read by persons with normal eyesight. Thus a vision of 10/200 would mean that the big C, which ought to be read at 200 feet, cannot be seen at a greater distance than ten feet. A vision of 20/10 would mean that the ten line, which the normal eye is not ordinarily expected to read at a greater distance than ten feet, is seen at double that distance. This is a standard commonly attained by persons who have practiced my methods.

Children under twelve years who have not worn glasses are usually cured of defective eyesight by the above method in three months, six months, or a year. Adults who have never worn glasses are benefited in a very short time—a week or two—and if the trouble is not very bad, may be cured in the course of from three to six months. Children or adults who have worn glasses, however, are more difficult to relieve, and will usually have to practice the various methods of gaining relaxation which have been presented from month to month in this magazine and will be described in more detail in my forthcoming book, *The Cure of Imperfect Sight by Treatment without Glasses.*

It is absolutely necessary that the glasses be discarded. No half-way measures can be tolerated, if a cure is desired. Do not attempt to wear weaker glasses, and do not wear glasses for emergencies. Persons who are unable to do without glasses are not likely to be able to cure themselves.

Modern Natural Vision Improvement teachers state that reduced, weaker eyeglass lenses can be worn, but only when necessary. In later years Dr. Bates stated glasses can be worn if absolutely essential but, glasses will slow vision improvement.

Children and adults who have worn glasses will have to devote an hour or longer every day to practice with the test card and the balance of their time to practice on other objects. It will be well for such patients to have **two test cards, one to be used at the near-point, where it can be seen best, and the other at ten or twenty feet. The patient will find it a great help to shift from the near card to the distant one, as the unconscious memory of the letters seen at the near-point helps to bring out those seen at the distance.** (Switching close and far. Shift on the E on the close card. Switch to the distant card. Shift on the E on that card. Then back to the close card. Repeat. Remember, imagine the E clear.)

If the patient can secure the aid of some person with normal sight, it will be a great advantage. In fact, persons whose cases are obstinate will find it very difficult, if not impossible, to cure themselves without the aid of a teacher. The teacher, if he is to benefit the patient, must himself be able to derive benefit from the various methods recommended. If his vision is 10/10, he must be able to improve it to 20/10, or more. If he can read fine print at twelve inches, he must become able to read it at six, or at three inches. He must also have sufficient control over his visual memory to relieve and prevent pain.

Parents who wish to preserve and improve the eyesight of their children should encourage them to read the Snellen test card every day. There should, in fact, be a Snellen test card in every family; for when properly used it always prevents myopia and other errors of refraction, always improves the vision, even when this is already normal, and always benefits functional nervous troubles. Parents should improve their own eyesight to normal, so that their children may not imitate wrong methods of using the eyes and will not be subject to the influence of an atmosphere of strain.

December, 1919

1 - Report on the Influence of School Books upon Eyesight, second revised edition, 1913.
2 – Pollock: The Education of the Semi-Blind, Glasgow med. Jour., Dec, 1915.
3 – Bates: The cause of myopia, N.Y. Med. Jour., March 10, 1912.
4 – School hygiene, in System of Diseases of the Eye, edited by Norris and Oliver, vol. II, P. 353.
5 - An instrument for viewing the interior of the eye. When the optic nerve is observed with the ophthalmoscope, movements can be noted that are not apparent when only the exterior of the eye is regarded.

11 years, 132 Monthly Better Eyesight Magazine Issues in text & the Original Antique Print, printable in a PDF E-book -Free - mclearsight@aol.com - www.cleareyesight-batesmethod.info

Read, learn from Dr. Bates, the Best, Original Natural Eyesight Improvement Teacher

From this page onward; the pages, page numbers and 'refer to page number' notes are from the large Textbook edition of Perfect Sight Without Glasses. Added to this book to include extra training. Some page numbers are omitted due to pages being added from different chapters of the Textbook. The Textbook will be free in PDF on the website, Googlebooks and Archive.org in 2016.

Suggestions

By EMILY A. BATES

1. If the vision of the patient is improved under the care of the doctor, and the patient neglects to practice, when he leaves the office, what he is told to do at home, the treatment has been of no benefit whatever. The improved vision was only temporary. Faithful practice permanently improves the sight to normal.
2. If the patient conscientiously practices the methods, as advised by the doctor, his vision always improves. This applies to patients with errors of refraction, as well as organic diseases.
3. For cases of squint we find that the long swing is beneficial to adults and to children.
4. When a patient suffers with cataract, palming is usually the best method of treatment, and should be practiced many times every day.
5. All patients with imperfect sight unconsciouly stare, and should be reminded by those who are near to them to blink often. To stare is to strain. Strain is the cause of imperfect sight.

The following rules will be found helpful if faithfully observed:—

6. While sitting, do not look up without raising your chin. Always turn your head in the direction in which you look. Blink often.
7. Do not make an effort to see things more clearly. If you let your eyes alone, things will clear up by themselves.
8. Do not look at anything longer than a fraction of a second without shifting.
9. While reading, do not think about your eyes, but let your mind and imagination rule.
10. When you are conscious of your eyes while looking at objects at any time, it causes discomfort and lessens your vision.
11. It is very important that you learn how to imagine stationary objects to be moving, without moving your head or your body.
12. Palming is a help, and I suggest that you palm for a few minutes many times during the day, at least ten times. At night just before retiring, it is well to palm for half an hour or longer.

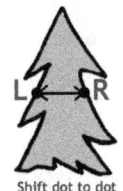

Shift dot to dot

Clarification for #11; The head moves with the eyes (most all of the time) when the eyes-vision move 'shifts' part to part on an object and from object to object.

Imagine and SEE opposite movement, 'The Swing'; Shift left and right on a distant tree and see it appear to move opposite the shifting movement of the eyes;

Shift left to right > - The tree moves < left
Shift right to left < - The tree moves right >

Moving the head with the eyes, in the same direction improves this movement, makes it easy and relaxed.

#11 is saying; the swing of opposite movement should also occur 'be seen' during times when the head and body are not moving. It's healthy to move. Most of the time the head and body move with the eyes.

Read the e-books for more examples of eye movement 'shifting', head, body movement and the appearance of opposite movement of stationary objects.

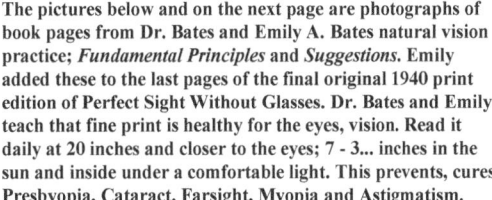

The pictures below and on the next page are photographs of book pages from Dr. Bates and Emily A. Bates natural vision practice; *Fundamental Principles* and *Suggestions*. Emily added these to the last pages of the final original 1940 print edition of Perfect Sight Without Glasses. Dr. Bates and Emily teach that fine print is healthy for the eyes, vision. Read it daily at 20 inches and closer to the eyes; 7 - 3... inches in the sun and inside under a comfortable light. This prevents, cures Presbyopia, Cataract, Farsight, Myopia and Astigmatism.

CHAPTER XXXIII

HOW TO DEMONSTRATE THE FUNDAMENTAL PRINCIPLES OF TREATMENT

THE object of all the methods used in the treatment of imperfect sight without glasses is to secure rest or relaxation, of the mind first and then of the eyes. Rest always improves the vision. Effort always lowers it. Persons who wish to improve their vision should begin by demonstrating these facts.

To demonstrate the strain lowers the vision, think of something disagreeable, some physical discomfort, or something seen imperfectly. When the eyes are opened, it will be found that the vision has been lowered. Also stare at one part of a letter on the test card, or try to see the whole letter all alike at one time. This invariably lowers the vision, and may cause the letters to disappear. Another symptom of strain is a twitching of the eyelids which can be seen by an observer and felt by the patient with the fingers. This can usually be corrected if the period of rest is long enough. Many persons fail to secure a temporary improvement of vision by closing their eyes, because they do not keep them closed long enough. Children will seldom do this unless a grown person stands by and encourages them. Many adults also require supervision.

CLOSING THE EYES

The simplest way to rest the eyes is to close them for a longer or shorter period and think about something

Helpful Suggestions

agreeable. This is always the first thing that I tell patients to do and there are very few who are not benefited by it temporarily.

PALMING

A still greater degree of rest can be obtained by closing and covering the eyes so as to exclude all the light. The mere exclusion of the impression of sight is often sufficient to produce a large measure of relaxation. In other cases the strain is increased. As a rule, successful palming involves a knowledge of various other means of obtaining relaxation. The mere covering and closing of the eyes is useless unless at the same time mental rest is obtained. When a patient palms perfectly he sees a field so black that it is impossible to remember, imagine, or see anything blacker, and when able to do this he is cured. It should be borne in mind, however, that the patient's judgment of what is a perfect black is not to be depended upon.

THE LONG SWING

Demonstrate—That the long swing not only improves the vision, but also relieves or cures pain, discomfort and fatigue.

Stand with the feet about one foot apart, facing squarely one side of the room. Lift the left heel a short distance from the floor while turning the shoulders, head, and eyes to the right, until the line of the shoulders is parallel with the wall. Now turn the body to the left after placing the left heel upon the floor and raising the right heel. Alternate looking from the right wall to the left wall, being careful to move the head and eyes with the movement of the shoulders. When practiced easily, continuously, without effort and without paying any attention to moving objects, one soon becomes conscious that the long swing relaxes the tension of the muscles and nerves.

Stationary objects move with varying degrees of rapidity. Objects located almost directly in front of you appear to move with express train speed and should be very much blurred. It is very important to make no attempt to see clearly objects which seem to be moving very rapidly.

The long swing seems to help patients who suffer from eyestrain during sleep. By practicing the long swing fifty times or more just before retiring and just after rising in the morning, eyestrain during sleep has been prevented or relieved. It is remarkable how quickly the long swing relieves or prevents pain. I know of no other procedure which can compare with it. The long swing has relieved the pain of facial neuralgia after operative measures had failed. Some patients who have suffered from continuous pain in various parts of the body have been relieved by the long swing, at first temporarily, but by repetition the relief has become more permanent. Hay fever, asthma, sea-sickness, palpitation of the heart, coughs, acute and chronic colds are usually relieved by the long swing.

MEMORY

When the sight is normal the mind is always perfectly at rest, and when the memory is perfect the mind is also at rest. Therefore it is possible to improve the sight by the use of the memory. Anything the patient finds it agreeable to remember is a rest to the mind, but for purposes of practice a small black object, such as a period or a letter of fine print, is usually most convenient. The most favorable condition for the exercise of the memory is, usually, with the eyes closed and covered, but by practice it becomes possible to remember equally well with the eyes open. When patients are able, with their eyes closed and covered, to remember perfectly a letter of fine print, it appears, just as it would if they were looking at it with the bodily eyes, to have a slight movement, while the openings appear whiter than the rest of the background. If they are not able to remember it, they are told to shift consciously from one side of the letter to another and to consciously imagine the opening whiter than the rest of the background. When they do this, the letter usually appears to move in a direction contrary to that of the imagined movement of the eye, and they are able to remember it indefinitely. If, on the contrary, they try to fix the attention on one part of the letter, or to think of two or more parts at one time, it soon disappears, demonstrating that it is impossible to think of one point continuously, or to think of two or more points perfectly at one time, just as it is impossible to look at a point continuously, or to see two points perfectly at the same time. Persons with no visual memory are always under a great strain and often suffer from pain and fatigue with no apparent cause. As soon as they become able to form mental pictures, either with the eyes closed or open, their pain and fatigue are relieved.

IMAGINATION

Imagination is closely allied to memory, for we can imagine only as well as we remember, and in the treatment of imperfect sight the two can scarcely be separated. Vision is largely a matter of imagination and memory. And since both imagination and memory are impossible without perfect relaxation, the cultivation of these faculties not only improves the interpretation of the pictures on the retina, but improves the pictures themselves. When you imagine that you see a letter on the test card you actually do see it, because it is impossible to relax and imagine the letter perfectly, and, at the same time, strain and see it imperfectly. The following method of using the imagination has produced quick results in many cases. The patient is asked to look at the largest letter on the test card at the near-point, and is usually able to observe that a small area, about a square inch, appears blacker than the rest, and that when the part of the letter seen worst is covered, part of the exposed area seems blacker than the remainder. When the part seen worst is again covered, the area of maximum blackness is still further reduced. When the part seen best has been reduced to about the size of a letter on the bottom line, the patient is asked to imagine that such a letter occupies this area and is blacker than the rest of the letter. Then he is asked to look at a letter on the bottom line and imagine that it is blacker than the largest letter. Many are able to do this, and at once become able to see the letters on the bottom line.

FLASHING

Since it is effort that spoils the sight, many persons with imperfect sight are able, after a period of rest, to look at an object for a fraction of a second. If the eyes are closed before the habit of strain reasserts itself permanent relaxation is sometimes very quickly obtained. This practice I have called flashing, and many persons are helped by it who are unable to improve their sight by other means. The eyes are rested for a few minutes, by closing or palming, and then a letter on the test card, or a letter of fine print, if the trouble is with near vision, is regarded for a fraction of a second. Then the eyes are immediately closed and the process repeated.

READING FAMILIAR LETTERS

The eye always strains to see unfamiliar objects, and is always relaxed to a greater or less degree by looking at familiar objects. Therefore the reading every day of small familiar letters at the greatest distance at which they can be seen is a rest to the eye, and is sufficient to cure children under twelve who have not worn glasses, as well as some older children, and adults with minor defects of vision.

CENTRAL FIXATION

When the vision is normal the eye sees one part of everything it looks at best and every other part worse in proportion as it is removed from the point of maximum vision. When the vision is imperfect it is invariably found that the eye is trying to see a considerable part of its field of vision equally well at one time. This is a great strain upon the eye and mind, as anyone whose sight is approximately normal can demonstrate by trying to see an appreciable area all alike at one time. At the near-point the attempt to see an area even a quarter of an inch in diameter in this way will produce discomfort and pain. Anything which rests the eye tends to restore the normal power of central fixation. It can also be regained by conscious practice, and this is sometimes the quickest and easiest way to improve the sight. When the patient becomes conscious that he sees one part of his field of vision better than the rest, it usually becomes possible for him to reduce the area seen best. If he looks from the bottom of the 200 letter to the top, for instance, and sees the part not directly regarded worse than the part fixed he may become able to do the same with the next line of letters, and thus he may become able to go down the card until he can look from the top to the bottom of the letters on the bottom line and see the part not directly regarded worse. In that case he will be able to read the letters. Since small objects cannot be seen without central fixation, the reading of fine print, when it can be done, is one of the best of visual exercises, and the dimmer the light in which it can be read and the closer to the eye it can be held the better.

THE EFFECT OF LIGHT UPON THE EYES AND SUN TREATMENT

Although the eyes were made to react to the light, very general fear of the effect of this element upon the organs of vision is entertained both by the medical profession and by the laity. Persons with normal sight have been able to look at the sun for a short length of time without any discomfort or loss of vision. Immediately afterward they were able to read the Snellen test card with improved vision, their sight having become better than what is ordinarily considered normal. Some persons with normal sight do suffer discomfort and loss of vision when they look at the sun; but in such cases the retinoscope always indicates an error of refraction, showing that this condition is due, not to the light, but to strain. It has been my experience that all persons who wear dark glasses sooner or later develop inflammation of their eyes. The human eye needs the light in order to maintain its efficiency. The use of eye-shades and protections of all kinds from the light is injurious to the eyes. Sunlight is as necessary to normal eyes as is rest and relaxation. If it is possible, start the day by exposing the closed eyes to the sun. Just a few minutes at a time will help. Get accustomed to the strong light of the sun by letting it shine on your closed eyelids. It is good to move the head slightly from side to side while doing this in order to prevent straining. One cannot get too much sun treatment

BRAIN TENSION

The brain has many nerves. Part of these nerves are called ganglion cells and originate in some particular part of the brain. Each has a function of its own. They are connected with other ganglion cells and with the aid of nerve fibres are connected with others located in various parts of the brain as well as in the spinal cord, the eye, the ear, the nerves of smell, taste, and the nerves of touch. The function of each ganglion cell of the brain is different from that of all others. When the ganglion cells are healthy, they function in a normal manner.

The retina of the eye contains numerous ganglion cells which regulate special things such as normal vision, normal memory, normal imagination and they do this with a control more or less accurate of other ganglion cells of the whole body. The retina has a similar structure to parts of the brain. It is connected to the brain by the optic nerve.

Many nerves from the ganglion cells of the retina carry conscious and unconscious control of other ganglion cells which are connected to other parts of the body.

When the ganglion cells are diseased or at fault, the functions of all parts of the body are not normally maintained. In all cases of imperfect sight, it has been repeatedly demonstrated that the ganglion cells and nerves of the brain are under a strain. When this strain is corrected by treatment, the functions of the ganglion and other cells become normal. The importance of the mental treatment cannot be over-estimated.

A study of the facts has demonstrated that a disease of some ganglion in any part of the body occurs in similar ganglion in the brain.

Brain tension of one or more nerves always means disease of the nerve ganglia. Treatment of the mind with the aid of the sight, memory and imagination has cured many cases of imperfect sight without other treatment

Fine Print for Relaxation

The Bible has been reduced from $4.00 to $2.50. Read what Dr. Bates says about fine and microscopic type, then get a Bible. This unique book measures only one by one and a half inches, and contains the Old and New Testament.

The Booklet

of fine print contains three chapters from the small Bible, together with "The Seven Truths of Normal Sight" as discovered by Dr. Bates. Instructions are also printed in the front of the book. Price 25c

Shift part to part on fine print letters, words. Even if they are blurry; just relax and move the vision upon them. Blink. Look at the white spaces between sentences. See the white closest to the black print 'glow' bright white. A thin white line is under the sentence. Look at, shift on the black print. Think something pleasant. Move the page a bit in the hand; left and right, up, down and in any direction. This prevents staring, it activates eye movement. Look at the white space and thin white line again, move along it. When the print flashes clear; read it. When the eyes-brain see the words clear; the brain moves the vision quickly along the sentences. Thoughts, mental pictures of the subject being read also create automatic eye movements. The vision remains clear.

Introduction, Directions, Dedication Continued

Dedication
To Ophthalmologist William H. Bates

William H. Bates, Ophthalmologist discovered and perfected Natural Eyesight Improvement, 'The Bates Method'. He discovered the natural principles, true, normal function of the eyes (visual system) and applied natural methods, relaxation to return the eyes, eye muscles, nerves, mind/brain, thought patterns, body (entire visual system) to natural, normal function with healthy eyes and clear vision.

The Bates Method of Natural Eyesight Improvement.
He cured; unclear close and distant vision, astigmatism, crossed, wandering eyes, cataracts, glaucoma, and other eye conditions. Natural Eyesight (Vision) Improvement was practiced years before Dr. Bates discovered it. It is the normal, natural function of the eyes. Hidden from the public by eye surgeons, optometrists, optical businesses for over 100 years because this method works, is easy, anyone can learn, teach it, including children. It produces healthy eyes, clear vision and frees the patient from the need to purchase eyeglasses, drugs, unnecessary eye surgery. Yes, it can and has reversed cataracts!

Dr. William H. Bates
Ophthalmologist - M.D.
Eye, Ear, Nose & Throat.
Discovered the Principles of Eye Function-Natural Eyesight Improvement.

Dr. Bates worked his entire life treating people successfully with Natural Eyesight Improvement. When he cured the eyes, vision of many patients, medical students and other doctors in the hospital where he worked with natural treatments, without use of eyeglasses, surgery, drugs and proved his method is fact and that some of the old theories of eye function are incorrect, only theories; the doctors, eye surgeons that preferred to sell eyeglasses, surgery, drugs became angry and expelled him. (See: 'Reason and Authority' and 'Dr. Bates Lecture' in Better Eyesight Magazine: November, 1919, April, 1923 and Articles in his book.)

Fig. 37. Myopic Astigmatism comes and Goes According as the Subject Looks at Distant Objects With or Without Strain

No. 1.—Patient regarding the Snellen test card at ten feet without effort and reading the bottom line with normal vision.
No. 2.—The same patient making an effort to see a picture at twenty feet. The retinoscope indicated compound myopic astigmatism.

Dr. Bates then opened his own office, a Clinic in Harlem, New York City. He treated thousands of people by natural methods, including many of the poor people that had little money. He kept his price for medical treatment low and also provided no charge office visits 'Free Clinic Days' for people that could not afford to pay for a visit to an Ophthalmologist. His treatments were successful. He cured the young and old, people of all ages, nationalities, cured a variety of eye conditions.

The Bates Method is so simple and effective that many of his cured patients, 'often children' then went on to cure their friends, family, parents, teachers and other children of defective vision including crossed, wandering eyes. Read the 'true story of the two little girls that restored a blind mans eyesight' in the Oct. 1925 Magazine Issue. Read Dr. Bates full story in 'Better Eyesight Magazine' and his book 'The Cure of Imperfect Sight by Treatment Without Glasses'.

Fig. 43
Patient with atrophy of the optic nerve gets flashes of improved vision after palming.

Dr. Bates recorded 11 years of work in his clinic, his patients and their varied treatments in his Better Eyesight Magazines, Books and Medical Articles. Dr. Bates Better Eyesight Magazines contain many Natural Treatments, a variety of Activities, Directions, Articles describing how Dr. Bates, Emily Lierman Bates, (his Clinic assistant, wife) and other eye Doctors, School Teachers, Bates Method Students, Bates Teachers, Children and Parents used Natural Treatments to remove, correct, prevent many different eye problems: unclear close and distant vision (nearsight, myopia, farsight, presbyopia), astigmatism, cataracts, glaucoma, conical cornea, cornea ulcers & scars, retinitis pigmentosa, wandering/crossed eyes (strabismus), amblyopia and other eye conditions. Done without eyeglasses, surgery, drugs. Dr. Bates used surgery, drugs only when necessary, (Eye injury, infection...).

The magazines contain `True Life Stories' of the doctors, assistants, patients, treatments. Interesting, entertaining, fun to read. A History book, life in the early 1900's. Vision improvement based `Fairy Stories' and other articles for children are included. The stories produce a positive, relaxed state of mind, activate, improve the memory and imagination, teach Natural Eyesight Improvement, normal, correct eye functions. This improves the eyesight.

Dr. Bates discovered Natural Eyesight Improvement over 100 years ago - Started around the year 1886. Dr. Bates Better Eyesight Magazines, books are the original source of The Bates Method and true Natural Eyesight Improvement. The Original Better Eyesight Magazine collection is proof that Ophthalmologist William H. Bates discovered the Bates Method, Natural Eyesight (Vision) Improvement and is the True Author of the Magazine.

The Optical, Medical Industry/Association and most Eye Doctors, Opticians have hidden Dr. Bates work, magazines, books, articles, Natural Eyesight Improvement from the public for over 100 years because: The Bates Method improves the clarity of vision, eye function, Dr. Bates writings are proof that Natural Eyesight Improvement works, produces clear vision, healthy eyes, it describes, teaches people how to apply Natural Eyesight Improvement & obtain clear vision 'on their own' and prevents the need for purchasing eyeglasses, contact lenses, sunglasses, eye surgery and drugs. The Bates Method is safe, healthy for the eyes, reverses and prevents vision impairment.
After Dr. Bates death, the Optical Industry, Medical Doctors/Association destroyed Dr. Bates magazines, books, articles, removed them from libraries, schools, colleges, bookstores in an attempt to hide the truth about Natural Eyesight Improvement from the public, prevent people from curing their eyesight.
They bribed dishonest politicians, judges to pass laws preventing the public from teaching Natural Eyesight Improvement. They passed a law stating that only an eye doctor can teach the Bates Method. Most doctors refused to teach it. Ophthalmology, Optometry, Optician Colleges hid it, refused to teach it and Eye Doctors were taught in College to ignore the Bates Method. Honest eye doctors were afraid to teach it, were told that they would lose their medical license if they used it in their practice.

A few honest Eye Doctors, Bates Teachers, Students, Libraries from the 1900's - present have preserved and republished Dr. Bates magazines, books and continued to teach the Bates Method despite harassment from the Optical, Medical Industry: Emily Lierman/Bates, Dr. Harold Peppard, Cecil S. Price, Dr. William B. MacCracken, Bernarr MacFadden, Clara Hackett, Margaret Corbett, Aldous Huxley, Dr. Clara & Emery Ingham and others. (See the case of Margaret Corbett and Aldous Huxley, New York City, USA; The Optical/Medical Industry, Association brought her to court, accused her of practicing Optometry without a license. She won all cases brought against her and cured the eyesight of many people that were in the courtroom. Aldous Huxley (famous Author) was a witness for Margaret Corbett, proved to the court how she reversed his near blindness, improved his eyesight. He later wrote the book: 'The Art of Seeing'. Many people cured of unclear eyesight, cataract, forms of blindness, other conditions were witnesses.

The Optical, Medical and Drug Industry prefers to sell eyeglasses, contact lenses, dangerous destructive cornea laser eye surgery, cataract lens surgery, other eye operations and drugs. They continue to suppress, hide the Bates Method from their patients, the public.
Dishonest Eye Doctors prescribe stronger and stronger eyeglass lenses, bifocals, unneeded astigmatism sections in the eyeglass lenses, tinted/UV blocking lenses & sunglasses knowing that this causes and increases vision impairment, eye muscle tension, abnormal pressure, tension on/in the eye, retina, lens.., dependence on stronger eyeglasses and leads to development of cataracts, detached retina, other eye health impairment and thousands of dollars profit from performing cataract, retina, cornea... surgery. I suspect that some Opticians, Optometrists that sell stronger and stronger eyeglasses receive money, 'kickbacks' from eye surgeons when the business sends a patient that has developed a cataract or other eye problem, 'advanced and ready for surgery', to the eye surgeon for a operation.
Senior citizens are their main victim, 'customer', abused by their doctors, told to wait for surgery until the cataract grows large enough while the doctor sells stronger and stronger eyeglass lenses, bifocals, unnecessary astigmatism sections in the glasses, sunglasses... knowing that this practice will cause more vision impairment, increase, speed the growth, development of the cataract and prevent a natural reversal, cure of the cataract. Reading glasses, astigmatism sections in the lenses are a main cause of cataract.
A sales pitch for laser eye cornea surgery is often done after the patient's eyesight is greatly impaired from being prescribed addictive, stronger and stronger eyeglass lenses, bifocals and astigmatism lenses. When the patient feels helpless, scared, they are pressured into agreeing to eye cornea laser surgery.
Laser cornea eye surgeons destroy the health, structure of the eyes cornea knowing it will lead to a variety of eye, vision impairments, sale of eyeglasses, more eye surgery. Many patients have experienced extreme, disabling vision problems, eye pain and blindness has occurred. Patients have committed suicide, explaining to their family they would rather die than live with the greatly impaired vision, pain and poor quality of life that the laser cornea eye surgery caused. See the FDA 'Cornea Surgery Side Effects Warning' links at http://www.fda.gov & YouTube: https://www.youtube.com/watch?v=lXzqwzQo0Oc
http://www.lasikcomplications.com. The law states that eye doctors do not have to tell their patients all the dangers, side effects of cornea eye surgeries. Laser surgery destroys the cornea's health, function and often results in more eye surgeries 'trying' to correct damage done by the first laser surgery. Even though the TV

news stations and newspapers receive a lot of money for advertising laser surgery, they do post reports on laser and other cornea eye surgery side effects. But the reports of eye injuries are usually hidden.

An honest eye doctor prefers to get the patient to stop use of eyeglasses, <u>will not</u> prescribe strong eyeglasses, bifocals, tinted, colored, UV blocking lenses, sunglasses, destructive astigmatism sections, laser... cornea eye surgery and other unnatural methods. He/she teaches the patient how to reverse, prevent unclear vision, astigmatism, cataracts and other abnormal eye, vision conditions.

Due to the truth about Natural Medicine being available to the modern public, interest in Natural Cures; Dr. Bates Better Eyesight Magazines, books, work has been recovered from individual owners, re-published and brought back to the public. Many Ophthalmologists, Optometrists are now learning, teaching the Bates Method and monitoring, recording their patients' Natural Eyesight Improvement progress.

Dr. William H. Bates Life & The Bates Method History

Dr. Bates started his career as an orthodox ophthalmologist following the old unnatural way, rules of the practice; prescribing eyeglasses... *This 100+ years harmful method was and still is the only thing taught in eye doctor colleges.*
During his practice, working with different patients, eye conditions he realized that unclear close, distant vision, astigmatism and other eye-vision states often cured itself, reversed back to clear vision, especially when his patients stopped wearing their eyeglasses. He noticed that wearing glasses strained the eyes, mind and lowered the vision resulting in stronger and stronger eyeglass lens prescriptions being needed in order to see clear through the glasses. He began his own studies on the eye and it's function. This led him to discover that many of the old ophthalmology, optometry 'supposed facts' about the eye, lens, their function and the cause of unclear vision... are incorrect. Dr. Bates began teaching his patients to avoid eyeglasses, he removed their glasses. He taught them natural methods, including relaxation, correct use of the eyes, practice of normal, natural eye-vision function to see perfectly clear. Dr. Bates cured his own eyesight, close vision 'presbyopia'. Distant vision also clear. He wrote an article in his book, magazine describing how he did it with Memory, Imagination, Relaxation. He controlled, changed the focus of light rays in his eyes with his mind.

Dr. Bates performed experiments on the eyes, eye muscles of animals, observed the function of thousands of animal & patient's eyes under different conditions, situations, state of mind, body, thoughts and emotions. He used the retinoscope to see the refraction, focus of light rays in the eye under these various conditions. He proved that the refraction, clarity of vision changes often. When the eyes are left alone, eyeglasses avoided; the refraction, clarity returns to normal, clear vision. He proved that the state of the mind, thoughts change the refraction of the eye, clarity of vision. Example; when the mind, body is relaxed, positive, happy thoughts, emotions; the refraction is normal and vision is clear. When the mind, body is under stress, strain; the refraction is abnormal and vision is unclear. Dr. Bates discovered that the main cause of unclear vision and other eye problems is; Wearing Eyeglasses, Mental Strain, Mental-Visual Effort to See, Incorrect Vision Habits (squinting, staring, trying hard to see clear, not shifting, lack of central-fixation, low memory, imagination...). <u>Perfect Sight occurs only with Perfect Relaxation</u> (deep or active-dynamic relaxation; See Aldous Huxley's book; T*he Art of Seeing*). <u>Relaxation occurs first</u> and <u>then the eyesight becomes clear</u>.

Dr. Bates experiments on the outer eye muscles proved that tension in these muscles disrupts their function, the eyes' movement *shifting*, accommodation, convergence, un-accommodation, divergence, causes pressure, tension on/in the eye, alters the eyes' shape, (and lens' shape, movement), disrupts focus of light rays on the retina and lowers the clarity of vision. Circulation in the eyes is also affected.

Mental strain, stress in the mind, negative thoughts, emotions cause eye muscle tension. Neck muscle tension causes eye muscle tension. Neck tension is caused by mental strain, negative thoughts, emotions, incorrect posture, immobility, injury; vertebrae out of alignment. Inner eye muscle tension; ciliary/lens, iris, tear gland, blinking muscles... also occurs. When the mind is strained-tense, the brain and retina do not communicate, function together at optimum level. Function of the retina and vision is lowered.

Dr. Bates proved that MENTAL STRAIN causes unclear vision. RELAXATION of the mind produces clear vision. Dr. Bates used his retinoscope to show that the refraction/focus of light rays in the eye are disrupted resulting in unclear vision when a person lies. Lying causes a bit of mental strain. When the person tells the truth, no strain occurs, the refraction is perfect and vision clear. Many things can cause mental strain. Avoid eyeglasses, remove the stress, strain and vision returns to clear. Practice of Natural Eyesight Improvement can uncover old, forgotten stressful experiences, resulting in strong emotions, feelings being remembered, activated. When the memory, feelings are acknowledged, released and new positive thoughts, emotions placed into the brain, system; often the vision immediately returns to normal 20/20 and clearer. No other practice is needed. The eyes relax, move, 'shift'... correct <u>on their own</u>.

Dr. Bates published Medical Articles, Books describing his experiments on the eyes, eye muscles, the effect of memory on the eyes, vision and the effect of the clarity of vision on the memory: 1891 'A Study of

Images Reflected from the Cornea, Iris, Lens, and Sclera' & 'Memory as an Aid to Vision'. These Articles and others are placed in his 1920 book: The Cure of Imperfect Sight by Treatment without Glasses, Better Eyesight Magazine and his Medical Articles E-Book.
Dr. Bates created Natural Treatments, Activities to cure: reverse, correct and prevent unclear vision and other eye conditions based on his discoveries. This became know as 'The Bates Method'. Glaucoma, cataracts and other eye conditions were also reversed successfully with Dr. Bates Natural Treatments.

>He made other discoveries, eye surgery inventions. Later, after he discovered the natural function of the eyes, vision, he stopped use of certain surgeries and cured the eyes-vision with his natural method.

Dr. Bates History - Dates

1860 - Born December, 23rd - New Jersey, USA.

1881 - Graduate - B.S. (Bachelor of Science) Agriculture - Cornell University in New York.

1885 - Graduate - MD (Medical Degree - Doctor of Medicine) - College of Physicians & Surgeons - Columbia University, New York.

1886 - Invented new operation for a type of deafness by incising the ear drum membrane and published article.
Published more articles on the Eye, Eye Muscles, Lens, Cornea, Cataracts, Accommodation, Myopia... from this date onward.
Discovered and published Article on properties of the aqueous extract of the suprarenal capsule, 'Adrenalin'.

1886 - <u>First Natural Eyesight Improvement Application - Dr. Bates cures a medical student of unclear distant vision, 'Myopia' without eyeglasses, surgery, drugs.</u>

1886 -1902 - Eye surgeon - Instructor of Ophthalmology - New York Postgraduate Medical School, Hospital. Dr. Bates teaches the other doctors, medical students to stop wearing their eyeglasses and how to cure their eyesight, myopia with Natural Methods. Dr. Bates natural treatments were successful. He states, proves the natural cure for Myopia, unclear distant vision.
  (1891 - Dr. Roosa, the chief director of the institution, expelled Dr. Bates in an attempt to hide Natural Eyesight Improvement from the public and maintain the practice of solely prescribing eyeglasses, surgery and drugs.) Dr. Bates was curing patients naturally with success. Dr. Roosa tried to prevent this.
  Dr. Bates then opens his own office, clinic and works for better hospitals.

Attending Physician, Surgeon, Clinic Assistant - Manhattan Eye & Ear hospital, Bellevue hospital, New York Eye Infirmary-Northern, Northeastern, Northwestern dispensary & Harlem Hospital.
Invented Astigmatic Keratotomy, an operation to correct astigmatism. <u>He discontinued applying this operation after he realized through further study of Natural Eyesight Improvement that the operation eventually impairs the eyes function, cornea, vision, health. It works against the natural function of the eye.</u>

Dr. Bates discontinued his hospital schedules for a while and started experimental work, studied the eyes natural function at the laboratory at Columbia University.., Research at the Pathology Laboratory of Dr. Pruden at the College of Physicians and Surgeons, Columbia University.

Dr. Bates goes to Grand Forks, North Dakota, (Medical License) and teaches his Natural Eyesight Improvement Method, correct natural use of Snellen Eyecharts in the schools, brings clear vision to the children and teachers. Elected president of the Grand Forks district Medical Society.

Back to New York, worked as Attending Physician - Harlem Hospital in New York City. Teaches his method, use of Snellen Eyecharts in the schools, brings clear vision to the children and teachers in New York City.

1911+ - Met Emily C. Lierman. Dr. Bates cured her eyesight, then hired her as his assistant clinic nurse -They worked his experiments in the Physiological Laboratory at the College of Physicians and Surgeons in New York and treated patient's eyesight with natural methods in the Harlem Hospital, Clinic. Many years giving <u>free treatments</u> to the Public. They Married in 1928.
  Dr Bates performs experiments on the eyes of Animals, Fish proving that the outer eye muscles when tense can alter the shape of the eye, lens and cause unclear vision, cataracts and other conditions. He proves the outer eye muscles, oblique can accommodate the eyes for clear close vision.

1918 - Course, booklets 'Strengthening the Eyes' by Bernarr Macfadden & Dr. William H. Bates - Physical Culture Publishing Co. In later book editions, Only MacFadden's name, picture was listed on/in the book.

1919 -1930 - Dr. Bates Published his Monthly 'Better Eyesight Magazine' - Central-Fixation Publishing Co. - 11 Years - 132 Issues recording a variety of Natural Treatments that Dr. Bates, Emily Lierman-Bates and other doctors, teachers... used to treat many different eye-vision conditions of their patients. A Gold Mine, History of Natural Eyesight Improvement Methods, Applications.

1920 - Dr. Bates published his book: 'The Cure of Imperfect Sight by Treatment Without Glasses'. (Perfect Sight Without Glasses). Advertised in Better Eyesight Magazine in 1919.

Medical Article - The American Journal of Clinical Medicine 'A Clinical and Experimental Study of Physiological Optics with a view to the Cure of Imperfect Sight Without glasses'. Information, directions on The Bates Method.
Many Medical Articles proving the effectiveness of The Bates Method were published though the years.

Elected Vice President of Allied Medical Associations of America.

Stopped work at Harlem Hospital, Clinic and starts work and Free Clinic treatments day at new location.

1926 - Emily C. A. Lierman (Bates) writes, publishes the book: 'Stories From The Clinic' describing The Bates Method, various natural treatments Dr. Bates and Emily applied to cure many different eye conditions for patients in their Clinic. Also listed in Better Eyesight Magazine. The book has a few different sentences...

1931, July 10th - Dr. Bates Deceased, age 70 at his home in New York City.
Emily Lierman/Bates, Dr. Harold Peppard, Dr. William B. MacCracken, C.S. Price, Clara Hackett, Margaret Corbett, Aldous Huxley and others continue to teach The Bates Method. Dr. Bates Better Eyesight Magazine and Books, Articles were Preserved. Bates Teachers work in Cities in the U.S.A., England, Germany, Spanish Teachers, South Africa...

1940 - Emily Lierman, Bates re-published Dr. Bates book with an additional chapter teaching The Bates Method's Application: The Fundamental Principles of Treatment. (The list of treatments is placed in this book, derived from the 1940 edition, Better Eyesight Magazine, June, 1921, other issues and Dr. Bates 1920+ editions). Eyechart training, appreciation letters... included. During her teaching profession Emily and others continued to bring the Bates Method to California and other states, countries. Thousands of people's eyesight was cured naturally. Emily and other teachers created and showed movies teaching The Bates Method. It is hard to find.

1940 - 1941+ - Natural Eyesight Improvement Teachers brought to court by the Optical, Medical Industry, Association in an attempt to stop them from teaching The Bates Method. (See Margaret Corbett, Aldous Huxley case in this book.) Optical Industry, AMA, Eye Doctors destroy Dr. Bates Books, Magazines, Articles, remove them from Schools, Colleges, Libraries, Bookstores... Bates teachers, honest doctors and others hide-preserve the books...

1943 - Emily Lierman/Bates re-publishes Dr. Bates book with a new title 'Better Eyesight Without Glasses'. The word *Perfect*, many treatments, all pictures are removed. The Bates Method is often mis-understood. People confuse Natural Eyesight Improvement with Eye Exercises. (The Bates Method uses relaxation of the mind, body, eye muscles and eyes. <u>Exercise, force, effort is not applied.</u>) Emily published this new limited book to avoid law suits, abuse, imprisonment by the medical people (eye surgeons, optical industry, AMA...) that prefer to continue selling harmful-addictive eyeglasses, eye surgery, drugs and hide Natural Eyesight Improvement from the public.
Emily and other Natural Eyesight Improvement Bates Teachers, a few honest eye doctors secretly preserved Dr. Bates Original Book, Medical Articles, 132 Better Eyesight Magazine Issues in the U.S.A. and other countries.

Bates teachers state; near the end of Dr. Bates' life the eye doctors that wanted to hide The Bates Method, to sell only eyeglasses, eye surgery and drugs ganged together, were taking Dr. Bates to court in an attempt to stop him from teaching Natural Eyesight Improvement. They wanted to take away his ophthalmology-medical license. Dr. Bates died before the court date. Was the cause of his death natural-really the flu or was it a conspiracy. Was he murdered by 'certain organizations' who feared that Dr. Bates would win the case? Businesses selling unnatural eye-eyesight treatments, some drug companies and corrupt politicians would have been happy to help, possibly expose Dr. Bates to a 'mysterious virus'.

Teaching, working under these adverse conditions, harassment for years must have been challenging. It was suggested that Dr. Bates had a type of amnesia. Was this just another lie created by the organized eye surgeons? People stated that Dr. Bates received *death threats*. Dr. Bates may have relocated, in full control of his mind searching for a *safe* place to work, practice his natural Method. Dr. Bates disappeared, reappeared, worked in different locations, hospitals. He learned, taught much in his travels and found friends, support among other honest eye doctors.

After Dr. Bates passed away and time went by, people could not find his original unedited magazines, books, articles and other books he and Emily may have or had been in process of creating. See Better Eyesight Magazine - April, 1930; "... Dr. Bates and Mrs. Bates to devote more time to the writing of new books on treatment alone for which there has been a very great demand during the past year". Dr. Bates stated in Better Eyesight Magazine - May, 1927 that they were showing training movies in California; "*Mrs. Lierman is delivering lectures throughout California and is showing moving pictures which illustrate the Bates Method of curing imperfect sight.*" ('Showing' = the movies were already created and were being shown?) No one has published the movies or new books... to this date. Were they destroyed? Are they being hidden by people afraid to come forward? Were people threatened? Are some vision teachers hiding the movies, books due to ego, a power-control type of mindset? Where are Dr. Bates' years of patient medical records? I appeal to your conscience, heart and humanity's education; come forward, preserve this great work. Do it anonymously if privacy, safety is the issue. If I find them I will place on YouTube and publish the books free in PDF e-book and paperback.

Dr. Bates life, work time-line originally researched
by a variety of Bates Teachers, news reporters, writers.

This book is also dedicated to the following persons: (Dedicated in Historical order.)
They worked with Dr. Bates & Emily and/or continued their work and wrote books on Natural Eyesight Improvement. This book (or the E-Book) contains a chapter providing more information on teachers, their books and links to websites.

+Emily C. A. Lierman, Bates- Dr. Bates assistant and wife. Dr. Bates cured her vision. Emily then worked with Dr. Bates in his clinic and continued his work after his death. She wrote a book; 'Stories From The Clinic' containing true articles, stories of the patients, natural treatments she and Dr. Bates applied to cure a variety of eye conditions.

Her stories are also in Dr. Bates monthly Better Eyesight Magazine. The book contains a few additions to the stories. With her kind manner she easily cured children, adults naturally of unclear vision, crossed, wandering eyes, cataracts and other conditions.

+William B. MacCracken M. D. - Medical Doctor - Trained with Dr. Bates and cured his patient's eyesight with the Bates Method. Wrote 2 books.

+Harold M. Peppard - Optometrist - Also trained with Dr. Bates and continued Bates' teachings. Book: Sight Without Glasses.

+ Cecil S. Price - Trained by Dr. Bates - Book : The Improvement of Sight by Natural Methods.

+Clara Hackett - One of the first, best Bates Method Natural Eyesight Improvement Teachers. Books.

+Bernarr A. MacFadden - Physical Fitness, Natural Eyesight Improvement. Studied Bates Method with Dr. Bates. Wrote a course, book with Dr. Bates. Only MacFadden's name was listed on later book versions.

+Margaret Corbett - Famous Bates Teacher. Saved writer Aldous Huxley from blindness. The Optical/Medical Industry brought her to court in an attempt to stop her from teaching the Bates Method. She won all cases. Wrote 4+ books: Help Yourself to Better Sight, How to improve your sight. Simple daily rules in relaxation....

+Aldous Huxley - Famous writer, cured of near blindness by Margaret Corbett, he then wrote; 'The Art of Seeing'. See his photo on the right; from the back of his book. A Natural Eyesight Improvement Book that has helped many people achieve clear vision. My first Bates Teacher, by book at age 17. Cured my distant vision.

+John N. Ott - Studied and wrote books on the health benefits of sunlight. He proved with his experiments the healthy effects sunlight produces for the body, brain, eyes, vision. Dr. Bates proved that lack of sunlight causes unclear vision, cataracts, many eye diseases.

+Jacob Liberman, Optometrist - http://www.jacobliberman.org/ - Bates Method, Natural Vision Improvement Optometrist – Books, Sunlight benefits for health of body, brain, eyes, Vision Training System using Moving Colored Light. Similar to John Ott's work with sunlight.

+Paul E. Dennison and Gail E. Hargrove – http://www.braingym.com - Left and Right Brain Hemisphere Activation and Integration Treatments. Method also improves eyesight and strabismus.

+Thomas R. Quackenbush – http://www.naturalvisioncenter.com - This is one of my 1st Natural Vision Improvement Teachers. He is the first Bates Teacher, the Pioneer (after Dr. Bates) that brought Better Eyesight Magazine to the modern public in the United States. See his books: 'Better Eyesight - The Complete Magazines of William H. Bates' & 'Relearning to See - Improve Your Eyesight Naturally'. The books contain the original and up to date Bates Method.

Modern Teachers before him did not make the magazines known and available to their students. This true source of the Bates Method was hidden. Why?, because it is free in a few libraries in the U.S and Europe and the method is simple, easy, people do not have to pay money to learn, apply and teach it. Mr. Quackenbush's books enable people that are low income, cannot travel, to have access to the best, <u>complete</u> and low cost Natural Vision Improvement Training. I was able to study his books and the original Better Eyesight Magazines and learn which old treatments have been changed, improved and new treatments added to the Bates Method. Taking his course resulted in clearer than 20/20 close and distant vision, improved my ability to relax, my state of mind, self-esteem, emotions, intelligent and creative thinking. I quit a dangerous job at a hotel, quit drinking beer using Rational Recovery, 'The Small Book' by Albert Ellis Ph.D. and Jack Trimpey and found an <u>honest</u> chiropractor that cured my neck/dizziness after taking Mr. Quackenbush's class.

+ All Bates Method Natural Vision Improvement Teachers, Bates Method Behavioral Optometrists, Ophthalmologists.

There are many more teachers in the U.S. and overseas and I apologize that I have not been able to list them all. Spanish, German, Italian, African, Chinese teachers... I have listed the teachers that I have taken in person & home study classes from and/or studied their books. Links to other teachers are in this book. All teachers books not listed here are in chapter 2 of the main Paperback book or PDF.

I have not listed teachers that are greedy, charge an extremely high price for Student and Teacher Training, hide Dr. Bates work, magazines and refuse to give out free vision improvement help to the public.

(Students must avoid Teachers that sell, advise referrals to eye doctors selling unhealthy, dangerous Plus Lens Eyeglass Therapy, any type of Contact Lenses, Laser Cornea Eye Surgery Treatments.)

The subject of seasickness was then discussed. Dr. Bates said this also is caused by strain. People who relax and allow their bodies to sway with the movement of the boat never become sick. A sailor's walk is spoken of as a "rolling gait." If he were to stand stiff, stare at the waves, and strain to resist the movement of the ship he would never become a sailor.

Dr. Bates told the story of one of his patients who would never ride in an elevator if she could avoid it. She detested going into the modern office buildings because the elevators were so swift and the buildings so high that she became ill before she was half way up. She told Dr. Bates she had to steel herself to the ordeal of boarding one, and at the end of the trip felt as though she had just crossed the Atlantic Ocean in a rough voyage.

When Dr. Bates invited her to go with him for a ride in the elevator of his building she opened her eyes in amazement, thinking he lacked sympathetic qualities. He explained to her that steeling herself to take a ride was wrong, in addition to being a dreadful strain. He told her to look at the operator and not at the walls gliding past. This helped her to such an extent that she insisted upon riding up and down several times to see if the cure was permanent. It was, just so long as she did not strain to hold the floors stationary.

A wonderful report was received from the superintendent of nine schools who installed this method in his classes. This proved without a doubt the value of Dr. Bates' method, especially with children. The report will be read at the September meeting of the League. We hope all the members may be able to attend, because the report of the summer work will be worth-while and helpful.

The September meeting will be held on the second Tuesday, as usual, which falls on the ninth.

Chief Four Eyes
By Emily A. Meder

A LADY called at the office and introduced herself. She was one of our regular correspondents and I remembered her name because she had such a great deal of trouble with her thirteen-year-old son, Dick. She explained in her last letter that he is a normal, active boy who finds more enjoyment in playing baseball and leapfrog than doing his home work. As Dick wouldn't wear glasses she decided to see what Dr. Bates' method accomplished.

There is a vacant lot near her home, used by a band of "wild Indians," with her son as "Chief." The band, however, objected to a leader with glasses, and Dick became quite ingenious in inventing ways to wear them and still not wear them. She said she watched him continually. He walked innocently past her with the glasses gracefully perched on his nose, but in some mysterious way they disappeared before he reached the sidewalk. This became a nervous game of hide-and-seek between them. He said he would not be called "sissy," and she was equally sure that he would have to wear glasses in order to be cured.

About this time news of Dr. Bates' work reached the mother's ears and she wrote to us for information. She bought the book and told Dick that if he did as she instructed he could leave his glasses off for two weeks. At the end of that time she found that he could not only go without his glasses but his sight had improved.

Dick enjoyed the palming, much to her surprise, and he did not have to be told to do it when his eyes felt strained. He is proud of his test card and his "Indians" try to outdo each other in reading it at the farthest distance. It has become a modern Indian rite.

"The best of it," Mrs. Jamison said, "is that I can look at my boy now without the suspicion usually attached to a murderer, and he lost the hatred nickname of 'Chief Four Eyes'."

Better Eyesight

The Mind's Eye

By Edith McNamara

Do you enjoy your mind's moving pictures or your mental pictures? I do. I get four times the value of a trip to the country or any place else by remembering the mental pictures of it perfectly.

I was not conscious at the time that while my physical eye was seeing everything around me my mind's eye was making a mental picture of it to be brought back later with the help of a perfect memory. After a few experiments with perfect mental pictures I came to the conclusion that I could only imagine what I remembered. It was impossible to imagine an object unless I could remember it perfectly. If I could not remember it perfectly it became only a jumbled up, hazy recollection of something.

I think its lots of fun playing tag with the memory or mental pictures. I like to dig out of my memory all the perfect mental pictures I can—one by one—for Central Fixation plays a big part in mental pictures, remembering one thing best at a time.

Having once been to Canada my favorite way of getting relaxed is to go there by mental pictures. I go along a beautiful country road, remember a lake that had impressed me, visualize it with my mind's eye and so on. Sometimes I skip a couple of towns and arrive in Canada very quickly and other times I get enough relaxation by just staying in one town for a while.

Why don't you try this? Perhaps someone will tell you a story that will remind you of an incident which happened years ago. Follow it up with the help of your memory and see how perfect a mental picture you can obtain. I am sure that you will find pleasure and relaxation in so doing. If you have to make an effort to form this mental picture let it alone for a while and then go back to it again and start where you left off. This will benefit you in your palming.

In the Office

By Emily A. Meder

THE Central Fixation office is a busy one. The regular routine is continually being interrupted by telephone calls, and personal visits from people who demand first-hand information.

One of our recent visitors was a writer who wore very heavy glasses. What I first noticed was that, while I was speaking, she would stare out of the window, as though in a trance, and slowly nod her head from time to time. This was to give me the impression that she was deeply interested in what I was saying, and carefully weighing each statement.

Staring, I told her is bad (I had noticed her doing this so dropped a little hint). She broke forth in smiles and made the astonishing remark that she thought it was bad also, and that she never stared. I politely told her she did, and how.

Our little black circular has been distributed quite widely throughout the United States. The first issue contained testimonials from book readers who were benefited and desired to help others. Owing to the fact that our work is so revolutionary, a great many people think we are boasting when we happen to print a few of these. Here's what one man answered:

"I am glad to advise you that for twenty-one years I have been stone blind in my right eye and the left has been removed and a glass eye placed in the socket. After reading four pages of Perfect Sight Without Glasses the vision in my right eye has become normal, and I can count my fingers at four feet with my glass eye."

Our business of explaining Perfect Sight Without Glasses is a serious one, but as shown above, it has its amusing side.

Perfect sight is natural and a normal condition, and those who have bad vision sometimes instinctively do those things which help them and improve their sight.

The meetings are proving so helpful and officers so enthusiastic that we extend a warm invitation to all those who are interested in this work.

Helpful Hints from Correspondents

These are extracts from letters received from book readers and others. They might suggest new ways of improving your vision.

"I AM proud of my ability to eliminate headaches, fatigue and even nausea resulting from eyestrain. I formerly retired to my room when one of my severe headaches came on, and required the entire household to be absolutely quiet. Now, if my head or eyes pain, I go to my room, palm for a few minutes, swing the card, and feel rested. The headaches usually disappear when I am relaxed. Another discovery! The headaches only come when I do something wrong. The last one was caused by late shopping, rushing to put the house in order, and cooking the whole dinner myself. When I slowly did the long swing (with the broom in one hand and a duster in the other), I grew calm enough to greet my guests pleasantly."

"I was shocked to discover that I was a starer. I knew that Dr. Bates advocated blinking to prevent the stare, and thought that I blinked and shifted constantly. Upon watching myself, however, I found that I only blinked when I remembered to do it consciously. I have made it a rule now to blink my eyes at the end of each line. This compulsory rule is becoming easier, and I believe that it will become a good habit real soon."

Margaret Corbett - Los Angeles, California - Defending *The Bates Method*

Margaret Corbett, famous Bates teacher. Trained directly by Dr. William H. Bates and Emily A. Bates. In the 1940's, eye doctors, opticians in Los Angeles, California tried to stop her from curing people's eyesight naturally. Other teachers were attacked. Later, laws were passed in New York City to block knowledge, teaching of The Bates Method. Eventually the laws were lifted as Bates teachers proved Dr. Bates' Method is safe, effective, natural. It is not medical treatment-practice of optometry. Picture, event date; 1941. Press photo. Stamp on back - NEA;ACME. Margaret is one of the first teachers to call central-fixation centralization and centralizing. A way to prevent staring by inducing the thought of movement 'eye-vision shifting' combined with central-fixation. See pg. 64 in her book *Quick Guide To Better Vision*.

Dedication to persons that directly and indirectly helped me to write this book

Robert Monroe - www.monroeinstitute.org
Author of Journeys out of the Body, Far Journey's, and Ultimate Journey.

THE MONROE INSTITUTE
365 ROBERTS MOUNTAIN ROAD
FABER, VA 22938
866-881-3440 See his YouTube videos; http://www.youtube.com/watch?v=VoZWOLWnQkw

Read more about Robert Monroe in the Authors Natural Eyesight Improvement Experience below.

Dedication to My Mom

Mom at Christmas

To Mrs. Nancy Oliver, Wilder. For raising me alone without a father, working for minimum wage in a hot laundry mat for years while we lived in a small apartment. We often did not have enough food. I would sneak outside and dig for empty soda bottles to cash in for money to buy crackers. I remember the day a man at the recycling store yelled at me, stating I cannot bring him bottles from the trash! Men would be cruel to Mom, try to corrupt her, but she would not break from her Catholic faith and favorite Saint, St. Anne. Mom saved her money and bought a Art Instruction Schools Course for me when I was 7 years old.
(The school that is advertised on matchbook covers and in TV Guide.) I remember thinking how boring it was to draw the stick figures of people, thinking its not helping my ability to draw and I wanted to go back to just copying cartoon pictures of Moose Miller, Fred Flintstone, Bugs Bunny, Donald Duck, Popeye, Dr. Strange... from the comics. I now realized at age 53 that the course helped me to draw the pictures in Better Eyesight Magazine and other books.
My Aunt Betty is a very good artist, used to draw lifelike pictures of baseball players, boxers, my grandfather when he was a Middle Weight Champion Boxer, Police Sergeant in New England, Massachusetts. She also drew cartoons and now paints. She helped to teach me how to draw. I cannot draw as well as most artists, but the basic skills helped to create this book.

The Author's Experience with Natural Eyesight Improvement

In 4th grade Elementary School I had to wear eyeglasses to see the blackboard from the back of the classroom. Mom bought the eyeglasses for me though she could not afford to spend the money. Stress can cause unclear vision. I was in constant fear at school due to a large boy that would bully me every day, wait to scare me, threaten to beat me up after school at the end of a long dirt road. I can still see him standing there, picking out kids to bully, knowing I was next along the line.
I do not remember him actually hitting me, mainly just coming up to me and acting like he was going to in order to scare me. Frazzled my nerves daily. During childhood and adult life I was hit in the head, face a few times by other children and adult men. (Snow, ice balls, and violent people.) I know this contributed to unclear vision, and a very slight wandering eyes condition. Neck vertebrae, collarbone or skull, eye socket, joints, bones misalignment?
My teacher also wore glasses. Children pick up eyestrain, incorrect use of the eyes, tension and lowered vision from being around people that wear glasses and stressful experiences in school... I hated the glasses and threw them out in a couple weeks. I sat closer to the blackboard and this prevented strain, effort to see and the vision returned to clear. I could then see clear from the back of the class when necessary. Mom made friends with the bully's family, then he decided to be my friend. We played 'The Long Ranger' make believe game together.
Mom could not afford to pay for the glasses but was kind and let me go without wearing glasses. My vision remained about 20/20-20/40 for years and it never bothered me. (Wish I knew The Bates Method back then, would have had 20/20 and clearer vision.)
In 10th grade high school Mom had to buy glasses for me again to read the distant blackboard in school. Learning Algebra and French, did not like these subjects. I threw the glasses out after 2 days. At this time I found Aldous Huxley's book: 'The Art of Seeing' in a old bookstore in Brookfield, MA and practiced Switching

and <u>Shifting</u> on objects at close and far distances with: both eyes together, one eye at a time, both eyes together again. My left eye needed more vision improvement than the right so I practiced extra time with the left eye. Shifting was combined with the Switching. I understood and practiced a little <u>Central-Fixation</u>. The first time, few seconds that I shifted on an object, distant tree, my vision improved. Within only 5 minutes my vision improved to 20/20 and in 2 days was perfect, clear. Vision was so clear in both eyes that I could not remember which eye used to have less clear vision. My mind felt more balanced, relaxed. It is often easy for children, young people to improve their vision.

Practicing the Bates Method, having the power to improve my vision <u>on my own</u> resulted in an improvement in my mental, emotional state. It was easy to learn, remember at school, my grades improved, I gained confidence. The Bates Method activates, integrates, improves functions of the left and right brain hemispheres, all brain functions. I left a gang of kids that were a destructive influence and learned to have compassion for others and respect myself. I realized the mind has more functions, abilities, 'power' than we are taught in school, including college. Went into study of Psycho-Cybernetics, other science and spiritual subjects. (Human potential seems to be suppressed by our leaders. Politicians and some religions are trying to remove history and other books from libraries, bookstores, schools, the Internet.)

My vision remained about 20/20-20/30 for years and it never bothered me. Mainly 20/20, sometimes clearer.

In the U.S. Army I was forced to wear glasses: distant eyesight 20/40 at times. (It's normal for vision to fluctuate. Glasses prevent natural fluctuation back to clear vision.) I refused to wear the glasses. One day while in a foxhole shooting my rifle at the distant target, the Sergeant made me wear the glasses. I could not hit the target after many shots while wearing the glasses. I got mad and took off the glasses and threw them in the dirt. Then aimed the rifle and hit the target easily for the remaining shots. Sargent then allowed me to permanently discontinue use of the glasses.

Did not need glasses for the rest of my life until age 40, Year 1997 – unclear close vision –
In the year 1995 the author of this book was listening to Robert Monroe's relaxation tapes. I worked a very high stress job in a old hotel dealing with violent, abusive people, life and death situations. I suffered with dizziness from an assault, neck injury. Drank too much beer at times to block out the stress. The tapes produced a great amount of relaxation and also teach a variety of tools to improve function of the brain, body. At the time I was reading Aldous Huxley's book 'The Art of Seeing' to try and improve my close vision & remove eye floaters at age 40. Practiced Bates Method activities: shifting, central-fixation, switching... at close distances. Also read fine print in the sunlight with relaxation, shifting, central-fixation, memory, imagination. It worked!

One night after falling asleep listening to Monroe's tape 'Focus 10', I heard a man's voice in a dream say; "Write a book on Natural Eyesight Improvement". The dream seemed very real and it woke me up. I remembered the man's voice and thought later that it would be a good idea to write a book on my experience with distant and close vision improvement for 30 years. I began writing the book: 'Do It Yourself – Natural Eyesight Improvement' and searching for more Bates Method Natural Vision Improvement books to study. This led me to teachings of Janet Goodrich, Martin Sussman-Cambridge Institute-The Program for Better Vision course *(I use only some of his methods)*, Carrie Anderson training at the Learning Annex, then in person training course and books by Thomas Quackenbush in San Francisco, CA, and further study of Dr. Bates Better Eyesight Magazines and other books. Distant and close vision improved to 20/20 and clearer.

Robert Monroe's tapes teach spiritual development, sprit travel and improvement of brain, body functions and produce natural states taught by Natural Vision Improvement Teachers: Deep, perfect relaxation in the beta, alpha, theta, delta brain wave states, dynamic relaxation, left and right brain hemisphere activation/integration, visualization of clear mental pictures, color treatment, creativity, imagination, memory, release of negative thoughts, emotions, energy strengthening, circulation, control. The activities on the tapes improve all functions of the brain.
All of these conditions improve the clarity of vision. Listening to his tapes improved my ability to write and create pictures for this book. Many famous scientists, artists speak of entering into a deep relaxed state, contacting the subconscious mind to obtain greater power of the brain, improve skills, solve scientific theories, formulas... Monroe's tapes activate this state. (See books by Dion Fortune for further study.)

In Oct., 2009 I experienced a neck injury from a dishonest, *very bad* chiropractor in Worcester, MA. It affected my vision: double vision, eyes' divergence, converge, balance, hearing impaired, astigmatism... All from misaligned neck vertebrae and neck, back injury. Neck is healing with new doctor's treatment for 15 months and use of Natural Eyesight Improvement, Bates Method has returned the vision to clear. Occasional slight fluctuations in vision to 20/30 and eye movement problem returns a little when the neck injury flares up, sinus congestion in air polluted city. Neck muscle relaxation, Physical Therapy, Home 'do it yourself' non-invasive chiropractic, less computer work, clean air in Boston, MA by the sea, and the Bates Method always returns the vision to 20/20 and clearer. In Mar., 2016, age 59; still some neck, back injury effects, but vision remains clear. I know from experience that the Bates Method works, even during difficult conditions!

Dedication To:

To Don Dixon - Best friend, Retired Air Force Pilot. Neighbor, landlord for 9 years in San Francisco Bay Area. Thanks for the Pilot Wings and taking me over the Golden Gate Bridge to the Marin Flea Market where I bought an Antique French Military Rifle.

Greg Dean and his Mom, Dad - Art and Jackie.
Truly rare, strong, great people, best friends. RIP Greg. See you up there eventually. Stay out of trouble; 'or not' - Ha-Ha!

To Richard Hess, 'Best friend' Cherokee, German at the Metro.

To all the Senior Citizens and Young People in California.
I learnt many things from the diversified personalities in Los Angeles, San Diego, San Mateo, South San Francisco, San Francisco! Farmers Market Bar on Main Street, Broadway, Watts in Downtown Los Angeles and all the wild, fun American Indians, Vets, Old Italian Men, ladies in Daly Cit, CA,The Homeless. Learning from a variety of people makes a person grow on all levels, strengthens the personality, mind, sprit.

Thank you to Barbara Gibbons at the Metropolitan Hotel in South San Francisco for a great place to live, work and write!

Picture = Christmas Tree on San Bruno Mountain- South San Francisco, CA - View from room #40, Metropolitan Hotel.
I used to watch my TV reflected in this window at night and 'switch' to the distant mountain and watch 'shift' on the Christmas Tree, cars moving along the hill, lights in the houses, stars, planes in the sky, people in the buildings, street lights, people walking on Grand Avenue, good looking Italian Man working at the Liquor store.

At this time even though the job was stressful, I was very happy, lots of friends, jokes, active. A positive mental, emotional state has a major beneficial effect on the clarity of vision. Relaxed, positive mind=clear vision. Physically active job, good posture. My vision was improved to better than 20/20 close and far while living here. Thomas Quackenbush, Natural Vision Improvement Teacher's School was over the mountain in San Francisco near the beach and Golden Gate Park.

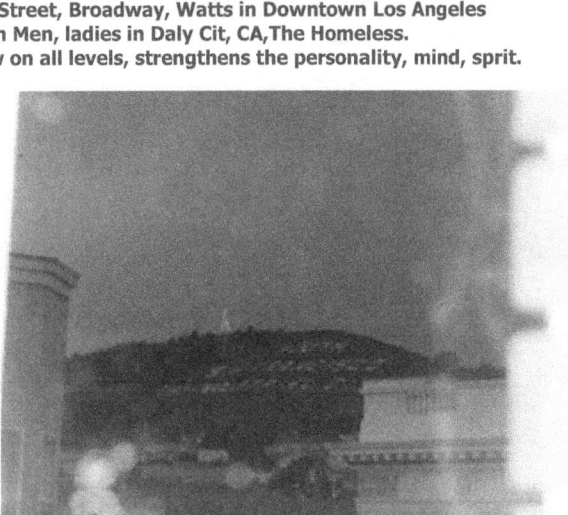

Moving objects on the TV screen reflected in the window also keeps the eyes moving, shifting easy, relaxed, vision clear.

How to Use The E-Book

This is a Natural Eyesight Improvement Paperback and Adobe Reader/Kindle PDF E-Book consisting of 1700+ pages. Chapter, Sub-Chapter, Title Navigation Bookmarks, Page Thumbnails, Multiple Pages view are on the left side of the E-book and a linked Chapter Index for moving quickly to any page, section of the book. A + sign is to the left of the main bookmarks; click it to reveal more bookmarks, books, pages, chapters.

Word Search for all 20 E-books; Type in a word, Example; Cataracts, Nearsight, Myopia, Farsight.., and all areas of the book that provide information on cause/cure of these eye conditions will be listed. Example; If Nearsight or Myopia is typed; 50+ different treatments to cure unclear distant vision will be listed with chapter, article title, page number. Click a link to go directly to a page, treatment.

Adobe Reader & Kindle read aloud for persons with low vision, blindness. Language conversion, translates to Italian, Spanish, German... Click the View Tab in Adobe. Kindle and Adobe print can be enlarged for the visually impaired.
Special Note for Kindle, PDF Computer, Mobile Book Readers; Voice, Read Aloud Option is Best for the Blind, Visually Impaired and for all people, to avoid reading on electronic screens all the time. Like carrying a small lightweight radio that speaks, reads to you. I read on PDF and Kindle occasionally. I prefer to sit back, relax

at the beach or under a tree and use the Audio Function. Print the Kindle, PDF E-Books on paper. Reading on r
paper, in the sunlight is most healthy for the eyes; true dimension, distance, shadow, contrast, texture and de

http://www.adobe.com/products/reader/languages/ See the E-Book videos for directions on how to use the E-books & free Natural Eyesight Improvement Training videos at; www.cleareyesight.info & YouTube; http://www.youtube.com/watch?v=WO9AS4A8f_c http://www.youtube.com/watch?v=5E5lBZ0BQuY

E-Books are the new 'Do It Yourself ' way to buy books at a decent price. No expensive publishers, printers, bar-codes, shipping, no censorship by governments, corporations, businesses… The reader can view the book on computer, laptop, Kindle other small electronic devices without Internet connection and the E-Book moves faster than highest speed Internet. Carry the book on a disk or in your pocket on a tiny computer chip disk, view it on any local library, hotel… computer.

This book is unlocked, no security. The reader can copy, paste, print and change the size of the print. **Print your own book** with home computer/printer or copy the book to a CD and bring it to a printer for printing, book binding. Print in color or black ink. Any size paper. Choose spiral binding so the book opens fully when set on a book holder - prevents the need to hold the book open with the hands for relaxed arms, shoulders, neck when reading.

Adobe can print in large, medium, small, fine & microscopic print. Fine print is healthy for the eyes, cures unclear close and distant vision when read correct with relaxation, shifting, central-fixation. Set Adobe Reader to print 2 or more pages per page for small print. 4 to 6… pages per page for a fine and microscopic print for perfect central-fixation, saccadic shifting, fine detailed vision at close and far distances. The Zoom Function also changes print size.

Create mini fine and microscopic print booklets to read in the sunlight daily. Practice the treatments described to prevent unclear vision, cataracts and other eye conditions.

In the Adobe Reader Print Setup: Select % of normal size, a number less than 100% or use page scaling. This will fit all text, pictures onto the paper, reduce the size to create a margin on the edge of the page for binding a printed book. Or print normal size 100% on larger paper.

Select 'Print Document and Comments/Markups' in the Adobe print box to print all page numbers on the upper right corner and text boxes in the book. Print pictures large for kids to color or to hang on a wall for Natural Vision Improvement Training. Adobe Acrobat 30 day Free Trail can be downloaded free from http://www.adobe.com to arrange the book pages as preferred.

For Better Eyesight Magazine

This book contains all publications of Dr. Bates Monthly 'Better Eyesight Magazine' – Unedited, everything included, July 1919 - June 1930, all of his original treatments and modern versions of older treatments.

+ Text in light blue are comments added by author Clark Night, Bates Method Natural Eyesight Improvement, Graduated Student, to clarify Modern Natural Eyesight Improvement versions of a few older methods described and to correct a few spelling errors in the original magazines.
+ Print in bold, black specifies Bates Method Natural Eyesight Improvement treatments for a variety of eye conditions, military articles, and other items of importance.
+ Print in bold, dark navy blue are specific Bates treatments, activities, steps for vision improvement.
+ This book contains 500 pictures placed on the right margin of the magazine pages to help the reader quickly understand every Bates Method treatment described.
+ The First Article and usually the 2nd article of each monthly Better Eyesight Magazine and other articles not labeled by author are written by Ophthalmologist Bates.
+ The First Article on page 2 (inside cover in the original magazines) consists of some of the best treatments, activities taught by Dr. Bates, specific directions for a Bates Method Natural Eyesight Improvement treatment.
Example; **July 1919 magazine PAGE TWO - Do You Read Imperfectly?**

Do you read imperfectly? Can you observe then that when you look at the first word, or the first letter, of a sentence you do not see best where you are looking; that you see other words, or other letters, just as well as or better than the ones you are looking at? Do you observe also that the harder you try to see the worse you see?

Now close your eyes and rest them, remembering some color, like black or white, that you can remember perfectly. Keep them closed until they feel rested, or until the feeling of strain has been completely relieved. Now open them and look at the first word or letter of a sentence for a fraction of a second. If you have been able to relax, partially or completely, you will have a flash of improved or clear vision, and the area seen best will be smaller.

After opening the eyes for this fraction of a second, close them again quickly, still remembering the color, and keep them closed until they again feel rested. Then again open them for a fraction of a second. Continue this alternate resting of the eyes and flashing of the letters for a time, and you may soon find that you can keep your eyes open longer than a fraction of a second without losing the improved vision.

If your trouble is with distant instead of near vision, use the same method with distant letters.

In this way you can demonstrate for yourself the fundamental principles of the cure of imperfect sight by treatment without glasses.

If you fail, ask someone with perfect sight to help you.

Dr. Bates Instructions on PAGE TWO

+The original photo copies of Better Eyesight Magazine are included with this book so the reader can verify the modern version, treatments in this book with the original printed magazines from the 1900's.
See original sample page on the right >, previous pg.

Dr. Bates 'Better Eyesight Magazines' contain hundreds of different natural treatments that he and his assistant Emily Lierman/Bates and other eye doctors applied to cure: unclear distant and close vision, (nearsight, farsight) astigmatism, cataracts, glaucoma, cornea scars, wandering/crossed eyes, amblyopia and other eye problems. A few Eye Doctors, Ophthalmology College Libraries have preserved these magazines. See Monroe J. Hirsch O.D. Ph. D.

Pictures in This book

A main Bates Method activity to relax the mind, body, eyes and bring clear vision is to improve the memory, imagination of mental pictures. This is a normal function of the eyes, brain, visual system to produce clear vision. A baby (and adults) see a unfamiliar, new object clear by first 'shifting on it' (looking at different parts, moving the visual attention part to part on the object, examining small details). The object becomes clear, familiar, memorized, a clear memory picture of the object is stored in the brain. The next time the baby looks at the object it is familiar, remembered clear and the brain quickly activates the correct eye movements on the object, no effort to see it, relaxation occurs and it is seen clear.
This process is done for every new object encountered. The brain stores thousands of pictures of objects. Example:

A baby sees an apple for the first time and it may be imperfectly clear due to it being a unfamiliar, new object. At first, the baby's eyes move, 'shift' slowly on the apple part to part as the baby's eyes, brain investigate the new object, become familiar with it. The baby's eyes, visual attention move from part to part on the apple, the brain registering, storing a image of each part the eyes look at. A image of the apple forms in the brain, memory each time the baby sees the apple again. Each time the apple is seen, a clearer and clearer, more familiar mental, visual picture of the apple is created and stored in the brain, memory and it is easier to see; the brain activates eye movement, shifting on the round, red object easy, relaxed and the eyes movement is improved, quicker. Smaller saccadic eye movements occur. A perfectly clear image of the apple is stored in the brain, memory and it is now a familiar object. When the baby looks at it, the brain moves the eye muscles, eyes correct, quick and easy, part to part on the apple and it remains clear.

When the brain remembers, imagines, creates, stores clear pictures in the mind, in color, motion like a real life movie: the mind, body, eyes relax, eyes move easy and vision is clear. (Even a stationary object appears to move, with 'oppositional movement' (The Swing) as the eyes shift part to part on it.)

Blind people use mental pictures, touch... and other senses. One treatment to help cure blindness, near blindness is to improve the memory, mental pictures of objects. Improve the memory, imagination, clear mental pictures to obtain clear vision. Read Helen Keller's story in Better Eyesight Magazine Illustrated with 500 Pictures.

The pictures, true life stories and fairy tales in Better Eyesight Magazine cause the person to create clear mental pictures, like an active motion 'movie' picture occurring in the mind. The stories are entertaining, interesting and fun to read.
This relaxes the mind, eyes, brings the mind to a positive state. All these keep the vision clear.

When the mind is positive, relaxed, vision clear: the memory and imagination improve and the improved memory, imagination further improve relaxation and the vision. Then the clearer vision further improves the memory, imagination, relaxation. More vision improvement occurs. Ability to remember, imagine and <u>see</u> a object clear is greatly improved. It's easy, relaxing to remember, imagine a clear object. Practice imagining, remembering objects clear. All functions of the visual system are connected. Improve one and all improve.

700+ pictures are placed in the main E-book and in Better Eyesight Magazine to help the reader easily see/imagine in the mind, learn and apply each treatment, activity Dr. Bates describes. Less reading, fast eyesight improvement.
Each picture teaches a Natural Eyesight Improvement treatment. Read the print below the picture for a quick lesson.

Remembering, imagining, creating clear mental/visual pictures is a main Natural Eyesight Improvement treatment, normal function of the visual system. The brain works with the eyes to produce clear vision.

Babies, children and adults learn to see clear by first shifting on a new object: moving the visual attention, central field from part to part on the object, becoming <u>familiar</u> with it, the brain visualizing, creating, storing a clear mental and visual picture of the object in the memory. In this way, the object is seen clear by the function of the brain activating, retrieving the clear memory picture of the object each time the eyes look at the object. The brain works with the eyes, eye muscles to move the eyes, (visual attention) on the object correct and see it clear. The object becomes familiar, easy to see and the brain, eyes relax, function perfect,

the object is seen clear.
Familiar objects are easy to see, relax the mind, eyes, produce clear vision.
The imagination also works with the memory to produce clear objects, vision.

The pattern of eye movement can change, move freely, vary each time the eyes look at the object but the brain will also produce certain eye movements for that specific object; the brain knows how to move the eyes, visual attention on that objects specific shape; Example: The brain moves the eyes, visual attention on a round object in a different pattern than when moving on a square object; The eyes, visual attention (center of the visual field) move in a certain basic pattern on the round shape, areas of a apple: the center, areas within the circular shape, along curved edges, top, bottom, sides…
If the eyes, visual attention try to move on the apple as if it has a square shape, squared edges and other shapes… (as in the middle picture, painting hanging on the wall), then the eyes will be moving, looking out into space sometimes, away from the apple (see 3rd picture). This will be diffusion, eccentric fixation, no central-fixation because the eyes are not on the object when looking away from it. Moving the visual attention, center of the visual field along, around the edge of an apple is different than moving along the edge, corner of a square. (See example; looking at the #7 on the bus in the Memory, Imagination chapter.)
A memorized, familiar object activates easy, mentally stored eye movements, shifting part to part, perfectly, automatically on the object. Perfect central-fixation, the object is seen clear. New, different eye movements are also added for each individual object and each time the object is viewed again because the eyes move freely and the eye movements on the object, scenery is also affected by thoughts in the mind, what the brain is thinking about the object or other subjects, the distance, angle the object is at, lighting, contrast, size…

Familiar objects are easy to see, relax the mind, eyes and produce clear vision. This is why Dr. Bates advises keeping a familiar, memorized Eyechart in the classroom to practice on, keep the children's vision clear.

Books that contain entertaining, interesting pictures improve the brain, visual systems memory, imagination of clear pictures of objects. This improves eye function with the brain and clarity of vision. Children enjoy books with pictures. The small pictures in the book can be printed larger for children to assemble into a coloring book. The child will learn the Bates Method as the parent describes what each picture is.
Coloring - eyes moving with the crayon, filling in small details, using a variety of colors activates eye movement 'shifting', central-fixation, relaxation, positive mind, left and right brain hemisphere activation, integration. These are Bates Method natural eye functions that produce clear vision and straight eyes.
Reading Comic books improve the clarity of vision due to the many colorful action pictures, interesting, fun to read stories engaging the memory and imagination. Eye movement, shifting is activated, improved as the eyes, mind look at a picture and move from picture to picture and on the bubbles of printed words.

The small pictures in this book prove that Natural Eyesight Improvement works! Most pictures in this book are drawn by the author. As stated earlier, the author of this book attained clear close vision at age 40 by using Aldous Huxley's book and taking a Bates Method Natural Vision Improvement course from Thomas Quackenbush in San Francisco, CA. At age 59 my close and distant vision is still clear. 500+ pictures were drawn by hand, in small size 1½ inches height/width using my memory, imagination as I read each article in Better Eyesight Magazines. Pictures were drawn on paper, then traced over on a window pane two times, sunlight shining through the window, looking at the pictures 1 inch to 6-20 inches and up to 5 ft. from the eyes seeing the fine details of pictures clear on paper.
Pictures were then scanned into a computer, refined again in Microsoft Digital Image and Photoshop. All this was done without eyeglasses or magnifiers. The Bates Method works!!

Clark Nights E-books are allowed to be distributed free by 4 Bates Teachers and all book customers. Be aware that a few photograph and other pictures in the book were taken from the Internet, Microsoft Free Clipart, historical sources that gave permission to use the pictures, Dr. Bates books, Articles and other old copyright free books. They stated the pictures are 'royalty free' but I did not get this in writing, only by phone and E-mail. I take full responsibility for all pictures in my books. 95% in the 2 main books are drawn, copyright by Clark Night.

The Natural Eyesight Improvement student must get an eye exam, to check the health of the eyes, preferably from an eye doctor experienced with the Bates Method of Natural Eyesight Improvement. A eye exam from a natural based eye doctor that performs exams without constant use of eye drops, without drugs, machines, time limits for reading charts is most healthy for the eyes and will result in the best, accurate prescription, not over prescribed/too strong in eyeglass strength.
Looking into a machine, mechanical or electronic device to test the clarity of vision blocks many natural eye functions, can cause temporary: increased visual blur, stiff neck, block relaxed, normal eye movements and result in a unnecessary eyeglass prescription and too strong prescription. This will maintain, increase vision impairment and interfere with application of Natural Eyesight Improvement, prevent the eyes from returning to normal function, clear vision. I do not trust the new 'Eye Scan Machines. Artificial light… into the eyes, directly on the retina.
An old fashioned paper eyechart hung on a wall with sunlight on the chart, no glare, used when the eyes, mind are relaxed, no pressure to hurry is the best way to test for the true level of visual clarity, along with the old time

retinoscope and other harmless instruments to look into, inspect the eye. Natural Bates Method Eye Doctors will do this. They give the patient time to read the chart.

Eye drops are used to widen the eyes pupil so the doctor can look into the eyes and completely check the eyes health. This may be necessary to insure a though eye exam but constant use of eyedrops on every exam can impair the eyes health. The eyedrops cause; a paralyzed eye muscle, widened pupil, blurred vision, light sensitivity... I personally will not allow eyedrops when taking an eye exam. The drug companies are placing harmful and unnecessary chemicals, toxins in the eyedrops, various drugs for the eyes, tear production drugs and drugs for other medical conditions. This causes eye, vision, health impairment. Toxins, chemicals are placed in vaccines, flu shots, even our food, water supply. Contact lens solutions have been contaminated with bacteria resulting in eye infections, blindness. Chemicals in Sinus, Nasal sprays cause Glaucoma, Cataracts, vision impairment. Modern Natural Eye Doctor's are seeking a safe alternative to eyedrops, drugs.

Disclaimer

The Author of this book; (Do It Yourself – Natural Eyesight Improvement – Original and Modern Bates Method & Better Eyesight Magazine Illustrated with 500 Pictures, EFT and all books by the Author) must place a disclaimer in this book to protect herself from lawsuits, imprisonment, destruction of this book by the Medical Association, Drug/Optical Industries, corrupt politicians, fraudulent vision improvement teachers that attempt to prevent the public from acquiring free, authentic Natural Eyesight Improvement information, training;

The author, publisher, (Clark Night-Pen Name) Mary I. Oliver www.cleareyesight.info mclearsight@aol.com
Clearsight Publishing Co. - Do it yourself - Natural Eyesight Improvement is not responsible for the readers use, misuse, misunderstanding of the information in this book and website. The author does not claim/promise to diagnose, treat, cure eye problems, disease, medical conditions. The reader agrees that he/she does not have a personal or professional relationship with the author. The author is not an eye doctor or medical doctor.
This book and other books, videos, website by the author consist solely of Educational Information for improving the clarity of vision and health/function of the eyes along with the student's communication with an Optometrist, Ophthalmologist. Always obtain an eye exam by an Ophthalmologist and medical exam by a Medical Doctor.

Choose a Bates Method Behavioral Ophthalmologist, Optometrist and Medical Doctor that prefers natural health treatment, prefers to teach Natural Eyesight Improvement, discontinue use of eyeglasses, keep the eyes healthy and prevent use of eye surgery, drugs. Avoid eye doctors selling laser and other eye cornea surgeries, drugs that are not needed, unnecessary lens removal/surgery, eyeglasses (especially strong over-corrected eyeglass lenses), unnecessary, addictive astigmatism sections in the glasses, contact lenses, bifocals, mono-vision lenses, plus lens treatment, tinted, colored lenses, sunglasses and all types of eyeglasses.
(Legal 20/40 reduced, weaker eyeglass lenses can be used temporarily, only if needed for driving, work... safety as the vision is improving. See a Behavioral Optometrist and on-line mail order low cost optical stores.)

An experienced eye doctor can detect health of the eyes and body by examining, looking at and into the eyes. Blood pressure, sugar levels, injury, stroke and many health conditions are reflected in the eyes, often in an early reversible stage.

An eye doctor experienced in iridology can determine health of organs, systems in the body.
See the story of Ignatz Von Peczely, Physician, a man that cured a injured owl and noticed that the owls eyes, iris was altered when the bird was sick, injured and it returned to normal as the birds health healed.

Children - Read/use this books contents only with direction of, supervised by parents and a Bates Method Eye Doctor. Children and adults: do not us the Sunglass and other methods that are for application only by an experienced Bates Method Ophthalmologist. If in doubt about how to apply a method; ask a Bates Teacher and Bates Method Eye doctor. See 'Better Eyesight Magazine Illustrated with 500 pictures'.

Natural Eyesight Improvement normalizes, corrects the eyes pressure. If a person is taking drugs, eye drops... for Glaucoma, eye pressure or other eye conditions; to lower or raise the pressure; ask your eye doctor's advice first before applying Natural Eyesight Improvement. The drugs strength, amount to take, may need to be changed or the drug may need to be discontinued. The doctor must monitor the eyes pressure as the person practices Natural Eyesight Improvement. Natural Eyesight Improvement also changes the eyes, corneas shape; back to normal, healthy shape. If the eye, cornea, retina has been operated upon, surgery; speak to your eye doctor first before applying Natural Eyesight Improvement to be sure it does not interfere with the surgery. Detached retina surgery... Read the laser cornea surgery articles in this book. I have communicated with Natural Eyesight Improvement Students that had; cataracts, glaucoma, holes, fluid leaking in the eyes retina, retinitis pigmentosa, other conditions and they have only benefited, regained good eye health and clear vision from practicing Natural Eyesight Improvement, The Bates Method and working with a Bates Method Ophthalmologist.

The Following Words Describe Eye Conditions Listed in This Book

+**Emmetropia**=Normal Round Eye=clear distant vision.

Dr. Bates states that the eye lengthens slightly (due to action of the outer oblique eye muscles) to produce accommodation for clear close vision. Other eye doctors state that the lens, or lens and eye, change shape (lens; due to action of the ciliary, inner eye muscle) to produce accommodation, others theorize the lens may move, as in a camera. The iris, pupil size, iris muscle also affects the function of the eye, light rays.., clarity of vision.

+**Myopia**=Nearsighted=abnormally lengthened eyeball=unclear distant vision.

+**Hypermetropia**=Hyperopia=Farsighted=abnormally shortened eyeball=unclear close vision.

+**Presbyopia**=abnormally shortened or greatly lengthened eyeball due to outer eye muscle tension, and/or the lens is inflexible, ciliary muscle stiff=unclear close 'Reading' Vision. <u>Extreme neck muscle tension, arthritis</u> lowering blood, oxygen, nutrient flow to the head, eyes, retina, lens and causing neck muscle tension to travel into the outer and inner eye muscles can cause unclear close, distant vision, cataracts and other eye problems.
   The Bates Method, nutrition, sunlight, posture, movement.., corrects this condition.
   Reading fine print cures presbyopia. See the Close Vision chapter and Better Eyesight Magazine.

+**Astigmatism**=irregular, abnormal cornea, lens, eye shape, due to outer, inner eye muscle tension, dysfunction.
   Vision/objects are distorted, blurred, unclear in various areas of the visual field at close and/or far distances. Headaches, dizziness can be experienced due to distortion of objects in the visual field. Objects can appear to move, produce a variety of visual effects when the eyes move and the astigmatism area of the eyes cornea passes over objects. It is usually the eye and cornea that have the abnormal shape, not often the lens.
   Headaches, sinus congestion, pressure can also affect the eyes nerves, muscles, eye movement, entire eye, eye shape and cause unclear vision, astigmatism, a variety of visual disturbances. Check with your doctor if a sinus infection is suspected. Usually is harmless but occasionally infection can travel. See the Nutrition Chapter for natural prevention of sinus congestion, infection. Extreme neck muscle tension, misaligned neck vertebrae can affect eye muscle, nerve, ear, sinus... function causing many different eye, vision problems.
   Relax the neck, stay healthy, use the Bates Method to avoid astigmatism, blur, eyeglasses.

+**Amblyopia**=Amblyopia Ex Anopsia=Dim, low, no vision or less clear vision in one eye, often in a wandering/crossed eye due to lack of use of the eye or the brain shutting off the image in the wandering/crossed eye to prevent double vision. Can occur in both eyes. Can occur in an eye with very unclear, blurry vision.

+**Squint**=Strabismus=Wandering/Crossed/Lazy Eye - Dr. Bates uses the word 'Squint' to describe this condition.
   A tense outer eye muscle pulls the eye in, out, up, down... causing strabismus, slow, stiff, un-coordinated eye movement, imperfect convergence, divergence, double vision. The state of convergence, for close vision, divergence for distant vision functions with and affects accommodation for clear close vision, un-accommodation for clear distant vision.
   Strain in the mind, left and right brain hemisphere imbalance, one hemisphere or part of the brain not working correct with a eye muscle, not activating its movement or partially activating it can cause strabismus, imperfect eye movement. Exercises, games, Bates Method corrects this condition.

Imperfect Left and right brain hemisphere function, imbalance, interfering with a baby's crawling, natural walking stage, use of baby walkers, (This disrupts natural left and right brain hemisphere development, activation & integration as the baby grows, learns to craw and walk. The brain, hemispheres work with the eyes, eye muscles, eye development, clarity of vision.), injury from forceps birth delivery, (incorrect handling of the baby at birth, doctors forcing mothers to avoid natural, healthy instincts of safe ways to massage, caress the baby's body, head that naturally insures perfect skull bone alignment after passing through the birth canal, 'like animals do with their tongue'), misaligned skull & eye socket bones and/or neck, back vertebrae, collarbones, other bones, pressure, pulling on nerves, muscles in/along the spine, neck, skull, eye socket can also cause eye muscle tension, eye/eye muscle dysfunction, strabismus, blur, astigmatism and other eye problems.   Usually;
   Mental strain, eye muscle tension, eyestrain, staring, not shifting, lack of central-fixation and other incorrect use of the eyes, wearing eyeglasses, sunglasses, lack of sunlight, using incorrect posture, is the cause of defective vision; blur, astigmatism, strabismus...
   Stress, negative emotions, thoughts, experiences can also strain, tense the mind/brain, eye muscles, cause Brain Hemisphere imbalance and un-coordinated eye muscle function, vision impairment. Stress can temporarily shut off part of the brain, lower certain brain functions, communication with the eyes, eye muscles, retina.   Computer use; looking all day at that one close distance, at the artificial 3-D images on the screen can tense up the eye muscles and eye movement in one or both eyes, cause one brain hemisphere to be dominant and one eye to be dominant at close distances, less clear vision at other distances... Divergence when looking to the distance after hours on the computer can be slow, double vision, one or both eyes movement almost frozen for close distance. (Looking at print, images, videos on the computer screen is different than looking at real print, pictures on a piece of paper. The computer screen strains the eyes when overdone.) Diet also affects the eyes health and vision.

Dr. Bates proved that all these eye conditions are most always caused by mental strain, incorrect use of the eyes and outer eye muscle tension placing pressure, pulling, stretching, tension on/in the eye, cornea, lens, retina, distorting their shape, function, disrupting the focus of light rays in the eye, on the retina, impairing blood, oxygen, nutrient, fluid, energy circulation to, in, out of the eyes and tear production. (Tears contribute to clear vision by acting as a natural contact lens and keeping the cornea, eye healthy. People state their vision improves to clear, even cataracts clearing from the eyes after crying. Crying improves eye circulation, cleansing inside and outside the eye, and stretches, relaxes the muscles in the eyes, head, neck, shoulders.) Sunlight on the eyes, no eye or sun-glasses cures many eye problems, improves the clarity of vision. <u>Outer</u> & <u>Inner</u> eye muscle tension affects eye, lens, iris/pupil, tear... function, health of the eye, clarity of vision.

Neck, shoulder muscle tension is a major cause of eye muscle tension, eye muscle and eye nerve dysfunction, impaired circulation in the head, eyes and unclear vision. Extreme neck muscle tension can pull or tilt a neck vertebra temporarily out of alignment, placing pressure, pulling on the nerves in the neck that travel to/connect to the brain stem, brain, eyes, retina, eye muscles, ears. (Eyes, ears, balance and vision are connected, work together.) Blood, lymph vessels can be affected. Neck muscle tension alone can do this to a lesser degree.

The Author, assembler (Clark Night) of this book experienced a crossed/wandering eye condition with astigmatism, double vision, sinus inflammation, congestion, ear ringing, balance impairment from a neck injury, misaligned vertebrae, torn muscles, ligaments, injured nerves in the neck from a dishonest chiropractor. The Bates Method and a new, good chiropractor corrected the eye, vision, sinus condition.

Natural Eyesight Improvement, Dr. Bates Method relaxes the mind/brain, body, eye muscles, eyes, neck, returns all parts of the eye to normal shape, function, circulation, correct focus of light rays in the eyes for healthy eyes and clear vision at all distances.

BETTER EYESIGHT

A MAGAZINE DEVOTED TO THE PREVENTION AND CURE OF IMPERFECT SIGHT WITHOUT GLASSES

Copyright, 1919, by the Central Fixation Publishing Company
Editor—W. H. BATES, M.D.
Publisher—CENTRAL FIXATION PUBLISHING CO.

Vol. 1   OCTOBER, 1919   No. 4

SIMULTANEOUS RETINOSCOPY

Much of my information about the eye has been obtained by means of simultaneous retinoscopy.

The retinoscope is an instrument used to measure the refraction of the eye. It throws a beam of light into the pupil by reflection from a mirror, the light being either outside the instrument—above and behind the subject—or arranged within it by means of an electric battery. On looking through the sight-hole one sees a larger or smaller part of the pupil filled with light, which in normal human eyes is a reddish yellow, because this is the color of the retina, but which is green in a cat's eye, and might be white if the retina were diseased. Unless the eye is exactly focussed at the point from which it is being observed, one sees also a dark shadow at the edge of the pupil, and it is the behavior of this shadow when the mirror is moved in various directions which reveals the refractive condition of the eye. If the instrument is used at a distance of six feet or more, and the shadow moves in a direction opposite to the movement of the mirror, the eye is myopic. If it moves in the same direction as the mirror, the eye is either hypermetropic or normal; but in the case of hypermetropia the movement is more pronounced than in that of normality, and an expert can usually tell the difference between the two states merely by the nature of the movement. In astigmatism the movement is different in different meridians. To determine the degree of the error, or to distinguish accurately between hypermetropia and normality, or between the different kinds of astigmatism, it is usually necessary to place a glass before the eye of the subject.

This exceedingly useful instrument has possibilities which have not been generally realized by the medical profession. It is commonly employed only under certain artificial conditions in a dark room; but it is possible to use it under all sorts of normal and abnormal conditions on the eyes both of human beings and of the lower animals. I have used it in the daytime and at night; when the subjects were comfortable and when they were excited; when they were trying to see and when they were not; when they were lying and when they were telling the truth. I have also used it, under varying conditions, on the eyes of many cats, dogs, rabbits, birds, turtles, reptiles and fish.

Most ophthalmologists depend upon the Snellen test card, supplemented by trial lenses, to determine whether the vision is normal or not, and to determine the degree of any abnormality that may exist. This is a slow, awkward and unreliable method of testing the vision, and absolutely unavailable for the study of the refraction of the lower animals and that of human beings under the conditions of life. The test card can be used only under certain favorable conditions, but the retinoscope can be used anywhere. It is a little easier to use it in a dim light than in a bright one, but it may be used in any light, even with the strong light of the sun shining directly into the eye. It is available whether the subject is at rest or in motion, asleep or awake, or even under ether or chloroform. It is also available when the observer is in motion. It has been used successfully when the eyelids were partly closed, shutting off part of the area of the pupil; when the pupil was dilated; also when it was contracted to a pin-point; when the subject was reading fine print at six inches, or at a greater distance; and when the eye was oscillating from side to side, from above downward, or in other directions.

It takes a considerable time, varying from minutes to hours, to measure the refraction with the Snellen test card and trial lenses. With the retinoscope, however, the refraction can be determined in a fraction of a second. With the Snellen test card and trial lenses it would be impossible to get any information about the refraction of a baseball player at the moment he swings for the ball, at the moment he strikes it, and at the moment after he strikes it. With the retinoscope, however, it is quite easy to determine whether his vision is normal, or whether he is myopic, hypermetropic, or astigmatic, when he does these things; and if any errors of refraction are noted, one can guess their degree pretty accurately by the rapidity of the movement of the shadow.

With the Snellen test card and trial lenses conclusions must be drawn from the patient's statements as to what he sees; but the patient often becomes so worried and confused during the examination that he does not know what he sees, or whether different glasses make his sight better, or worse; and, moreover, visual acuity is not reliable evidence of the state of the refraction. One patient with two diopters of myopia may see twice as much as another with the same error of refraction. The evidence of the test card is, in fact, entirely subjective; that of the retinoscope is entirely objective, depending in no way upon the statements of the patient.

SAVE A TREE – PLEASE PRINT THIS BOOK ON 100% RECYCLED PAPER WITH ORGANIC ENVIRONMENTALLY SAFE INK

Better Eyesight

The following poem was taken from a current magazine, but its discrepancies were so apparent that I could not pass it unchallenged.

E. A. M.

MY EYEGLASSES

Little helpmates yoked together,	Many days have laboring men
Twin-born servants of mine,	In mines across the sea
How your presence helps and cheers me,	Spent searching for the components
You barriers of time.	To solve your mystery.
Glistening eyes and dainty rims,	Sometimes I lay you out of labor,
Exquisite mountings, too,	A place I cannot see,
What dreary days of solitude	And then it seems part of myself
Had I not met with you.	Has gone away from me.
And then I pause to wonder how	I have no means to show the depth
You ever could be here,	Of my gratitude to you.
What genius burned the midnight oil	My eyes will flood with burning tears
To make your portals clear.	When your services are thru.

I herewith seal this solemn vow
That henceforth you will be
Kept clean from dust and fingerprints
While you are serving me.

My Eyeglasses
By EMILY A. MEDER

THE sentimental poem given above evidently required a good deal of forethought and concentrated effort to devise. We wonder, however, if this anonymous genius had spent the time taken to create this gem, by reading Dr. Bates' book, and practicing the method as outlined by him, whether he would not have written a masterpiece. He would have discarded his "twin-born servants," attained better eyesight, and we know, would have been benefited physically.

With apologies to the author, I am going to dissect this "child of his brain" to see what it is made of. As the surgeons say, this might be painful and uncomfortable, but it is for the patient's eventual good.

Like a great majority of people this man believes that glasses have to be put on when one has attained a certain set age. I suppose that we must be grateful that theorists have not ordained that we place splints on our arms and legs to prevent old age attacking them prematurely. However, as all know, who have read Dr. Bates' book, and who have been treated by him, the eyes are no more delicate than any other part of the anatomy. When we read the sentence, "You barriers of time," it seems as ludicrous to us as the opinion people held in the olden days when they ridiculed Columbus for thinking the earth round. We might fittingly change that sentence to read "You hasteners of time."

The author continues to relate the labor men were put to, "to make these portals clear." We admit that a great deal of time was spent to make the glasses ornate. But this did not in any material way add to their usefulness and value. We know that when people purchase glasses they spend a good deal of time making eyes that they look well in them. There is always a heated and lengthy debate as to whether tortoise shell or gold is more studious looking, or whether rimless glasses add to one's dignity. Men may have exhausted their energy in "mines across the sea," and I have a mental picture of them using their life forces to attain—nothing. It makes me think of the squirrel on a revolving wheel. The faster he works, the more energy he uses, and he is eventually exhausted, getting nowhere. The trouble with the old oculists is that they were started on the wrong track, and stayed there, without looking for an avenue of escape. Like the labyrinth in mythology, they walked and walked and went back and forward, in a ceaseless round, with no one to show them the one way out. To follow the metaphor you may remember the story of the cruel giant who put all the fair young maidens in the labyrinth and left them to die. But one maiden obtained a ball of twine and fastened it to the entrance of the cavern. As she was lead deeper and deeper into the intricate passages, she let out the cord. Upon being left alone, she called all the unfortunate prisoners to her, and they followed the right path back, as indicated by the ball of twine. This story always occurs to me when I think of Dr. Bates' work. As all the others are lost in a maze of theories, his wonderful truth is the string of hope to cling to when escaping the awful giant—bad sight and glasses.

Natural Eyesight Improvement After Unsuccessful Eye Cornea Surgery - Is it Safe? Can it Reverse the Cornea Damage, Vision Impairment Caused by the Cornea Surgery?

Often, people that have had eye cornea laser and other surgery develop unclear vision and/or astigmatism, light sensitivity and other types of vision impairment. This can occur immediately after the surgery or weeks, months, a year or more after surgery. They ask if Natural Eyesight Improvement can restore the vision?

The cornea, in some ways is like the human liver and skin: it can repair itself. Eyes with cornea injuries, scars can repair naturally, the cornea heals as the skin heals from a cut and clear vision returns. See Dr. Bates 'Better Eyesight Magazine'.

Cornea surgery removes part of the cornea, weakening it. The cornea might repair itself after surgery if Natural Eyesight Improvement is used but this is not definite. The cornea might be able to re-grow, return to full normal thickness, strength and shape.

Natural Eyesight Improvement relaxes tense eye muscles and returns the eyes shape to normal but this might interfere with the surgically altered cornea which has been formed by the surgery to work with an abnormal eye shape, function existing at the time of the surgery. Cornea surgery, alteration, removal of part of the eyes cornea is done to match the abnormal eye shape, state of eye muscle tension causing the abnormal eye shape existing at the time of the surgery. The eye and muscles must remain in this abnormal state for the eye to see clear through the surgically altered cornea. A surgically altered cornea is like an eyeglass lens constructed for a specific abnormal eye/vision state. If the state/shape of the eye changes; becomes more impaired or improves; the eye can no longer see clear through that eyeglass lens prescription. Eyeglass lens strength can be changed: reduced, increased but the surgically altered cornea cannot be changed. Some surgeons attempt this resulting in more vision impairment.

Natural Eyesight Improvement might help the cornea rebuild its structure and work with the eye producing clear vision as the Bates Method returns the eye to normal shape or:

The improved eye shape occurring from practice of the Bates Method might pull on the surgically weakened cornea, as the weakened cornea un-successfully tries to change shape with the eye as the eye changes back to normal shape. This results in impaired cornea function: waves, tears in the cornea, blur, astigmatism...

A patient might develop increased eye muscle tension (which increases abnormal eye shape) after the cornea surgery or, less muscle tension occurs (which changes the shape of the eye toward a normal shape). As the surgically altered cornea tries to reform to fit the changing eye shape, this results in unclear vision;

Eye muscles more tense=more impaired eye shape=more impaired cornea shape=blur.

Eye muscles less tense, relax=eye shape returns to normal but cornea cannot return to normal shape with the eye=cornea and eye do not fit/work together=blur.

If the cornea can return to normal shape with the eye, without tension, injury, then vision will be clear.

If the surgically altered cornea cannot return to the correct shape to fit the changing eye shape, vision can blur and astigmatism and other vision impairment can occur.

The right amount of practice of the Bates method might help the eye/cornea stay within a workable state: the right amount of balance, amount of eye muscle relaxation with improved eye shape, but not too much all at once, and then, if the cornea can rebuild itself, in the future it might be able to fully, safely change shape with the eye into a state of complete, perfect eye/cornea shape, perfect muscle relaxation and clear vision.

If a Cornea Surgery Patient is getting clearer vision with the Bates method and does not feel, see any problems with the cornea, it may be alright to continue. If the cornea feels like it is pulling, stretching... or things get really blurry, increased astigmatism..., take a break and let the cornea have a chance to catch up to the improvement in eye shape. **Check with your eye doctor.**

Fluctuations in the vision are normal for everyone, and some slightly double 'astigmatism like effect' or blur can occur as the vision is improving, reversing back to normal eye/cornea shape, clear vision and this may not be a problem with the cornea. It would be normal and it clears up quickly with relaxation and Bates Method practice.

When the cornea is weakened, parts removed, due to laser surgery: the cornea, eyes natural protection, tolerance to sunlight is impaired. The cornea and lens protect the eye from over-exposure to sunlight.

I do not know if Sunning is safe if the eyes have been treated with cornea surgery. If the cornea does not get some natural full spectrum sunlight, it will not stay healthy and growth, repair may be blocked. Closed Eye Sunning only and some sunlight exposure by taking a walk outside daily wearing a hat with a brim, worn on and off may help. Check with your eye doctor first.

AVOID LASER CORNEA EYE SURGERY AND OTHER CORNEA SURGERIES. LASER AND OTHER CORNEA EYE SURGERIES CAUSE EYE HEALTH IMPAIRMENT, UNCLEAR VISON, A VARIETY OF VISION PROBLEMS INCLUDING BLINDNESS

Eye surgeons advertise expensive cornea surgery to improve the clarity of distant and close vision but are not required to warn the patient about all of the side effects the surgery causes. The eye surgeon does not tell the patient the truth; that many different types of vision impairment and blindness can, has and will occur due to cornea laser surgery.
A woman on a television news show described how laser cornea surgery has caused her to be blind at night and in low light. She cannot go outside at night due to extreme glare, halos from lights. Other vision impairments have developed, unclear daytime vision, reading vision. This condition is permanent. The woman says the cornea surgery has ruined her life.

In 2008 - Television news broadcast - a father telling about how his son was so depressed, his life miserable due to the incurable eye problems, near blindness, eye pain he suffered caused by laser cornea eye surgery. The son committed suicide.
Many people have impaired vision due to cornea surgery.
Read Laser surgery side effects warning - FDA; www.fda.gov Click medical devices, lasik.

See YouTube videos on eye/vision impairment caused by lasik.
Type in 'laser surgery, suicidal patients'. http://www.youtube.com/watch?v=97609G6Dno0

Also see website, YouYube videos: www.lasikcomplications.com
Many patients are developing cataracts after laser cornea surgery.

Some of the side effects of laser and other cornea surgeries are;
The surgery destroys, weakens the cornea's structure. Part of the cornea is permanently removed.
Cornea injury, ulcers, scars, infection in the cornea and eye, waves, uneven and torn areas in the cornea and other impairments occur resulting in; vision less clear than it was before surgery at close and far distances, double, triple vision, astigmatism, dizziness, cloudy, dull vision, haze, spots in the visual field, impaired tolerance to light and large halos, glare from indoor lights, from sunlight and from lights at night resulting in night blindness and low daylight vision.
The peripheral field of vision is lowered and the central field becomes unclear.
Increased cornea structure impairment occurs. Many people have become blind right after the surgery or a short time into the future after the surgery. The permanently weakened cornea is easily injured and the person must avoid certain activities, sports, climates, altitudes... for life. Even a soft touch of the hand, a blanket, sleeve... to the cornea can injure it. Cornea injury can occur from a light blow to the body, head. Pilots, various government, military persons and people in certain occupations are not allowed to have cornea surgery.
Some surgery results in clearer than 20/20 vision but this is temporary and the clarity of vision goes below 20/20 in a short time. Most people still need eyeglasses after cornea surgery.
Cornea surgery causes the eyes to feel tired and the clarity of vision to lower during the day and become more unclear at night. Most cornea surgery patients need permanent use of eyeglasses at night and in dim light. The eyeglasses then cause and increase eye muscle tension, abnormal eye/cornea shape and vision impairment resulting in eyeglass prescriptions for the day and night at close and far distances. More vision impairment occurs and stronger and stronger eyeglass prescriptions are prescribed causing increased eye muscle tension, abnormal eye shape with pulling, stretching, tension on/in the eye, cornea. The surgically weakened cornea develops waves, tears, ulcers. Multiple eye problems develop. Cornea transplants and other eye surgeries are needed.

The eyes cornea and lens absorb/control the amount of sunlight and UV light that enters the eye, protecting the eye from over exposure to sunlight, UV light. Cornea surgery; removing part of the cornea destroys this natural eye function. Cornea surgery leaves the cornea, iris/pupil, lens, retina overexposed to sunlight/UV light and overexposed to unhealthy partial spectrum artificial light.
This can result in impaired eye health, damage to the cornea, lens, retina... causing pupil malfunction, cataracts, macula degeneration, and other retina damage, unclear vision and other eye problems, including blindness.
Abnormal pupil enlargement in sunlight, artificial light and in dim light occurs. This also causes a abnormally large amount of sunlight and unhealthy partial spectrum light to enter the eyes.

DANGERS OF LASER AND OTHER CORNEA EYE SURGERIES

LASER AND OTHER CORNEA EYE SURGERIES CAUSE CORNEA INJURY, UNCLEAR EYESIGHT AND OTHER EYE PROBLEMS

1 NORMAL ROUND EYE SHAPE.
CORNEA NORMAL, NO CORNEA SURGERY.

LIGHT RAYS FOCUS CORRECT ON THE RETINA.
DISTANT VISION IS CLEAR.
THE EYE LENGTHENS <u>SLIGHTLY</u> FOR CLEAR CLOSE VISION.

---

2 ABNORMAL LENGTHENED EYE SHAPE DUE TO OUTER EYE MUSCLE TENSION. NO CORNEA SURGERY.

LIGHT RAYS FOCUS INCORRECT BEFORE THE RETINA.
DISTANT VISION IS UNCLEAR.
CLOSE VISION ALSO BECOMES UNCLEAR IF INCREASED EYE MUSCLE TENSION AND LENGTHENING OF THE EYE OCCURS.

---

3 AFTER CORNEA SURGERY.
EYE SHAPE STILL ABNORMAL, LENGTHENED.
EYE MUSCLES STILL TENSE.

CORNEA MADE SHORTER, PART OF CORNEA REMOVED BY SURGERY

PART OF THE EYES CORNEA HAS BEEN PERMANENTLY REMOVED BY LASER OR OTHER SURGERY. THE CORNEA IS SHORTENED IN AN ATTEMPT TO MAKE THE EYE CLOSER TO A ROUND SHAPE TO IMPROVE FOCUS OF LIGHT RAYS IN THE EYE. LIGHT RAYS FOCUS BETTER, CLOSER TO THE RETINA, BUT OFTEN FOCUS IMPERFECT. DISTANT VISION IS CLEARER BUT NOT PERFECT.

4 5 MONTHS AFTER CORNEA SURGERY. VISION IS MORE IMPAIRED THAN BEFORE SURGERY.

IN DIAGRAM # 4 IT IS 5 MONTHS AFTER CORNEA SURGERY.
THE EYE MUSCLES HAVE RELAXED, NATURALLY AND THE EYE HAS RETURNED TO NORMAL SHAPE..
THE LIGHT RAYS SHOULD FOCUS CORRECT AND DISTANT VISION SHOULD BE CLEAR, BUT, THE CORNEA HAS BEEN PERMANENTLY SHORTENED, IMPAIRED BY SURGERY AND THE CORNEA CANNOT RETURN TO NORMAL SHAPE WITH THE EYE.
THIS CAUSES THE EYE TO BE TOO SHORT CAUSING LIGHT RAYS TO FOCUS INCORRECT BEYOND /BEHIND THE RETINA.
DISTANT AND CLOSE VISION ARE UNCLEAR.
THE CORNEAS STRUCTURE IS ALSO WEAKENED AND EASILY INJURED, INFECTED, SCARRED RESULTING IN ASTIGMATISM, HAZE, BLIND SPOTS, OTHER VISION PROBLEMS INCLUDING BLINDNESS.
THE CORNEA, IRIS, LENS, RETINA IS ALSO OVEREXPOSED TO LIGHT DUE TO IMPAIRED STRUCTURE, FUNCTION, SIZE, THICKNESS OF THE SURGICALLY ALTERED CORNEA. CATARACTS, MACULA DEGENERATION AND OTHER EYE INJURY OCCURS.
LASER AND OTHER CORNEA SURGERIES CANNOT BE REVERSED.

Eye muscle tension causes abnormal eye/cornea shape; incorrect focus of light rays in the eye and unclear vision. See picture # 2.
Natural Vision Improvement relaxes the eye muscles and returns the eye/cornea to normal shape with correct focus of light rays in the eye with clear vision at close and far distances without use of surgery, eyeglasses. The cornea remains whole, strong and healthy. See picture # 1.
A normal round eye shape, relaxed eye muscles keeps normal pressure/circulation in the eye, retina, lens, cornea... resulting in healthy eyes and prevention of cataracts, macula degeneration, glaucoma and other eye problems.

Contact lenses also impair the shape and health of the cornea.
Read more in the introduction, beginning of this book.

This causes the eye problems listed above. Cornea surgery impairs the eyes natural tolerance to sunlight and artificial light. The eyes hurt, are sensitive in all types of light. This causes the person to wear sunglasses, tinted and UV blocking eyeglass lenses which are addictive, cause and increase vision impairment, close and distant blur, and causes more abnormal pupil enlargement, further impairs the eyes tolerance to light. The enlarged pupil increases the eyes exposure to unhealthy partial spectrum light that passes through the sunglasses, tinted, UV blocking lenses.
All eyeglasses, contact lenses; plain, tinted, UV blocking, dark, colored...cause partial spectrum light to enter the eyes, brain, body, cause abnormal pupil enlargement and impair the eyes tolerance to light.

The sunglasses, tinted, UV blocking lenses also block out full spectrum sunlight causing a constant flow of unhealthy partial spectrum sunlight and even more unbalanced partial spectrum artificial light to enter the

eyes, brain, body. Health and function of the eyes, brain, body become impaired.
Cataracts, macula degeneration, detached retina and other eye problems occur.
Sunglasses, tinted, UV blocking lenses and plain eyeglasses cause and increase vision impairment resulting in prescriptions for eyeglasses.

The cornea and lens refract, bend, focus light rays in the eyes. <u>Cornea - 80% Lens - 10%</u>.
Removing part of the cornea by surgery impairs the corneas natural focus of light rays.

Outer eye muscle tension can cause a abnormal eye/cornea shape with incorrect focus of light rays in the eyes and unclear vision. When the eye muscles relax due to natural causes; relief of stress and mental strain, improved diet and health, good posture, relaxation of the neck.., use of Natural Eyesight Improvement; Correct Vision Habits, relaxation... the eye returns to normal shape with correct focus of light rays and clear vision.
(Correct Vision Habits and other Natural Eyesight Improvement states can occur automatically, without the person learning, consciously using Natural Eyesight Improvement because; <u>it is the normal function of the eyes. The visual system always returns the eyes to normal correct function</u>.)

Cornea surgery does not correct the cause of unclear vision. Cornea surgery does not relax tense eye muscles, does not remove; stress, mental strain, use of Incorrect Vision Habits, does not return the eye to normal shape, does not remove abnormal pressure, tension, pulling, stretching on/in the eye, retina, lens, cornea, does not improve circulation to, in the eye.

Example; the eye surgeon cuts off part of the eyes cornea in an attempt to make the shape of the eye closer to a normal round shape with better focus of light rays in the eye for clearer distant vision.
(see picture)

<u>If, in the future, after cornea surgery, the eye muscles relax</u> due to natural conditions; relief of stress, strain, improved diet, health, better job, life situation... using the eyes correct with relaxation, Correct Vision Habits, Natural Eyesight Improvement, correct posture, relaxed neck and other natural causes and the eye returns to normal shape; <u>the surgically altered, impaired cornea will be too flat and cannot return to normal shape and function with the eye. This causes the eye to be too short</u>.
(see picture 4) Focus of light rays in the eye are now more impaired than before surgery. Light rays focus beyond the retina resulting unclear close and distant vision.
The weakened, impaired cornea stretches, pulls, experiences tension, pressure as it tries to return to normal shape with the eye. This causes the cornea to develop waves, uneven areas, ulcers. Infection in the cornea and eye, scars occur resulting in unclear vision, astigmatism, blind spots, large halos, glare from lights and other eye problems.

The cornea also changes shape with the eye when the eye lengthens slightly when looking at close distances and returns to a round shape when looking at far distances. The surgically weakened, impaired cornea will not be able to change shape perfectly with the eye-the cornea will stretch, pull, develop waves, uneven areas causing blur, astigmatism, glare and other eye problems.

It is normal for the shape of the eye and cornea to change, fluctuate slightly and this can occur often; within a second, minute, hour, day...causing the clarity of vision to fluctuate slightly and temporarily; clear, little less clear and back to clear. A surgically altered cornea will cause the temporary state of less clear vision to be increased. The vision is much more unclear.
When the cornea is normal, not altered by surgery, temporary states of less clear vision are slight and are usually not noticed. The clarity of vision always fluctuates back to normal when eyeglasses, surgery are avoided.

Natural Eyesight Improvement keeps the vision clearer than 20/20; to 20/15, 10, 5, 40/20...
When temporary fluctuations of clarity occur, vision goes from 20/5, 20/10 to 20/15, 20/20, occasionally to 20/30, 40 and then returns back to clearer than 20/20.
Vision rarely goes less clear than 20/20, 20/30.

Cornea surgery does not remove the underlying cause of unclear vision; does not remove eye muscle tension, mental strain, use of Incorrect Vision Habits, neck tension... and abnormal eye shape.

<u>After cornea surgery eye muscle tension may increase,</u> causing the shape of the eye to become more abnormal. This will also impair focus of light rays in the eye and result in unclear eyesight.
(Example; cornea surgery was done for a eye that is abnormally lengthened. The eye surgeon cut, shortened the shape of the cornea to fit that specific eye shape. If, after surgery, the eye muscle tension and abnormal

eye shape increases: the surgically altered cornea will not fit the eye, cannot change shape with the eye.) Increased pulling, stretching on the cornea occurs resulting in cornea injury and vision impairment as described previously.

Wearing eyeglasses after cornea surgery will increase the eye muscle tension, abnormal eye shape (increased lengthened, shortened, irregular shape), vision impairment and cornea, eye injury. Stronger and stronger lenses are prescribed causing more vision impairment.

(Contact lenses must never be worn after cornea surgery because the contacts easily injure and infect the weakened cornea. Contacts cause injury even to a healthy, strong non-surgically altered cornea.)

The same side effects occur due to cornea surgery to steepen, (raise, lengthen) the cornea in an attempt to improve close vision and altering the shape of the cornea to treat astigmatism.
All these surgeries involve permanently removing part of the cornea, removing a healthy, normal part of the eye. This is poor medical practice, breaks a medical law: 'Do not harm, destroy healthy tissue'.
   Notice that cornea surgery applied in an attempt to obtain clearer distant vision is done to make a lengthened eye more round and, that, cornea surgery to obtain clearer close vision is done to make a shortened eye longer but; eye doctors, surgeons refuse to admit that a abnormally lengthened or shortened eye/cornea shape is caused by outer eye muscle tension and that the eye muscles can be relaxed naturally with Natural Eyesight Improvement enabling the eye, cornea to return to normal shape with clear close and distant vision, thus avoiding cornea eye surgery.

(Cornea surgery is necessary sometimes for treating a eye cornea injury, possibly infection... if other, preferably natural methods, cannot save the eye, vision.)

Natural Eyesight Improvement (no glasses, no surgery) relaxes the eye muscles and returns the eye to normal healthy shape with clear vision at all distances.

Natural Eyesight Improvement may improve the clarity of vision by relaxing the eye muscles if the eye muscles have become <u>more tense</u> after cornea surgery, but may result in <u>less clear vision</u> if the eye muscles <u>completely relax</u> and returns the eye to normal shape because the surgically impaired cornea will not be able to return to normal shape with the eye.
   Increased eye muscle tension, further impairing the shape of the eye, cornea also can result in more vision impairment after cornea surgery. See Article below:

CONTACT LENSES CAUSE EYE INJURY

Cornea injury and vision impairment occur often due to wearing of contact lenses;
It is normal for the shape of the eye/cornea to change often, naturally, on its own. The shape of the eye/cornea can change, fluctuate in a second, minute, hour, day... It is impossible to prescribe a exact size/fit for contact lenses because the size, shape of the cornea is always changing. The contacts will never fit the cornea and will scrape, infect, injure, scar the cornea and eye.
Contact lenses enable bacteria, and a variety of germs to grow on the cornea and on/in the eyes.
Contact lens solutions often contain bacteria, viruses and other contaminants that cause frequent cornea/eye infection and can and has caused blindness, loss of the infected eye.

ORTHO-KERATOLOGY; Fitting the eyes corneas with contact lenses that are a different size/shape than the cornea, to be used as braces on the corneas to try to force the cornea to change shape in an attempt to remove close and distant blur, astigmatism results in frequent cornea injury.

Because Natural Eyesight Improvement causes the shape of the eye and cornea to change as the eye muscles relax and the eye/cornea returns to normal shape; <u>contact lenses must never be worn before, during and after use of Natural Eyesight Improvement</u> - the contacts will not fit the changing cornea shape.
Never wear contacts at night, during sleep; the shape of the eye/cornea changes during sleep. The contacts will injure the eyes corneas during sleep. Any injury to the cornea can result in infection which can go into the eye and cause cornea/eye damage, vision impairment and blindness.
   The eye, cornea changes shape often, a natural, normal function, with or without Natural Eyesight Improvement. This makes it impossible to prescribe a correct contact lens size.

ORTHO C-ORTHOCULOGY - A new method using contact lenses to force the cornea, lens, eye to change shape, force some eye muscles to become tense, stretch, and other eye muscles to un-contract in a abnormal state. This is unnatural and dangerous. People selling this method warn the patient that there are risks; cornea, eye infection, injury, permanent damage, abnormal eye and eye muscle function, dependence on the method and other eye, vision impairment.
Avoid these and all unnatural methods.

The Bates Method teaches that all the eye muscles must relax, function together, contracting and un-contracting in a coordinated, relaxed state. The eye, cornea, lens returns to normal shape on its own.

Contact lenses impair the shape of the eyes cornea causing a uneven cornea shape and astigmatism.
A uneven cornea is easily scraped, injured by contact lenses.
Contact lenses must not be worn when the cornea/eye contains astigmatism.
Astigmatism is caused by a uneven area in the cornea and abnormal eye/cornea shape.
The degree, type, shape, and placement of the astigmatism/abnormal eye/cornea shape/wave causing the astigmatism changes frequently.
Contact lenses will never fit the changing cornea shape.
Contacts often injure the cornea that contains astigmatism.

Contact lenses impair tear production, coating of tears over the eyes/corneas, cause abnormal pupil enlargement, impair tolerance to light, block oxygen, nutrient flow to the cornea. The cornea becomes dry, weak and injured. All contact lenses; soft, flexible, night wear... cause eye injury and act as eyeglasses causing increased vision impairment leading to prescriptions for stronger and stronger contact lenses and eyeglasses. Contact lenses impair; balance, coordination, blinking, shifting and other Correct Vision Habits. Contact lenses completely block out all full spectrum sunlight causing the eyes, brain, body to be constantly exposed to unhealthy partial spectrum light. UV blocking, tinted and colored contacts cause light to be more unbalanced and increase abnormal pupil enlargement.
   Eyeglasses allow some full spectrum sunlight to enter around the edges of the frames.
No eyeglasses is best.

Avoid all cornea surgeries, contact lenses and eyeglasses.
Use natural eyesight improvement to relax the eye muscles and return the eye, cornea to normal shape with correct focus of light rays in the eye, clear eyesight at all distances and healthy eyes.

The Bates Method of Natural Eyesight Improvement cures many different eye problems. Natural Eyesight Improvement relaxes the outer and inner eye muscles causing the eye, cornea, lens to return to normal healthy shape, function. This condition along with neck muscle relaxation, movement improves circulation in the eye and normalizes eye pressure. This can reverse and cure glaucoma, cataracts and other eye problems.
   (If taking drugs, eye drops to lower eye pressure to treat glaucoma, check with your eye doctor. As Natural Eyesight Improvement normalizes eye pressure, the drug may have to be reduced or discontinued.) Check with your Ophthalmologist if you have had or are going to have any eye surgery or are being treated with drugs for a eye condition and let him/her know you plan to apply Natural Eyesight Improvement. Most eye doctors prefer to sell surgery, drugs, eyeglasses and contact lenses. Find an eye doctor that teaches the Bates Method of Natural Eyesight Improvement and prefers to avoid surgery, drugs, eyeglasses, contacts.

Avoid Sunglasses. Sunglasses cause eye sensitivity to light, lowers natural light tolerance, lowers, impairs use of sunlight by the eyes, brain, body, causes watering, burning eyes, eye infections, sties, unclear vision, cataracts, and other eye diseases, impairs vitamin D and other nutrient absorption, hormone balance, sleep cycle and other functions. Sunglasses cause unbalanced, partial spectrum light to enter the eyes, brain, body. Sunglasses block healthy full spectrum sunlight.
Impairment of the health and function of the eyes, eye muscles, lens, retina, brain, left and right brain hemispheres and body occur due to lack of full spectrum sunlight and exposure to the unhealthy, unbalanced light entering the eyes through the sunglasses.

MENTAL STRAIN, EYE MUSCLE TENSION, ABNORMAL EYE SHAPE CAUSES UNCLEAR EYESIGHT
Dangers of, Vision Impairment Caused by; Laser Cornea Eye Surgery, Eyeglasses and Contact Lenses

Strain, tension in the mind, visual system, incorrect posture, shoulder, neck muscle tension, Incorrect Vision Habits cause eye muscle tension. Myopia, Fasight, Presbyopia... occur.

Tension in the outer eye muscles places pressure on/in the eye causing abnormal eye shape, incorrect focus of light rays in the eye and unclear vision. Muscles inside the eye (ciliary...) also become tense; function of the lens, iris, retina are impaired.

+Picture # 1 shows the Normal Round Eye Shape.
Eye muscles are relaxed.
Light rays focus correct on the retina.
+ The central light ray focuses on the center of the fovea centralis in the macula, in the center of the retina.
This produces the exact center of the visual field.
+ Peripheral light rays focus on the peripheral areas of the retina (all areas around, near and away from the macula and fovea) which produces the peripheral field of vision. Distant vision is clear.

Dr. Bates states; The oblique muscles around the outside of the eye contract to slightly lengthen the eye to accommodate, focus divergent light rays on the retina for clear close vision. (like a camera.) They un-contract, return the eye to a round shape for clear distant vision.

+Picture # 2 shows a Abnormal Lengthened Eye Shape.
The eye is lengthened too much and is kept in this state due to tension in the oblique outer eye muscles.
Light rays do not focus on the retina.
Light rays focus incorrect before the retina causing unclear distant vision.

Close vision may be clear if the eye is not lengthened too much, but it is never perfectly clear when the distant vision is unclear.

Increased eye muscle tension causes increased lengthening of the eye resulting in unclear distant and close vision.

Addiction to eyeglasses is the main cause.

Caused and increased by - minus lens distant vision eyeglasses.

+Picture # 3 shows a Abnormal Shortened Eye Shape.
Caused by tension in the recti outer eye muscles pulling back on the front of the eye.
Light rays focus incorrect beyond the retina.

In early stages of eye muscle tension the eye may stay in a round shape unable to lengthen slightly when looking at close distances, and the lens' normal full movement is blocked resulting in unclear close vision.

Distant vision may be clear, but it is never perfectly clear when the close vision is unclear.

As eye muscle tension increases, the eye is pulled into a shortened shape causing unclear close and distant vision.

Addiction to eyeglasses is the main cause.

Caused and increased by + plus lens close vision eyeglasses.

+Picture # 4 shows a Irregular, Uneven Eye Shape.
Caused by tension in one or more outer eye muscles, oblique and/or recti. The shape of the cornea is also uneven. Astigmatism, unclear vision result. This condition can occur with a abnormal lengthened or shortened eye shape.
Light rays focus incorrect; all or some light rays focus incorrect before and/or beyond the retina.

Uneven lens shape or dust, dirt... on the cornea, sinus pressure, incorrect posture, neck tension can also cause astigmatism. Addiction to eyeglasses is the main cause.

Eyeglasses, contact lenses CAUSE and INCREASE; strain, tension in the mind, eyes, eye muscles, abnormal eye shape, all the conditions listed in # 2, 3 and 4. Leads to detached retina, cataract, glaucoma and other conditions.

Caused and increased by - minus lens distant vision and/or + plus lens close vision eyeglasses.
A uneven long or short eye occurs.

OUTER EYE MUSCLES
RECTI - # 1, 2, 3, 4
OBLIQUE - 5, 6

Incorrect vision habits, strain, eye muscle tension, abnormal eye shape cause; The central ray focuses incorrect onto the peripheral area of the retina. Peripheral rays focus incorrect onto the fovea centralis in the center of the retina. This impairs both central and peripheral vision, causes astigmatism and unclear vision at close and/or far distances. Eye movement 'shifting and convergence, divergence' are also affected by the conditions shown in pictures 2, 3, 4. The eyes lens' function, movement-shape can be affected. Incorrect focus of central and peripheral light rays onto the peripheral and central areas of the retina can occur when the eye is abnormally lengthened, shortened with or without a uneven shape.

Diagrams of abnormal eye shapes are accentuated for easy view.

STOP STARING

It can be demonstrated by tests with the retinoscope that all persons with imperfect sight stare, strain, or try to see. To demonstrate this fact:

Look intently at one part of a large or small letter at the distance or nearpoint. In a few seconds, usually, fatigue and discomfort will be produced, and the letter will blur or disappear. If the effort is continued long enough, pain may be produced.

To break the habit of staring:

(1) Shift consciously from one part to another of all objects regarded, and imagine that these objects move in a direction contrary to the movement of the eye. Do this with letters on the test card, with letters of fine print, if they can be seen, and with other objects.

(2) Close the eyes frequently for a moment or longer. When the strain is considerable, keep the eyes closed for several minutes and open them for a fraction of a second—flashing. When the stare is sufficient to keep the vision down to 2/200 or less, palm for a longer or shorter time; then look at the card for a moment. Later mere closing of the eyes may afford sufficient rest.

(3) Imagine that the white openings and margins of letters are whiter than the rest of the background. Do this with eyes closed and open alternately. It is an interesting fact that this practice prevents staring and improves the vision rapidly.

Note for #1; If you cannot see a letter, it is unclear; shifting on it from one blurry part to another, and looking for the contrary (opposite) movement improves the clarity of the letter.

BETTER EYESIGHT
A MAGAZINE DEVOTED TO THE PREVENTION AND CURE OF IMPERFECT SIGHT WITHOUT GLASSES

Editor—W. H. BATES, M.D.
Publisher—CENTRAL FIXATION PUBLISHING CO.

Vol. VI.   JANUARY, 1922   No. 1

BE COMFORTABLE
By W. H. BATES, M. D.

IT can be stated without fear of successful contradiction that persons with perfect sight are always comfortable, not only as to their eyes, but as to the rest of the body. As soon as they cease to be so, it can be demonstrated, by examination with the retinoscope, that their sight has ceased to be perfect. They become nearsighted, farsighted, or astigmatic. The art of learning to use the eyes properly, is, in short, the art of learning to be comfortable. Even the memory of comfort improves the sight, while the memory of discomfort lowers it. Persons with imperfect sight often say and think that they are perfectly comfortable; but invariably such persons experience a feeling of relief when they close their eyes, demonstrating that they were not perfectly comfortable before, but had merely formed a habit of ignoring that discomfort. Persons with perfect sight, on the other hand, can immediately produce discomfort by producing imperfect sight, or even by remembering or imagining it, and persons with imperfect sight can produce a degree of discomfort that cannot be ignored by making their sight worse.

Copyright, 1922, by the Central Fixation Publishing Company

Suggestions to Patients
By Emily C. Lierman

(1) Palm in the morning while in bed.
(2) Take sun treatment for twenty minutes or longer every day.
(3) Mentally or physically, keep up that pendulum-like motion.
(4) After sitting in the sun, hold the small card and flash the white spaces.
(5) What you do not see immediately, do not worry about.
(6) While practicing with the Seven Truths of Normal Sight, always move the card slowly from side to side as you hold it six or eight inches from your eyes.
(7) To induce sleep when suffering from headache or nervous strain, close your eyes, remember the small F or T of the ten line of the test card and imagine it is moving slightly, about one-quarter of an inch, either up and down or to the left and right.
(8) There is a right way and a wrong way to blink the eyes while practicing. Children like to hold up their two hands about ten or twelve inches apart, looking first at one hand and then at the other. In this way one blinks when looking at the right hand and again when looking at the left hand. The head should turn in the same direction with the eyes.
(9) Near-sighted patients sometimes get along faster in the cure of their eyes by using two similar test cards at the same time while practicing. One card is held in the hand while the other is five or ten feet away. The patient looks at a letter up close and imagines he sees the same letter on the distant card. Then the patient closes his eyes and imagines that letter perfectly. Having seen it perfectly up close, he becomes able by practice to see it just as well on the distant card.

A Case Report

(Report of a man, 63 years old, who has worn glasses for a great many years. He improved his own vision merely by following directions. Others can do the same.)

I WILL be 63 years old in July and have not worn lenses since reading "Perfect Sight Without Glasses"; it will be two years the latter part of next July.

I have had monocular vision all my life, congenital convergent squint of left eye producing what has always been called "partial blindness from disuse." I could always see parts of everything but nothing distinctly; enough to get around if I closed my good eye, but could never see to read any printed matter with it.

At first I could not see the big "C" at any distance with the left eye. Now I can see its whole outline at about six inches and all of the letters on line ten at three or four feet.

In scanning even fine print I can now discern lines and spaces and almost distinguish the letters by holding it close up.

I should add that I have not been at all diligent nor faithful in using Dr. Bates' methods and am surprised at the results obtained by me in spite of that fact. With more devotion I am sure I will get better results.

One patient, a woman of 25 or 30, had worn glasses seventeen years. She was myopic with astigmatism, seeing about half the distance with the left eye as with the right. She had frequent headaches, could not go to the "movies" without great distress. She spent $300 or more on glasses, had no comfort with them and could not see well with or without them.

She was induced to buy Dr. Bates' book last March. She laid aside her glasses and began to work according to the method, wholly by herself, with most satisfactory results.

Very gratefully yours,
Fred W. Morris, D.O.,
Ridgewood, N. J.

Sunning, Sun-Gazing For Healthy Eyes, Mind, Body and Clear Eyesight

Sunning

Face the sun with the eyes closed and move the eyes, head/face & body slowly side to side, left and right.

Two little girls that learnt the Bates Method, obtained clear eyesight teach the Bates Method to a blind homeless man they found living outside under a bridge.
They cure the blindness, his eyesight and health are restored.
Treatment: Sunning, sunlight, palming, shifting and switching on letters on identical close and distant eyecharts, swinging, central fixation...
Children are often the best Natural Vision Improvement teachers.

His blindness cured, he now reads the newspaper, walks the city on his own, looks for a job and continues to practice the Bates Method.

Persons with normal sight can look directly at the sun without injury or discomfort. Note that the eyes are wide open, with no evidence of pain and no watering.

Emily C. Lierman (A. Bates) looking at the sun; Sunning with relaxation, shifting and blinking.

Most modern teachers advise only closed eyes sunning. Others allow the original open eyes method shown above by Emily C. Lierman. (Emily A. Bates, Dr. Bates Wife, Assistant in his New York City Clinic.) The eyes are kept in constant movement; eyes, head/face moving side to side and in other directions. Shift the eyes and blink when facing the sun. Blink often, relaxed, easy. Circle the sun counter-clockwise and clockwise, draw the Figure Eight, do the Sway, Long Swing. Close and open the eyes. Palm. See Dr. Bates Better Eyesight Magazine and the E-books for more pictures, directions for Sunning, Sun-Gazing, 'Saccadic Sunning' and drawing the Figure Eight correct.

The eye evolved in sunlight. The eyes and entire body; brain, all organs, systems, skin... need <u>pure full spectrum sunlight</u>, all frequencies, light waves to remain healthy, function correct, produce clear eyesight. Mood, sleep, absorption, creation and use of nutrients, chemical, hormone production-regulation, energy, chi, aura.., memory and all brain, body functions need full spectrum sunlight. Sunlight and raw organic apple cider vinegar and honey cures arthritis. Eyeglasses, sunglasses, tinted, colored, UV blocking eyeglasses, windows, all glass, plastic... blocks out part of the sun's light spectrum causing partial spectrum, unbalanced, unhealthy light to enter the eyes, brain and body. This lowers health and eyesight. Contact lenses completely seal over the cornea-pupil blocking out all full spectrum light.

Full spectrum sunlight destroys harmful bacteria, germs, mold.., protects the cornea, sclera, eyes from infection.

Picture below; Emily C. Lierman, A. Bates sunning her eyes.

From *Strengthening The Eyes*, the 1918 book-course by Dr. William H. Bates and Bernarr A. MacFadden.

Picture on right > From the early 1920 red and maroon editions of Dr. Bates book Perfect Sight Without Glasses.

Demonstrating again that the normal eye can regard the orb of day without injury. With the sun shining almost directly into her eye, the subject reads the Snellen test card with normal vision.

ARTIFICIAL LIGHT MAY BE BENEFICIAL

Like the sun, a strong electric light may also lower the vision temporarily, but never does any permanent harm. In those exceptional cases in which the patient can become accustomed to the light, it is beneficial. After looking at a

Additional page, photo from another 1920 edition.

WOMAN READING THE SNELLEN TEST CARD WITH NORMAL SIGHT WHILE THE SUN IS SHINING ALMOST DIRECTLY INTO HER EYE

strong electric light some patients have been able to read the Snellen test card better.

It is not light but darkness that is dangerous to the eye. Prolonged exclusion from the light always lowers the vision, and may produce serious inflammatory conditions. Among young children living in tenements this is a somewhat frequent cause of ulcers upon the cornea, which ulti-

light is one of the best curative agents we can employ for the eye. Persons with weak and defective eyes should gaze up in the direction of the sun every day, until they are able to look straight at it without pain or injury.

If the eyes are sensitive to sunlight from wearing eyeglasses, contact lenses, addiction to tinted or UV blocking lenses, sunglasses or just lack of sunlight exposure; start sunning with closed eyes. Then sun with one eye at a time. Equal time for each eye, alternating. When the eyes are comfortable in the sunlight; sun with both eyes together to keep the treatment, vision balanced.

Sunlight kills germs, bacteria, mold, heals injuries... It keeps the eyes healthy. A healthy diet improves the eyes, body's use of sunlight. Sunlight improves absorption of nutrients. Sunlight contains healthy natural vitamin D.

Artificial light is not as healthy as natural full spectrum sunlight. For indoor light; get sunlight into the room and use full spectrum light bulbs.

It is not light but darkness that is dangerous to the eye. Prolonged exclusion from the light always lowers the vision, and may produce serious inflammatory conditions. Among young children living in tenements this is a somewhat frequent cause of ulcers upon the cornea, which ultimately destroy the sight. The children, finding their eyes sensitive to light, bury them in the pillows and thus shut out the light entirely. The universal fear of reading or doing fine work in a dim light is, however, unfounded. So long as the light is sufficient so that one can see without discomfort, this practice is not only harmless, but may be beneficial.

DR. BATES SUNLIGHT TREATMENTS
(As described in Better Eyesight Magazine)

Shining direct sunlight on the sclera, the outer white part of the eye is a old treatment Dr. Bates applied to bring life, health, activity to the retina and its cells, cones, rods, nerves, blood vessels. Dr. Bates cured unclear vision and other eye problems, diseases with this treatment. People that were blind or almost blind would begin to see light and obtain clear vision as result of this treatment and other Bates activities.

Directions

Sunlight on the Sclera

Face the sun,
the eyes pupil directed away from the sun.

1 - Face the sun with the <u>eyes pupil directed away from the sun</u>. Allow full spectrum sunlight to shine directly on the sclera, (white part of the eye) by <u>pulling the upper eyelids up while looking down</u>. The sun shines on the upper white area of the eye. The eyes pupil is down, under the lower eyelid to prevent direct sunlight from shining into the pupil.

Move the eyes and head/face side to side to move the sunlight over the entire sclera and retina, lens through the sclera. Keep the sunlight moving on the sclera for a few seconds. Then stop, rest. Repeat if comfortable. Do not overdo it. Movement of the eyes, light places sunlight on all areas of the eye, retina, improves absorption, use of the light, activation of the retinas cells, light receptors... and prevents overexposure, concentration of the light, sunburn on the eye.

1 - Pull the upper eyelid up and look down.
Sunlight shines on the upper area of the Sclera.
Sunlight does not shine into the pupil.

When pulling the eyelid; do not touch the eye or eyelid. Pull on the skin above the eyelid. Keep fingernails very short. <u>Wash your hands first</u>. Avoid chemical based soap.
Do both eyes at the same time; left thumb pulls left lid, right thumb pulls right lid. Pull gently.
This treatment also helps the eye build normal tolerance to sunlight, improves health and color of the sclera, perception of light, color, clarity of vision.

2 - Pull the lower eyelid down and look up.
Sunlight shines on the lower area of the Sclera.
Sunlight does not shine in the pupil.

2 - Now, direct the sunlight onto the bottom of the sclera; <u>Pull the lower eyelids down, move the eye/pupil up in the opposite direction</u> so the sun shines on the lower area of the sclera and not directly into the pupil.

Expose left and right eyes to the sun at the same time.
Move the eyes left and right enabling the sun to shine/move on all areas of the Sclera.

Move the eyes, head/face side to side. Keep the sunlight moving on the sclera for a few seconds. Then stop, rest. The head/body may need to be tilted back a bit to keep sunlight on the lower sclera and away from the pupil. Practicing this treatment repeatedly can tense the eye muscles and the pull of the fingers can irritate the eyelids, skin. Use it occasionally.

Sun-Glass Treatment

Dr. Bates cured advanced eye problems, blindness by the sunlight methods and, also applying the use of the Sunglass to increase the strength of the sunlight on the eyes sclera and retina through the sclera. He moves the sunlight through the Sunglass quickly over the sclera for only a second, few seconds. He also moves the sunlight through the Sunglass on/over closed eyelids. <u>Light is not directed into the pupil</u>. Light on closed eyelids is done first. <u>The light is kept in movement</u> and <u>moved quickly on the sclera</u> and <u>not for too long; only a few seconds</u> in order to prevent over concentrating sunlight on any one or more areas of the eye, to prevent overexposure, sunburn on/in the eye. <u>Distance of the glass must be correct or the eye can be burned</u>.

The patient is exposed to plain sunlight first, without the glass to get the eyes adjusted to the light before using the sun-glass.
<u>Do not do this at home without an eye doctor's direction. Done incorrect, it can burn the eye.</u>

Concentrating the rays of the sun upon the eyeball with a lens or "burning glass," demonstrated to be an effective curative measure in conjunctivitis, iritis, ulcers of the cornea and other diseases of the eyes.

Closed-Eyes Sunning, then the Sunlight on the Sclera treatment (see picture top of page), then Open-Eyes Sunning are done first to adjust the eyes to bright light. Palm. THEN; CLOSED-EYES Sun-Glass Treatment is done FIRST before Open-Eyes Sun-Glass.
See the following pages for entire Closed and Open-Eyes Sunning, Sun-Glass directions. Find a Bates Method Ophthalmologist if you need the Sun-Glass treatment. If the eyes have been treated with surgery, medicine, drugs for the eyes, mind, body, any medical treatment; the patient may not be able to do certain sunlight treatments. Lasik and other cornea surgeries, possibly some lens surgeries impair the eyes' natural light refraction, control, absorption and use of sunlight. Sunlight can help some surgeries heal.

The Sun-Glass (Burning-Glass) Treatment is only for the blind, cases of advanced vision impairment. The sun-glass can burn the eye if done incorrect. It is a magnifying glass, it can set objects on fire! The sun-glass is a small convex lens ( ) magnifying glass, plus diopters. The eye doctor uses a specific size-number. When used correct it activates, brings function, life to the eye's retina, light receptors, nerves, lens... Closed Eyes Sun-Glass Treatment is applied first. It is the safest way to do the treatment and is often completely effective along with the other sunlight treatments without applying the Open-Eyes Sun-Glass. For both closed eyes and open eyes sun-glass treatment; precautions must be taken. Only an Ophthalmologist trained in this method should apply it. *All these conditions must be exact so the light emitted from the glass does not burn the eye;* Size, (length across the center of the circular glass from one side to the other), strength-diopter, thickness-amount of curvature of the convex magnifying glass, amount of magnification of the glass, the placement and angle of the glass and the distance the glass

Circle of light exiting the glass must be small enough to move upon the eye's sclera but not too small-bright or it will increase concentration of the light-heat and burn, injure the eye. A specific strength of light is needed to be effective, produce optimum benefit.

Only a Bates Method experienced Ophthalmologist should apply this treatment and determine the exact distance of the glass, it's size, strength, the size, strength of the light spot when shining the light on the eye's sclera to heal the eyes, vision. The correct treatment brings life, function to the cells, light receptors... in the eye of the blind and visually impaired.

Light circle exiting and focusing under the glass changes size; large, small, large... as the glass is moved far and close from the object the light rays are being placed upon. A smaller-brighter size 'usually' increases the heat, potential to burn the eye. This is a convex glass, plus lens of low diopters-strength.

is placed from the eye, size and strength of the light spot on the eye (sclera), how strong must the light be to be effective but also safe, not too hot. Do not use the sunglass in very strong sunlight. The brightness, strength of the sun speeds and increases the heat of the light through the sunglass posing a risk of burning the eye. Strength of the sun-time of day, area on planet, ozone layer state and other conditions affect the heat of the light spot, it's potential to burn, injure the eye. Precision, perfect application must be applied. After distance of the glass is determined, then the doctor determines placement of the glass; above the eye by the forehead, eyebrow or top sclera. Do not shine the light into the eye's pupil! When applying Open Eyes Sunglass (One eye at a time. Patch the other eye.); the eye looks far down with the pupil protected, covered by the lower eyelid. The upper eyelid is lifted. The Sun-glass light spot is then moved quickly, continuously for only a few seconds on the upper white area of the eye, on the sclera only. Keep the glass moving-the light spot in **constant rapid movement** upon the eye's sclera for a short time; **Open Eyes; only a few seconds; 2- 3 seconds, Closed Eyes; part of a minute; 10-15 seconds.** Movement of the light helps prevent heat, burns and activates all parts of the sclera and inside the eye, retina... PREVENT HEAT but get a good beam of light, not too strong but effective enough to activate the cells, light receptors... in the eye. Avoid placing strong, concentrated light on the cornea. See pictures > **(Read entire tests, directions below before using sunglass.)**

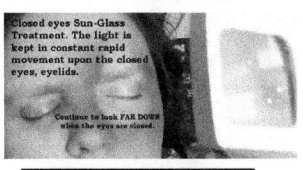

TEST the light strength, distance of the magnifying glass first; Test the strength of the sunlight 'heat' through the glass on a piece of paper first, then on the hand's skin to determine the distance the glass is to be placed to control the strength of the light, avoid heat so it does not burn the skin. The distance of the glass changes the size of the spot of light emitted from the glass. The distance of the glass, size, brightness of the light spot circle affects the strength-intensity of the light, heat and the speed that the light spot becomes hot, can set things on fire. This is concentrated energy.., light waves. Test the distance; move the glass far away from the paper; the light is big and not very strong. When the glass is moved closer to the paper, the light spot turns into a small very bright circle of light and is very hot, burns the paper and hand quickly. This is the dangerous light. At very close distances, 1½... inches, the circle becomes large again, the heat is reduced but still burns the hand. Give it time on the paper, then hand/skin to be sure of the distance; Test, find the distance with the sun-glass light immobile on the hand without burning it, feeling no heat for 30 seconds. Then test at the same distance on the hand 1 minute with the glass-light moving. If no heat, no burn when it is immobile for 30 seconds and when moving it for 1 minute; that might be the safe distance to use the sunglass on the eye (sclera) for a few seconds. This is only a home test. The Ophthalmologist will measure it perfectly.

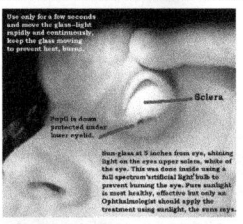

I prefer a small round glass for an even circle of light as shown in Dr. Bates sun-glass picture on the right. > For the experiment below and above I used a small square magnifier. Below; test with pure sunlight. Above; example using a light bulb. Other size, strength magnifiers will act differently. More information with large color pictures are in the free PDF E-books. Picture below on the far right > shows a test using a full spectrum light bulb, closer glass, smaller stronger light spot on closed eyes. The light bulb is not completely natural, it is less beneficial than pure sunlight. Read the Sunglass, Partial Light warning on the following pages.

(In the experiment below for this glass; 5-4 inches might be the correct light, distance. See large pictures on the next page.)

   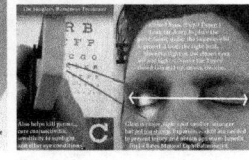

1st tests; in pictures #1 to 5 above (light immobile) were done in Worcester, Massachusetts, USA on April 24th, 2013 at 5:30-6:00 PM on a sunny day, no clouds. When the light was immobile it burned the hand on some tests-distances, mainly with the smaller, brighter lights.
2nd tests; #1 to 5; the light was moving continual, rapidly on the hand for 10 seconds; I felt heat (mostly from the smaller, brighter lights) but it did not burn my hand.

THE EYE WILL BE MORE SENSITIVE to the light, heat so additional adjustments are needed to prevent injury when the light shines on the white area of the eye and also when shining the light on closed eyelids. Do not allow heat to occur because it can quickly turn to fire. You want only the concentrated 'but not too concentrated, not too strong' light beam circle on the eye's sclera. (Test the strength of the moving light on the forehead, then closed eyelids first before moving the light on the open eye's sclera.) Time the light is on the eye affects intensity of the heat; Short time=less heat. Rapid continual movement of the glass-keeping the light spot moving on the sclera helps prevent heat. Pictures are a basic example. Ask the eye doctor for the exact distance, placement... of the glass. Practice the entire Bates Method to gain clear eyesight. Do not rely solely on the sun-glass, sunning.

For picture on the far right > bottom page; When using the sunglass on closed eyes; continue to look FAR DOWN under the closed eyes to protect the pupil. Adjust sunglass distance to reduce strength-heat of the light. The light can be moved back and forth in small circles across both eyes when the eyes are closed.

Larger *Sun-Glass* Pictures-Directions. For Ophthalmologist Only to Treat the Blind, Semi-Blind.

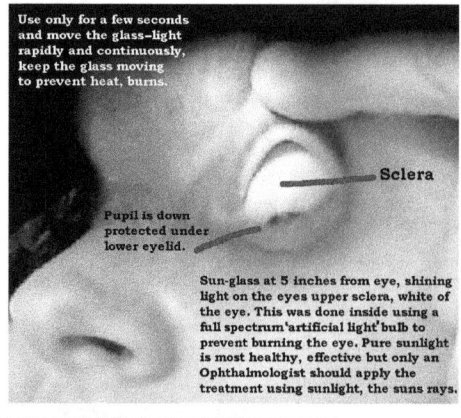

Use only for a few seconds and move the glass-light rapidly and continuously, keep the glass moving to prevent heat, burns.

Sclera

Pupil is down protected under lower eyelid.

Sun-glass at 5 inches from eye, shining light on the eyes upper sclera, white of the eye. This was done inside using a full spectrum 'artificial light' bulb to prevent burning the eye. Pure sunlight is most healthy, effective but only an Ophthalmologist should apply the treatment using sunlight, the suns rays.

Done inside with a full spectrum light bulb as a source of light in place of the sun to help prevent heat, burns. Pure sunlight is best, healthiest for the eyes.
Only a Bates Method Ophthalmologist should apply this treatment.
Using sunlight, it can cure blindness, eyelid, iris, cornea, eye inflammation, cataract, glaucoma and other conditions.

The light spot is smaller and the light is stronger when the glass is closer to the eye. Requires precision, expert application to prevent burns.

Look far down, pupil under the lower eyelid, protected from the light.

Sun-glass is closer in this picture – 4 to 4½ inches. This makes the light spot smaller, easier to shine only on the sclera but the light is stronger. Precision must be used to prevent burning the eye. Keep the glass moving to avoid heat, burns. Use only for a few seconds and move the glass, light rapidly and continuously to prevent heat, burns.

1
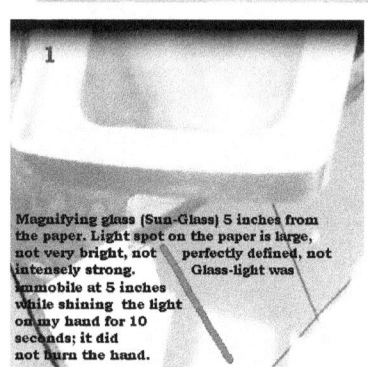

Magnifying glass (Sun-Glass) 5 inches from the paper. Light spot on the paper is large, not very bright, not perfectly defined, not intensely strong. Glass-light was immobile at 5 inches while shining the light on my hand for 10 seconds; it did not burn the hand.

A bigger, stronger glass will burn the hand. If the glass, light is constantly moved; that helps to prevent heat, but heat, burns can still occur depending upon the glass strength, size, distance...

2
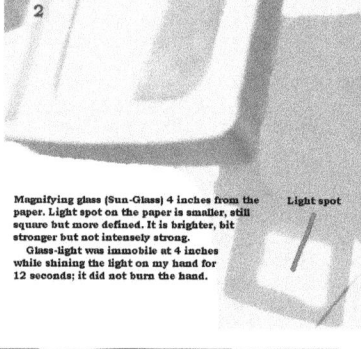

Magnifying glass (Sun-Glass) 4 inches from the paper. Light spot on the paper is smaller, still square but more defined. It is brighter, bit stronger but not intensely strong.
Glass-light was immobile at 4 inches while shining the light on my hand for 12 seconds; it did not burn the hand.

Light spot

3

Magnifying glass (Sun-Glass) 3 inches from the paper. Light spot on the paper is much smaller, more defined, starting to form a circle. It is much brighter, stronger.
Glass-light was immobile at 3 inches while shining the light on my hand for 3 seconds; it burned the hand.

At 2½ inches the light became smaller, turned into a very bright circle and burned my hand quickly before 3 seconds.

Light spot

For this magnifier; this begins the danger distance; here and closer the light can burn, injure the eye. (Farther distances at 3½ to 5, 7... inches can still burn the eye. Strength of the sun effects the heat.)

4

Magnifying glass (Sun-Glass) 2 inches from the paper. Light spot on the paper is very small, defined, formed into a small circle. Light is very bright, strong.
Glass-light was immobile at 2 inches while shining the light on my hand for 3 seconds; it burned the hand before 3 seconds, more than at 2½ inches. Heat, burn was more intense, quick.

Light Spot

5

Magnifying glass (Sun-Glass) 1¾ to 1 inch from the paper. Light spot on the paper turns into a large well defined square as the glass moves closer. The light is bright, still strong but less strong than at 3 to 2 inches. It is stronger and smaller than the square at 5 inches.
Glass-light was immobile at 1 to 1¾ inches while shining the light on my hand for 10 seconds; it started to burn the hand at about 10 seconds.

Light spot

Do not place the sunglass-light on the eye at any close, warm-hot distances. Even though the light, heat is less strong at certain distances it can still burn, injure the eye.

Move the eye-pupil more downward than shown in this picture. It is best for the lower eyelid to completely cover the eyes pupil. Picture may have a defect making it 'appear' that part of the pupil is exposed or this way is safe because the light is at an angle not shining into the pupil.

The Sunglass, Blindness Treatment

Closed Eyes. (Pupil Down.)
Look far down to place the pupil down, under the lower eyelid to protect it from the light-heat.
Move the light on the closed eyes; left and right < > over the 2 eyes closed lids and up, down, circular.

Also helps kill germs., cure conjunctivitis, sensitivity to sunlight and other eye conditions.

Glass is closer, light spot smaller, stronger but not too strong. Experience, skill are needed to prevent injury and obtain optimum benefit. Find a Bates Method Ophthalmologist.

Closed Eyes (Pupil down) Sun-Glass Treatment
Move the light on the closed eyes.

Glass is closer, light spot smaller, stronger but not extreme. Experience, skill are needed to prevent injury.

Closed eyes Sun-Glass Treatment. The light is kept in constant rapid movement upon the closed eyes, eyelids.

Continue to look FAR DOWN when the eyes are closed.

< Picture left; Sun-glass example using light from a full spectrum light bulb on closed eyes.
For the sun; move the glass farther away, making the light circle lighter, bigger, weaker strength.
Albinos; check with your medical and eye doctor first before trying any sunlight treatment.

Directions, Examples from Dr. Bates Better Eyesight Magazine;

THE normal eye needs light in order to maintain normal health and normal sight. People who do not see the sun always have eye trouble. Miners working in the dark all day long, and never seeing the sun, all have trouble with their eyes. Children living in dark tenement houses acquire a great sensitiveness to the light, and spend most of their time holding a cloth up to their eyes, or they bury their heads in a pillow, shutting out all light. They acquire many kinds of inflammation of the eyelids, and of the eyeball. The burning glass has a very wonderful effect on some of these cases. I remember one man who had not been able to do any work because of the sensitiveness of his eyes to the light. He was very promptly cured by a few minutes exposure of the eyeball to the strong light of the burning glass.

In using the burning glass, it is well to prepare the eyes of the patient by having him sit in the sun with his eyes closed. Enough light shines through the eyelid to cause some people a great deal of discomfort at first, but after a few hours' exposure in this way, they become able to gradually open their eyes to some extent without squeezing the lids. When this stage is reached, one can focus with the burning glass, the light on the outside of the eyeballs, which at first is very disagreeable! When the patient becomes able to open the eyes, he is directed to look as far down as possible, and this can be done in such a way that the pupil is protected by the lower lid. It is not well to use the burning glass when the patient squeezes the eyelids shut. As long as the light is focused on the white of the eye, and is done quickly, all heat is avoided. The length of time devoted to focusing the light on the white part of the eye, is never longer than a few seconds, moving the light from side to side, up and down, or in various directions.

WITHIN the past few months we have received innumerable inquiries regarding the use of the burning glass. It is well known that the sun strengthens the eyes, and with the aid of the burning glass the direct rays of the sun are focused on the sclera.

By persistence in looking at the sun, a person with normal sight soon becomes able to do so without any loss of vision; but persons with imperfect sight usually find it impossible to accustom themselves to such a strong light until their vision has been improved by other means. One has to be very careful in recommending sun-gazing to persons with imperfect sight; because, although no permanent harm can result from it, great temporary discomfort may be produced, with no permanent benefit. In some rare cases, however, complete cures have been effected by this means alone.

In one of these cases the sensitiveness of the patient, even to ordinary daylight, was so great that an eminent specialist had felt justified in putting a black bandage over one eye and covering the other with a smoked glass so dark as to be nearly opaque. She was kept in this condition of almost total blindness for two years without any improvement. Other treatment extending over some months also failed to produce satisfactory results. She was then advised to look directly at the sun. The immediate result was total blindness, which lasted several hours; but next day the vision was not only restored to its former condition, but was improved. The sun-gazing was repeated, and each time the blindness lasted for a shorter period. At the end of a week the patient was able to look directly at the sun without discomfort, and her vision, which had been 20/200 without glasses and 20/70 with them, had improved to 20/10, twice the accepted standard for normal vision.

Have you ever noticed that upon emerging from a dark room into a strongly lighted one, or from the dark movies into the sunlight, that you are temporarily blinded? This should not be. The normal eye accommodates to the varying conditions, and if it fails to do so the vision is defective. The burning glass accustoms the patient to the strong sunlight, and strengthens the eye.

Q—Is the effect of the burning glass and that of sunshine falling on closed eyelids different, so that one needs both kinds each day?
A—The sun treatment with the burning glass is more intensive than without it. At first, patients become accustomed to strong light by sitting in the sun and allowing the sun's rays to shine directly on the closed eyelids, as they slowly move their heads a short distance from side to side. Then, with the burning glass, the strong light of the sun is focused on the closed eyelids, and when the eyes are accustomed to that, one can consider the advisability of focusing the direct rays of the sun upon the eyeball, itself. This is done by lifting the upper lid while the patient looks down. When the sun is focused upon the naked eyeball, one should keep moving the glass from side to side, and for a short time only, so as not to produce discomfort from the heat.

Note by Clark Night; I notice in some doctors' directions for using the sun-glass with CLOSED EYES; they do not say to look far down. I advise looking far down for safety, even when the eyes are closed. Allowing the eyes to look to another direction when they are closed; up, down, sideways, corners... enables the sun-glass light to shine through the closed eyelids onto more areas of the sclera; top, bottom, sides.., but; NEVER place the light on the eye's pupil (even when the eyes are closed). If the doctor prefers to also move the closed eyes to a new position; remove the sun-glass. Then use the sun-glass-apply the light AFTER the closed eyes are in the new position and the pupil is covered-protected. Never place the sunglass and it's light in front of-on the eye's pupil when the eyes are closed or open. Look far down when using the sun-glass with the eyes open. No other direction.

When the eyes are inflamed from disease of the eyelids, the cornea, the iris, the retina, the optic nerve, from glaucoma and other inflammations, the use of the burning glass (sun-glass) has been followed immediately by a lessening of the congestion and a decided improvement in vision.

Many people ask the question: "How long does it take to obtain a sufficient benefit to be noticeable?" When the sun treatment is employed, the improvement in the sight may be demonstrated in a very short time. The sun treatment improves the vision of all patients who are wearing glasses for the relief of pain, fatigue, and imperfect sight, no matter what kind of glasses are worn or how strong they may be. (Do not wear eyeglasses, contact lenses, sunglasses... during any type of sunlight treatment.)

The direct sunlight focused on the white part of the eye is a benefit in many cases of blindness with hardening of the eyeball (glaucoma), or softening of the eyeball (cyclitis), also in cases of cataract, and of opacities in other parts of the eye. It was interesting to observe the improvement in a large number of patients blind from scar tissue on the front part of the eye, the cornea. They were benefited so much that their sight became normal. (Be careful using telescopes, binoculars... My friend burned his cornea, developed a cornea scar that blocked part of his vision due to looking at the bright sky, near the sun with a telescope. The previous user forgot to place the eye protection piece back into the telescope.)

One of the best treatments is to focus the strong light of the sun on the white part of the eye with the aid of a burning glass (sun-glass), which is kept moving from side to side to prevent the discomfort of the heat, while the patient is looking far down. In many cases treatment has accomplished in a few minutes a complete cure of sensitiveness to light. Paul was a boy who came for treatment. His father telephoned before sending his son, telling me that the school authorities had insisted very strongly that he get glasses for Paul, but the father refused to submit to such a thing, until he was sure that nothing else could be done. Paul had never worn glasses and when they were suggested to him, if Dr. Bates could not help him, he wept bitter tears and at times was disobedient, which sometimes called for punishment. Paul came with a written statement from his mother, saying that at the age of five years, he was taken ill with measles and after that sties appeared at intervals, causing an almost constant inflammation of the eyelids. Because Paul had played with a child who was supposed to have an incurable eye trouble, Paul's mother feared that he had acquired this incurable disease also. His eyelids were itchy most of the time and at the advice of an eye doctor a solution of boric acid was used and a medicine called "mecca" was also applied. Paul found some relief from the use of these applications, but the sties appeared just the same and he noticed that the letters on the blackboard at school became less distinct at such times. In 1928 he had scarlet fever, and pink eye began three months previous to his visit to me. Paul's vision with each eye was 10/10 but he strained to see as he read the smaller letters of the test card. The sun was shining through the windows in the room where I was treating him. I placed him in the sun with his eyes closed and used the sun-glass rapidly on the edge of his eyelids as well as on the upper and lower lids. This was about midday, and the sun was rather hot so I had to use the glass very *rapidly* in order to avoid any discomfort or burning of the lids. His elder brother who came with him remarked how well the eyelids looked after the sun treatment. This was accomplished in less than an hour's time. After the sun treatment, I placed the test card ten feet. He read the smallest letters without any effort or strain. Again I placed him in the sun and taught his elder brother how to use the sun-glass while I was occupied with something else. We had to keep Paul busy while he was resting this way, because he was restless and being a perfectly normal healthy boy did not like being quiet. He told me a funny tale and then in turn I told him one and in this way we passed the time away. Finally after another half hour of sun treatment, Paul read all the tests cards with different letters at fifteen feet from his eyes without any trouble whatever. The irritation of the eyelids had disappeared and the itching had stopped, but Paul was told that this might be only a temporary relief and that he would have to take a good deal of sun treatment before he was finally rid of his trouble. He promised to take all the sun treatment he could possibly get by placing himself in the sun, and raising his head so that the sun could shine on his closed eyelids. He was given a test card to practice with daily and to use to show his mother how far away he could read it while blinking and swaying his body from side to side to avoid the stare. Paul and his brother promised to notify Dr. Bates if he needed further help, or if he had any further discomfort with his eyes. Two weeks later, his elder brother came to report that apparently Paul was cured in one treatment because no further complaints came from the school about his having to wear glasses nor did the irritation of the eyelids reappear. I am sure that Paul himself takes time enough for the sun treatment whenever there is sun, because he promised me faithfully that he would do so without troubling any member of his family.

Question - a - How often should the sun-glass be used? **b** - How long on the closed lids before using it on the eyeballs themselves? **c** - Can one use the sunglass on one's own eyes? **Answer - a** - Daily for two or three minutes. (Clarification; minutes are too long for open eyes. Do two or three *seconds* at a time for open eyes; apply, rest one minute, apply. Applying the sunglass for only a few seconds prevents burning the eye. On closed eyes the time can be increased to part of a minute, 5-10 seconds at a time; apply, rest 30+ seconds, apply. Dr. Bates' answer; "two or three minutes" means *the total daily combined time for the closed and open eyes sunning* in intervals; seconds, rest, seconds.) **b** - Usually for several weeks on the closed lids before using it on the eyeballs themselves, although the length of time varies with each individual case.
c - Some people can, but it is rather difficult and awkward to do. In my experience, the wearing of dark glasses or the use of other methods to reduce the glare of strong daylight or artificial light is an injury rather than a benefit. One of the best methods to relieve or prevent the intolerance of all kinds of light is to encourage the individual to become accustomed to strong light. **Sunglass - A convex glass of about 18 D** is very useful in these cases. One way to use the glass is to have the patient look far downwards while the instructor lifts the upper lid of the eyeball with the help of the thumb. This procedure exposes a considerable amount of the sclera.

The strong light of the sun is now focused on the white sclera for only *short periods of time* to prevent the heat produced by the strong glass from causing discomfort. (To be safe, I use a much lower D. 'diopter' than 18 D. Check with a professional Bates Method Ophthalmologist)

Dr. Bates examined a patient with the ophthalmoscope and found Keratitis, or inflammation of the front of the eyeball of the left eye. The right eye was normal. While the examination was going on, Albert's sister was weeping. She tried very hard to conceal her tears but in vain. They had been to other doctors and were told that Albert would always have to wear glasses to save the right eye; nothing more could be done for the left eye. The last oculist they consulted said the left eye had cataract and as there was no sight, there was no use to operate. What a shock it was to his family!

I placed Albert in the sun and focused the sunglass on his closed eyelid. Then I raised the upper lid and quickly focused the strong light of the sun on the white part of the eye as he looked down. Immediately he called out to his sister: "I see the light. I can see a sort of web inside of my eye when the light is focused on it." This made me very happy indeed. I knew then that Albert could be benefited.

The light through the sunglass is constantly moving and is used for a short time to prevent the sun from burning the eye.
(Closed eyes sun-glass treatment can be longer; part of a minute. Open eyes sun-glass treatment on the sclera is always only for a few seconds. The light is always moved rapidly and continuously on closed eyes sclera and on the open eyes sclera.)

Another one had irritated eyelids, the appearance of which was worse than the discomfort or pain that the boy experienced. He blinked more rapidly than the normal eye does unconsciously. Sun treatment was given to him also. When the mother saw that he had obtained a noticeable amount of relief from the first treatment, she purchased a sunglass and under my supervision she learned how to use the glass on his closed eyelids and in this way all he needed was the one treatment. Note by Clark Night; People use the glass with their family due to most eye doctors hiding this cure.

Dr. Bates discovered many years ago the benefit of strong light on the eyes and I have seen many patients cured by the sun treatment alone. Some of these cases were seriously affected because of their inability to stand even the rays of the sun. It is curious but true that this patient has been benefited mostly by a magnifying glass which focused the light on the white part of each eye as he looked down while the upper lid was raised. In the beginning of his treatment the mere mention of light would make him frown and shrink with fear. Now he enjoys sitting in the sun all day long and realizes that it gives him the greatest benefit. He is steadily improving. While he is not entirely cured, he reads the bottom line of the test card occasionally at ten feet.

Sun treatment is an immediate benefit to many diseases of the eye. Before the treatment, take a record of your best vision of the Snellen test card with both eyes together and each eye separately without glasses. Then sit in the sun with your eyes closed, slowly moving your head a short distance from side to side, and allowing the sun to shine directly on your closed eyelids. Forget about your eyes; just think of something pleasant and let your mind drift from one pleasant thought to another. Before opening your eyes, palm for a few minutes. Then test your vision of the test card and note the improvement. Get as much sun treatment as you possibly can, one, two, three or more hours daily. When the sun is not shining, substitute a strong electric light. A 1,000 watt electric light is preferable, but requires special wiring. However, a 250 watt or 300 watt light can be used with benefit, and does not require special wiring. (Full spectrum bulbs, no fluorescent) Sit about six inches from the light, or as near as you can without discomfort from the heat, allowing it to shine on your closed eyelids as in the sun treatment. (Warning; light bulbs can suddenly burn out and break throwing glass into the eye. Avoid other people, pets, clutter so the bulb is not accidently broken by people, pets running by... Do not practice during a lighting storm which can blow out, shatter the electric bulb. Avoid high heat bulbs... that can burn the eyes, skin. NO tanning booths!)

The strong light of the sun focused on the sclera, or white part of the eyeball, with the sun-glass, also improves the vision. After the eyes have become accustomed to the sunlight with the <u>eyes closed</u>, focus the light of the sun on the <u>closed eyelids</u> with the sun-glass. <u>Move the glass rapidly from side to side while doing this for a few minutes.</u> *NOTE: When looking down, pupil protected under the eyelid; do it gently. No force!*

Then have the patient <u>open his eyes</u> and <u>look as far down as possible</u>, and in this way, <u>the pupil is protected by the lower lid</u>. Gently lift the upper lid so that only the white part of the eye is exposed, as the sun's rays fall directly upon this part of the eyeball. The sun-glass may now be used on the white part of the eye for a *few seconds*, moving it quickly from side to side and in various directions. Notice that after the use of the sun-glass, the vision is improved. When the light is on the sclera, it is normal to see a reflection of the blood vessels in the eye.

Whenever possible she was placed in the sun, and the sunlight was focused on her closed eyelids with the sun-glass. This always improved her vision. When there was no sun, I placed her close to a strong electric light for a half hour or longer. She liked this treatment because the sunlight was so restful to her, and she could read the test card at ten feet. *More of Dr. Bates sun-glass, sunlight articles can be found in his Better Eyesight Magazines by searching in the PDF for; Sunglass, Sun-Glass, Burning Glass, Sun Treatment.*

The Eye is a Natural Sun-Glass

Plain sunlight, closed and open-eyes sunning and sunlight on the sclera <u>without the sun-glass</u> is all that is needed in most cases to return the vision to perfect clarity with healthy eyes. Plain open-eyes and closed-eyes sunning, daily sunlight with the natural eye is the healthiest way to obtain sunlight. The eyes' lens is a double convex ( ) lens. See picture on right. >
It is a perfect, natural, safe sun-glass (burning glass)! The eyes' cornea is also convex. The cornea, aqueous, lens, vitreous... control the amount, focus of light entering and in the eye. The cornea, lens, eye... are the exact shape, thickness, curvature, (diopters) strength, distance, position to perfectly focus-refract, concentrate sunlight in the eyes and on the retina.

For Sun-Gazing, Sunning, Sunlight Practice (No Sun-Glass) ;

Tension, strain can lower the eyes' natural function with sunlight. The mind, body, eyes must be relaxed, happy positive thoughts. Keep good and easy relaxed posture. Avoid twisting the neck, tilting the head to one side. Avoid tensing the face, head, neck muscles. No squinting, staring. Relax, allow movement. Teeth apart-not clenched together. Deep but relaxed, comfortable abdominal breathing. Nose in and out breathing is most relaxing, beneficial. If it is more comfortable; breathe out through the nose and mouth. Yawn to stretch, relax the neck, head... muscles and produce healthy tears. Deep breathing, yawning induces relaxation and brings oxygen, blood, lymph, energy flow to the head, eyes, body.
The brighter the sunlight, the more it relaxes the eyes, mind and body. The best, brightest sunlight is when it's strong, high in the sky; 11am-1pm, but sunburn occurs faster at this time. Also, the head has to be tilted up more and this can tense the neck, unless you sit or lay back. Sunning is best with bare feet on the bare dirt or grass ground because this connects the body with the planet's energy. Native Americans lean against a tree to connect with it's energy into the earth and up into the sky, heaven. Deep breathing strengthens the energy. Sunlight is energy. Full spectrum sunlight contains all colors, frequencies, energy of the light spectrum even more than seen in the rainbow. See the E-book color chart chapter for chi energy circulation, strengthening, movement. Area of the planet, ozone layer should be considered when sunning when the sun is brightest, strongest. When sunning (open and closed eyes), move the head and eyes side to side, up and down... and; see oppositional movement 'the swing' of the sun; the sun appears to move opposite of the direction the eyes, head move to. Shift and blink. Shift the eyes, head across the sun left and right, up, down, diagonally from one side of the sun to the other. Shift to the left and right, top, bottom... area of the sky around the sun. Do the long swing and sway at sunrise and sunset; swing, rock left and right and see the sun appear to move opposite. This helps blind people regain their vision. Practice swaying with the sun shining through a fence to activate massage and saccadic eye movements. (see e-book) Do the figure eight.

Avoid staring at the sun. Do not keep the eyes 'vision' on one area of the sun longer than a fraction of a second. Always keep the eyes (and head with the eyes) moving 'shifting' to a new part of the sun or to the sky every fraction of a second. A continual easy movement. Keep the eyes (where you are looking) moving on and across the sun and sky. Look away from the sun to the sky often. Blink, blink, blink. Staring 'eye immobility' causes eyestrain, eye muscle tension and unclear vision. When the eyes are strained, stare immobile; sunlight feels uncomfortable, is over concentrated on the retina and causes colored light-spots in the visual field lasting for a while. If the sun makes the eyes feel like they need to close 'sleepy'; close the eyes, take a break. Do closed eyes sunning. Take your time building tolerance to open-eyes sunlight. Note; *Sun-Gazing* does NOT mean to stare at the sun, eyes immobile. Always keep the eyes, head moving and look away from the sun often. Limit time the eyes look directly at the sun to a few seconds.

Sun-Glass Basic Directions Page

THE USE OF THE SUN GLASS

In using the sun glass, it is well to accustom the eyes of the patient to the strong light by having him sit in the sun with his eyes closed, and at the same time he should slowly move his head from side to side, in order to avoid discomfort from the heat. Enough light shines through the eyelid to cause some people a great deal of discomfort at first, but after a few hours' exposure in this way, they become able to gradually open their eyes to some extent without squeezing the lids. When this stage is reached, one can focus, with the aid of the sun glass, the light on the closed eyelids, which at first is very disagreeable. When the patient becomes able to open the eyes, he is directed to look as far down as possible, and in this way the pupil is protected by the lower lid. Then by gently lifting the upper lid, only the white part of the eye is exposed, while the sun's rays strike directly upon this part of the eyeball. The sun glass may then be used on the white part of the eye. Care should be taken to move the glass from side to side quickly. The length of time devoted to focusing the light on the white part of the eye is never longer than a few seconds. After such a treatment the patient almost immediately becomes able to open his eyes widely in the light.

Most Modern Natural Eyesight Improvement Teachers do not apply the Sunglass Treatment -(Mainly due to fear of the AMA.) Ophthalmologist Bates cured many vision problems, eye diseases, various types of blindness with the Sunglass and Sunlight, Sunning Treatments. Try plain Sunning, Sunlight first.

The Sun-Glass Treatment is to be done by an experienced Bates Method Ophthalmologist, only if necessary in cases of blindness, advanced vision impairment and only after closed eyes and open eyes sunning, daily sunlight exposure; eyes open, looking at, shifting on the bright sunny sky, clouds, trees and other Bates Method Treatments have been tried first.

(Never stare at the sun. See entire directions for the different sunlight treatments in this book.)

If these have not brought light perception, complete vision improvement; the Sun-Glass Treatment may.

Caution; Be aware that certain types of glass... act as a magnifying glass. The sun-glass is a magnifier. Sunlight through the Sun-glass <u>can burn the eye</u> if applied wrong.

Only a professional should apply this method;

The glass is never still; the glass is moved continually side to side... causing the light to move quickly on the top white area of the eye. A short time; only a few seconds of light is placed on the eye. Do one eye at a time.

(Patch the eye not being treated with a thick white eyepatch to prevent the eye, pupil from contact with the light of the Sun-glass. Keep the patch open on the <u>outer face side away from the glass</u> to allow plain daylight into that eye to keep both brain hemispheres, eyes active.)

Do not wear any type of eyeglasses, contact lenses, sunglasses, tinted, colored, UV blocking lenses when using the Sun-Glass, open and closed eyes Sunning.

Distance of the glass from the eye must be exact, a specific distance. The time the light is on the eye (white area, <u>sclera only</u>, through eyelids or eyes open) must be brief, a few seconds so the eye is not burned.

It is a certain type of magnifying glass; type, size, thickness, curvature... of the glass, distance, angle from the eye, strength of the sun affects the strength, intensity, concentration of the light rays beam, heat of the sunlight through the glass. The heat increases when the time the light is on the eye increases. The correct amount is relaxing, healthy for the eyes and improves the vision.

<u>The light must never shine on/into the eyes' pupil.</u> Keep the light away from the pupil, iris. Keep the eye, pupil far down, under the lower lid to prevent the light beam from shining into the pupil. Do not move the eyes when the Sun-glass light is on the eye's sclera.

DO NOT BURN THE CORNEA! Keep the light away from it.

Test the intensity of the light, heat, distance of the glass... on the hand, then forehead, then closed eyelids first. <u>Then: Start with eyes closed</u>, look <u>far down</u>. Bring the glass-light beam close, but a safe distance from the eye. <u>Move the light beam</u> on the white area of the eyeball through the closed eyelids. The movement helps to prevent heat. Through closed eyes; notice the size of the light spot on the eye and the blood vessels... in the eye's sclera, retina. Keep the light moving, move it quickly on the upper sclera for a few seconds. (Light is kept *away from the eye's pupil*. Yes, even when the eyes are closed; look far down and keep the light far away from the pupil.)

When the *eyes are closed*; do one eye at a time, and then the light may also be moved over both closed eyes together; side to side, up, down, diagonally, small circles. Also get some light on the eyelids and eyelash area.

<u>Then: Use the Sun-glass with the eyes open;</u> still looking <u>far down</u>, eyes' pupil under the lower eyelid, protected from the light. Do one eye at a time; lift the upper eyelid and move the light quickly side to side, small circles... a few seconds on the white area, upper sclera of the eye. Then repeat the steps with the other eye.

The Sun-glass is a glass. As described on other pages, chapters; all glass, plastic... eyeglasses, windows, sunglasses, contact lenses block out part of the sun's light spectrum causing unhealthy partial spectrum, unbalanced light to exit the glass and travel into the eyes, brain and body. Abnormal energy, chemical reactions also occur. This impairs health, function of the eyes, brain, body and lowers the clarity of vision. For this reason the sun-glass is only used to get the cells, light receptors, capillaries... in the eye, retina, lens back to full life, activity, to bring the vision back. Then the sun-glass is not used. Plain sunlight not passing through glass, plastic is used by practicing open and closed eyes Sunning as described in this chapter.

Sunlight relaxes the eye muscles. Relaxed eye muscles move the eyes easy, <u>perfect shifting</u> and returns the eyes to normal shape with correct focus of light rays on the retina. Sunlight can be a quick cure, speeds eyesight improvement but it is essential that all of Dr. Bates practices are studied and applied to maintain clear eyesight.

Read more directions for Sunning, Sun-Gazing, Sun-glass Treatments in the Natural Eyesight Improvement E-book; Ophthalmologist Bates 'Better Eyesight Magazine' describes this treatment. See; Better Eyesight Magazine; April, May, June, August, October, December, 1926 and November, 1924 and other

'Use of the Sun-Glass, Burning Glass' articles. Better Eyesight article June, 1926 in original antique print is shown on the previous page.

I place the instructions here due to the many cures Dr. Bates, Emily Lierman/Bates and other doctors obtained with the Sun-glass and to enable people to know if their eye doctor is doing the treatment correct and safe. *If a blind person cannot find a doctor; his-her family may learn to apply it and cure the blindness.*

Sun-Gazing; Looking into the sun with the eyes open, while moving the eyes, head/face side to side, keeping the eyes, head/face in movement 'shifting' is still done by some people in various countries, cultures. For sun-gazers that look at the sun with the eyes open; Practice only for 5-10 seconds at a time, always moving the head/face, eyes; shifting side to side, top and bottom... across the sun. Blink often.
Never stare into the sun. Application time may vary with certain cultures, countries, treatments by experts.

Avoid areas where the sunlight is concentrated-very strong and where the ozone layer is depleted. Looking at the sun at sunrise, sunset in safe areas of the planet is allowed as long as staring, over-exposure is avoided. People have been looking at the sky, sunrise, sunset for millions of years with benefit.

Due to depletion of the ozone layer, Modern Bates Teachers do not advise looking into the sun with the eyes open. <u>Closed Eyes Sunning only is practiced</u>. Albinos; check with your doctor first for all sunlight treatment.

Looking at the bright areas of the sky, clouds, tree tops <u>with the eyes open</u> on a sunny day is allowed.
Do not look at or near the sun during a solar eclipse of the sun.
Reflections of sunlight off snow, water and high altitudes increase the sun's strength and chance of eye, skin sunburn. Get used to stronger light a little at a time. Build tolerance. Native African's don't wear sunglasses! Their vision is clear, skin normal. Redheads-light skin needs clothing skin protection, a gradual exposure.

Good nutrition is necessary to maintain the eyes' natural protection-tolerance to sunlight. Sunlight through the eyes and on the skin is necessary to enable the body to absorb, create, function with nutrients, vitamin D, other vitamins, calcium.., minerals and protect the eyes, skin from sunburn, over-exposure to sunlight and to produce-balance-control hormones, chemicals in the brain, body, organs, systems, including melatonin for a normal sleep cycle and serotonin, tryptophan... for a positive state of mind, good mood, happy thoughts, emotions. The eyes need sunlight to remain healthy, keep the vision clear. Most drugs and some herbs impair the vision, eyes' health and natural use of light, light tolerance, protection from over-exposure to sunlight.

Chi, the body's electrical-magnetic energy flow is strengthened by sunlight.
Sunlight contains all colors, frequencies, energy of the light spectrum.

People that had eye surgery (the eye's lens altered, removed, replaced, prescription implants), cornea surgery (part of the cornea removed or altered) or other eye surgeries might not be able to practice certain types of sunlight treatments, *especially the sun-glass*. Plain closed-eyes sunning, possibly some open-eyes sunning and daily sunlight with open eyes not facing the sun might be practiced. But, check with your eye doctor first because; <u>the cornea.., iris, lens, vitreous control the amount of sunlight entering the eyes, prevents over-exposure</u>. An artificial or altered lens in the eye might not function perfectly correct with sunlight as the eye's natural lens. Prescription in the eye is like wearing glasses. A partial and/or altered cornea will not function completely correct with sunlight. Sunlight is necessary to keep the eyes, cornea, iris, lens, retina... healthy. It can help eye, vision problems, surgery to heal. It fights infection. Sunglasses, eyeglasses and avoiding sunlight leads to eye problems, blindness. Use the Bates Method to prevent eye, vision impairment and surgery.

SUN TREATMENT. The eyes need sunlight. People who work in mines, where there is no sun, sooner or later develop inflammations of the interior of the eyes. The cloudiness of the lens from cataract is lessened by exposing the eye to the direct rays of the sun. When using the sun treatment, it is best to let the eyes become accustomed to the sun by mild treatment at first. Have the patient sit in a chair with his eyes closed and his face turned toward the sun. He should slowly move his head a short distance from side to side. The movement of the head prevents concentration of the sun's rays on one part of the eye. After some days of treatment, or when the patient becomes more accustomed to the light, one may use the sun-glass with added benefit. Direct the patient to look far down and while he does this, lift the upper lid gently, exposing to view the sclera or white part of the eye. Now, with the aid of the sun-glass focus the sunlight on the forehead or on the cheek, and then rapidly pass the concentrated light over various parts of the sclera. This requires less than a minute of time. It is

Aspirin, tobacco, some herbs, chemicals and *phony* natural ingredients in skin, hormone creams.., sinus sprays, soap, food impair the body, eyes' health, vision and raise-lower eye pressure to abnormal levels.

Better Eyesight

not well to be in a hurry. One should wait until the patient becomes sufficiently accustomed to the sun to permit the upper eyelid to be raised while he looks far down, exposing the sclera only. It is important that the patient be cautioned not to look directly at the sun.

Prognosis

The cure of cataract is usually accomplished more quickly than the cure of some other diseases of the eye. My assistant, Emily C. Lierman, has had unusual success in treating cataract cases, as she adapts my methods to each individual case. In her book, "Stories from the Clinic," the treatment is described in detail.

Better Eyesight - June, 1920 - SUN-GAZING; *Light is necessary to the health of the eye, and darkness is injurious to it. Eye shades, dark glasses, darkened rooms, weaken the sight and sooner or later produce inflammations. Persons with normal sight can look directly at the sun, or at the strongest artificial light, without injury or discomfort, and persons with imperfect sight are never permanently injured by such lights, though temporary ill effects, lasting from a few minutes to a few hours, days, weeks, months, or longer, may be produced. In all abnormal conditions of the eyes, light is beneficial. It is rarely sufficient to cure, but is a great help in gaining relaxation by other methods.*

Note; The eyes, mind and body are relaxed and benefited by *NATURAL* darkness obtained by closing and Palming the eyes and sleeping at night in normal darkness; television, lights turned off. (moonlight is ok.) It is the darkness, abnormal light produced by sunglasses, tinted lenses, eyeglasses and constant artificial light and avoiding the natural sunlight of the day that injures the eyes, vision and body's health.

The Sun Treatments - For Healthy Eyes, Body & Clear Eyesight

Treatment can also help the blind, advanced vision impairment, cataract, glaucoma, people very sensitive to sunlight due to living in low light, darkness, addiction to sunglasses or many years wearing eyeglasses. Practice in a state of mind-body relaxation. The body, eyes must be free of drugs, medications, eye drops, chemicals. A good diet, nutrition maintained. Avoid eating soy, tofu, certain herbs. They impair the vision, thyroid, hormones and some eye, light functions. (Epileptics affected by flashing, moving light cannot do parts of this practice; 'Saccadic Sunning' with the tree leaves, fence, hands... See the E-books. If the eyes had surgery; see the copyright-directions pages beginning of this book and previous sunlight pages.)

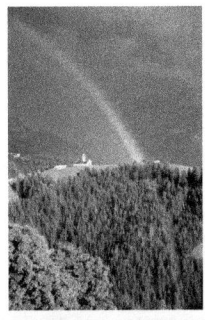

Sunlight, Closed and Open-Eyes Sunning, Sunlight on the Sclera and the Sun-Glass Treatment are applied in this way, order; # 1 to 8b. (Take your time. # 7 to 8b can be practiced in the future after the eyes build tolerance to sunlight.)

1 - Expose the open eyes to natural full spectrum sunlight outside. No sunglasses, tinted, colored, UV blocking... lenses. No eyeglasses or contact lenses. No sunscreen, UV blocking skin creams. Bare feet, stand on the earth's land when sunning.
    Start by walking around in partial shade under a tree. Wear a white hat with a wide brim if the light feels too strong.

2 - Face the sunlight under the tree, then face directly at the sun through the tree leaves. Blink and move 'shift' the eyes and head/face with the eyes side to side; left, right, left, right, then; up, down... Relaxed, easy, slowly. Then; work your way into the sunlight with, then without the hat. Walk around in the sunlight, look at the tree tops, clouds. Blink, eyes shifting.

3a - Face the bright sky, then sky near the sun with eyes closed. Head, eyes moving. Then with eyes open. Blink, eyes shifting.
    Then; close the eyes and face directly at the sun with the hands a few inches in front of the eyes. Do Saccadic Sunning; Open the fingers and move the hands-fingers across the eyes-face; left and right, up and down, diagonally... allowing sunlight and shadows to shine, move upon the closed eyes. The eyes, head move side to side as the hands, fingers move in various directions in front of the eyes. Blink. See the Saccadic Sunning picture, directions with the tree, hands on this page, bottom right >.
    3b - Repeat # 3a with eyes open. Blink frequently, keep the eyes, head moving, shifting. Rest.

4 - Practice Open-Eyes Sunning, briefly, for a few seconds. (no hands) Face the sun. Keep the eyes and head moving; eyes shifting, blink frequently. Then stop. Rest and Palm. Repeat, then Rest and Palm.
    Saccadic Sunning; move the hands-open fingers up and down, left and right, diagonally... in front of the eyes while facing the sun; eyes open, then closed, then open. Eyes, head moving. Blink.
    When facing the sun, sunning; a white cloth mask with non-obstructed eyeholes (and nose-mouth breathing holes) is worn to protect the face from sunburn. Get some sunlight on the skin for vitamin D... production and top of the head (no hat) to strengthen chakras, chi energy centers, flow. (When sunning, moving the head, eyes; see the sun 'Swing' opposite.)

5 - Practice the Sunlight on the Sclera 'white of the eye' Treatment. Face the sun. Eyes open. Look down, the eyes' pupils under the bottom eyelids. Pull both eyes' top eyelids up and move the eyes, head side to side to move sunlight upon the top of the eyes' sclera. Then look up and do the bottom sclera. (See directions on previous pages.) Stop the sclera treatment. Rest.

6 - Practice Closed-Eyes Sunning. Face the sun. Move the closed eyes, head/face side to side-left and right, up, down, diagonally, circle the sun counter-clockwise, clockwise, draw the Figure Eight. The head moves with the eyes in the same direction. Face the sun, sky, sun... Closed eyes sunning can be done for 10-30... minutes. (No sunglasses, eyeglasses..!)

7 - Practice Open-Eyes Sunning, briefly, a few seconds. Keep the eyes and head moving. Head moves with the eyes, in synchronization. Shift on the sun and shift left and right... across the sun to the sky. Blink frequently. Then stop. Rest and Palm. Repeat, then Rest, Palm. Open-eyes sunning can be practiced for a bit longer time as the eyes get used to the sunlight.
    If you see a light-spot in the visual field (like a temporary after-image seen after looking at a light bulb or a neon sign at night); stop, limit open-eyes sunning exposure time until the eyes build more tolerance to the sun. Light-spots are red, yellow, green, blue, purple, pink, white, other colors and change color, size as they fade away. Light-spots disappear in a short time. When the eyesight, eyes, mind-visual system are functioning normal, relaxed, healthy, no tension, strain, the vision is clear; there is no sensitivity to sunlight, light-spots are few and fade away quickly. Light spots and other effects can last for months if sunning is done wrong and/or there is tension, strain in the visual system. Limit eye exposure to a few seconds at a time.
    Improve adjustment of the eyes, vision, retina, visual purple production, iris-pupil reaction-size to light and dark by alternating; Palming-Sunning-Palming-Sunning. Sunlight, Sunning with Palming improves day and night vision. Sunlight relaxes the mind, body, eyes and eye muscles. The clearer the vision is = the less sensitivity to sunlight.

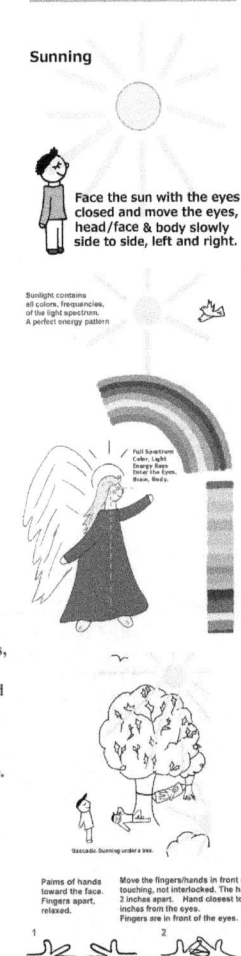

8a - Use the Sun-Glass Treatment on Closed Eyes. Do one eye at a time. (See entire directions, placement, distance of the glass, heat tests... on previous and next pages. Use only if necessary.) Look far down, the eye's pupil is under the lower eyelid to keep the sun-glass light away from the pupil. Keep the eyes closed. The 'light spot' through the sun-glass is moved rapidly and continuously side to side... 10-15 seconds on the closed eyelid, upon the eye's upper sclera 'white' area, through the eyelid.
    Then do the other eye. Alternate on left and right eyes. The eyes can be moved up, down, left, right as long as they stay closed and light does not shine on the pupil. (read previous pages; don't move the eyes when the sun-glass light is on the eyes.) The light shines on many areas of the sclera, helps the entire eye through the closed eyelid. Rest. Palm. Repeat if comfortable.
    The sun-glass can also be used on both eyes together when the eyes are closed. Light on the closed eyelids IS effective.

8b - Use the Sun-Glass Treatment on Open Eyes. (See complete directions, placement, distance of the glass, heat tests... on previous and next pages. Use only if necessary.) Do one eye at a time. The eyes look far down, the eye's pupil is under the lower eyelid to keep the sun-glass light away from the eye's pupil. Sunlight through the glass must NOT shine into the pupil! (Patch the other eye.) Lift the upper eyelid of the non-patched eye. The light spot exiting the sun-glass is moved rapidly and continuously for only 2-3 seconds on the eye's upper sclera 'white area' of the eye. Stop, rest. Switch the eyepatch to the eye you just treated. Do the sun-glass treatment on the other eye. Stop the sun-glass treatment. Rest and Palm. Walk around in the shade under a tree, alternating to full sunlight. Do a few seconds of open-eyes sunning (no sun-glass); blink and shift the eyes across the sun to get balanced, full spectrum sunlight into the eyes, because; a negative effect of the sun-glass is that it emits unbalanced light. (See next page.) If blind; watch for moving light, shadow when doing sunlight treatments. Watch for flashes of clear or partially clear vision immediately or as time passes. Moving the hands in front of the eyes when facing the sun helps activate the retina, cones, rods, nerves, lens and brain's function with the eyes and appearance of moving light which leads to a return of the vision. (The Sun-Glass Treatment is used only if necessary, temporarily and is applied only by an experienced Bates Method - Natural Eyesight Improvement Ophthalmologist with many excellent patient references.)

Precautions, Benefits For the Sun-Glass, Sunlight Treatments

This is an old-time Bates Method treatment. It can heal some types of blindness, advanced eye problems, cataract, glaucoma, help heal the optic nerve... It must be preserved, but; it must be **applied correct**. Complete old-original and modern directions, warnings must be taught for safety of the Sun-Glass (Burning Glass) because it is a magnifying glass and sunlight passing through a magnifying glass can burn, blind the eye. Dr. Bates is not here now to apply it, teach us how to use it correct. It must not be advised for, given out carelessly to every student.

The Sun-Glass is not needed except sometimes in advanced cases of vision impairment, blindness and should be done only by an expert eye doctor, Ophthalmologist experienced in the Bates Method and only after other Bates' Method practices are tried first. This type of doctor is hard to find so people often apply this method on their own or with a friends' help. Be careful! Study the directions completely and **be sure you can trust the friend**. Experts with clear enough eyesight and/or **perfect** perception of the location of the light can do it themselves, but that is still not perfectly safe.

The Sun-Glass is a magnifier, a glass and similar to a strong reading eyeglass prescription; sunlight passing through it becomes very unbalanced, no longer full spectrum, it converts to partial spectrum light and abnormally focused light which is not healthy, it's not the beneficial full spectrum sunlight we get when it's not passing through glass, plastic, windows, eyeglasses... People that use the Sun-Glass every day or weekly... are placing unbalanced, partial spectrum light on their eyes. This continual exposure to unbalanced sunlight waves, frequencies, altered energy is unhealthy. Avoid teachers who advise this overuse of the Sun-Glass. Some teachers use it to appear professional, mysterious, as a tool to attract people as paying customers. Even monthly or less often can be harmful. It is only needed for treating blindness.., some types of eye infections.., and must be a **temporary** practice! Only an eye doctor or medically trained professional should be in charge of it, apply it. This will prevent misuse.

Using the Sun-Glass inside under artificial light bulbs (which produce unbalanced light) makes the light through the Sun-Glass more unbalanced, unnatural, removes more of the light spectrum, impairs the eyes, retina, lens'... health, function and clarity of vision. Even if you use the best full spectrum light bulb, lamp; the light is not 'perfect' full spectrum as healthy natural pure sunlight not passing through a glass is. A safe type of **full spectrum lamp** (no fluorescent, no types that are too hot) is good for indoor light and can be used for sunning the eyes when stuck working inside and in low sunlight areas of the planet. But; passing this light through the Sun-Glass makes it partial, unbalanced, unhealthy. The full spectrum lamp can be used with the Sun-Glass for some benefit to the blind if pure sunlight is unavailable. Open all the windows, get a lot of sunlight inside the house.

Used correct, **temporarily** by an Ophthalmologist, the Sun-Glass treatment with pure sunlight can bring back the eyesight, the eyes' health. **But**; it's a temporary treatment and is combined with permanent use of the Bates Method and natural full spectrum sunlight NOT passing through the Sun-Glass. The Sun-Glass and Open-Eyes Sunning are not needed for most cases. I DO endorse some open-eyes sunning; few seconds occasionally. It is healthy. Due to depletion of the planet's ozone layer from pollution; Open-Eyes Sunning (and the Sun-Glass Treatment) must be done with care, detailed instructions, precautions must be given. Some areas of the planet have better ozone protection. (The Sun-Glass is NOT Sunglasses.)

Colored spots in the visual field lasting for days, months is a side effect when these treatments are done wrong. Open-eyes sunning can be done safely and with great benefit to the health of the eyes, mind, body and vision. Sunlight is a natural antidepressant, a healer. Vision becomes clear, eyes healthy with use of the Bates Method, avoiding eyeglasses and obtaining natural exposure to normal sunlight by just walking outside daily, looking at the bright sky, clouds, trees, moving the eyes, head/face across the sun with blinking for short periods and using Closed-Eyes Sunning.

I repeat; (The Sun-Glass light never shines on, in the eye's pupil. It shines only on the sclera, white area of the eye.) Do not wear any type of eyeglasses, sunglasses, tinted, colored, UV blocking lenses, contact lenses... while sunning, sun-gazing, applying sunlight on sclera, using the Sun-Glass, any sunlight treatments. Eyeglasses, lenses can act as a magnifying glass causing sunlight through the eyeglass lens to burn the eyes, even when the eyes are closed. The eyeglasses, all lenses impair the natural structure of the suns' light rays causing unbalanced, partial spectrum, unhealthy light to enter the eyes, visual system resulting in eye, vision, health impairment. Do NOT use binoculars, telescopes, magnifiers when facing the sun!

I prefer direct, pure full spectrum, balanced sunlight on the sclera 'white of the eye' (pulling the eyelids up, down while looking in the opposite direction with the eyes' pupils away from the sun. See directions, pictures on previous pages.) without the light passing through the Sun-Glass or any type of glass, plastic, eyeglasses, sunglasses... I also use closed eyes sunning and a bit of occasional open-eyes sunning done correct; look directly at the sun, **always with eyes-head moving, keep the eyes shifting, blink often, avoid staring**. Move the head/face with the eyes; at the same time, in the same direction. Limit eye exposure time. Protect the skin from sunburn. Avoid skin UV blocking... sunscreen creams. They disrupt the sun's rays.

Do the long swing, sway, figure eight facing the sun and see the illusion of opposite movement 'The Swing'; The sun appears to move opposite of the direction the eyes, head, body move to. Practice it with the eyes **closed**, **open**, **closed**. Try saccadic sunning; face the sun under a tree or in front of a picket or wire fence with openings and rock left and right; see flickering light and shadows. Or, move the hands/fingers in front of the eyes.

I like to watch, copy animals, birds' natural reaction to the sun, their instincts. Some have additional eye-vision functions. Many birds' vision is better than humans, see more light waves... Healthy eyes work best with healthy *full spectrum* sunlight; Good nutrition, diet, no drugs, chemicals...

SUN TREATMENT

Most ophthalmologists prescribe dark glasses to nearly all of their patients who suffer from the brightness of light. This practice, in my opinion, has been overdone. I remember one patient who was in the hospital for two years in a dark room, with both eyes bandaged with a dark binding day and night continuously. When she left the hospital she was in a very pitiable condition. She was practically blind in the bright sunlight. She went to a great many clinics and eye doctors and all they did for her was to give her stronger dark glasses. In time these dark glasses did not give her any relief. Instead of being helpful to her weak eyes, the glasses had the effect of making them more sensitive to the light than they had ever been before. It has been my experience that all persons who wear dark glasses sooner or later develop very serious inflammation of their eyes. The human eye needs the light in order to maintain its efficiency. The use of eye-shades and protections of all kinds from the light is very injurious to the eyes.

Sunlight is as necessary to normal eye as is rest and relaxation. If it is possible, start the day by exposing the eyes to the sun—just a few minutes at a time will help. Get accustomed to the strong light of the sun by letting it shine on your closed eyelids. Later, when you can look down sufficiently, by gently lifting the upper lid the white part of the eye can be exposed, while the sun's rays strike directly on it. It is good to move the head slightly from side to side while doing this, in order to prevent straining. One cannot get too much sun treatment.

By Dr. Bates; *Looking at the sun, while slower in its results, has often been sufficient to effect permanent cures, sometimes in a very short time. There is a right way and a wrong way to do this. Persons with imperfect sight should never look directly at the sun at first, because, while no permanent harm can come from it, great temporary inconvenience may result. Such persons should begin by looking to one side of the sun, and after becoming accustomed to the strong light, should look a little nearer to its source, and so on until they become able to look directly at the sun without discomfort.*

This book includes all of Dr. Bates treatments and gives exact directions. If advanced treatment is needed; ask an experienced Bates Method Ophthalmologist. Parts of the sunlight chapter of this book is repetitive. This is to ensure that people learn how to apply the practice correct, safely. Repetition improves the memory, perfect application.

Read the free PDF E-book; '*Do It Yourself - Natural Eyesight Improvement - Original and Modern Bates Method*' for directions on how to reduce the strength of eyeglass lenses 'wear weaker and weaker lenses' and permanently discontinue use of eyeglasses. Glasses are worn only if absolutely necessary for driving, safety at work... Not wearing eyeglasses is the fastest, easiest way to obtain perfect clear 20/20 and better vision at all distances, close and far.

AVOID EYEGLASSES, SURGERY AND DRUGS.
EYEGLASSES, SURGERY AND DRUGS CAUSE AND INCREASE EYE MUSCLE TENSION, MENTAL STRAIN, ABNORMAL EYE SHAPE, UNCLEAR VISION, CATARACTS AND ALL EYE PROBLEMS.

The Bates Method relaxes the eye muscles, returns them to normal function, coordination. If strengthening is needed it will happen automatically when the muscles function correct. Sometimes people misunderstand Natural Eyesight Improvement, they think the Bates Method consists of strict Eye Exercises. In the article on the right > the words strengthening, exercise are used. The Bates Method is not eye exercises. The Bates Method consists of relaxation of the <u>mind</u>, body, eye muscles, eyes and practicing 'imitating' correct relaxed function, use of the eyes-vision, 'the visual system'. Blinking is rapid but it is done soft, easy, frequent, same as a person with clear eyesight blinks. The lover looking at the photo will not stare, not strain the eyes if she-he shifts upon the picture while thinking happy thoughts.

Bring your mind out into the world, enjoy looking at things; investigate the type of wood a staircase banister is made of. It's color, design, age. Watch birds, bees in the garden. They move often. Follow their flight. This gets your mind off your eyes, off the clarity of vision. Note how the eyes move natural *on their own* when you do not try to control the eyes' movement, clarity; you just relax and enjoy looking at things. This is when you see most perfectly clear 'without effort'.

Imperfect Sight Can be Cured **Without Glasses**
You Can Cure **Yourself**
You Can Cure **Others**

Better Eyesight

A MONTHLY MAGAZINE DEVOTED TO THE PREVENTION
AND CURE OF IMPERFECT SIGHT WITHOUT GLASSES

Vol. III   SEPTEMBER, 1920   No. 3

Make Your Sight Worse
This is an excellent method of improving it

Experiences with Central Fixation
By M. H. Stuart, M.D.

How I Improved My Eyesight
By Pamela Speyer

Sleepiness and Eyestrain
By W. H. Bates, M.D.

Stories from the Clinic
By Emily C. Lierman

$2.00 per year   20 cents per copy

Published by the CENTRAL FIXATION PUBLISHING COMPANY
342 WEST 42nd STREET   NEW YORK, N. Y.

Now Cross-Eyed Tommy Looks Straight At Future

EYES RIGHT for Caroline Gowdy as she performs eye muscle strengthening exercise. As the instructor (left) moves the the string fastened between two pencil-like tubes. Caroline follows it with her eyes. The exercises is designed to help the eyes co-ordinate.

By FRED ZAVATTERO
NEA Staff Correspondent

SEATTLE, Wash. —(NEA)—"Yah! Yah! Cross-eyed can't be on our side."

For 15 years Tommy suffered while his schoolmates poked fun at him for his crossed-eyes and thick-lensed glasses. But now Tommy has taken off his glasses. He doesn't need them. His eyes are straight.

To the boy and his parents, it's unbelievable. But to the men and women who developed the technique of correcting eye defects without the use of glasses, it's just a sample of what can be achieved by a new system for correcting vision.

A New York oculist, Dr. W. H. Bates, gave up his practice in the early part of this century to seek a new way of treating his patients. Eyeglasses, he knew, don't always help. Bates found another way.

After a number of experiments, Bates discovered that vision defects were often caused by the habitual improper use of the eyes.

He also found that this improper usage was related to mental and emotional strain. By easing the strain and teaching the eyes to see in a relaxed way, a large percentage of his patients regained normal vision.

Since his death in 1931, the doctor's work has been carried on by the American Association for Eye Training, Inc., under the direction of Mrs. Clara Hackett.

Several methods have been developed for relaxing the eyes. "Palming," or covering the eyes with the palms of the hands at regular intervals, is restful. Blinking rapidly is helpful.

Exposing the eyes to the sun —"sunning"—has helped to correct eye ailments. "Dark glasses may give you Hollywood glamor, but they don't do the eyes any good," reports one instructor.

"Above all," eye trainers caution, "use your eyes and keep them in motion. The lover who stares for hours at the picture of his heart's desire may satify his soul, but he's ruining his eyes."

School children, who worry about their lessons, often develop nervous tension which creates eye strain. Once their worries are relieved, their vision improves.

In spite of active opposition from some groups, the Bates method is arousing interest and has chalked up some successes.

A 24-year-old woman who wore glases for 11 years now has normal vision without glasses. She has been training her eyes less than two months.

After six weeks' work, an eight-year-old girl, near-sighted and crossed-eyed, now has normal vision. Her schoolwork has improved along with her sight.

The best record in Seattle was achieved by a 63-year-old man who wore glasses for 50 years. With only light perception in one eye and only 25 per cent vision in the other when he started, he has gained almost normal sight in less than two years. His instructors think he will recover completely within another year.

Some Seattle schools use the Bates method to prevent eye tension and fatigue in their pupils. A large number of teachers have been able to give up wearing glasses.

More pictures, true stories are in Dr. Bates Better Eyesight Magazine and Medical Articles. Where are Dr. Bates' patient medical, office records? Were they destroyed by dishonest people who want to hide his effective natural method? Did honest doctors or Bates teachers preserve his records; all the different eye-vision conditions he treated, the natural treatment, practices he applied. Are they hidden in Ophthalmology colleges or... due to laws, doctors still trying to hide the Bates Method?

Glasses are often prescribed unnecessarily or 'too strong' (over-corrected) due to temporary nervousness, pressure to hurry, limited eye, head, neck, body movement, looking into test equipment during an eye exam. Eye doctors also prefer to prescribe an 'extra strength' to the eyeglass lenses. All eyeglasses, especially strong eyeglass lenses cause fast, increased vision/eye impairment and prescriptions for stronger and stronger lenses.

Some years ago an English gentleman wrote to me that his glasses were very unsatisfactory. They not only did not give him good sight, but they increased instead of lessening his discomfort. He asked if I could help him, and since relaxation always relieves discomfort and improves the vision, I did not believe that I was doing him an injury in telling him how to rest his eyes. He followed my directions with such good results that in a short time he obtained perfect sight for both the distance and the near-point without glasses, and was completely relieved of his pain. Five years later he wrote me that he had qualified as a sharpshooter in the army. Did I do wrong in treating him by correspondence? I do not think so.

After the United States entered the European war, an officer wrote to me from the deserts of Arizona that the use of his eyes at the near-point caused him great discomfort, which glasses did not relieve, and that the strain had produced granulation of the lids. As it was impossible for him to come to New York, I undertook to treat him by correspondence. He improved very rapidly. The inflammation of the lids was relieved almost immediately, and in about four months he wrote me that he had read one of my own reprints—by no means a short one—in a dim light, with no bad after effects; that the glare of the Arizona sun, with the Government thermometer registering 114, did not annoy him, and that he could read the ten line on the test card at fifteen feet almost perfectly, while even at twenty feet he was able to make out most of the letters.

A third case was that of a forester in the employ of the U. S. Government. He had myopic astigmatism, and suffered extreme discomfort, which was not relieved either by glasses or by long summers in the mountains, where he used his eyes but little for close work. He was unable to come to New York for treatment, and although I told him that correspondence treatment was somewhat uncertain, he said he was willing to risk it. It took three days for his letters to reach me and another three for my reply to reach him, and as letters were not always written promptly on either side, he often did not hear from me more than once in three weeks. Progress under these conditions was necessarily slow; but his discomfort was relieved very quickly, and in about ten months his sight had improved from 20/50 to 20/20.

In almost every case the treatment of cases coming from a distance is continued by correspondence after they return to their homes; and although the patients do not get on so well as when they are coming to the office, they usually continue to make progress till they are cured.

At the same time it is often very difficult to make patients understand what they should do when one has to communicate with them entirely by writing, and probably all would get on better if they could have some personal treatment. At the present time the number of doctors in different parts of the United States who understand the treatment of imperfect sight without glasses is altogether too few, and my efforts to interest them in the matter have not been very successful. I would consider it a privilege to treat medical men without a fee, and when cured they will be able to assist me in the treatment of patients in their various localities.

The Main Natural Eyesight Improvement Practices. Fast Clear Eyesight.
Easy to learn with pictures, quick directions.
Practice the 10 steps and see clear, often in a few minutes to 1-2 days.

 1-Relaxation
 2-Shifting
 3-Central Vision
 4-Blinking
 5-Breathing

 6-Movement (with Opposite Swing)
 7-Memory, Imagination
 8-Switching
 9-Sunlight

10-Fine Print   Read Fine Print   Microscopic print

PALMING

TO COVER THE CLOSED EYES WITH THE PALMS OF THE HANDS WHILE RELAXING AND THINKING SOMETHING PLEASANT.

RIGHT EYE RIGHT HAND

LEFT EYE LEFT HAND

THE FINGERS OF THE RIGHT HAND CROSS OVER, ON TOP OF THE LEFT HANDS FINGERS, IN THE CENTER OF THE FOREHEAD.

THIS PICTURE SHOWS THE LEFT AND RIGHT HANDS/EYES OF A PERSON FACING THE READER.
TO SEE HOW THE READERS HANDS ARE PLACED; VIEW THIS PICTURE IN A MIRROR OR PLACE THE PICTURE OUTWARD ON THE CHEST AND LOOK DOWN AT THE PICTURE FOR A SECOND.

PALMING RELAXES THE MIND, BODY, NECK, EYE MUSCLES, EYES, AND WHEN COMBINED WITH SUNNING IMPROVES THE EYES/RETINA, BRAIN AND BODY'S ACTIVATION/REACTION TO SUNLIGHT AND ABSORPTION, USE OF SUNLIGHT. THIS IMPROVES FUNCTION, HEALTH OF EYES, BRAIN, BODY.

THE LONG SWING

TURN AND SWING RIGHT   CENTER   TURN AND SWING LEFT.

See the free E-books for more Long Swing & Sway (Rock) Examples-Directions.

SHIFTING 'EYE MOVEMENT' - The Eyes (Visual/Mental Attention) SHIFT 'MOVE' continually from part to part on a object and from object to object. It is easy to see clear by shifting from <u>one small part to another small part</u> on an object, seeing one small part at a time clearest as the eyes, (macula/fovea in the center of the retina, 'the central field') move upon each part, one at a time. Blink, Breathe, and Relax. The macula/fovea contains many cones 'light receptors' which produce very clear vision. In reality; The EXACT CENTER OF THE VISUAL FIELD, the eyes *FOVEA's center* moves POINT TO POINT upon the object as the eyes shift from part to part. This occurs subconsciously, automatic and enables the eyes to see very tiny parts, fine details crystal clear at any distance, close or far. Use it consciously, relaxed, without effort to improve the vision. The fovea may be on a small part (point) for only a fraction of a second before moving to another part. During that time, that part is in the central field and seen clearest. The eyes shift continually, easy moving the macula/fovea (central field) from object to object, part to part on an object causing the entire visual field, all objects, all parts of objects to appear perfectly clear. In reality, the part the eyes are looking directly at, in the central field is most perfectly clear, better than 20/20. The part of the macula, fovea around the fovea's center produce the central area of the visual field that is very close to the exact central field. Those areas are also very clear. The eyes-brain pick it up along with the entire visual field. *The fovea, exact center is most clear.* Look at a street sign 100 feet away. Look 1 foot to the side of it; it's not perfectly clear. Look directly at it; it's seen perfectly clear. Shift.

   Shifting is combined with Central-Fixation. Look at a tiny object; a small letter E. Notice the eyes (fovea) continue to move 'shift' upon that small E. Try keeping the eyes immobile (staring) and note that tension begins, leads to strain and unclear vision. Let the eyes (where you are looking) move. Blink. Note relaxation and clarity occurs. See the central best! Read about Central-Fixation in this book.

   Practice shifting.., then DONT PRACTICE; Let the eyes move, function completely natural <u>on their own</u>. Notice vision is very clear when you are not thinking about the eyes, clarity of vision. Practice Dr. Bates methods relaxed, no effort. Eyes-vision work as the sense of touch, taste, as the heart beats, lungs breathe automatic 'on their own'. This is the optimum visual system, *eyes, mind, body* function.

SHIFT ON THE HOUSE, DOT TO DOT.

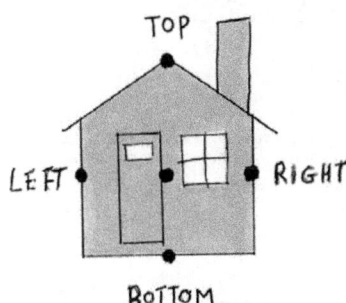

SHIFT IN ANY DIRECTION/PATTERN.

Shifting on the dots in the pictures is only to learn shifting. When looking at real objects; do not imagine dots on the the object. Shift on the object in any direction, pattern from one small part to another small part. Blink and relax.

THE DIAGRAM ABOVE SHOWS A EXAMPLE OF THE NATURAL SHIFTING PATTERN OF THE EYES.. NOTICE THE EYES MOVE FREELY ON THE HOUSE IN A VARIETY OF PATTERNS, DIRECTIONS.

Shift dot to dot (part to part) on the E.

Shift dot to dot on the Tree.

Blink, Relax

Shift dot to dot on the Dog.

SHIFT, TRACE, CENTRAL-FIXATION WITH THE NOSEFEATHER

THE NOSEFEATHER

Trace directly *on* the edge of the object for perfect *Central-Fixation*. Tracing combines Shifting with Central-Fixation.

Shift part to part on the house. Shift on small parts; the window, window pane, door, small window on top of the door, chimney... Practice shifting from dot to dot on the picture. Blink, a few gentle relaxed deep breaths.

The dots on the green house are only to learn, practice *shifting with central-fixation* (fovea vision). Do not imagine dots on objects when practicing shifting on real objects or pictures without dots printed on them. Shift on your own, without the dots from <u>one small part to another small part</u>. Shift on other pictures and objects in your environment. If shifting on a black object or letter; you can imagine it is composed of hundreds of tiny black dots and shift from dot to dot.

THE MAN IS TRACING AROUND THE EDGE OF THE TREE WITH THE IMAGINARY NOSEFEATHER.
THE END OF THE FEATHER EXTENDS OUT FROM THE END/CENTER OF THE NOSE AND BENDS UP TO EYE LEVEL TO TOUCH THE PART OF THE OBJECT THE EYES ARE LOOKING AT IN THE <u>CENTER</u> OF THE VISUAL FIELD.
THE FEATHER IS VERY THIN AND THE END FORMS A VERY SMALL POINT WHICH IS THE SIZE OF THE EXACT CENTER OF THE VISUAL FIELD PRODUCED BY THE FOVEA CENTRALIS IN THE MACULA, CENTER OF THE EYES RETINA.
MOVE THE POINTED END OF THE NOSEFEATHER AROUND THE EDGE OF OBJECTS AND PARTS OF OBJECTS.
THE EYES, END OF THE NOSEFEATHER, HEAD/FACE AND BODY MOVE TOGETHER, IN SYNCHRONIZATION; SAME TIME, SAME DIRECTION.
THE NECK IS RELAXED AND MOBILE.
BLINK, BREATHE ABDOMINALLY, RELAX. **Trace relaxed, easy, loose. Don't force perfection. Avoid tension, immobility.**
THE NOSEFEATHER IS ALSO USED TO SHIFT FROM POINT TO POINT (SMALL PART TO SMALL PART) ON A OBJECT.
THE NOSEFEATHER IS USED TO SWITCH FROM CLOSE OBJECTS TO DISTANT OBJECTS AND DISTANT TO CLOSE, MIDDLE...
THE FEATHER BECOMES LONGER WHEN LOOKING TO THE DISTANCE AND SHORTER WHEN LOOKING AT CLOSE OBJECTS.
THE NOSEFEATHER ACTIVATES EASY USE OF CORRECT VISION HABITS; SHIFTING (EYE MOVEMENT), CENTRAL FIXATION, MOVEMENT OF THE HEAD/FACE, BODY WITH THE EYES, RELAXATION AND MOVEMENT OF THE NECK.
THE FEATHER CAN BE IMAGINED AS BEING INVISIBLE.
THIS ALLOWS THE BRAIN TO IMAGINE, REMEMBER THE OBJECT THE EYES ARE LOOKING AT CLEAR WITHOUT BEING DISTRACTED BY THE IMAGE OF THE FEATHER.

The Big Fluffy Nosefeather sweeps upon objects. The person just relaxes and sweeps the feather over trees, houses, scenery... This brings movement to the eyes, head, neck, body. Great relaxation of the mind, eyes, neck and body. Option; to use a tiny pointed end of one 'central piece' of the feather to touch, shift, trace on objects with Central-Fixation or let the eyes do central-fixation on their own.

Try imagining a nose pencil or light ray beam. Choose a lightweight, soothing, easy moving object.

Middle size Nosefeather with Central-Fixation point on the end.

Trace, Shift, Central-Fixation with the Nosefeather

Practicing shifting, central-fixation and all Correct Vision Habits is the act of _imitating normal eye, vision function._ With a little practice the eyes do this 'on their own', automatically and vision is clear. Practice, then don't practice; let the eyes work _Completely Natural, On Their Own_ for perfect Vision.

Practice Shifting, Tracing, Central Fixation on Yellow Kitty.

Tracing with the eyes/nosefeather near but away from the edge of the object or part of a object is incorrect, causes diffusion, strain, prevents central fixation. Use <u>central fixation</u> = look at, trace <u>directly on</u>, along the edge of the object or parts of the object. (See dots in picture.)

Trace Yellow Kitty.
Trace with the eyes (vision) and end of the nosefeather.
Trace exactly <u>on</u> the edge of the cat and parts of the cat for perfect central fixation and shifting/eye movement. Trace the head, body, tail, eyes, nose... Follow the dots in any direction. Blink, relax. Shift part to part, point to point.
The central field of vision traces (moves on/along) the edges of the cat.

Relax. Let the mind, 'mental attention' move from part to part, dot to dot (true eyes function is moving point to point). Then the eyes, 'center of the visual field, visual attention' will move automatically with the mind. This is a way to 'forget about the eyes', don't try to shift/move the eyes. Let the mind/brain, eyes, visual system work completely natural, on their own. Vision becomes clear without trying. No effort, no strain=no blur.

For Clear Close Reading Vision;

Shift on a Small Part of a Fine Print Black Letter;

Shift tiny point to tiny point on a imagined black period on a part of a fine print letter, and remember, imagine and see it dark black and clear. Practice with the eyes open, then closed using the memory, imagination, then open again. Example; imagine a black period on a fine print letter r; the top right curved part of the letter that looks like a period. Imagine the black period on it. Shift on that small part. Blink. Bring the r closer and closer to the eyes as it becomes clear at closer distances. Keep shifting on it. Blink. Shift on the entire letter. Then move back to the part.

Practice shifting on a black dot, then smaller dot, smaller... to period size. Then fine and microscopic print size. Blink. See pictures below. Start on larger letters, then practice on the smaller and fine, microscopic print letters.

Place two dots side by side . .   Look at and shift on the dot on the < left. Notice it is darkest black, clearest. The dot on the right is also clear but not as perfectly clear as the dot directly regarded. This is Central-Fixation; the dot the eyes are looking directly at is most clear because it is in the exact central field. Next; look at, shift on the dot on the right >. Now this dot is darkest black and clearest. Try it on dots closer together . .   . . Shift and blink.

This can also be done on far objects.
See chapter XI - Central-Fixation.

**Remember, imagine and shift on a small black dot with the eyes closed.
With practice it can also be remembered with the eyes open and the vision becomes clear.**

Central Fixation- Look directly at the dot on the left and see it clear. Look away from it and see it less clear in the peripheral field.

Shift on the dots on the E; left and right, top and bottom, middle. See one dot at a time clearest, darkest black in the central field. Move the central field onto each dot you look at. Next; Imagine the E consists of many small black dots. Shift from small dot to small dot upon the E. Blink. Imagine smaller dots and shift on them. Imagine tiny dots.

Next; practice on the smaller E's; imagine dots on the E and shift dot to dot.

Do not imagine parts of the dots are off of the E, as in the picture of the largest E. The large dots on that picture are just for learning this practice. The true practice does not place parts of the dots outside of the E because; the eyes must use central-fixation *look directly at the object*. Not away from it. When imagining dots on the E, the dots must be on/in the E, the entire dot in the black ink.

Can you see one part of the tiny dot darkest black and clearest?
Yes = you have perfect Central-Fixation.

WATCH YOUR STEP

WHEN you know what is the matter with you it is possible for you to correct it and bring about a cure. If you do not know what is wrong with you the cure of your imperfect sight is delayed. Some persons have been cured quickly when they were able to demonstrate that to see imperfectly required a tremendous effort, an effort which was very difficult. Some persons are cured in one visit and they readily demonstrate that imperfect sight or failure to see is difficult. Others require weeks and months to demonstrate the facts. Perfect sight is quick, comes easy and without any effort whatever. Imperfect sight is slow, difficult. One cannot consciously make the sight worse as readily as it can be done unconsciously. There is no danger in demonstrating the facts.

Look at a small letter on the Snellen test card which can be seen clearly at ten or twenty feet, a letter O for example. When the letter is seen quite perfectly it is usually seen without any apparent effort. However, by looking intently, staring at it and making an effort to improve it the letter blurs. It can always be demonstrated that the effort to see very soon blurs the letter. Now close the eyes and rest them for a part of a minute or longer and then glance at the letter again. It will usually be as clear as it was before. Again by straining, making an effort, the letter becomes blurred. One can readily demonstrate that to make the sight worse requires an effort, a strain.

Many obstinate cases have obtained a permanent cure only after learning how to make the sight worse consciously. In my book are published Seven Truths of Normal Sight. Prove the facts by demonstrating that the sight becomes imperfect when one or all of them is made imperfect by a strain.

The Combinations Test Type as Suggested by Chas. Wray.

Practice shifting on the house; shift 'move' the eyes (vision-where you are looking) from dot to dot (small part to small part). Start by shifting back and forth; left, right, left, right, then top and bottom, corner to corner, and to-from the middle dot to any dot. Then shift on the dots in any direction, order. Don't try to control the eyes. Let the eyes move freely. They will move automatically with the mental attention, to 'where you look'. Blink and relax. Shift on small parts of the house; the door, chimney, a window, window pane... Practice shifting part to part without the dots. See small parts clear as the eyes shift from one tiny part to another tiny part on a small part. Blink. Shift on the T-bear. Move from one small part to another small part, another, another... on his face, nose, eyes, fuzzy ears. His red tie, arms, feet, tummy. Shift on the stars and stripes on the United States flag. Shift on the Scottish plaid cloth.

Next; practice on real objects at close and far distances; a far house, tree, airplane, sign. A close flower, leaf, stone. (Do not imagine dots on the objects. The dots on the picture are only to practice, learn shifting.)

Shifting is the natural way to see any object clear. Try it on a letter on a distant eyechart, then on a tiny fine print letter up close.

Then; <u>Don't practice</u>; let the eyes, mind drift freely from object to object and part to part on objects. Enjoy the scenery, investigate things as the eyes shift <u>completely natural</u> on their own, automatically moving with the mind's interest. Relax, deep easy breaths, blink. Forget about the eyes. Use your mind and vision. Bring your thoughts out into the world and enjoy what you see. The end of this book and the E-books contain more pictures, examples of shifting, central fixation and other practices.

Human Eye

All labels with a number 2 indicate the part is also on the opposite side of the eye...

See a small branch on the top of a dead tree far away in the mountains; The top of the tree has a tiny branch that bends out to the right. > It is smaller, thinner than in the picture, barely visible. It is seen perfect, with better than 20/20 vision when the vision moves (eyes are shifting on it automatically), the mind and eyes are relaxed, looking at the branch without trying to see it clear. No effort. Looking at things for fun, entertainment, interest. Aldous Huxley calls it; *spontaneous attention*.

Practice shifting on the branch. Then; see it *completely natural* by spontaneously looking at it during your day when active, running around or relaxing in a chair...

Practice; Look at the top bent branch of the tree. Shift on that tiny part; use central-fixation 'centralizing'. Place the exact central field on it and shift point to point on the tiny branch; left and right, up and down. Move freely to any part, direction. Then, shift up and down the tree and on other branches. Shift on the tiny top branch again.

Then; <u>pass over it out into the sky</u>; sweep over it left and right, top and bottom, diagonally, in any direction into the sky. Look at the sky on the left side of it, then the right, above it, below... The vision moves over the sky, then branch, then sky as you move from one part of the sky, over the branch and out to another part of the sky. The exact central field (fovea) and inner and outer central moves over the branch as you pass over it. The branch is seen most perfectly clear when the exact central is moving over it. Shift on the branch for a while. Practice the eyes' fine detail *point to point* exact central field 'fovea' shifting. The eyes' fovea (exact central) moves around on it without 'trying' to shift. Avoid trying to see. Let the vision move. When looking at a tiny part; shift on it. Blink. Shift along the entire tree from part to part. The central field-fovea automatically moves to the part you are looking at. The eye movements are perfect, vision moves nice and easy, continually, drifting, flowing, shifting *without effort*. The tiny branch on the top of the tree flashes clear and remains clear! Blink, breath and move. <u>Note</u>; the clarity is lost, tension occurs if the eyes lock onto the branch/stop shifting. Movement 'shifting' prevents staring, tension and blurry vision. Let the vision move freely on the branch, with *complete relaxation*. Move back to the sky, then to the branch, then sky... Think something happy, or engaging. Look for a bird... in the tree.

Top of the tree bends to the right. >
A <u>very small</u> branch. See it with central-fixation
(centralizing) and shifting on and across it.
Keep *moving*.

If the eyes, head, neck feel tight, vision blurs
when shifting on tiny parts; it indicates effort is
occurring and it is interfering with mobility.
Let go, relax and float. Let the eyes-vision shift,
do central-fixation (centralizing) *on their own*.

Imagination Helps

A mental picture of a letter can, as a rule, be made to swing precisely as can a letter on the test card. Occasionally one meets a patient with whom the reverse is true; but for most patients the mental swing is easier at first than visual swinging; and when they become able to swing in this way, it becomes easier for them to swing the letters on the test card. By alternating mental with visual swinging and shifting, rapid progress is sometimes made. As relaxation becomes more perfect, the mental swing can be shortened, until it becomes possible to conceive and swing a letter the size of a period in a newspaper. This is easier, when it can be done, than swinging a larger letter, and many patients have derived great benefit from it.

All persons, no matter how great their error of refraction, when they shift and swing successfully, correct it partially or completely, as demonstrated by the retinoscope, for at least a fraction of a second. This time may be so short that the patient is not conscious of improved vision; but it is possible for him to imagine it, and then it becomes easier to maintain the relaxation long enough to be conscious of the improved sight. For instance, the patient, after looking away from the card, may look back to the big C, and for a fraction of a second the error of refraction may be lessened or corrected, as demonstrated by the retinoscope. Yet he may not be conscious of improved vision. By imagining that the C is seen better, however, the moment of relaxation may be sufficiently prolonged to be realized.

When swinging, either mental or visual, is successful, the patient may become conscious of a feeling of relaxation which is manifested as a sensation of universal swinging.

Different Types of Shifting - Eye Movements;

<u>Shifting</u>; Shifting object to object, part to part on objects. Point to point (tiny part to tiny part) central-fixation with shifting.

<u>Saccade (Saccadic) Shifts</u>; Tiny and microscopic shifts; automatic high frequency, optical drift, healthy tremors, jerking movements...; like a fine tuned car motor humming along. Keeps the eyes in constant movement, relaxed eyes, eye muscles, mind. The fovea is always moving. Many movements are so small they cannot be seen or felt. The nerves in the retina vibrate, especially the fovea centralis keeping it in movement, maintaining clear vision. To see some of the tiny shifts; relax and watch for a tiny opposite swing caused the tiny eye shifts in various directions.

<u>Scanning</u>; Enjoying the scenery, moving on-through it, looking at any objects. Example; moving the vision along the mountains, trees, through a park, city. Saccadic movements occur. Scanning, saccades also occur when looking at a object, it's parts. A tiny high frequency tremor keeps the eyes-fovea in rapid movement, moving every fraction of a second and seeing the point the fovea is on clearest. This is central-fixation with shifting. The brain creates mental pictures of every tiny part of the object by using the fovea centralis, exact central field; it moves rapidly upon the object, putting together all the tiny parts into a perfect clear picture. Similar to the many tiny pixels combined to make a perfect clear picture in a book, movie. The images are stored in the memory for future use. If shifting, scanning, saccades stops; the vision blurs, the eyes' health is impaired.

<u>Searching</u>; Similar to scanning. The mind-eyes are looking for something specific; a bluebird... in the trees, sky. A person, building or street sign in a crowded city. Baseball in the grass. Looking for boats moving on the ocean, islands. Seashells on the beach. Saccadic movements occur. When the object is located; the eye movements center onto that object and more small, tiny movements occur; shifting, scanning, saccades...

<u>Tracking</u>; Eyes-vision on-and moving with a moving object; bird, plane flying over-along the mountains, moving across the sky left or right, diagonally or away from or toward you. A moving football, baseball, tennis ball, racing car. Both eyes move together perfectly, synchronized, equally; the eyes' foveas on the same point, moving together on/with the object and looking at/shifting on parts of the moving object.

Scientists state; tracking signals for eye movements are controlled in the brain and in the eye, retina. The eye is an extension of the brain. The eyes, brain also calculate the next position of the moving object; Example; a object flying in the sky; where its next placement ahead of it will be.

If trying to hit, catch a moving object; the brain, eyes calculate its speed, position, future position.., look to it's present and future placement. Another example of a moving object; a squirrel jumps into your peripheral field. Which nerve signal is quickest to make the eyes turn to look at it; the nerve signal from the brain or nerve signal directly from the eyes-retina, or both? Automatic and controlled movements from eyes and brain.

<u>Convergence, Accommodation and Divergence, Un-accommodation</u>; Looking close and far. Control of the central ray, visual axis's. Balanced eyes.

These 6 eye movements are a combination of automatic eye shifts and conscious-controlled (the brain sending the eyes-central vision to where you decide to look) eye shifts. Scanning, saccades are mainly automatic. Imitate the eye movements to return their automatic, perfect function.

CENTRAL-FIXATION   SUNNING

BIRD IS SEEN CLEAR BY PLACING IT IN THE CENTER OF THE VISUAL FIELD

Sunning

Face the sun with the eyes closed and move the eyes, head/face & body slowly side to side, left and right.

White cloth over the head, face with eye, nose, mouth holes. For sunning without getting a sunburn on the face.

When looking at the bird;
Place it in the center of the visual field.
Shift part to part on the bird, moving the exact center of the visual field part to part.
Do this for any object the eyes look at; shift part to part on the object. Blink, relax.
Move the head/face, body with the eyes, in the same direction.
The center of the visual field moves with the eyes from object to object, part to part.
Use perfect, exact central fixation; shift <u>small point to small point</u> on objects and small parts of objects.

MEMORY AND IMAGINATION – CLEAR MENTAL PICTURES

REMEMBERING, IMAGINING OBJECTS CLEAR IMPROVES FUNCTION OF THE BRAIN WITH THE EYES AND CLARITY OF VISION.

EYES OPEN
APPLE SEEN UNCLEAR.
APPLE IN MIND,
IMAGINATION IS CLEAR.

EYES CLOSED
APPLE IN MIND,
IMAGINATION IS CLEAR.

EYES OPEN
APPLE IS SEEN CLEAR
APPLE IN MIND,
IMAGINATION IS CLEAR.

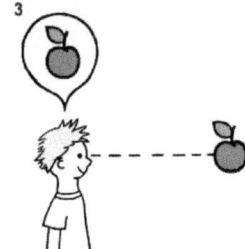

REMEMBER, IMAGINE THE APPLE CLEAR.
SHIFT FROM PART TO PART ON THE UNCLEAR APPLE AND REMEMBER, IMAGINE THE APPLE CLEAR.

SHIFT FROM PART TO PART ON THE APPLE IN THE MIND, IMAGINATION AND REMEMBER, IMAGINE THE APPLE CLEAR.

SHIFT FROM PART TO PART ON THE APPLE AND REMEMBER, IMAGINE AND SEE THE APPLE CLEAR.
REPEAT STEPS # 1,2,3.

USE THE IMAGINARY NOSEFEATHER WITH STEPS # 1,2,3.   (SEE NOSEFEATHER, CHAPTER ---)
REMEMBER, IMAGINE, SEE THE APPLE CLEAR WITH THE EYES OPEN, CLOSED, OPEN WHILE SHIFTING FROM PART TO PART ON THE APPLE WITH THE NOSEFEATHER. TRACE AROUND THE EDGES OF THE APPLE, STEM, LEAF WITH THE END OF THE FEATHER. TRACE SMALL PARTS OF THE APPLE.
PRACTICE STEPS # 1,2,3 WITH BOTH EYES TOGETHER, THEN ONE EYE AT A TIME, THEN BOTH TOGETHER AGAIN.
PRACTICE ON ANY SIZE OBJECT; LARGE, MEDIUM, SMALL, TINY AT CLOSE, MIDDLE, FAR DISTANCES.

Remembering, imagining any pleasant object, scene, happy memory, fantasy relaxes the mind, body, eye muscles, eyes resulting in clear vision.
Remembering, imagining the objects, scene clear while relaxed, easy, without effort improves the clarity of vision.
If the boy remembers, imagines a different object, any happy memory, image, scene (playing baseball, a favorite adventure...) with the eyes open looking at the apple, shifting on it and when the eyes are closed shifting on the imaginary image: when the eyes are opened - the apple will be seen clear.   He can remember, imagine the apple or any pleasant object clear, shift on it in his mind and the apple will be seen clear.
Palming with the eyes closed combined with the memory imagination activity brings clear vision.

Memory
By W. H. BATES, M.D.

When the sight is normal, the memory is perfect. The color and background of the letters or other objects seen, are remembered perfectly, instantaneously, and continuously.

Central-Fixation-Central, 'Fovea' Vision

CONES - LIGHT RECEPTORS IN THE RETINA. PRODUCE VERY CLEAR FINE DETAILED VISION AND BRIGHT COLOR PERCEPTION.

RODS - LIGHT RECEPTORS IN THE RETINA. PRODUCE LESS CLEAR VISION. RODS PERCEIVE LIGHT/ DARK, BLACK/GREY AND WHITE COLOR. RODS DETECT MOTION, OBJECTS MOVING IN THE VISUAL FIELD. EXAMPLE: A OBJECT (BIRD....) MOVES IN THE PERIPHERAL FIELD, THE RODS DETECT IT AND THE PERSON TURNS AND LOOKS DIRECTLY AT THE BIRD, PLACING IT IN THE CENTER OF THE VISUAL FIELD TO SEE IT CLEAR. RODS ALSO CONTINUE TO FUNCTION IN VERY DIM LIGHT, ALMOST COMPLETE DARKNESS.

FRONT VIEW OF THE BACK OF THE EYES RETINA, LOOKING IN THROUGH FRONT OF THE EYE.

OUTER PERIPHERAL FIELD OF RETINA. MANY RODS - NO CONES. PRODUCES MOST UNCLEAR VISION IN THE OUTER PERIPHERAL FIELD. ONLY GREY/BLACK/WHITE COLOR PERCEPTION.

MIDDLE PERIPHERAL FIELD. CONES AND RODS - MORE RODS, LESS CONES. PRODUCES CLEARER VISION THAN THE OUTER PERIPHERAL FIELD AND LESS CLEAR VISION THAN THE CENTER OF THE VISUAL FIELD.

INNER PERIPHERAL FIELD CONES AND RODS - MORE CONES. VISION CLEARER THAN THE OUTER AND MIDDLE OF PERIPHERAL FIELDS BUT NOT AS CLEAR AS THE CENTER OF THE VISUAL FIELD.

MACULA - CENTER OF THE RETINA. MANY CONES - FEW RODS PRODUCES VERY CLEAR VISION, CLEARER THAN 20/20 AND BRIGHT COLOR IN THE OUTER AREA OF THE CENTER OF THE VISUAL FIELD.

FOVEA CENTRALIS - CENTER OF THE MACULA IN THE CENTER OF THE RETINA. MANY CONES - VERY FEW RODS. PRODUCES VERY CLEAR VISION, CLEARER THAN 20/20, (CLEARER THAN THE MACULA PRODUCES) AND BRIGHT COLOR IN THE CENTER OF THE VISUAL FIELD.

CENTER OF FOVEA CENTRALIS MANY CONES - HIGH CONCENTRATION OF CONES. NO RODS. PRODUCES THE CLEAREST VISION, MUCH CLEARER THAN 20/20; 20/10, 20/5, 40/5 ... AND BRIGHT COLOR IN THE <u>EXACT</u> CENTER OF THE VISUAL FIELD.

Central Fixation and Shifting.
The center of the visual field moves, shifts with the eyes, point of visual attention.

Looking at the center of the tree. Center of visual field moves here.

Looking at the top of the tree. Center of visual field moves here.

Eyes, center of visual field move up.

Looking at the bottom of the tree. Center of visual field moves here.

Eyes, center of visual field move down.

The head/face body move with the eyes, same time, direction.

Since small objects cannot be seen without central fixation, the reading of fine print, when it can be done, is one of the best of visual exercises, and the dimmer the light in which it can be read and the closer to the eye it can be held the better. Read fine print in the sunlight daily. No eyeglasses!

I think its lots of fun playing tag with the memory or mental pictures. I like to dig out of my memory all the perfect mental pictures I can—one by one—for Central Fixation plays a big part in mental pictures, remembering one thing best at a time.

Having once been to Canada my favorite way of getting relaxed is to go there by mental pictures. I go along a beautiful country road, remember a lake that had impressed me, visualize it with my mind's eye and so on. Sometimes I skip a couple of towns and arrive in Canada very quickly and other times I get enough relaxation by just staying in one town for a while.

The eyes face directly at the object of visual attention, placing the center of the fovea centralis/visual field directly on the part of the object the eyes are looking at.
The eyes, head/face, center of visual field are directed at the part of the object the eyes are looking at.
The center of the visual field moves with the eyes (& head, face) as the eyes move 'shift' from part to part on the object and from object to object.
The Central light ray from the part of the object the eyes are looking directly at/center of visual field focuses on the exact center of the fovea centralis in the center of the macula, eyes retina.
Peripheral rays focus on the peripheral areas of the retina.
Vision is perfectly clear.

Palming

Palm and remember, shift on a favorite object: flower, colorful stone, jewelry, tree, land, old house... Improving the memory, imagination of clear mental pictures relaxes the mind, body, eyes and improves the vision.

Palm and imagine drifting down a river. See objects in color, clear, motion. Movement of the boat, water, birds flying, sun shining, sparkling on the river, animals walking on the shore, colorful dragonflies... Imagine all the senses; touch, warmth of sun, feel the breeze, hear the water, birds, wind, taste your favorite drink...

Palm and remember a sunset, blue sky, white cloud... and shift part to part on the objects and from object to object. Then, it is easy to remember a clear, black letter o. Place the o on the white cloud and shift on the o and see it move, 'swing' opposite the shift of the eyes. Open the eyes, vision is clear.

Remember pleasant objects, favorite scene, adventure, activity... Remember, imagine objects clear, in color, motion: Birds, butterflies flying about, wind blowing the tall grass, flowers, sun sparkling on the mountain tops, river. Shift on the objects. Shift on, see in the mind small fine details clear.

Sunlight and Sunning daily
Sit in the sun, eyes open looking at the bright sky, then eyes closed facing the sun and move the head side to side, up and down...

Kitty

Doll

Remembering, imagining clear mental pictures improves the memory, imagination, relaxation and clarity of vision.
The girl palms and thinks of her doll, (a favorite thing), remembers, imagines, shifts part to part on her doll seeing one part best at a time (Central Fixation). Doll is imagined clear, in color. This improves the memory, imagination and clarity of vision for other objects.
Remembering mental pictures of a pleasant object, subject relaxes the mind, eyes, improves the vision.
She shifts on a clear mental image of her kitty cat.
Sees it in motion, playing.

Shift left and right on the E and see it move in the opposite direction.
+Shift to the dot on the left, The E moves right.
+Shift to the dot on the right, the E moves left.

E

Palming
Palm and imagine black or any pleasant object, scene... Think happy thoughts. Shift on objects in the mind, see them clear, in color, motion.

Girl palms and remembers her doll, color of its dress... Opens the eyes and Eyechart letters are seen clear.

E

Perfect mental pictures, relaxation=clear vision.

Sway, dancing to music improves clarity of vision and straightens the eyes, gets them moving together.

CENTRAL-FIXATION – Seeing Clearest with the Center of the Visual Field

GIRL LOOKING AT BLUEBIRD.
BIRD IS IN THE CENTER OF THE VISUAL FIELD.

Videos;
https://www.youtube.com/watch?v=-HcAMLGptHo
https://www.youtube.com/watch?v=YVQ6pWHcO78

Central-fixation is a Correct, Natural Vision Habit, (the normal, relaxed function of the eyes) that produces very clear fine detailed vision.
Central-fixation = to see clear by using the center of the visual field.
To place the object the eyes are looking at in the center of the visual field.
   The center of the visual field is between the left and right eyes, at eye level.
The center is the clearest area of the visual field, clearer than 20/20.
The center of the visual field is produced by the fovea centralis, macula in the center of the eyes retina. The fovea and macula produce the clearest vision, clearer than 20/20.
   The center of the visual field, (central Field) moves with the eyes, visual attention; from object to object and part to part on objects. See one small part of a object clearest at a time, in the center of the visual field. Move the central field from part to part. Each new part the eyes shift to, look at is in the center of the visual field and is seen clearest. The new part is clearest while the central field is on that part. Then, when the eyes (central field) move to a new part, that part will be seen clearest. The eyes move continually from part to part, seeing one part at a time clearest, in the central field.

In the picture above the girl is looking at the bluebird in the tree.
The bird is in the center of the visual field and is seen clear.
Relaxation, shifting and central-fixation are the 3 main Correct Vision Habits that keep the vision clear. Practice them in a relaxed, easy, effortless manner.
Avoid staring, eye immobility, becoming stiff, immobile when placing a object in the center of the visual field. Relax, blink and move.

Central-fixation is combined with shifting = shift, move the eyes (visual attention, center of the visual field) from part to part on the object. The eyes, head/face, neck and body are relaxed and move freely. Blink, relax and move. The entire visual field is seen by the eyes, brain. The central field is clearest.

Move the head with the eyes; eyes, head/face move together, at the same time, in the same direction.

SWITCHING, SHIFTING CLOSE, MIDDLE AND FAR

Switching Close, Middle, Far on objects at different distances is a type of Shifting that improves the clarity of vision at all distances.

Switching; to switch (change) the visual attention from one distance to another distance.

Example;
+Look at a object at a close distance, the cat on the fence. Shift part to part on the cat. Blink, Relax.

+Then switch to a object at a far distance - trees, mountains, sky. Shift part to part on the far objects.

+Then switch back to the close object - cat. Shift part to part on the cat.

+Switch back and forth; cat, trees, mountains, sky, cat, trees, mountains, sky, cat... Shift on each object the eyes look at, one object at a time.

+Switch to the middle distance; cat to house, house to cat, cat to house... house to trees, mountains, back to house, trees...

Switch back and forth on any objects, any distances, close, middle, far, in any order.
Let the eyes move, shift freely from object to object and part to part on objects; shift along the fence, grass, flowers, truck, dog, house, owl, trees, mountains, sky, birds. Shift on small parts, tiny details on objects; shift part to part on the windows in the house, window panes, chimney, bricks in the chimney. Shift on the owls face, eyes, ears, wings, claws. Central-fixation: shift point to point on tiny parts. No effort to see. Blink, breathe deep, relax.
Trace on/along the edge of objects, parts of objects with the Nosefeather; mountains, hills, trees, house, fence, any object.

Switch on objects at close, middle, far distances that are in a <u>straight line, row with eachother</u>.

In the picture of the kitty on the fence, house, mountains; To practice switching, shifting on the objects; the person stands with the cat, fence at eye level. Height of the cat, fence is in front of the persons face. This causes some distant objects (house, trees...) to be directly beyond the cat, fence. The objects are aligned with eachother. Placing a few objects in a straight line with eachother greatly improves accommodation, un-accommodation and convergence, divergence when looking close, middle and far, switching back and forth on the cat, house...

Practice with; both eyes together, then one eye at a time. If the vision is less clear in one eye; do an extra 20-30 seconds switching, shifting practice with that eye. Then practice with both eyes together again.

Shift on the kitty, then on the distant moon, then on the kitty, then moon, kitty... Blink, relax.

This improves the clarity of vision.
Example: See the picture of the kitty and moon. The kitty and moon are in a row, aligned.
Shift part to part on the kitty, then switch to the distant moon and shift on the moon, then back to the kitty, then moon, kitty... See the pictures below; The man switches, shifts close, middle, far on 5 telephone poles aligned with eachother, in a straight line down the side of the street. He shifts, traces on the poles, one at a time.

Switch, Shift, Trace on objects at <u>different distances in a straight line with eachother</u> to perfect: accommodation, un-accommodation, convergence, divergence, clarity of vision. Practice with: both eyes together, then one eye at a time, then both eyes together again.

Switch, shift, central-fixation on objects at different distances; close, middle and far, in a straight line with each other. This perfects convergence, divergence, accommodation, un-accommodation for clear eyesight at all distances.

He then does the Rock; moves the eyes, head, face, body side to side and notices oppositional movement of the poles; Poles at different distances appear to move against eachother in opposite directions as he rocks side to side. The close pole moves opposite his eyes, head, body moment and the far distant pole appears to move with him in the same direction.

He also switches, shifts on the houses along the side of the street. He gets a good view of the houses aligned by standing where the kitty is by the edge of the house.

The 2 other pictures show more objects in a straight line.

Example: Shifting part to part on the Pete's brewery sign, then on the truck beyond it, then back to the sign, then to the truck, then to the trees, back to the truck, then trees, sign, trees, truck... Switch to and shift on the fields, mountains, airplane, parachute, birds. Switch to any object, any order and shift on it.

(Switching is not done only on objects in a straight line. Switching is also practiced on objects at a variety of locations; left, right, up, down, diagonally... to give the eyes complete freedom of shifting movement. This is the normal, natural function of the eyes. Straight line switching is only practiced a short time to 'tune up' the eyes function, visual clarity.) More examples for switching in a straight line are in the 'Pens in a Row' section in this chapter.

Switching, shifting... at night video;
http://www.youtube.com/watch?v=r5JxOFVi3hc

Switch back and forth on objects at different distances, in line with eachother. Shift part to part on objects.

Practice switching, shifting, central fixation... on real objects in your environment. (Switching cannot be done on these pictures because they are on a flat surface, all are at one distance so changes in convergence, accommodation, divergence, un-accommodation do not occur when looking at objects that appear at different distances on the paper.) Shifting, central-fixation can be done on the pictures with benefit.

When looking at a object; shift on it, even when looking at the object for only a few seconds. Shift from part to part.

Central-fixation - keep the object the eyes are looking at in the center of the visual field. The center of the visual field is clearest, clearer than 20/20. Placing the object (part of the object) the eyes are looking at in the center of the visual field keeps the object clear.
The center of the visual field moves with the eyes as the eyes move, shift from part to part on a object and from object to object keeping every object, every part of a object the eyes look at perfectly clear.
The head, face and body move with the eyes, at the same time, in the same direction.
The eyes, head/face, neck and body are relaxed and move freely, easy. Blink and relax.

Keep the eyes moving, shifting easy, relaxed from part to part and object to object. Look at a object and shift on it. Then look at a different object, shift on it, then look at another object, shift on it.
Eye movement keeps the mind, eyes relaxed and vision clear.
With practice the eyes shift '<u>on their own', automatically</u>, without the person thinking about it, the true natural function of the eyes.

Practice switching back and forth on objects at <u>close</u>, <u>middle</u> and <u>far</u> distances with;
<u>**Both eyes together**</u>**, then with** <u>**one eye at a time**</u>**, then,** <u>**both eyes together again**</u>**.**
<u>**If vision is less clear in one eye, practice a little more with that eye**</u> to get the vision equal and perfectly clear in the left and right eyes at all distances. When the vision is equal in the left and right eyes, the vision quickly improves to perfect clarity. The memory, imagination, left and right brain hemispheres work with the eyes. Their function improves when the vision is equal in the left and right eyes. Brain function with the eyes, visual system, all brain functions and clarity of vision improve.

Keep the objects in the center of the visual field, between the left and right eyes, at eye level when using both eyes together and when using one eye at a time.

The eye that is <u>not in use</u> is covered with a eye patch and the eye is kept <u>open</u> under the patch. (Closing one eye causes eye muscle tension and blur so keep both eyes open when using one eye at a time). Both eyes close when the eye in use is closed. Leave a little space between the eye and patch so some light gets in to keep both eyes, left and right brain hemispheres activated.

Practice switching, shifting, tracing, central fixation on objects, parts of objects with the Nosefeather.

Switching improves convergence and accommodation of the eyes when looking at objects at close distances - (20 feet and closer) for clear close vision and improves un-convergence (divergence) and un-accommodation when looking at objects at far distances (about 20 feet and farther into the distance) for clear distant vision.

The author of this book learnt switching and shifting from reading Aldous Huxley's book 'The Art of Seeing' in high school, 1974 and regained 20/20 clear distant vision in 5 minutes and clearer vision in one day and threw away her glasses. Close and distant vision continues to be clear at age 58 in Mar., 2015. I practice with fine and micro print.

Window pane bars (wood surrounding a window pane) can be used to practice switching close and far.

The bar is the close object. The objects outside the window (tree, birds, house...) are the distant objects.
Switch back and forth, close and far, on a window bar and a distant object <u>in line with the bar</u>.
Then, move the eyes, (visual attention) throughout the scene, looking at, shifting on any objects, at any location. Shift on the close and far objects, use central-fixation, shift on small objects, parts. Blink.
Practice with; <u>both eyes together</u>, then <u>one eye at a time</u>, then <u>both eyes together again</u>. <u>Extra practice with a eye that has less clear vision.</u>

Place a close and far object in the central field-between the eyes. When looking at the far object; the close object in line with it appears double, its 2 images appearing in the peripheral field on the left and right sides of the far object. The images are equally spaced. When looking at the close object; the far object appears double.

A open window is best, bringing full spectrum sunlight onto the face, eyes and a perfect view, unobstructed by glass. Open the window and hang a pencil vertically on a string in the center of the window for the close object. (Cap the pointed end of the pencil for safety.)

Switch, shift back and forth on the pencil and distant objects beyond the pencil.
Hang a few more pencils or other objects in the window so the eyes, head/face, body have more movement, more close objects (pencils...) to look at.
Objects can be hung on a rope at close, middle, far distances outside in the sunlight.

See The Illusion of Oppositional Movement

Rock the body side to side, left and right, while facing the window bar and distant objects and see oppositional movement, 'The Swing';

+ When the eyes, head/face, body move to the <u>left</u> <
  the window bar (close object) appears to move in the opposite direction, to the <u>right</u>. >
+ When the eyes, head/face, body move to the <u>right</u> >
  the window bar appears to move in the opposite direction, to the <u>left</u>. <
+ Notice that the house (distant object) appears to move with the eyes, head/face, body in the same direction.
+ Notice that the window bar (close object) and the house (distant object) appear to move <u>against eachother, in opposite directions</u>.

Do not lock the eyes/visual attention on any objects when moving left and right; just relax and let the objects move. Don't try to see anything clear.
This activity relaxes the mind, body, eye muscles, eyes and improves the clarity of vision.

When the eyes can move, shift on small and tiny objects and see oppositional movement-the eyes function is perfect and vision is most clear; Practice shifting on and seeing 'The Swing' of a small tiny object=fine print letter or tiny flower.

Shift <u>left to right</u> > on the letter - the letter moves, 'swings' to the <u>left</u> <.
Shift <u>right to left</u> < on the letter- the letter moves, 'swings' to the <u>right</u> >.
Blink and relax. No effort to see the letter or the swing. This brings very clear, fine detailed vision.

Practice shortening the rock, eye, head/face, body movement; shift on a small object; letter, fine print and see a small swing of oppositional movement. This activates saccadic eye movements, perfect central fixation and very clear vision. Small eye shifts, seeing tiny details clear with relaxation.

Switching, shifting on objects and seeing oppositional movement can be done most anywhere throughout the day and at night. There are always close and far objects in the visual field to practice on. Just a little practice, couple minutes a day or two, three days week will improve the vision. Once vision is clear, practice only if needed to bring the vision clearer than 20/20 in times of normal fluctuations. Keep natural, normal eye, visual system function as a healthy habit.

The business cards showing the San Francisco Bridge in California, USA and the field, trees can be given to people that need vision improvement. Pictures on the cards are pleasant to look at, induce a positive, happy state of mind, relax the mind, body and eyes. The person presenting the card can be a Natural Vision Improvement Teacher and give the person a quick, easy lesson by describing how to switch the visual attention back and forth on objects at close, middle and far distances; bridge at close distance, sea at middle distance, city of San Francisco and skyline, clouds far distance. Describe shifting from object to object in the visual field, shifting part to part on objects, moving the head/face, body with the eyes, central-fixation; placing objects, parts of objects in the center of the visual field, seeing the central field clearest, seeing small fine details clear at close and far distances, relaxation, memory, imagination. Place your website, contact information on the card for in person training.

Close the eyes and imagine looking close and far; shift on a close object, then a far object, then close, far... The eyes converge inward when looking close and diverge out when looking far *even when practicing using the memory-imagination with the eyes closed*. This can also help the blind; get the lens and eyes moving. When the eyes accommodate (look close) the lens and eye change shape to focus light rays correct. As the lens changes shape, the eye lengthens. When looking far the lens returns to its previous shape and the eye returns to its round shape. The movement keeps the lens flexible, hydrated, nutrients flow in, waste moves out. Circulation in the eyes is improved. This can help to reverse cataract, unclear eyesight.

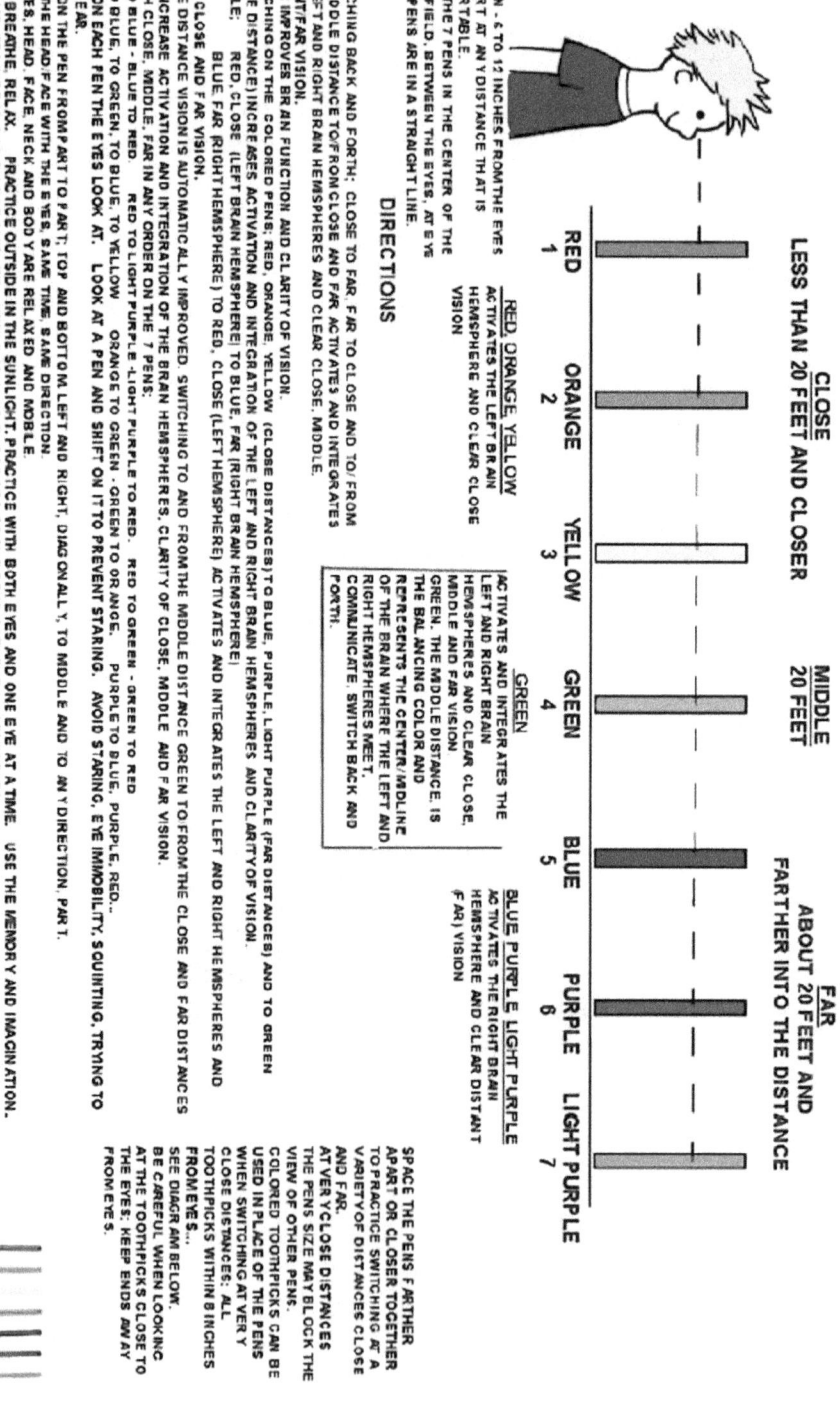

SWITCH ON THE SEVEN COLORED PENS PLACED AT CLOSE, MIDDLE AND FAR DISTANCES

RED 1	ORANGE 2	YELLOW 3	GREEN 4	BLUE 5	PURPLE 6	LIGHT PURPLE 7

CLOSE
LESS THAN 20 FEET AND CLOSER

MIDDLE
20 FEET

FAR
ABOUT 20 FEET AND FARTHER INTO THE DISTANCE

RED, ORANGE, YELLOW
ACTIVATES THE LEFT BRAIN HEMISPHERE AND CLEAR CLOSE VISION

GREEN
ACTIVATES AND INTEGRATES THE LEFT AND RIGHT BRAIN HEMISPHERES AND CLEAR CLOSE, MIDDLE AND FAR VISION GREEN, THE MIDDLE DISTANCE, IS REPRESENTS THE CENTER/MIDLINE OF THE BRAIN WHERE THE LEFT AND RIGHT HEMISPHERES MEET, COMMUNICATE, SWITCH BACK AND FORTH.

BLUE, PURPLE, LIGHT PURPLE
ACTIVATES THE RIGHT BRAIN HEMISPHERE AND CLEAR DISTANT (FAR) VISION

DIRECTIONS

RED PEN - 6 TO 12 INCHES FROM THE EYES OR START AT ANY DISTANCE THAT IS COMFORTABLE. PLACE THE 7 PENS IN THE CENTER OF THE VISUAL FIELD, BETWEEN THE EYES, AT EYE LEVEL. PENS ARE IN A STRAIGHT LINE.

+SWITCHING BACK AND FORTH: CLOSE TO FAR, FAR TO CLOSE AND TO/FROM THE MIDDLE DISTANCE TO/FROM CLOSE AND FAR ACTIVATES AND INTEGRATES THE LEFT AND RIGHT BRAIN HEMISPHERES AND CLEAR CLOSE, MIDDLE, DISTANT/FAR VISION.

COLOR IMPROVES BRAIN FUNCTION AND CLARITY OF VISION.

+SWITCHING ON THE COLORED PENS; RED, ORANGE, YELLOW (CLOSE DISTANCES) TO BLUE, PURPLE, LIGHT PURPLE (FAR DISTANCES) AND TO GREEN (MIDDLE DISTANCE) INCREASES ACTIVATION AND INTEGRATION OF THE LEFT AND RIGHT BRAIN HEMISPHERES, CLARITY OF CLOSE, MIDDLE AND FAR VISION. EXAMPLE: RED, CLOSE (LEFT BRAIN HEMISPHERE) TO BLUE, FAR (RIGHT BRAIN HEMISPHERE)

BLUE, FAR (RIGHT HEMISPHERE) TO RED, CLOSE (LEFT HEMISPHERE) ACTIVATES AND INTEGRATES THE LEFT AND RIGHT HEMISPHERES AND CLEAR CLOSE AND FAR VISION.

MIDDLE DISTANCE VISION IS AUTOMATICALLY IMPROVED. SWITCHING TO AND FROM THE MIDDLE DISTANCE GREEN TO FROM THE CLOSE AND FAR DISTANCES WILL INCREASE ACTIVATION AND INTEGRATION OF THE BRAIN HEMISPHERES, CLARITY OF CLOSE, MIDDLE AND FAR VISION.

SWITCH CLOSE, MIDDLE, FAR IN ANY ORDER ON THE 7 PENS:
RED TO BLUE - BLUE TO RED   RED TO LIGHT PURPLE - LIGHT PURPLE TO RED   RED TO GREEN - GREEN TO RED
RED TO BLUE - TO GREEN, TO BLUE, TO YELLOW   ORANGE TO GREEN - GREEN TO ORANGE,   PURPLE TO BLUE, PURPLE, RED...
SHIFT ON EACH PEN THE EYES LOOK AT. LOOK AT A PEN AND SHIFT ON IT TO PREVENT STARING. AVOID STARING, EYE IMMOBILITY, SQUINTING, TRYING TO SEE CLEAR.

SHIFT ON THE PEN FROM PART TO PART; TOP AND BOTTOM, LEFT AND RIGHT, DIAGONALLY, TO MIDDLE AND TO ANY DIRECTION, PART.
MOVE THE HEAD/FACE WITH THE EYES, SAME TIME, SAME DIRECTION.
THE EYES, HEAD, FACE, NECK AND BODY ARE RELAXED AND MOBILE.
BLINK, BREATHE, RELAX.   PRACTICE OUTSIDE IN THE SUNLIGHT. PRACTICE WITH BOTH EYES AND ONE EYE AT A TIME. USE THE MEMORY AND IMAGINATION.
SEE COMPLETE DIRECTIONS ON TOP PICTURE.   TRACE AROUND THE EDGES OF THE PENS WITH THE NOSEFEATHER.
SWITCHING, SHIFTING ON THE PENS AND USE OF CENTRAL FIXATION KEEPS THE EYES RELAXED, IMPROVES CONVERGENCE, ACCOMMODATION AT CLOSE DISTANCES, UNCONVERGENCE, UNACCOMMODATION AT FAR DISTANCES.
CENTRAL FIXATION: PLACE THE PART OF THE PEN THE EYES ARE LOOKING AT IN THE CENTER OF THE VISUAL FIELD, BETWEEN THE EYES AT EYE LEVEL. THE CLEAR CENTER OF THE VISUAL FIELD MOVES WITH THE EYES AS THE EYES SHIFT FROM PART TO PART ON THE PENS.

SPACE THE PENS FARTHER APART OR CLOSER TOGETHER TO PRACTICE SWITCHING AT A VARIETY OF DISTANCES CLOSE AND FAR.
AT VERY CLOSE DISTANCES THE PENS SIZE MAY BLOCK THE VIEW OF OTHER PENS.
COLORED TOOTHPICKS CAN BE USED IN PLACE OF THE PENS WHEN SWITCHING AT VERY CLOSE DISTANCES; ALL TOOTHPICKS WITHIN 8 INCHES FROM EYES...
SEE DIAGRAM BELOW.
BE CAREFUL WHEN LOOKING AT THE TOOTHPICKS CLOSE TO THE EYES; KEEP ENDS AWAY FROM EYES.

COLORED TOOTHPICKS

234

A case of divergent vertical squint ultimately cured by educational methods. In the picture at the left the right eye turns out and up, while the left eye looks straight. At the right the patient has learned to look straight with the right eye, while the left turns down and out.

A part of the treatment. The patient has learned to turn both eyes in by looking at a pencil held over the bridge of the nose. Later she became able to turn them in without the pencil, or to turn either eye in while the other remained straight.

The same patient after a complete cure had been effected. All four pictures were taken within fifteen minutes of each other, the patient having learned to reproduce the conditions represented voluntarily

1-Both Eyes   2-Right Eye   3-Left Eye

4-Right Eye   5-Left Eye   6-Both Eyes

See complete practice on the right >

After using the pen, practice with any close object; a t-bear, ring, flower in your garden...

Plain, Basic Switching;

A - <u>Eight Steps for Switching Close and Far with Both Eyes Together and One Eye at a Time with the Pen and Far Object Between the Left and Right Eyes, at Eye Level in the Two Eyes One Central Field</u>. Shift on the close object, then shift on the far, then close, then far... Shift on middle distance objects. Practice this with the 8 Steps below. (Picture is of a person facing you.) This person has 20/50 vision in the right eye and 20/100 (<u>less clear</u>) vision in the left eye. Practice brings the vision to equal, perfect 20/20 and clearer in both eyes at all distances. Practice with the close pen and far object at a variety of distances; 2 to 7 - 20 inches from the eyes. 2 feet to 5 - 10, 25, 40, 300... feet into infinity.

Do not wear eyeglasses, contact lenses, sunglasses.

See the main book chapters for descriptions, directions for Shifting, Switching, Central-Fixation...

Right Eye   Left Eye

1 #1 -Practice with both left and right eyes together. 30 seconds to 2 minutes... as is comfortable.

2 #2 -Practice with One Eye at a Time; Practice with the <u>Right</u>, clearest vision eye first to get the clearest visual, mental picture of the close and far objects stored in the brain, memory.
(Patch the Left eye)

3 #3 -Practice with the <u>Left</u>, less clear vision eye.
(Patch the Right eye)

4 #4 -Practice with the <u>Right</u> clearest vision eye again.
(Patch the Left eye)

5 #5 -Practice with the <u>Left</u>, less clear vision eye.
(Patch the Right eye)

6 #6 -Practice extra time 10 - 30 seconds... with the <u>Left</u>, less clear vision eye.
(Patch the Right eye)

7 #7 -Practice with the <u>Right</u>, clearest vision eye again, a short time, 2-5 seconds.
(Patch the Left eye)

8 #8 - End; Practice with both left and right eyes together again for equally clear, balanced vision in the left and right eyes at all distances-close, middle and far.

Repeat Steps # 1-8

B - Seven Steps - Secret Switching # 1
with Pen & Far Object in Front of One Eye

Switching Close & Far

The Pen and Yellow Kitty are aligned with eachother in the one eyes central field, in line with the eyes pupil.

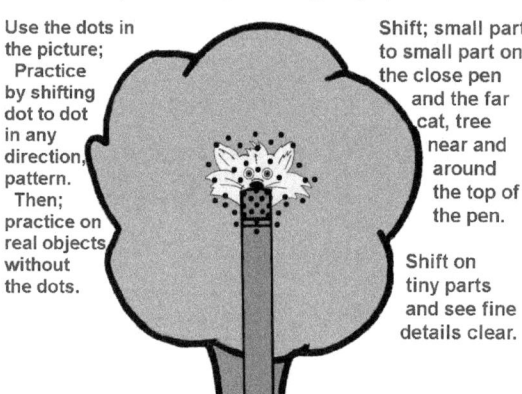

Use the dots in the picture; Practice by shifting dot to dot in any direction, pattern. Then; practice on real objects, without the dots.

Shift; small part to small part on the close pen and the far cat, tree near and around the top of the pen.

Shift on tiny parts and see fine details clear.

The pictures on this page show another type of Switching; 7 Steps for *Secret Switching #1*; changing 'switching' the eyes' focus, visual-mental attention back and forth on close and far objects with the close and far objects in front of one eye. *(Done only with one eye at a time. Never do this with the close pen and far object in front of one eye with both eyes together because that will disrupt convergence, divergence and cause crossed, wandering eyes and unclear vision*.)

Done correct, it specifically improves 'perfects' the eye's lens and eyeball's accommodation, un-accommodation (shape change), the lens and it's *ciliary* eye muscle function, outer eye muscle function, lens and eye circulation, central-fixation, shifting and clarity of vision to better than 20/20 in each individual eye. See picture above; Switching on the close red pen and far yellow kitty. Practice Steps # 1-6 on the right. >

Patch the eye not in use. Work with the non-patched eye; Place the red pen top and a far object (cat) in line with eachother, in front of the one eye, in front of the eye's pupil - in that one eye's exact central field. Move the pen top down a bit so you can see the far object. Shift part to part on the close pen top. Then switch to and shift on the far object (cat) that is in line with the pen top. Then back to the pen, then far again, then pen... Repeat. Blink and relax. Switch from the close and far objects to a middle distance object also in line with the eye, pen.

Next; practice with the other eye. (Use steps # 1-6 above.)

Step #7; <u>Begin</u> and <u>end</u> the practice with <u>*both eyes together, the pen and far object between the left and right eyes*</u>; repeat A - # 1-8 Steps on the previous page. All 8 Steps. The switching practices produce perfect clear eyesight in the left and right eyes at all distances and helps to correct strabismus (crossed, wandering eyes).

Right Eye | Left Eye

1 #1 - Practice with One Eye at a Time; Practice with the <u>Right</u>, clearest vision eye first to get the clearest visual, mental picture of the close and far objects stored in the brain, memory. (Patch the Left eye)

2 #2 - Practice with the <u>Left</u>, less clear vision eye. (Patch the Right eye)

3 #3 - Practice with the <u>Right</u> clearest vision eye again. (Patch the Left eye)

4 #4 - Practice with the <u>Left</u>, less clear vision eye. (Patch the Right eye)

5 #5 - Practice extra time 10 - 30 seconds... with the <u>Left</u>, less clear vision eye. (Patch the Right eye)

6 #6 - Practice with the <u>Right</u>, clearest vision eye again, a short time, 2-5 seconds. (Patch the Left eye)

7 #7 - End; Practice with both left and right eyes together again for equally clear, balanced vision in the left and right eyes at all distances - close, middle and far.

Pen and far object are always between the left and right eyes when using both eyes together.

Secret Switching #1 - Steps 1 to 6 above with one eye at a time. Pen and cat in the tree are in front of one eye.

Blink and relax. No tension. Do it nice and easy. Allow movement.

Using the Right > Eye. Eye, pen and cat are aligned in a straight line. Pen, cat are in front of the one eye's pupil.

Using the Left < Eye. Eye, pen and cat are aligned in a straight line. Pen, cat are in front of the one eye's pupil.

<u>Secret Switching #2</u> will be free in PDF on the website in 2016 in the *Perfect Sight Without Glasses* Teacher/Student Textbook edition.

Correct, Relaxed, Natural Vision Habits Card

PRACTICE CORRECT VISION HABITS #1 TO 8

NATURAL EYESIGHT IMPROVEMENT CORRECT VISION HABITS CARD

1 - RELAXATION

2 - BLINK

3 - BREATHE RELAXED, DIAPHRAGMATIC/ABDOMINAL

4 - SHIFTING - SHIFT ON THE LETTER E; SHIFT LEFT AND RIGHT, TOP AND BOTTOM, DIAGONALLY, TO THE MIDDLE AND TO ANY PART IN ANY DIRECTION.

5 - CENTRAL FIXATION - SEE THE CENTER OF THE VISUAL FIELD CLEAREST. PLACE THE PART OF THE E THE EYES LOOK AT IN THE CENTER OF THE VISUAL FIELD.
SEE ONE SMALL PART OF THE E CLEAREST AT A TIME IN THE CENTER OF THE VISUAL FIELD. SHIFT THE EYES/VISUAL ATTENTION FROM SMALL PART TO SMALL PART, RELAXED, SLOW, EASY, CONTINUALLY. THE CENTER OF THE VISUAL FIELD MOVES WITH THE EYES KEEPING EACH PART PERFECTLY CLEAR.

6 - MOVEMENT - MOVE THE HEAD/FACE AND BODY IN SYNCHRONIZATION WITH THE EYES, AT THE SAME TIME, IN THE SAME DIRECTION THE EYES SHIFT/MOVE TO.
THE EYES, HEAD/FACE, NECK AND BODY ARE RELAXED AND MOVE FREELY.
SEE THE ILLUSION OF OPPOSITIONAL MOVEMENT; THE E APPEARS TO MOVE IN THE OPPOSITE DIRECTION THE EYES SHIFT/MOVE TO.
SHIFT RIGHT - THE E MOVES LEFT
SHIFT LEFT - THE E MOVES RIGHT.
SHIFT UP - THE E MOVES DOWN.
SHIFT DOWN - THE E MOVES UP.

7 - MEMORY AND IMAGINATION - SHIFT ON A LETTER E AND REMEMBER, IMAGINE AND SEE THE E DARK BLACK AND CLEAR.
DO THIS WITH THE EYES OPEN, THEN CLOSED, THEN OPEN.
REMEMBER, IMAGINE AND SEE THE WHITE GLOW ON THE WHITE PAPER SURROUNDING/AROUND THE E..
PRACTICE PALMING AND REMEMBER, IMAGINE, THINK POSITIVE, PLEASANT THOUGHTS AND SEE OBJECTS IN THE IMAGINATION PERFECTLY CLEAR, IN COLOR, MOTION. IMAGINE USING CORRECT VISION HABITS; SHIFTING ON THE CLEAR OBJECTS IN THE MIND.

8 - SWITCHING - SWITCH BACK AND FORTH; CLOSE, MIDDLE, FAR ON THE 3 E'S #1,2,3 TO IMPROVE CLARITY OF EYESIGHT AT 3 DIFFERENT CLOSE DISTANCES.
SHIFT ON EACH E THE EYES LOOK AT, ONE E AT A TIME.

PRACTICE SWITCHING AND SHIFTING ON THE 3 E'S WITH ONE EYE AT A TIME;
BOTH EYES TOGETHER, THEN ONE EYE AT A TIME -- ONLY LEFT, THEN ONLY RIGHT,
THEN PRACTICE WITH BOTH EYES TOGETHER AGAIN.
IF EYESIGHT IS LESS CLEAR IN ONE EYE, PRACTICE A LITTLE LONGER WITH THAT EYE.
PLACE A EYE PATCH OVER THE EYE NOT IN USE AND KEEP BOTH EYES OPEN.

TRACE THE E'S WITH THE NOSEFEATHER

PRACTICE CORRECT VISION HABITS 1 TO 8 ON SMALL AND FINE PRINT LETTERS.
SHIFT ON THE SMALL DOT BELOW THE E ON EACH POPUP SECTION.

IMPROVE THE CLARITY OF DISTANT EYESIGHT BY SWITCHING BACK AND FORTH CLOSE, FAR, CLOSE, FAR... ON ONE POPUP SECTION AND A DISTANT OBJECT; HOUSE, TREE IN THE DISTANCE, IN LINE WITH THE SECTION.

AVOID INCORRECT VISION HABITS; SQUINTING, STARING, TRYING HARD TO SEE CLEAR.
BLINK AND SHIFT TO SEE A LETTER CLEAR.
LOOK AT SOMETHING ELSE, THEN RETURN TO THE LETTER.

PRACTICE WITH THIS CARD OUTSIDE IN THE SUNLIGHT. OBTAIN FULL SPECTRUM SUNLIGHT DAILY.
READ THE FINE PRINT ON THE BACK OF THIS CARD IN THE SUNLIGHT, SUN SHINING OVER THE SHOULDER, ONTO THE CARD.

PRACTICE CORRECT VISION HABITS ON ANY OBJECT, AT ANY DISTANCE; CLOSE, MIDDLE, FAR.
WITH PRACTICE CORRECT VISION HABITS BECOME AUTOMATIC, OCCUR ON THEIR OWN, ALL THE TIME, RESULTING IN CLEAR EYESIGHT.

SWITCH BACK AND FORTH, CLOSE, MIDDLE, FAR ON THE THREE E'S PLACED AT THREE DIFFERENT CLOSE DISTANCES FOR CLEAR CLOSE EYESIGHT.

PRACTICE THE 8 CORRECT VISION HABITS ON THIS CARD WITHOUT EYEGLASSES.

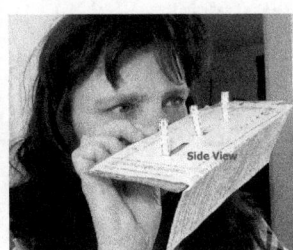

Side View

Presbyopia Cure - For Clear Close Reading Vision.

Maintains a healthy lens, perfect lens movement, accommodation, un-accommodation and the eyes' convergence, divergence.
Practice switching, shifting on the E's on the 3 pop-up sections. Place them in a straight line, between the left and right eyes, the 3 E's at eye level, in the central field.

Switch back and forth on the 3 E's. Shift on one E at a time. Then; shift, switch on the smaller E's. Then; on the small dot .

Use this card with *Plain-Basic Switching - Eight Steps*.

Shifting as a automatic relaxed habit, Switching, Reading Fine and Microscopic Print, use of the Correct Vision Habits Card is all I needed for 41 years (1974 to 2015+) to keep close and far eyesight 20/20 and clearer. Video; https://www.youtube.com/watch?v=knHMjB7T39A

The Duty of Parents

Parents who wish to preserve and improve the eyesight of their children should encourage them to read the Snellen test card every day. There should, in fact, be a Snellen test card in every family; for when properly used it always prevents myopia and other errors of refraction, always improves the vision, even when this is already normal, and always benefits functional nervous troubles. Parents should improve their own eyesight to normal, so that their children may not imitate wrong methods of using the eyes and will not be subject to the influence of an atmosphere of strain. They should also learn the principles of central fixation sufficiently well to relieve and prevent pain, in order that they may teach their children to do the same. This practice not only makes it possible to avoid suffering, but is a great benefit to the general health.

Bead String
Head is straight, bead string straight, aligned between the eyes at nose level or up toward eye level. Look at, 'shift and centralize' upon one bead at a time. Trace around the beads. Blink and relax

Bead String Directions for Chapter XXII
Bead String is at nose level. The eyes look down at the beads. It is best to place the string-beads up higher toward eye level, and still provide a good view of the string and beads. Looking down at nose level can tense the eye muscles if done excessively because; the face is forward while the eyes look down to the string at nose level. The head/face, eyes should be in the same direction. But, when using the bead string; the beads and X are easier to see with the string-beads a bit below eye level or at nose level. The head is straight, not tilted. The bead string is straight. Do not angle it up, down, left, right...

Using Both Eyes; When looking at a bead at about 21 to 23 feet; all beads beyond it farther into the distance (25 to 200 to 500+ ft.) do not appear double. The 21-23 ft. distance varies for some people.

Do not touch the end of the string to the nose. Move it out a few inches, away from the end of the nose to allow the head to move freely, relax.
The Bead String improves the eyesight and corrects strabismus (crossed, wandering eyes, amblyopia).
More Switching Close and Far practices are on the following pages.

SWITCH CLOSE, MIDDLE AND FAR ON THE BEADS

RED ORANGE YELLOW GREEN BLUE PURPLE
1   2   3   4   5   6   7

Shift on the beads; look at #1, red. Shift on it part to part. Blink, relax. Then 'Switch' to #7, purple bead. Shift on it. Then back to #1, red. Shift on it. Back to #7. Shift on it. Switch back and forth on any of the beads in any order, close, middle and far. Build strings of different lengths. The string/beads are placed between the left and right eyes, at eye level, center of the visual field. The string is moved down a bit toward the nose to enable a full view of the string, all beads. But; if this 'eyes look down' posture is maintained too long; tension sets in. The <u>Pens in a Row</u> switching practice shown previously places the pens at eye level. This is a completely natural way to place objects. That is good head/face with the eyes posture. The neck is straight, relaxed. Practice with the beads, then use the pens for extended practice. Blink, breath, relax. More examples are in the E-books.

**Bead String up ^
higher toward eye level.**

The Bead String is placed between the eyes, at nose level or up toward eye level. Look at, *shift and centralize* on one bead at a time. Trace around, on the edge of the beads clockwise, counter-clockwise. Blink, relax. Switch back and forth on the beads; Close red bead to the green or blue or purple bead. Yellow... Move back and forth on any beads, in any order.

Correct Images Seen
For the Beads and String.

   1   2   3
 CLOSE   MIDDLE   FAR

LOOKING AT BEAD 1
RED - CLOSE
The X crosses on the bead the eyes are looking at. Move from bead to bead and see the X move along the string over each bead.
Beads the eyes are not looking at appear double.

LOOKING AT BEAD 2
GREEN - MIDDLE
Practice with;
Both eyes together, then; One eye at a time. Keep the beads in the <u>central field</u>, between the eyes when using both eyes, and when using one eye. There are no double images of the beads, string when using one eye.

LOOKING AT BEAD 3
BLUE - FAR

The Bead String and Pens in a Row can correct Strabismus; crossed, wandering eyes. Additional practice with a moving light or colorful picture moved from the direction the eye is abnormally turned, (the eye looking at it, moving with it), to, onto the bead string in the central field of vision helps activate correct eye movement. See complete directions and eye patch use in this book and the e-books. Do not overuse one eye. The other eye must also be activated to keep a balance.

SWITCH BACK AND FORTH ON OBJECTS AT CLOSE, MIDDLE AND FAR DISTANCES WITH BOTH EYES TOGETHER, THEN ONE EYE AT A TIME, THEN BOTH EYES TOGETHER AGAIN TO IMPROVE CONVERGENCE, ACCOMMODATION FOR CLEAR CLOSE VISION AND UNCONVERGENCE, UNACCOMMODATION FOR CLEAR DISTANT (FAR) VISION.

A typical case of convergent squint or "cross eyes."

The same patient cured by rational methods of eye training.

TREATMENT. One patient, forty years of age, had been blind from birth. The corneas of both eyes were totally opaque, so that it was impossible to see the color of the iris. The patient was helpless on the street and required someone to lead him. Central fixation, the use of his memory and imagination, and other methods for the relief of eyestrain were practiced. The sun treatment was especially beneficial. The patient was taught to expose his closed eyelids to the sun for many hours daily.

At the end of a few months' treatment, he became able to recognize people on the street. He was taught the alphabet and the names of the figures. When his knowledge of the letters became perfect, he was able to read the Snellen test card, 20/20. He was also able to read fine print without glasses. After thirty-five years, his friends reported that his eyes were still normal.

Another case was that of a woman, aged seventy-five, who had to be led into the office. She had suffered from inflammation of the cornea of both eyes for many years, and had frequent attacks of ulcers. From time to time, these ulcers would heal, but they always left a scar.

When the patient was first seen, a scar tissue involved the whole cornea, so that one could not distinguish the colored part of the eye. I believe that eyestrain was the only cause of the trouble, because the sun treatment, palming and swinging, brought about an improvement so that the cornea became perfectly clear, and the vision of the patient for distant and near objects was normal.

The Blindness of Squint or Amblyopia Ex Anopsia

In cases of squint, the vision of the eye which turns either in or out is variable. In many cases, the squinting eye may have normal vision, but in the majority of cases, the vision may be very much lowered, and in rare cases, the squinting eye may be totally blind with no perception of light.

CAUSE. There have been many theories proposed to account for the blindness of squint. I have found, however, that the cause of the blindness is due to eyestrain.

TREATMENT. The vision of these cases is benefited by relaxation methods—palming, swinging, and the use of the memory or the imagination. A letter may be imagined perfectly or imperfectly. When imagined imperfectly, the vision is always lowered. When imagined perfectly, with the eyes open as well as with the eyes closed, the vision is always improved. By remembering or imagining a letter, with the eyes closed for half a minute or longer, one becomes able to imagine a letter quite perfectly with the eyes open for a few seconds. Repeat.

CASE HISTORY. In one case, a woman, about thirty years of age, was totally blind in the right eye which turned in, although the eye itself was apparently normal. That is to say, there were no opacities in any part of the eye, and the retina and optic nerve were normal.

With both eyes open, the vision was 15/20. By practice, with the aid of her memory and imagination, the vision, with both eyes, soon became normal without glasses, 15/10. Coincident with the improvement of the vision of both eyes together, which meant an improvement in the vision of the left eye, the patient gradually became able to distinguish light in the right or blind eye. In less than two weeks, after daily treatment, the vision of the right eye became normal and the eyes straight.

It seems curious that so many articles have been published on amblyopia (dim-sightedness) ex-anopsia (from lack of education or use of eye) without going further and studying the results of the opposite of ex-anopsia,— relaxation methods of treatment.

Sunning Examples

Face the sun with the eyes closed and move the head/face slowly, relaxed side to side; left, right, left, right... Feel and see the sun move across the face/closed eyes.
Then, move the head/face up and down, then circular; trace around the sun counter clockwise, clockwise.
The eyes, head/face (and body) move together, at the same time, in the same direction.

Do the rock while sunning; Face the sun with the eyes closed and rock the entire body side to side, left and right.
Do the long swing.

Sit facing the sun, relax, eyes closed and daydream pleasant thoughts. Occasionally move the head/face side to side.

THE FIGURE EIGHT

LEFT ↓   ↓ RIGHT
CENTER

FAR

CLOSE

Sway < left and right > and see the close chart swing opposite the movement of the eyes, head, body.
Notice the far chart appears to move in the same direction with you and against the close chart. Far objects shows less opposite swing. Close objects shows the most opposite swing.

Swing shorter and;

Switch, shift on letters on two **identical eyecharts** placed at close and far distances.

THE FIGURE EIGHT – INFINITY SWING

DRAW THE FIGURE EIGHT WITH THE EYES, HAND AND END OF THE NOSEFEATHER WHILE DOING THE LONG SWING.
FOLLOW THE ARROWS - START IN THE CENTER AND DRAW UP THE CENTER AND TO THE LEFT FIRST. DRAW THE LEFT SIDE AND BACK UP THE CENTER. THEN DRAW THE RIGHT SIDE. DRAW LEFT, RIGHT, LEFT, RIGHT...

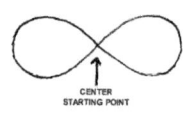

THE FINGERTIPS OF THE 3RD FINGER OF THE LEFT AND RIGHT HANDS TOUCH WITH THE PALMS FACING IN TOWARD THE FACE.
THIS IS THE START POSITION AT THE CENTER OF THE FIGURE EIGHT.

CENTER STARTING POINT

START IN THE CENTER
FRONT VIEW

DRAW THE LEFT SIDE FIRST WITH THE LEFT HAND.
SWING. TURN LEFT AND LIFT THE HEEL OF THE RIGHT FOOT.
EYES LOOKING AT/SHIFTING ON AND MOVING WITH THE CENTER FINGERTIP OF THE LEFT HAND AS THE HAND DRAWS THE EIGHT.
THE END OF THE NOSEFEATHER AND EYES (VISUAL ATTENTION) ARE ON AND MOVING WITH THE LEFT HANDS CENTER FINGERTIP.
PALM OF HAND IS FACING IN TOWARD THE FACE WHEN IN THE CENTER, THEN MOVES OUT STRAIGHT WITH THE ARM AS THE HAND DRAWS THE LEFT SIDE.

DRAW THE RIGHT SIDE WITH THE RIGHT HAND.
SWING. TURN RIGHT AND LIFT THE HEEL OF THE LEFT FOOT.
EYES LOOKING AT/SHIFTING ON AND MOVING WITH THE CENTER FINGERTIP OF THE RIGHT HAND AS THE HAND DRAWS THE EIGHT.
THE END OF THE NOSEFEATHER AND EYES (VISUAL ATTENTION) ARE ON AND MOVING WITH THE RIGHT HANDS CENTER FINGERTIP.
PALM OF HAND IS FACING IN TOWARD THE FACE WHEN IN THE CENTER, THEN MOVES OUT STRAIGHT WITH THE ARM AS THE HAND DRAWS THE RIGHT SIDE.

BACK VIEW
LOOK AT THE DIAGRAM AND FOLLOW THIS MOVEMENT

LOOKING, MOVING LEFT WHEN DRAWING THE LEFT SIDE ACTIVATES THE RIGHT BRAIN HEMISPHERE AND CLEAR DISTANT VISION.

LOOKING, MOVING RIGHT WHEN DRAWING THE RIGHT SIDE ACTIVATES THE LEFT BRAIN HEMISPHERE AND CLEAR CLOSE VISION.

MOVING BACK AND FORTH; LEFT, RIGHT, LEFT, RIGHT AND PASSING ACROSS THE CENTER OF THE EIGHT (MIDLINE/CENTER OF THE BRAIN AND BODY) ACTIVATES AND INTEGRATES THE LEFT AND RIGHT BRAIN HEMISPHERES, CLEAR CLOSE AND DISTANT VISION AND EQUALLY CLEAR PERFECT VISION IN THE LEFT AND RIGHT EYES.

DRAWING THE FIGURE EIGHT RELAXES AND BRINGS MOVEMENT TO THE EYES, HEAD/FACE, <u>NECK</u>, BACK AND BODY AND ACTIVATES CORRECT VISION HABITS.
THIS ALSO IMPROVES THE CLARITY OF EYESIGHT.

The Figure Eight - Infinity Swing

EYECHARTS

Letter size for the charts on the following pages are approximate; print from the PDF E-Book and resize with a copy machine for exact measurement. Print the 20/20 line 3/8 inches. When letters on that line and below are clear; vision is clearer than 20/20 for distant vision at 20 feet and farther. Print the charts small and fine print for close vision practice at 5 feet and up to 1 inch from the eyes.

Read, See Small letters Clear on a Familiar Eyechart Daily;
Both eyes together, one eye at a time, both eyes together again.

SNELLEN TEST CARDS

There should be a Snellen test card in every family and in every school classroom. When properly used it always improves the sight even when it is already normal. Children or adults with errors of refraction, if they have never worn glasses, are cured simply by reading every day the smallest letters they can see at a distance of ten, fifteen, or twenty feet.

For Sale By

The Central Fixation Publishing Company

Paper ....50 Cents

Cardboard (folding) ....75 Cents

DELIVERED

Back numbers BETTER EYESIGHT: single copies, 30 cents; first and second years, unbound, $3 each; bound in cloth, $1.25 extra. Photographic reductions of the Bible, $4. Ophthalmoscopes (best quality), $20. Burning glasses, $4. Reprints of articles by Dr. Bates in other medical journals, a limited number for sale. Send for list.

Eyechart Videos

Videos are on Youtube. Download with Real Player SP.
Watch on computer. Can also be converted for television.

http://www.youtube.com/watch?v=sM-EHgC-J6w&feature=channel
http://www.youtube.com/watch?v=863yFmc-Ius&feature=channel
http://www.youtube.com/watch?v=mYpsYPPV_hg&feature=channel
http://cleareyesight.info/id79.html

How to Use the Snellen Test Card
FOR THE
Prevention and Cure of Imperfect Sight in Children

The Snellen Test Card is placed permanently upon the wall of the classroom, and every day the children silently read the smallest letters they can see from their seats with each eye separately, the other being covered with the palm of the hand in such a way as to avoid pressure on the eyeball. This takes no appreciable amount of time, and is sufficient to improve the sight of all children in one week and to cure all errors of refraction after some months, a year, or longer.

Children with markedly defective vision should be encouraged to read the card more frequently.

Records may be kept as follows:

John Smith, 10, Sept. 15, 1918.
  R. V. (vision of the right eye) 20/40.
  L. V. (vision of the left eye) 20/20.

John Smith, 11, Jan. 1, 1919.
  R. V. 20/30.
  L. V. 20/15.

The numerator of the fraction indicates the distance of the test card from the pupil; the denominator denotes the line read, as designated by the figures printed above the middle of each line of the Snellen Test Card.

A certain amount of supervision is absolutely necessary. At least once a year some one who understands the method should visit each classroom for the purpose of answering questions, encouraging the teachers to continue the use of the method, and making a report to the proper authorities.

It is not necessary that either the inspector, the teachers, or the children, should understand anything about the physiology of the eye.

Man improves vision in his left eye, the eye with less clear vision.
+Shift on letters on the large distant card and close fine print card with the left eye. Blink.
+Shift on a letter with the eye open and remember, imagine it clear,
+Then: repeat in the imagination with the eye closed.
+Open, repeat.
+Look at and remember, imagine the white spaces between sentences, in and around letters pure, bright white with the eye open, closed, open.
+Then look at the black print and read it clear.
+Last: practice with the right eye, then left again, then both eyes together.

Shift on letters on a eyechart (test card) with
+both eyes together, then
+one eye at a time, then
+both eyes together again.

Place a eyepatch over the eye not in use and keep the eye open under the patch.

10 Ft. to 20+ ft.

20 FT. / 20 LINE

Read the test card daily in good light, sunlight is best. Shift on a letter and remember, imagine it clear, correct with the eyes open, then in the imagination with the eyes closed, then with the eyes open again. Repeat. Blink. Practice on smaller letters. Practice with both eyes together, one eye at a time, then both eyes together again. Practice with the chart at various distances 5 ft. to 200 ft.
+ Practice on fine print at 20 inches and closer to 3, 2, 1, inches from the eyes.

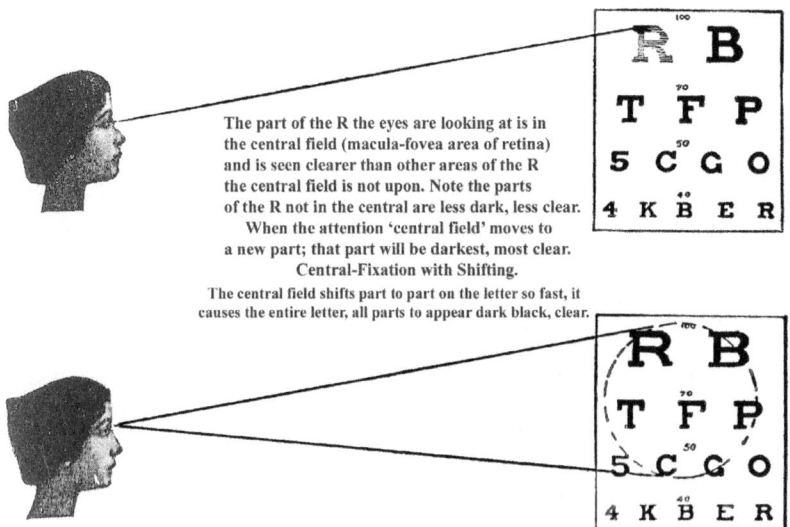

The part of the R the eyes are looking at is in the central field (macula-fovea area of retina) and is seen clearer than other areas of the R the central field is not upon. Note the parts of the R not in the central are less dark, less clear. When the attention 'central field' moves to a new part; that part will be darkest, most clear.
Central-Fixation with Shifting.
The central field shifts part to part on the letter so fast, it causes the entire letter, all parts to appear dark black, clear.

In the upper picture the sight is centered upon one spot, the upper left-hand corner of the letter R, which is seen more clearly and appears to be blacker than the rest of the field of vision. This is central fixation. In the lower picture the subject is endeavoring to see every part of her field of vision equally well at the same time. This is eccentric fixation and always accompanies eye strain.

Upper picture; the less black, less clear parts of the R <u>not</u> in the central field is accentuated to emphasize what central-fixation is. In reality those areas do not appear as light, blurred as in the picture.

Shift left and right, top and bottom and in any direction on the E.

Person is looking at, shifting on the middle part of the B. The middle of the B is in the center of the visual field, is seen darkest black, clearest. The center of the visual field is seen best, clearest.

Central Field

Peripheral Field - less clear.

Shift: ⟷
left and right, dot to dot on the o and see oppositional movement.

Look at/see clearest - one part (dot) of the C at a time, in the <u>center</u> of the visual field. The part (dot) in the peripheral field is less clear.

All parts of the B that are away from the middle part that the eyes are looking directly at and other letters around the B are in the peripheral field and are seen less clear. They are seen clearest only if the eyes, central field moves onto them.

Shift left and right, top and bottom, middle, diagonally and in any direction on the E and see it move in the opposite direction. Practice on the dots: shift dot to dot and see the E move.

Practice shifting on a familiar object - letters on a test card daily with;
Both eyes together, one eye at a time, both eyes together again.

Emily C. Lierman seeing the 20/20 line on the eyechart clear after her eyesight was cured by Ophthalmologist William H. Bates. She became his assistant, working in his Clinic in New York City for many years practicing, teaching patients Natural Eyesight Improvement, The Bates Method. They later married. Her name was changed to Emily A. Bates. She Authored the book; 'Stories From The Clinic'

20/20 Line

White Glow Around Letters

The fact is that it requires an effort to state what is not true, and this effort always results in a deviation from the normal in the refraction of the eye. So sensitive is the test that if the subject, whether his vision is ordinarily normal or not, pronounces the initials of his name correctly while looking at a blank surface without trying to see, there will be no error of refraction; but if he miscalls one initial, even without any consciousness of effort, and with full knowledge that he is deceiving no one, myopia will be produced.

CURED IN FIFTEEN MINUTES

Patients often ask how long it takes to be cured. The answer is that it takes only as long as it takes to relax. If this can be done in five minutes, the patient is cured in five minutes, no matter how great the **degree of his error of refraction, or how long its duration.** All persons with errors of refraction are able to relax in a few seconds under certain conditions, but to gain permanent relaxation usually requires considerable time. Some persons, however, are able to get it very quickly. These quick cures are very rare, except in the case of children under twelve; but they do occur, and I believe the time is coming when it will be possible to cure everyone quickly. It is only a question of accumulating more facts and presenting them in such a way that the patient can grasp them quickly.

A very remarkable case of a quick cure was that of a man of fifty-five who had worn glasses for thirty years for distant vision and ten years for reading, and whose distant vision at the time he consulted me was 20/200.

When he looked at the Snellen test card the letters appeared grey to him instead of black. He was told that they were black, and the fact was demonstrated by bringing the card close to him. His attention was also called to the fact that the small letters were just as black as the large ones He was then directed to close and cover his eyes with the palms of his hands, shutting out all the light. When he did this he saw a perfect black, indicating that he had secured perfect relaxation and that the optic nerve and visual centers of the brain were not disturbed. While his eyes were still closed he was asked:

"Do you think that you can remember with your eyes open the perfect black that you now see?"

"Yes," he answered, "I know I can."

When he opened his eyes, however, his memory of the black was imperfect, and though able to read the large letters, he could not read the small ones. A second time he was told to close and cover his eyes, and again he saw a perfect black. When he opened them he was able to retain complete control of his memory, and so was able to **read the whole card. This was ten minutes after he entered the office.**

Diamond type was now given him to read, but the letters looked grey to him, and he could not distinguish them. Neither could he remember black when he was looking at them, because in order to see them grey he had to strain, and in order to remember black he would have had to relax, and he could not do both at the same time. He was told that the letters were perfectly black, and when he looked away from them he was able to remember them black. When he looked back he still remembered them black, and was able to read them with normal vision at twelve inches. This took five minutes, making the whole time in the office fifteen minutes. The cure was permanent, the patient not only retaining what he had gained, but continuing to improve his sight, by daily reading of fine print and the Snellen test card, till it became almost telescopic.

One of the ways the eyes-brain see is by contrast of white-black and other colors, light-dark, shadows, texture... This relaxes the mind and eyes. Relaxation, variety brings clarity. Look at the white page, then at the white spaces between sentences, white area around and inside letters and words. Then look at the black letters. Look at the black edges of the letters, then at the white page <u>near</u> the letter's edge. The white area closest to the black edge appears brighter, whiter, it 'glows'. Move back and forth on the white glowing areas, the black letters and it's edges. Shift this way along the letters on the eyechart. The white glow on the page near the edge of the bottom of each black letter combines to create a <u>thin bright glowing white line</u> under sentences. The bright white line also appears along the top edge of the sentence. Look at the white line, then the letters, then line, letters... Blink. The glow is a natural illusion. The white relaxes the mind and eyes because it is a blank area; prevents using effort to see, squinting, tension. White also activates the retina, its cones, rods; as light does. Relaxation from the white, contrast and the activation by 'light' continues when looking at the black print. The letters are seen dark black and clear. Look at the print, read the letters, words, sentences easy, effortless. Blink, relax.

Looking back and forth on the white areas and black letters when reading the eyechart keeps the eyes-vision moving. This prevents staring, strain. Movement maintains relaxation and clarity. A entire eyechart is read in seconds. Eye movement *moves* light on the retina, is necessary to activate the cones, rods, nerves... in the retina, send energy, light-image signals to the brain. Note the chart is perfectly clear when glancing at it without thinking to 'test' the sight; when relaxed deeply, or active running around the house, yard and you suddenly look at the chart *without planning to*. It is seen clear because there is no feeling of a test to pass, no pressure to be perfect, no nervousness. Just relaxed, moving vision. Blink and shift. 4 Videos;

http://www.youtube.com/watch?v=sM-EHgC-J6w&feature=channel   http://www.youtube.com/watch?v=863yFmc-Ius&feature=channel
http://www.youtube.com/watch?v=mYpsYPPV_hg&feature=channel   http://cleareyesight-batesmethod.info/id79.html

EYECHARTS TO TEST AND IMPROVE CLOSE AND DISTANT EYESIGHT

SWITCH AND SHIFT ON LETTERS ON TWO IDENTICAL EYE CHARTS PLACED AT CLOSE AND FAR/ CLEAR AND UNCLEAR DISTANCES.

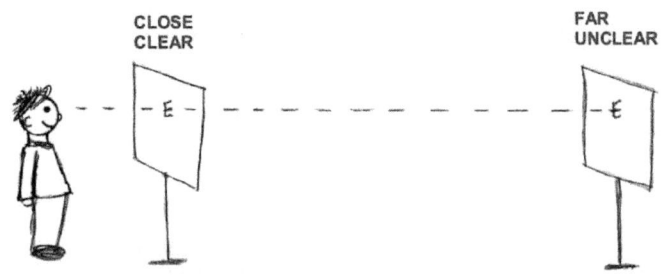

SHIFT FROM PART TO PART (DOT TO DOT) ON THE E'S

E — TOP AND BOTTOM
E — LEFT AND RIGHT
E — DIAGONALLY CORNER TO CORNER
E — MIDDLE
E — SHIFT FROM PART TO PART IN ANY DIRECTION

Videos - http://www.youtube.com/watch?v=863yFmc-Ius

Meaning of 20/20; (for Distant Vision)
+The top number indicates the distance the person is standing from the chart.
+The bottom number indicates the size of the letter, the line the eyes are looking at.
 A 20/20 letter is 3/8 inch. high.

E < This **E** is about 3/8 inch. on 100% computer screen.

+The bottom number also indicates the distance that a person with clear vision sees the letter clear.

Example; the 20/20 line on the test chart for distant vision;
+The top number, 20 indicates; the person is standing 20 feet away from the letter on the eyechart.
+The bottom number, 20 indicates the person is looking at the 20/20 line, 3/8 inch. letter and, that; a person with clear 20/20 vision can see the letter clear at 20 feet away.

The eyechart is placed at 20 feet to test distant vision because the eyes do not need to un-converge, un-accommodate any further when looking at about 20 feet and farther into the distance. If the letters are seen clear at 20 feet, they are seen clear at all distances beyond 20 feet.

At farther distances (300+ ft.) usually people move closer (200 to 40, 20 ft.) to see the medium, small letters, bottom 10 line and smaller. There are people with such perfect vision and relaxation that they can see small details at very far distances.

Here's another example; **20/200;**

+The top number (20) indicates the person is standing 20 feet away from the eyechart.
+The bottom number (200) indicates the size of the letter, line the person is looking at.
The 200 line letter is the largest letter on the top of the chart.
A 20/200 letter is 3½ inches high.
+The bottom number, (200) also indicates that a person with

Distant vision - Big C eyechart with a small 5 line added at bottom.

20/20 = 20 feet
20 = 3/8 inch letter - 20 line.
Normal, clear vision.

20/5 = 20 feet
5 = Smallest letter, bottom of chart - 5 line.
Clearer than 20/20.

40/5 = 40 feet
5 = Smallest letter, bottom of chart - 5 line.
Most clear vision, much clearer than 20/20.
Person sees 5 line at 40 feet away.

C L E A R

20/200 = 20 feet
200 = Largest letter, top of chart - 200 line.
Most unclear vision for this eyechart.

5/200 = 5 feet
200 = Largest letter, top of chart.
Vision more unclear.
The person must stand closer to the chart, at 5 feet, to see the 200 line letter clear.

20/300 = 20 feet
300 = Letter larger than 200 line.
More unclear than 20/200.
Person cannot see the 200 line clear.
A larger, 300 size letter is seen clear.
The 200 and other lines might be seen clear at closer distants to the chart.

U N C L E A R

Perfect eyesight; seeing the 20 line, the bottom 10 line and smaller letters clear at 20 feet and farther; 25, 30, 40... ft.

clear 20/20 distant vision can see the letter clear at 20 feet and up to 200 feet away and often farther.

A person with 20/200 distant vision can see the large 20/200 letter at 20 feet but cannot see it clear farther than 20 feet. It is usually also seen clear at distances closer than 20 feet. The person cannot see smaller letters below the 20/200 line clear at 20 feet and farther away.

20/200 vision is the most unclear level of vision on the eyechart, much less clear than 20/20.

Vision can be more unclear; 20/300, 5/200... Many people with 20/200, 300 and more unclear vision have attained 20/20 and clearer vision with practice of the Bates Method.

20/40 vision is clearer than 20/200 but less clear than 20/20. 20/40 is considered legal for driving in most states. 20/40 is close to 20/20 clarity and people can function comfortably with 20/40 vision without wearing eyeglasses. 20/30, 20/25 is clearer than 20/40, its almost 20/20.

Remember; vision fluctuates. Any level of unclear vision has moments of improved and sometimes perfect clarity. We learn to reproduce and maintain the conditions that bring the clear vision.

It's best to avoid wearing glasses. Eyeglasses maintain and increase eye muscle tension and blur. When glasses are avoided; the eyes, eye muscles, mind/brain (visual system) relax, correct natural vision habits are easily applied and clarity of vision improves. Lowering the eyeglass prescription, weaker and weaker is the next best option. See website; 20/40 to 20/50 legal-safe prescription clarity.

Close vision is tested with smaller letters with the eyechart placed at various distances closer than 20 feet. Reading vision is tested at 3 ft. to 6 inches and closer to the eyes with small and fine print. Seeing fine print clear at 5 to 1 to 1/4 inches from the eyes is very clear vision. Healthy for the eyes.

Relax and Shift, Blink when Reading the Eyechart. Use Central-Fixation

Does your boy squint?

1. This boy is reading the Snellen test card with normal vision. Note the absence of facial strain.
2. The same boy straining to see at a distance is producing myopic astigmatism in eyes previously normal.
3. In this picture the boy is making himself myopic by partly closing his eyes and making conscious effort to read the test card at ten feet.

Immediate Production of Myopia and Myopic Astigmatism in Eyes Previously Normal by Strain to See at the Distance;

Fig 1 - Boy reading the Snellen test card with normal vision. Note the absence of facial strain.
A boy with normal eyes reading the X line of the Snellen test card at 10 feet.
Notice the expression of the eyes with the focus completely relaxed.

Fig 2 - The same boy trying to see a picture at twenty feet. The effort, manifested by staring, produces compound myopic astigmatism, as revealed by the retinoscope. Simultaneous retinoscopy indicated compound myopic astigmatism. He was unconscious of the fact that his eyes were focused for a near point. Note the manifestation of effort by staring.

Fig 3 - The same boy making himself myopic voluntarily by partly closing the eyelids and making a conscious effort to read the test card at ten feet. Functional myopia produced voluntarily by partly closing the eyelids (squinting) and making an effort to read the Snellen test card at ten feet.

There are large and small close and distant eyecharts on the last pages of this book and in the PDF E-Books.

Creating the exact, correct letter size to fit the PDF and paperback book is difficult. Reprinting at larger or smaller setting corrects this. If the chart letters are too small, large; place it in a copier, printer, use the zoom setting until all letters print the correct eyechart size. Correct sizes are listed below. Smaller is better!

The Big C and E charts print out on 3 separate pages, 10 x 8 or 11 x 8½... inches, landscape. Tape them together on cardboard after printing. An exact size Big C chart as shown on the right > can be downloaded from the website.

If the print is too light; darken it to dark black with a black marker.

Chart letters can be reduced to small and fine print for testing, improving close vision and reading vision distances, 5 feet to 20 inches, 10, 6, 5, 3, 1... inches away from the eyes. Or use the small charts.

The charts can be printed from the PDF E-Book with white letters on a black, blue... background. White letters are easy to see and relaxing to the eyes, mind. Color, light activates, is healthy for the eyes, brain, visual system. White is a color, similar to sunlight. The eyes' fovea, it's cones seek light.

The reader can also create small charts as a identical copy of the big C, E charts. Place the identical copy at a clear close distance and look at the identical clear letters to strengthen the memory, imagination of the same letter on the distant chart. If preferred, use a large close and distant chart.

The Big C chart is the eyechart Ophthalmologist Bates refers to in his Better Eyesight Magazine, book. The large big letter E and C charts are for testing distant vision.

Fig. 43
Patient with atrophy of the optic nerve gets flashes of improved vision after palming.

Print the chart with correct letter size;

Start with the big letter E (or C) at the top of the chart - 20/200 line;

20/200 - 3 ½ inch. high
20/100 - 1 ¾ inch.
20/70 - 1 ¼ inch.   **All numbers above 20/20 indicate vision**
20/50 - 7/8 inch.   **less clear than 20/20.**
20/40 - 11/16 inch.
20/30 - 1/2 inch.
20/20 - 3/8 inch. ------------ **Normal clear vision at 20 feet away.**
20/15 - 1/4 inch.   **All numbers below 20/20 indicate clearer**
20/10 - 3/16 inch.   **than 20/20.**
20/5 - 3/32 inch.
20/4, 3, 2, 1... Letters are smaller. Very clear vision.

Standing farther away and seeing the letters clear; Example 40/5; standing 40 feet away and seeing the 20/5 - 3/32 inch. letter and smaller letters clear indicates very clear vision, much clearer than 20/20.

Snellen Test Cards

THERE should be a Snellen test card in every family and in every school classroom. When properly used it always improves the sight even when sight is already normal. Children or adults with errors of refraction, if they have never worn glasses, are cured simply by reading every day the smallest letters they can see at a distance of ten, fifteen, or twenty feet.

PAPER .... 50 CENTS
CARDBOARD (folding) . 75 CENTS
DELIVERED

Back numbers BETTER EYESIGHT............$ .30
Bound vols., 1st, 2nd and 3rd years, each.. 4.25
Photographic reduction of the Bible........ 4.00
Ophthalmoscopes, with and without Battery,
from .... 10.00 to 50.00
Retinoscopes 4.00
Burning glasses........................... 5.00
Reprints of articles by Dr. Bates in other medical journals: a limited number for sale. Send for list.

For Sale By
Central Fixation Publishing Company
300 Madison Avenue, New York City

Read, See Small Letters Clear on a Familiar Eyechart Daily; Both eyes together, one eye at a time, both eyes together again.

Due to page limit, book size; some pages are combined on one page so the book may contain more pictures, training. A blank page should be placed after eyechart pages in all editions so the chart may be extracted without removing other pages. I decided to place extra eyesight practices, pictures on the back of the eyecharts. Letter size for the charts are smaller than normal in most book editions. Seeing these smaller letters clear indicates better vision than indicated on a standard size chart. Print the charts with a scan/copy machine set to adjust each line of letters to correct size as listed in the directions above. Print the 20/20 line 3/8 inches high or a bit smaller. When letters on that line and smaller ones below are clear at 20+ feet; vision is clearer than 20/20 for distant vision (20 feet and farther). Also test, practice for every distance before 20 ft. Unclear vision can occur at a variety of distances. It can be clear at 100 feet and unclear at 50... feet. Clear at 20 feet, unclear at 5... feet. Improve vision at all distances.

Practice Shifting, Central-Fixation, Switching Close and Far on the Eyecharts

Print the Eyecharts.
Make two identical copies of the chart, place them at close and far distances. Practice Correct Vision Habits: shifting, central-fixation... on the charts one or two times per day.
Practice in the sunlight, sun shining over the shoulder onto the charts.

Shifting, switching on the two identical charts improves the memory, imagination, ability to remember, imagine and see the letters clear, improves the brain's function of storing clear images of objects in the memory. Memorize the letters.

The eyecharts become a familiar object. Familiar objects are relaxing to the mind, eyes and are easy to see clear. Prevents effort, squinting.

When a letter on the chart is seen clear at a specific distance; all letters, objects at that distance and often all other distances are clear.

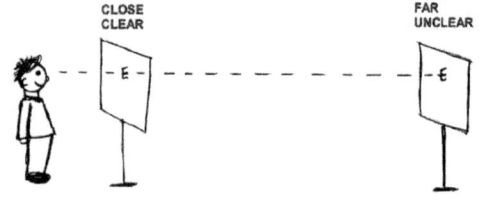

Practice Correct Vision Habits #1 to 10 on two identical eyecharts;   (Correct Vision Habits; see pictures previous pages.)
One chart is placed at a close distance.
The other chart is placed at a far distance. See picture. ^
Keep one chart at a clear distance, the other chart at a unclear distance.

When looking at a chart, place the chart at eye level, directly in line with the eyes, face. The letter the eyes look at is placed in the center of the visual field; between the left and right eyes, at eye level.
  Move the head with the eyes. Relax, allow movement. Avoid tension.
The far chart is placed about 1 foot to the left or right (alternate) so the close chart does not block the view of the far chart.
When looking at a chart, maintain central-fixation (central vision) ;
When looking at the close chart - stand directly in front of it.
When looking at the far chart - move and stand directly in front of it.
  See picture on the right. >

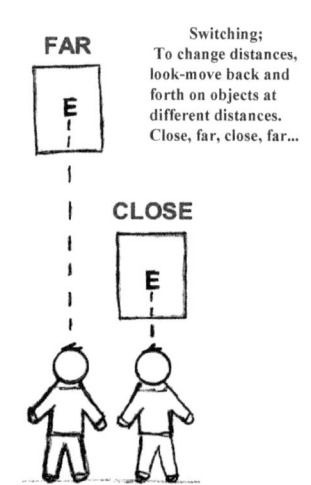

Shift on letters on the clear and unclear eyecharts and remember, imagine and see the letters **dark black** and clear.
Practice with the eyes open, then closed-use the mind-memory. Open again.
Practice with both eyes together, then one eye at a time, then both eyes together again. If vision is less clear in one eye, practice extra time with that eye. Then again a bit with the other eye, then both eyes together again to keep the vision balanced, equal in both eyes.
  Keep the letter between the eyes, at eye level 'center of the visual field' when using both eyes together and when using one eye at a time.
Do this without becoming stiff, immobile. Don't 'try' to be perfect. The eyes-vision will move the central field naturally, on its own as it shifts on a letter and from letter to letter. Blink, breathe and relax.

  Cover the eye not in use with a eyepatch and keep the eye open under the patch when the eye in use is open.

Example; Person needs distant (far) vision improvement.
Place one chart at a far, unclear distance.
Place the other identical chart at a clear close distance.
  Look at the letter **E** at the clear close distance; shift on the letter.
Remember, imagine and see the **E** dark black and perfectly clear.
Do this with the eyes open, then in the imagination with the eyes closed, then with the eyes open again.

Next; switch to the unclear far chart. Look at the identical letter **E**.
Shift on the **E** and continue to remember, imagine the **E** is dark black and clear. See it flash clear.
Practice with the eyes open, closed, open. With practice the far **E** will be seen clear.   (continued on next page.)

> Place two eyecharts in line with eachother at close and far distances; 5 feet and 20+ feet. Sway left and right 1 to 4 feet in front of the charts. See the close chart move opposite of your movement. The far chart moves in the same direction you move to. The far really moves opposite. But, when swaying; far objects show a smaller opposite movement. This causes the far chart to appear to move with you. The close chart's longer opposite movement increases the far chart's same direction appearance. Far away into infinity; far objects show the smallest opposite movement. The 2 charts also appear to move against eachother in opposite directions when swaying. The brain-eyes-vision use this to determine depth, distance, time, speed, location... It is also used to distinguish individual objects when the vision is very unclear, thus enabling and improving Central-Fixation.

Switch back to the <u>clear</u> close **E**.
Repeat; shift on the **E**, remember, imagine, see it dark black and clear.
Practice with the eyes <u>open</u>, <u>closed</u>, <u>open</u>.
   Looking at the clear close **E** reinforces the clear image of the **E** in the brain/memory. This helps the brain and eyes work together to produce a clear image of the **E** when it is seen at the far distance.

Switch back to the **E** at the far distance.
Shift on it, remember, imagine and see it dark black and clear.
Blink, breathe, relax.

For one eye at a time; start with either eye. But; it helps to start with the clearest vision eye first to get the clearest memory image of the E into the brain.

Practice switching, shifting on the close and far E's with <u>both eyes together</u>, then <u>one eye at a time</u>, then <u>both eyes together again</u> for perfect equally clear 20/20 and clearer vision in the left and right eyes at close and far distances. Example: <u>Both eyes together</u>. Then <u>one eye at a time</u>: start with either eye (or use the clearest first); left, then right, then left, right... <u>If vision is less clear in one eye; practice extra time with that eye</u>. Then; <u>end with both eyes together again</u>.

  Allow the eyes, head/face, neck and body to relax, move freely when looking at the letters. Relaxation and movement bring clear vision.
Eye, head/face, neck, body immobility, tension and staring, squinting, straining, trying hard to see the letters clear produces unclear vision.

Practice on other letters.   Move upon the chart nice and easy from letter to letter. Blink, shift.
Practice on smaller letters.
Practice at a variety of close, middle, far distances for clear vision at all distances.
   Practice on two identical fine print charts with medium, small, fine and microscopic size letters.
Place the charts at two different close distances.

Memorize the letters on the chart. Memorizing the letters causes the chart to become a familiar object, something that is easy to see. **Familiar objects** relax the mind, eyes and activates clear vision.
When the brain memorizes the letters, becomes familiar with them, there is no effort to see them, mental strain and eyestrain are avoided, the mind/brain, eye muscles, eyes stay relaxed when viewing the chart and the letters are seen clear *without trying to see.*
This relaxation and clear vision continues when looking at other objects.
   When taking a eye test at the eye doctors' office, the patient is often hurried, pressured to see the letters clear on a unfamiliar eyechart. Being hurried can tense and reduce the eyes' movements.
This causes <u>temporary</u> mental strain, leads to squinting, staring, effort to see the letters. This causes <u>temporary</u> eye muscle tension, slightly altered eye, cornea shape with incorrect focus of light rays in the eye causing <u>temporary</u> blur that results in a unnecessary prescription for eyeglasses and over-corrected lenses that are too strong and cause increased eye muscle tension, abnormal eye shape, mental strain, increased blur and future prescriptions for stronger eyeglass lenses.
   If the patient knew the letters on the chart and was allowed to relax, use Correct Vision Habits 'shifting, central-fixation...' on the letters; the mind, eye muscles, eyes would remain relaxed, the letters on the memorized <u>and unfamiliar</u> eyecharts would be seen clear and the eyeglass prescription would be avoided. A test on a familiar paper chart on the wall, with Dr. Bates' retinoscope detects true eye focus.
   Place a familiar eyechart in the home, work, school and shift on the letters occasionally.
Practice all Correct *Relaxed, Natural* Vision Habits on the letters;
Central-fixation; the letter the eyes are looking at is placed in the center of the visual field; between the eyes, at eye level. Look at and see one letter darkest black, clearest at a time in the center of the visual field. The letter the eyes are looking at is in the center of the visual field and is clearest. Other letters on the chart around and away from the letter are in the peripheral field and are less clear.
   Avoid staring, squinting, trying hard to see letters clear. Blink, relax and combine shifting with central-fixation; When looking at a letter; <u>shift</u> on it from small part to small part. Move the small exact center of the visual field point to point on a letter. Blink. Let the eyes <u>move</u>. Shift relaxed, easy, continually, restful. Shift letter to letter. The central field-eyes move *on their own* to where you (the brain) decide to look.

Shift on the letters, move along the chart letter to letter. As you move from letter to letter the head moves with the eyes, facing each letter you look at. The vision moves on the letter, head moving with the eyes-visions' shift. The more you relax and move, the clearer the sight becomes. Blink. Don't get stuck on a letter. Move on. You can return to it when relaxation is perfect.
  Try this method to bring relaxation, see letters clear; Pick a partly blurry letter on the far chart; the P on the 20/20 line. Close your eyes and imagine an object that begins with a P. Example; Piano. See the piano in the mind. Use the memory, imagination; it's a beautiful semi dark chestnut brown with the natural wood grain, shapes, colors in it. It is polished, shiny and reflective. See mirror like images in it. Look at the black and white parts of the keys, the design of the legs, who might be playing it. See the white paper with black music notes on top of the piano. The window is open, the long sheer white curtains are blowing. See the green grass, flowers, trees outside. Feel the relaxation. Open the eyes and look at the P; it will flash clear if you gained relaxation and easy use of the memory-imagination. Move to a smaller letter below; a D on the 15 line. Imagine, remember a object for the letter; Dog. A cute Golden Retriever puppy. See her in the grass, playfully edging up to you, tail wagging. The sun is out. You sneak her a snack. You become friends. She visits often and hangs out under the pine tree. Open the eyes, see the D Clear. Move to another letter anywhere on the chart. Try a smaller letter. Repeat using imagination.

(The point to point shifting practice imitates the eyes' exact central fields' function-movement. It does not need to be consciously practiced all the time. It occurs on its own as the eyes-vision move over an object.)

See Doctor Bates' directions in his articles in the Close Vision chapter in the E-Books and his Better Eyesight Magazine, Dec., 1919; 'The Menace of Large Print' and 'Think Right', Dec., 1921.

See the **'Illusion of Oppositional Movement'**; the letter appears to move opposite of the direction the eyes move to; a small, quick movement not longer than the size of the letter when shifting from one side of the letter to the other side. 'The Swing.' When shifting on a part of the letter; the swing is smaller; not longer than the shift on the part. See this book, Better Eyesight Magazine; The Long Swing, Rock, Short Swing.

When reading a eyechart;
Don't spend a long time looking at a letter if it's unclear. Avoid staring, squinting, straining, trying hard to see it. Shift on it, then move, shift to a new letter. Shift on that letter.
Blink, breathe abdominally, relax. Trace on-along the black edges of the letters.
Shift from letter to letter on the chart. Normal vision=the entire chart is read clear in a few seconds! It is ok to stay on a letter if relaxation, eye shifting occurs. Relax, shift point to point with the fovea to see tiny parts. Let the eyes (vision) move on the letter automatically, on their own.

The eyes, head/face, neck and body are relaxed and move freely. Move the head/face and body with the eyes, in the same direction when shifting on a letter and from one letter to another.

Central-Fixation (Centralizing); When moving to a new letter, move the head, body with the eyes and look-face directly at the letter. This improves central-fixation.
The center of the visual field is clearest. The center of the visual field moves with the eyes from letter to letter, placing each letter you look at, one letter at a time, in the center of the eyes' visual field, keeping each letter perfectly clear.
The exact center of the visual field is most clear. Place the part of the letter the eyes look at in the exact center of the visual field. The part you are looking at is *most dark black, most clearest.*
Shift the eyes (visual attention) from small part to small part, also moving the small exact center of the visual field '*fovea*' from tiny part to tiny part (point to point) on each part you look at, seeing one tiny part (point) of the letter **most darkest black, clearest** at a time in the exact center of the visual field. The part (point) of the letter the central field is on, 'moving upon it-over it' is darkest black, clearest while the central field is on that part. Then; the next part 'point' the central moves over is clearest.

Practice on small and fine print letters. Practice, then don't practice; let the eyes do the point to point shifting on their own. Many of the tiny shifts are saccades, very tiny and microscopic, automatic shifts.

The exact center of the visual field; produced by the fovea centralis in the center of the macula, in the center of the eyes' retina can be seen/measured by looking at a capitol letter E, 3/8" high, 20/20 line of the distant eyechart, from 20 feet away.
When looking directly at the E, the E occupies space in the center of the visual field produced by the macula and fovea. When looking at a small part of the E (Example; a part in the center of the E); that small part is in the exact center of the visual field produced by the fovea. The fovea is always moving.
+Light rays from this part of the E focus on the center of the fovea when looking at this part, placing it
   in the central field. Look at a even smaller part, a tiny point; that light ray goes to the most exact center of the fovea; the area that produces the most clearest vision, bright color!
+Light rays from other areas of the center of the visual field focus on the macula around the fovea.
+Light rays away from the E in the peripheral field of vision focus on the peripheral field of the retina around/away from the fovea and macula.
The fovea (especially the center of the fovea) produces the clearest vision, much clearer than 20/20. The outer fovea and macula also produce very clear vision, much clearer than 20/20, but not completely matching the most clear level of clarity produced by the center of the fovea.

The peripheral field of the retina, going outward farther away from the macula, away from the central field produces less clear vision. The far outer peripheral field is the most unclear.

Let the peripheral do it's own thing. It is also functioning with the brain-eyes-vision. The inner peripheral is clear, but the central *where you are looking* is the most clear, with brightest color, detail.

Remember; the eyes-vision move. Avoid locking the central on one part. Keep it moving 'shifting'. See a letter clear by placing it in the center of the visual field and then; use the exact center of the visual field; place one small part of the letter at a time in the exact center of the visual field and see it darkest black and clearest. Move continually part to part. Floating along nice and easy. Relax.
Avoid staring. Always shift to prevent staring, immobility. Shift 'move' the eyes-visual attention (center of the visual field) from small part to small part on the letter; top to bottom, side to side, corner to corner, middle; shift part to part in any direction on the letter. Blink. Practice the detailed tiny point to tiny point shifting. *This is the true function of the eyes.* Then; don't practice. Let the eyes, vision do all of this automatically, keeping perfect central clarity and optimum peripheral.

Example; shift from dot to dot on the letter E. See picture on next page. As the eyes-center of the visual field move from part to part (dot to dot); see one small dot at a time darkest black, clearest in the center of the visual field. The dot the central field is moving on is blackest, clearest.
The entire visual field moves with the eyes as the eyes shift from part to part, object to object.

Example;
Looking at the small part (dot) in the middle of the E.
This part is in the center of the visual field and is darkest black and clearest.
All other parts are in the peripheral field and are less clear.
Next; shift from that small part in the middle of the E to a small part (dot) on the top.
The small part on the top is now in the center of the visual field, its light rays are focusing on the fovea and it is seen darkest black and clearest.
   The previous part and all other parts of the E are in the peripheral field and are less clear.
Shift to a new small part; that new part is now in the center of the visual field and is darkest black and clearest. Blink. **(Try exact central field 'tiny point' shifting; look at a part of the dot the size of a tiny fine print period.)**
   The eyes can shift to a new part each second, fraction of a second. In that short time that a part is in the center of the visual field, it is seen darkest black and clearest. This is central-fixation.

   When you look at the part of the object you want to see using central-fixation (the exact center of the visual field); the exact center is very clear, <u>much</u> clearer than 20/20, and the outer center of the visual field is also very clear, clearer than 20/20. The peripheral field which is normally less clear is at it's maximum clarity and function of detecting movement, light...
   Seeing clear with central-fixation and shifting improves clarity and function of the entire visual field.

When the mind, body, eyes are relaxed the letters are clear.

ROCK LEFT AND RIGHT IN FRONT OF THE CHART
RELAX, DONT TRY TO SEE THE LETTERS CLEAR

   Do the rock and long swing in front of the eyechart and <u>do not</u> try to see the letters clear. Just relax, rock left and right and notice the soothing oppositional movement of the chart;
When the eyes, head/face, body move left <;
the chart appears to move right >.
When the eyes, head/face and body move right >;
the chart appears to move left <.

ROCK LEFT   ROCK RIGHT

Read about the Rock and Long Swing in this book.
(The Rock is also known as the Sway. A shortened version of the Long Swing). The eyes, head/face and body move <u>together</u> in the same direction. Relax and rock or swing left and right without looking at the letters. Don't stop to shift on them, don't try to see the letters. Just swing.
   Then; stop moving left and right. Keep some movement; shorten the rock to a few inches.
Look at the chart and shift on letters. Blink, breathe, relax. They will flash clear.
   When swaying left and right in front of a chart that is far away in the distance; the chart appears to move with you. Read more about the opposite and same direction movement of the far chart in this book.

'The Short Swing'

See the **'Illusion of Oppositional Movement'** of the letter when the eyes shift on it;
+Shift from the left side of the letter to the right side > ;
  the letter appears to move 'swing' to the left <.
+Shift from the right side of the letter to the left side < ;
  the letter appears to move 'swing' to the right >.
Shift up, down, diagonally, in any direction and see the letter appear to move in the opposite direction, 'opposite of the direction that the eyes *central field-where you are looking* move to.'
Practice shifting and seeing oppositional movement on large, medium, small and fine print letters at close, middle and far distances. The movement of the letter is short, less than the size of the letter. It can be equal to the letter's size; <u>to the shift of the eyes-central field</u> across the letter. It is never longer than the letter, shift. If shifting on part of a letter; it is not longer than the shift of the eyes on the part.

   If the swing is larger than the letter, larger than the eyes' shift, is stiff or shaky, does not occur; that is caused by eye muscle tension preventing perfect, flowing eye movements, central-fixations. As the mind and eyes, eye muscles relax; the vision improves. Then the eyes' shift and opposite swing are normal. Blink, breathe and relax. Seeing opposite movement of the letter relaxes the mind and eyes, improves the clarity of vision. Practice shifting on the letter and seeing the illusion of oppositional movement with; <u>the eyes open</u>, then, <u>with the eyes closed (using the memory, imagination)</u>, then, <u>with the eyes open again</u>.

   Shifting on a small letter produces a smaller opposite movement, a small **Short Swing.** Shift on this E
With practice; smaller shifts on small and tiny letters occur with small and tiny opposite movement of the letters. This greatly improves shifting, saccades, central-fixation resulting in very clear vision. E E .
   The Short Swing, small and tiny shifts, swings produce clearer, more detailed vision than the Long Swing, larger shifts, swings. All shifts, swings activate relaxation, movement and improve the vision.

The Long Swing and Rock are longer movements of the eyes, head, body and produce a longer appearance of oppositional movement 'swing' because the eyes are not shifting on objects. (unless doing a short rock when shifting on a object; then there is a short swing not longer than the shift of the eyes.)

Next; return to the rock or long swing. Don't shift on anything. Just relax and move.
The rock, long swing keeps the mind, body, neck, eyes relaxed, keeps the eyes moving and vision clear.
   Stop rocking, swinging left and right every once in a while, then; shift on the letters on the eyechart.
Notice they are seen clear now that the mind/eyes are relaxed. There is no effort to see.

Shorten the Rock for a Short Shift and Swing;
   Rock left and right 2 feet, then 1 foot, then 6 inches, 4,3,2,1, ½... inch. Rock with a small movement ½ to 1-2... inches left and right and shift on letters on the eyechart in synchronization; left, right, left, right with the movement of the rock. See a small opposite movement swing of the letters.
   The rock keeps the eyes, head/face, neck, body relaxed and moving when looking at a letter.
This prevents staring, strain and blur. The small shift, swing produces clear vision.
   Practice Dr. Bates method of 'Flashing the Letters' ; looking at, shifting on a letter for only a <u>fraction of a second</u>. Then, <u>look away to a different object, shift on that object</u>. Then, <u>return to the letter, shift on it for a fraction of a second</u>, then look away, return, look away...
   This prevents effort to see, prevents strain and blur; there is not enough time to 'strain, try' to see an object clear, so relaxation is maintained. Relaxation, no effort to see=clear vision.
   The normal eye moves continually, restful, it's fovea shifting easy from part to part, point to point.

Practice the Long Swing with Two Identical Eyecharts on the Left and Right Sides of the Body and 'Flashing' Shifting for a 'Fraction of a Second' on letters on the Eyecharts;

The Long Swing with Two Eyecharts
Identical eyecharts placed on left and right side of the body.
 Swing and turn left and right and 'Flash' glance at, shift on a letter on the eyechart for a 'fraction of a second':
Swing, turn <u>left</u> and 'flash' a letter on the <u>left</u> chart. Blink and shift quickly, easy on the letter. Do not stop swinging.
Swing, turn <u>right</u> and flash a letter on the <u>right</u> chart.
Keep swinging left and right, glancing at the letters.
   Relax, no effort to see - vision becomes clear.

Place 2 identical eyecharts on the left and right sides of the body.
Swing left and right and <u>flash</u> a letter on the eyechart for a <u>fraction of a second</u>;
+Swing left < ; shift on 'flash' the letter for a fraction of a second on the left chart. Blink.
+Swing right > ; shift on 'flash' the identical letter for a fraction of a second on the right chart. Blink.
Then swing back to the left side, flash the same letter again... Repeat right, left, right, left...
Do this <u>without stopping</u>; keep moving, swinging left and right. Do not stop swinging when looking at the letter. The eyes, head/face and body move-swing and turn left and right together, at the same time, in the same direction.
   The continual movement keeps the eyes, mind and body relaxed, left and right brain hemispheres integrated. The very short time the eyes, head, body are facing the chart prevents strain, staring at the letter. The eyes shift on the letter quick, easy, no attempt to see it clear. Relaxation occurs and vision becomes clear. Practice shifting on identical letters, then on any letters. Shift on small, tiny letters.
   'Flashing the letters' - *shifting on a letter for a fraction of a second* produces a 'Flash' of clear vision. The flash of clarity may last only a second. With practice, maintaining relaxation; the flashes occur more often, last longer and soon the vision remains clear. https://www.youtube.com/watch?v=TxRQ2Y-7nCM

See far objects swing opposite; Place an eyechart at 80 to 200 feet. Face it. <u>Shift</u> left and right on the chart; look at the left < side, then the right >, then left <, then right > and see the chart appear to move 'swing by' in the opposite direction. Move the head with the eyes. The head-face, body move in the same direction the eyes move to. Note; if you stop shifting on the chart and the eyes-head-body are just swaying left and right in front of the chart and other objects around it, not stopping to shift on them; the movement of the <u>far</u> chart changes; the chart now appears to move *with the eyes-head-body in the same direction.* Try it; face the far chart and sway left and right or walk sideways a few feet; the chart appears to move with you. If you shift on the chart, or a letter while <u>walking</u>; it's opposite movement will be seen, but the main movement appears to go with the direction you are moving to. (The head moves with the eyes when shifting on a object when walking.) Make it easy to see the far opposite movement; Stop walking. Face the chart, shift on it and <u>keep the head-body movement equal to the eyes' shift on the chart</u>; *not longer, not shorter than the length of the eyes (fovea-central field's) shift upon the chart from one part of the chart to another part.* Example; from the left side to the right side or bottom to top. See it swing opposite. Blink. Shift smaller, on a tiny letter on a far chart and see it move opposite with a tiny opposite swing. Perfect clarity! Practice with the chart at close and far distances; 3ft. to 300+ ft. Seeing the opposite and same direction swings relaxes the mind, eyes and brings clear vision. See it from a moving car's side window; let the different distances pass by. If you want to look at a moving object; turn to face it and shift on it.

Practice palming 'close, cover the eyes', then read, flash the letters on the eyechart. (See examples in this book & the Palming chapter in the E-books.)

+Palm for a while, relax.
+Uncover and open the eyes. Look at a letter on the chart.
+Shift on the letter for only <u>1-3 seconds or just a fraction of a second</u>. <u>No effort to see clear.</u>
+Then close, cover the eyes and palm again. Think pleasant thoughts. Remember, imagine shifting on the letter and see it dark black and clear in the mind. See the mental picture of the letter show opposite movement as the eyes shift on the letter in the mind.
+Uncover, open the eyes and shift on the letter again, fraction of a second.
+Close the eyes, palm again. Open, shift.
+Repeat palming, then flashing the letter-shifting on the letter for a fraction of a second.

This method keeps the eyes, mind relaxed, prevents effort to see, mental, visual strain and blur. Flashes of clear vision occur. When relaxation of mind, eyes continues, the letters and vision for all objects remain clear.

Shift top and bottom, left and right on the E. (Shift dot to dot). Blink.

Rock (sway) the body left and right in front of the eyechart placed at 5 to 20 feet and see the chart, letters move 'swing' in the opposite direction.

Next; reduce the length of the rock to 2-4 inches, moving left and right while shifting part to part on the letters. The eyes, head, body move in the <u>same direction</u>. Shift on the letter that is in front of the eyes as you rock and move over it. Then go to the next letter that you move in front of, then the next... The eyes 'vision' move freely to another letter, then another, another as you rock. As you move left and right; the eyes shift left, right, up, down, diagonally, in any direction on the letters as you move over them. The head, body moves left, right, up, down, diagonally... with the eyes. These small movements on the letters 'mix in' with the left-right movement of the rock. Blink. Move left and right along an entire line of letters; eyes, head, body moving together as the eyes shift about on the letters. Rock 4-10+ inches moving up and down the chart shifting on the letters. Zig-zag through the chart. Rock up and down on the toes 1-3 inches. Rock on the feet 1-2 inches forward and backward; heels, toes, heels, toes. Movement brings relaxation, clarity. No effort to see. Just relax, move, shift. Blink and breath.

Flash a letter -
+Shift on the E for a fraction of a second then
+look away from it to another object or close the eyes, palm and remember the E, shift on it in the mind. Or just think any pleasant thoughts with the eyes closed.
+Open, shift on the E fraction of a second,
+Close, repeat...

+Use the memory, imagination:
Remember, imagine the E is clear when the eyes are open and when closed. Practice on any objects, at any distance.

https://www.youtube.com/watch?v=863yFmc-Ius
https://www.youtube.com/watch?v=mYpsYPPV_hg
Click the links for YouTube Videos teaching Natural Vision Improvement with Eyecharts. ROCK LEFT   ROCK RIGHT

The pothooks eyechart is designed for children, adults that have not yet learned to read the alphabet. The person points their finger in the direction the E is pointing. The chart makes vision improvement easy;

Familiar objects relax the mind, eyes and keep the vision clear. This eyechart is easy to see clear because it is a <u>familiar object</u>: the person knows that every letter on the chart is an E. This makes it relaxing, easy when looking at a unclear small, tiny size E and using the memory, imagination to see the E clear. The person only needs to; shift on the E, guess-imagine which way the E is pointing. When the brain remembers, imagines a clear, dark black letter E and guesses, imagines the E pointing in the correct direction; the brain and eyes relax, the brain directs the eye muscles to move correct and the eyes to shift correct <u>directly on the letter E</u>, perfectly on it's parts. The E is seen clear.

If you guess an incorrect direction; the E remains unclear because; the eyes, brain are trying to shift on, see an incorrect image; trying to move 'shift' the eyes' fovea-central field on areas of the page away from the E's true placement, imagining parts of the E are there when in reality a different part or nothing is there. Confusion, strain in the mind-eyes occurs resulting in blur. (Read the example of using the memory and imagination in the *Do it Yourself-Natural Eyesight Improvement* E-book, Memory and Imagination chapter; Looking at, guessing the #7 on a city bus 10 blocks away.)

Pothooks, Tumbling, Inverted E Eyechart

Place a familiar eyechart in your home. Notice when you are not thinking about the eyes-vision and you unexpectedly look at the chart; the letters are clear, the eyes (vision) quickly move upon the chart and see the 20/20, 20/15 and bottom 10 lines perfectly clear at 20, 30, 40 feet! The entire chart is read in seconds. No effort to see=no tension=clear vision. Close the eyes and imagine a perfect dark black page. Or a wall, any black object. Relax. Open the eyes. The chart is clear, letters dark black. Repeat; imagine pure white, green, blue, any color. Practice Dr. Bates tiny black period relaxation method. Imagine it; . Shift left and right on it and see it swing opposite. (with eyes open, then closed, then open). Learn how to re-create and keep that relaxed state of mind, body that brings effortless clear eyesight.

20/200 at 200 Feet

E

20/100

F P

20/70

T O Z

20/60
P D C

20/50
L P E D

20/40
P E C F D

20/30
E D F C Z P

20/25
F E L O P Z D

20/20 Vision at 20 Feet
20/20 **D E F P O T E C**

20/15

L E F O D P C T

20/13

F D P L T C E O

20/10

P E Z O L C F T D

20/8

E D L T O Z F C P

20/6

L P C F E T O D Z

20/5

T F D O P Z L E C

Very Clear Vision, Small Print Clear at 20 Feet

Z C T L O P D F E

Exact standard letter size eyecharts can be printed using the directions in the eyechart chapter and by downloading the Big C chart in 3 pictures from the Eyecharts page on the website; http://cleareyesight-batesmethod.info/id25.html and the E-books page; http://cleareyesight-batesmethod.info/id148.html

It is the subtle, taken-for-granted habits of getting ready for every move that must be revealed and prevented. (Lifting a full suitcase that turns out to be empty, or stepping to an extra stair that does not happen to be at the top of the staircase, we are sometimes made acutely aware of these unconscious habits of readiness.)

The reader of this page is now asked to stand up for a moment. ... Stop! Before even starting to rise from your sofa or chair, did you perhaps begin to foreshorten the muscles at the back of your neck? If so, that constitutes a part of your particular 'set', or involuntary preparation for getting up. It is also an example of the kind of thing that you would gradually learn to prevent during lessons.

With this special form of cooperation from the student, the teacher then 'stands' him, 'sits' him, 'walks' him, encouraging the desired head-neck-torso relationship throughout the process. To the degree to which the student does not intrude any of his old habits, he allows the teacher's manual guidance to give him, over and over again, a new sensory experience of these common acts. And in his new movements, which might be called 'reflex facilitated'[1] rather than active or passive, there occurs a redistribution of postural tone. Finally, sitting, standing, walking *like this*—or engaging in no matter what activity *like this*—begins to 'feel right'. His neck feels free, his head feels as if it is going forward and up, and his torso feels as if it is lengthening and fanning out toward the shoulders. Between lessons, he will continue saying 'no' to his old movements, actively permitting their replacement by the new ones acquired during lessons.

Lessons in the technique form a gradual process with a fascination of its own. The end result is that, in time, the special requisite head-neck-torso pattern is established and continues as the major feature in all of our activities. Nothing static: nothing 'postural'. Head, neck and torso—like every other part of the body—are freely and independently movable at all times. There persists, however, a certain dynamic relationship among them. And it is this relationship, presumably, which allows the greatest lengthening of the spine as 'the true and primary movement in each and every act'.

There are an overall flexibility and tonic ease of movement, greater freedom in the action of the eyes, less tension in the jaws, more relaxation in the tongue and throat, and deeper breathing because of the effect of the new alignment on the diaphragm. There are also a sense of weightlessness and a diminution of the effort previously thought necessary to move one's limbs. Activity is now more free and flowing—no longer jerky and heavy with strain.

This lighter-than-air effect must not, at all costs—as Alexander insisted—be confused with what is usually meant by 'relaxation'. John Dewey, in a letter, mentioned 'Alexander's point that when people are told to relax, they do so at one locus and tense themselves at another place.' This tendency, Dewey believed, might be tested objectively.

More importantly, however, Alexander was appalled by the customary approach to the problem. To relax, in his meaning of the word, does not mean that you should become a bag of bones. If one observes a cat or dog at rest, one will see what true relaxation is: the dog and cat are completely relaxed, yet they are still capable of making sudden and definite movements. Alexander deplored the lack of muscular tone in students who, in later years, came to him after having undergone the new relaxation training. The purpose of his technique, as he saw it, was not to get rid of tensions, but to reorganize them into a source of energy and satisfaction.

The question of breathing likewise receives unique emphasis in his work. Alexander, from the very start of his career, opposed the schools of 'deep breathing' then in vogue. He was interested, rather, in coaxing an awareness of breathing as it supports movement, and of movement as it reinforces breathing. The possibilities of orchestration between the two, in activity, are practically infinite. 'We never talk about breathing,' Alexander once cryptically informed a pupil, thus expressing his deep concern with it only as manifest in the precise exigencies of doing: it was to be seen only as a function of using oneself properly.

After all, one never has to worry about whether or not breathing is going on. The question is whether it is free or forced.

[1] For the important topic of antigravity reflexes, see Appendix III. The anatomical and physiological explanations put forward to account for the new facts of space medicine (for example, that skylab astronauts living without the effects of gravity gain inches in height and lose inches around the waist) are interesting in the present context.

Download Alexander's books free on GoogleBooks and www.cleareyesight-batesmethod.info

Move to See the Eyechart Letters Clear;

Look at the eyechart. Move the eyes (*vision*) left and right across the lines of letters. Sway left and right sweeping over the letters. Blink. The head-body moves with the eyes. Move through one line at a time.

Repeat. Then; shorten the movement to the size of a letter and shift on it. Move to another letter, then another. Blink. The head-body moves with the eyes. Size of the eyes' shift, head-body movement varies with the letter size. Avoid trying to see clear. Relax, relax, relax. No effort. The letters will flash clear. Think something happy, fun. It activates relaxation, natural automatic eye movement and clear vision.

Return to moving left and right sweeping across the lines of letters. Then; shorten movement to the size of a letter and shift on it. Move to another letter, then another. Blink. Then sweep left and right again.
Sweep diagonally, shifting over the letters as is done on the astigmatism chart end of this book.

Next; sweep up & down the chart while moving back and forth on 2 to 3 letters through the middle. Zig-zagging left and right as you go down, up, down, up... the chart. Blink. *Movement* prevents tension, blur.

Dr. Bates & Emily's *Memory-Imagination-Relaxation* Practice to See Letters Clear;

Start with a letter that is seen clear. If none are clear; move close or far and start with a letter seen best.

#1; Look at-shift on the letter. See and imagine it dark black and clear. (if blurry; just imagine it is clear.)

#2; Close the eyes (palm if you like) and remember, imagine the letter dark black and clear. Shift on the letter in the mind. Shifting part to part on the mental image maintains the clear picture in the mind.

When the letter is seen clear in the memory-imagination and relaxation occurs;
#3; Open the eyes and see the letter flash clear. Shift on it for a split second. Then quickly close the eyes to maintain the relaxation and clarity. Remember, imagine the clear letter in the mind. Shift on it using the imagination. (Quickly closing the eyes prevents strain and blur by avoiding effort to see, immobility.)

#4; Open the eyes and look at a smaller letter under the previous letter. See it flash clear. Shift on the letter. Quickly close the eyes and remember-imagine the clear letter. Shift on it using the imagination.

#5; Open the eyes, go to the next smaller letter under the previous letter-line. It flashes clear. Shift on it.
Repeat closing the eyes, remember-imagine the letter clear, shift on it, then open the eyes, move to the next smaller letter below, close the eyes again... until you get to the smallest letter on the bottom line.

Practice this across a line of letters; Look at, shift on and see clear the first letter on the < left. Close the eyes, then open and move right > to the last letter on the line. Try smaller lines. Do all the letters on a line, moving right or left, one letter at a time. Notice; when one letter is *perfectly* clear; all are clear.

Vary the distance, letter color. Use entertaining pictures, or s e n t e n c e s that are *easy to memorize*.

There are a variety of breathing techniques for relaxation & energy, oxygen flow to the head, brain, eyes, body and to improve lung function. Natural teachers prefer abdominal-diaphragm breathing; like a baby naturally breathes. Usually breathing is through the nose. Sometimes nose and mouth. Depends on the level of activity, method-exercise.
See the Free PDF E-books for natural breathing and breathing exercises.

< The Alexander Technique by Frederick Matthias Alexander. Teaches ways to correct movement, posture, cure *neck-head*, back tension and a variety of health problems with natural, safe methods. He cured his throat-voice. Books; 'Man's Supreme Inheritance'. 'The Use of Self-Its Conscious Direction in Relation to Diagnosis, Functioning and the Control of Reaction'. Wrote many books, articles, speeches.

Moshe Feldenkrais.
Books; 'Awareness Through Movement-Health Exercises for Personal Growth'. 'Body Awareness as Healing Therapy-The Case of Nora'. 'The Potent Self-A Study of Spontaneity & Compulsion'

Osteopathy (when done by a honest, experienced doctor) is a natural alternative to risky, often dangerous chiropractic. The bones, spine can be aligned using safe physical movements, massage and other natural ways to move the bones.
The original TRUE Osteopathy method and other old authentic, effective natural practices are free in PDF on GoogleBooks.

John E. Sarno, MD; Teaches how the emotions, thoughts, fear can cause pain and how the brain makes it move.

'Dr. B'; Fereydoon Batmanghelidj, M.D. Books, videos; 'You're Not Sick, You're Thirsty! - Water; For Health, for Healing, for Life' and many other books. Natural salt with water... (exact recipe) cures pain, injuries, disease. A secret doctors hide and some religions preserve. The first thing often given in the hospital is a salt and water... solution. The doctors then tell us to avoid salt. Many natural cures are hidden by the drug companies, doctors.

BETTER EYESIGHT
A MONTHLY MAGAZINE DEVOTED TO THE PREVENTION AND CURE OF IMPERFECT SIGHT WITHOUT GLASSES
June, 1921
By W. H. Bates, M.D.

Imagination - Imagination is closely allied to memory, for we can imagine only as well as we remember, and in the treatment of imperfect sight the two can scarcely be separated. Vision is largely a matter of imagination and memory. And since both imagination and memory are impossible without perfect relaxation, the cultivation of these faculties not only improves the interpretation of the pictures on the retina but improves the pictures themselves. When you imagine that you see a letter on the test card, you actually do see it because it is impossible to relax and imagine the letter perfectly and, at the same time, strain and see it imperfectly. The following method of using the imagination has produced quick results in many cases:

The patient is asked to look at the largest letter on the test card at the near point, and is usually able to observe that a small area, about a square inch, appears blacker than the rest, and that when the part of the letter seen worst is covered, part of the exposed area seems blacker than the remainder. When the part seen worst is again covered, the area at maximum blackness is still further reduced. When the part seen best has been reduced to about the size of a letter on the bottom line, the patient is asked to imagine that such a letter occupies this area and is blacker than the rest of the letter. Then he is asked to look at a letter on the bottom line and imagine that it is blacker than the largest letter. Many are able to do this and at once become able to see the letters on the bottom line.

One part of the letter is blacker because that is the part you are looking directly at; the central field is on that part. The central field produces the best vision and color. The peripheral field has less clarity and color, is most unclear in the far outer peripheral. As you reduce the size of the area you are looking at, covering the areas that are not as black (part seen worst), you are covering up the peripheral area of the object as you move closer and closer to the center of the visual field produced by the center of the retina 'macula-fovea'. The *exact* center has the very best clarity (much clearer than 20/20) and best color, fine detailed vision. Produced by the center of the fovea. It is very small. Prove it; reduce down to looking at 2 tiny black periods very close together and see the one the eyes (fovea-exact central field) are looking directly at, best, clearest and blackest. Shift back and forth on the 2 periods. This is perfect central-fixation, tiny shifting, it produces very clear eyesight. The eyes continue to move even when looking at a very small part; the fovea moves part to part on that very small part. Blink.

Flashing - Since it is effort that spoils the sight, many persons with imperfect sight are able, after a period of rest, to look at an object for a fraction of a second. If the eyes are closed before the habit of strain reasserts itself permanent relaxation is sometimes very quickly obtained. This practice I have called *flashing*, and many persons are helped by it who are unable to improve their sight by other means. The eyes are rested for a few minutes, by closing or palming, and then a letter on the test card, or a letter of diamond type, if the trouble is with near vision, is regarded for a fraction of a second. Then the eyes are immediately closed and the process repeated.

March, 1924 - Illusions of Normal Sight

AN illusion is defined by the dictionary to be something which does not exist.
Illusions are not seen, they are imagined. One cannot have perfect sight without illusions.

CENTRAL FIXATION - When the sight is normal one is always able to demonstrate that things regarded are seen best while those not regarded are always seen worse. With Central Fixation if one recognizes or sees a letter correctly, all other letters are seen worse. With the best vision that can be obtained it can be demonstrated that one cannot see a letter or any other object perfectly without seeing one part best. (Central-Fixation; the part of the object the eyes are looking directly at is in the central field; the macula-fovea's area of the retina. This area contains the most cones 'light receptors' that produce very clear detailed vision and bright color. The clearest vision. That central field moves part to part on the object, seeing one part at a time best-perfectly clear.) No matter how large or how small the letter or object may be, it is impossible to see it perfectly without Central Fixation. Many people believe that when they look at a small letter or a small period that they see it all at once; but, when you notice the facts, one finds that to see or to try to see a letter, a number of letters all perfectly, the vision becomes modified or imperfect. (Because the eyes are not using central-fixation and shifting, are not looking at-moving on one letter, one part of the letter at a time.) Some persons with unusually good vision can read the Snellen Test Card so rapidly that they have the impression that they see all the letters perfectly at the same time. It requires, in some cases, considerable trouble to demonstrate that this is impossible. In some obstinate cases it has required not only some hours but some days to prove that this is a fact. The letters of the Snellen Test Card are equally black. To see one blacker than the others, or a part of a letter blacker than the rest of it, is seeing something which is not so. The large letters and the small letters are printed in the same ink and all are equally black and although one cannot read the letters unless they see them by Central Fixation it is still, nevertheless, an illusion. One should emphasize the fact that it is possible to have illusions or that one cannot see perfectly unless the illusion of Central Fixation can be demonstrated.

SWINGING - When a small letter of the Snellen Test Card can be seen perfectly and continuously it can be demonstrated that the letter is moving from side to side about its own width or less or that it is moving in other directions. To look fixedly at a letter and try to imagine one point of the letter is seen continuously, can be demonstrated to be impossible. One cannot obtain perfect sight by staring or trying to see things or imagine things as stationary. I have never seen this truth stated in any publication. It is just as important an illusion as is CENTRAL FIXATION in order to have perfect sight continuously. It can be demonstrated that all persons with imperfect sight stare, concentrate or try to see letters stationary. The illusion that the letter is moving, when the sight is normal, is brought about by the normal eye to avoid the stare and the strain of seeing things imperfectly. The point of fixation changes continuously, easily.

When one looks to the right of the letter, the letter is to the left of where you are looking. If you look to the left of a letter the letter is to the right of where you are looking. Every time your eyes move to the right, the letter moves to the left. Every time your eyes move to the left the letter moves to the right and by alternately looking from one to the other side of a letter one becomes able to imagine the illusion that the letter is moving from side to side. When reading rapidly one does not have time to demonstrate that each individual letter is moving. Here again the imagination is responsible for the illusion of the swing. The letters do not really move, we only imagine it; and, unless we can imagine a letter moving continuously we are unable to see it with normal sight continuously. This is a truth; it has no exceptions. It is a necessary part of normal vision, and yet it has not, to my knowledge, been published in any book or periodical. People who write works on physiological optics have much to learn. So many of my patients who have been benefited by my methods have asked me: "Why didn't Helmholtz, Donders and all those other authorities publish the truths that you have discovered?" Nearly all ophthalmologists put glasses on people because that is all they know. I can recall the time when that was all I knew. If a patient left the office without a prescription for glasses it was not my fault. Now when persons with imperfect sight, wearing glasses, become able to practice CENTRAL FIXATION and the OPTICAL SWING in the right way, their vision becomes normal without glasses.

HALOS - When the sight is normal and when one regards a letter of the Snellen Card with a white center, the white part of the letter appears whiter than it really is and whiter than the rest of the card. I use the word Halos for this illusion. This is an illusion which can be demonstrated quite readily by covering over the black part of a letter with a screen with an opening slightly smaller than the white part of the letter, which permits the center of the letter to be observed. When this is done the white center of the letter is the same shade of whiteness as the rest of the card. Some people can imagine the illusion when it is described to them. When reading fine print the spaces between the lines appear whiter than the rest of the card, but only when the vision is good. As a general rule when one can imagine these white spaces between the lines are whiter than the rest of the card, Halos, the black appears more perfectly black and the letters can be read with normal vision. Halos are imagined, not seen. Imagination of the illusion of the Halos is a quick cure of myopia and astigmatism, farsight, presbyopia as well as other cases of imperfect sight. (The visual system creates the appearance of halos on the page near the black print, due to black and white contrast...)

All persons who have normal sight are always able to demonstrate the Halos. All persons with imperfect sight are cured, temporarily or permanently, when they become able to imagine the Halos.

20/200 Vision at 200 Feet

20/100

T F P 20/10

5 C G O 20/50

4 K B E R 20/40

Big C Chart
From Better
Eyesight
Magazine

C

R B

T F P

5 C G O

4 K B E R

3 V Y F P T

20/20   2 Q C O G D □ C

R Z 3 B 8 S H K F O

20/10   F T Y V P E C □ O B R K 5 6

**White Print Relaxes the Mind and Eyes,
Acts as Light-Activates the Retina**

20/20

```
            C

         R     B

        T  F  P

      5  C  G  O

     4  K  B  E  R

    3  V  Y  F  P  T

   2  Q  C  O  G  D  □  C

   R Z 3 B 8 S H K F O

   F T Y V P E C □ O B R K 5 6
```

Close Reading Vision

White print is as light to the eyes, easy, relaxing to read. Helpful for the blind,
people with low vision as they practice improving the sight back to clear.

THINK RIGHT

"As a man thinketh in his heart so is he," is a saying which is invariably true when the sight is concerned. When a person remembers or imagines an object of sight perfectly the sight is perfect; when he remembers it imperfectly the sight is imperfect. The idea that to do anything well requires effort, ruins the sight of many children and adults; for every thought of effort in the mind produces an error of refraction in the eye. The idea that large objects are easier to see than small ones results in the failure to see small objects. The fear that light will hurt the eyes actually produces sensitiveness to light. To demonstrate the truth of these statements is a great benefit.

Remember a letter or other object perfectly, and note that the sight is improved and pain and fatigue relieved; remember the object imperfectly, and note that the vision is lowered, while pain and fatigue may be produced or increased.

Rest the eyes by closing or palming, and note that the vision is improved, and pain and discomfort relieved; stare at a letter, concentrate upon it, make an effort to see it, and note that it disappears, and that a feeling of discomfort or pain is produced.

Note that a small part of a large object is seen better than the rest of it.

Accustom the eyes to strong light; learn to look at the sun; note that the vision is not lowered but improved, and that the light causes less and less discomfort.

Remember your successes (things seen perfectly); forget your failures (things seen imperfectly); patients who do this are cured quickly.

BETTER EYESIGHT

A MAGAZINE DEVOTED TO THE PREVENTION AND CURE OF IMPERFECT SIGHT WITHOUT GLASSES

Editor—W. H. BATES, M.D.
Publisher—CENTRAL FIXATION PUBLISHING CO.

| Vol. V. | DECEMBER, 1921 | No. 6 |

THE CORRECTION OF IMPERFECT SIGHT WITHOUT GLASSES

By Dr. Etha Marion Jones

THE correction of imperfect sight by Central Fixation, as taught by Dr. Bates, first came under my observation one year ago this September while assisting for a month in the practice of my friends, Drs. H. S. and Jennie K. Beckler, of Staunton, Virginia. I was astonished at the results they were obtaining in eye cases and at once began to study the system under their supervision.

About the same time I received a letter from a sister of mine, a teacher in the Detroit Public Schools, who had worn glasses for twenty years for myopia and astigmatism. She stated in her letter that she had discarded her glasses and was taking the Central Fixation treatment from an osteopathic physician in Detroit who had been a student of Dr. Bates. The treatment was continued during the winter, my sister keeping right on with her school work and doing extra reading at night without suffering with headaches as she had previously done. On seeing her this summer I was agreeably surprised at the change in her appearance. The strained look

Copyright, 1921, by the Central Fixation Publishing Company

about the eyes and face had given place to one of relaxation, the eyes were straight, and the nervous system had lost its tension and gained a poise formerly unknown. The retinoscope showed no errors of refraction in either eye.

Encouraged by this and other cases, I decided to prepare myself to specialize in this work. After studying the anatomy, pathology and physiology of the eye all last winter, and treating several patients as best I could with my limited knowledge of the system, I decided that what I now needed most was a course of personal instruction from Dr. Bates. I went to New York for this purpose a few months ago and spent a wonderful fortnight there. The course included work in Dr. Bates' clinic held three times a week in the Harlem Hospital. The hospital being in one of the colored sections of the city, many of the patients are negroes, and they are very appreciative, too; but both white and colored come in droves to be cured of all kinds of eye afflictions. Here I had a good opportunity to study eyes by means of the retinoscope and ophthalmoscope, and I observed the changes in the refraction and pathology as the treatment progressed. I can tell of only a few of the remarkable cases which I saw, for it would take days to tell about them all.

I was especially interested in a case of squint in a girl of fourteen, who had been attending the clinic about three months before I saw her. She had worn glasses since she was four years of age to correct the trouble, but had been growing gradually worse. When her sight was first tested she read 12/40 with her left or better eye. When asked to read the card with her squinting eye, she turned her head half way around to the left in trying to see it. Mrs. Lierman gave her one simple relaxing exercise to do and left her for a few minutes. At the next test she read 12/40 with the squinting eye without turning her head. Of course, that was temporary relief, as on straining again the squint would recur; but it showed what could be done by continuous treatment, and when I left New York the right eye was as straight as the left and did not change when the patient was excited or annoyed, or on reading or studying. She told me she could read or study for hours at a time without headaches or discomfort, while before coming to the clinic she could look at a book for only a few minutes at a time.

A negress, seventy-two years old, was responding wonderfully to treatment for cataract in the advanced stage. She had been in the clinic for two months. At first she could not distinguish the large C at the top of the test card. Before I left she could read 10/40 with both eyes.

A girl of twelve was suffering from retinitis pigmentosa, a condition generally pronounced incurable, in which spots of black pigment are deposited in the retina, parts of the retina destroyed and the nerve of sight diseased. On examination by the test card, the patient could read only the seventy line at five feet. Nystagmus was one of her worst symptoms, the eyes vibrating continually from side to side. She was extremely nervous, and very sensitive in regard to her condition, the slightest annoyance making her worse. At the first treatment, the nystagmus temporarily stopped, and she read the fifty line instead of the seventy at five feet. The last day I saw her at the clinic she could read the twenty line through at ten feet, and the nystagmus had entirely disappeared.

After seeing these things it would seem impossible for anyone to doubt that Dr. Bates' discoveries are bound, before long, to revolutionize the practice of ophthalmology. They offer hope to millions for whom formerly there was no hope, and I am glad to have a share in the wonderful work of making them available to the world of eye sufferers.

470 First Avenue, North, St. Petersburg, Fla.

Natural Eyesight Improvement astigmatism removal wheel

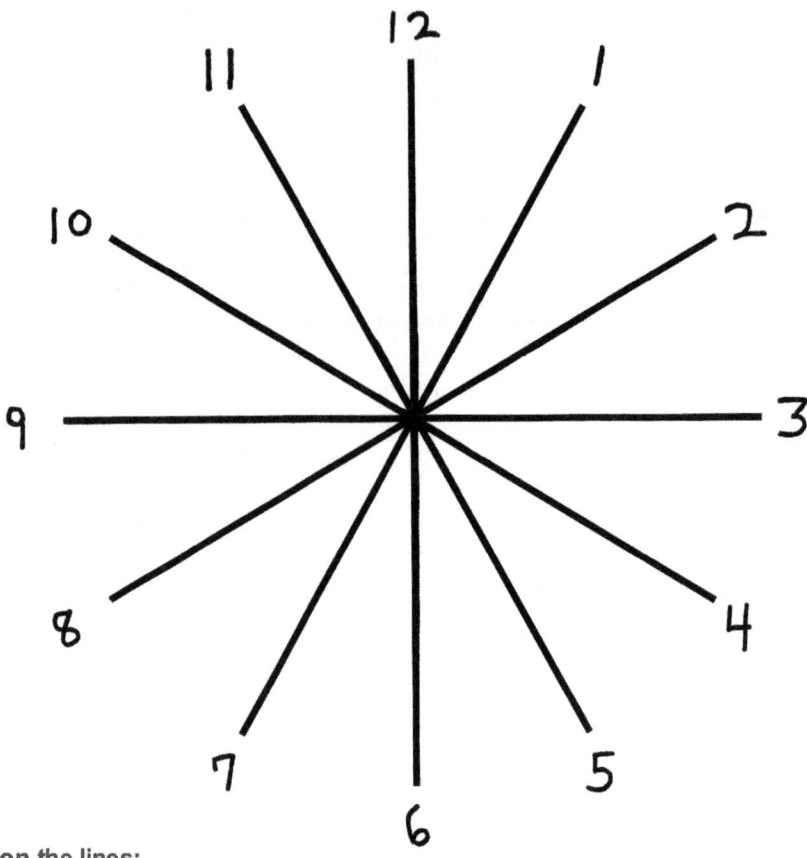

Shift on the lines;
Left and right - 9 to 3, 3 to 9
Up and down - 12 to 6, 6 to 12
Diagonally - 8 to 2, 2 to 8, 10 to 4, 4 to 10, 5 to 11, 7 to 1
Shift, trace on the lines in any direction; center to left or right, up, down, diagonally... and back to center.
Move the eyes/center of the visual field along the lines and remember, imagine, see the lines dark black and perfectly clear.
Central fixation; see one small part of a line clearest at a time in the center of the visual field and move the eyes/center of the visual field continually, easy, relaxed along the line from part ot part. Look at the white page, then black lines, then white, black... Blink. breathe slow, abdominally, relax.

Shift from line to line and part to part on lines. Combine shifting and tracing on lines. Practice with; <u>Both eyes together</u>, then with <u>one eye at a time</u>, then with <u>both eyes together again</u>.

Have You a Bible?

You all know fine print is beneficial.
Do you practice reading it?
Doctor Bates has proven that by reading a few lines of very fine print daily you are giving your eyes the relaxing "exercise" that will tend to prevent many common defects.

We publish a Bible that is printed in microscopic type, and measures one by one and a half inches and contains the new and old Testament.

Many patients past fifty have learned to read this with ease. Send for yours today.

Price $4.00

Snellen Test Cards

THERE should be a Snellen test card in every family and in every school classroom. When properly used it always improves the sight even when sight is already normal. Children or adults with errors of refraction, if they have never worn glasses, are cured simply by reading every day the smallest letters they can see at a distance of ten, fifteen, or twenty feet.

PAPER .... 50 CENTS
CARDBOARD (folding) 75 CENTS
DELIVERED

Back numbers BETTER EYESIGHT............$ .30
Bound vols., 1st, 2nd and 3rd years, each.. 4.25
Photographic reduction of the Bible......... 4.00
Ophthalmoscopes, with and without Battery,
from .... 10.00 to 50.00
Retinoscopes 4.00
Burning glasses 5.00
Reprints of articles by Dr. Bates in other medical journals; a limited number for sale. Send for list.

For Sale By
Central Fixation Publishing Company
383 Madison Avenue, New York City

How to Use the Snellen Test Card
FOR THE
Prevention and Cure of Imperfect Sight in Children

The Snellen Test Card is placed permanently upon the wall of the classroom, and every day the children silently read the smallest letters they can see from their seats with each eye separately, the other being covered with the palm of the hand in such a way as to avoid pressure on the eyeball. This takes no appreciable amount of time, and is sufficient to improve the sight of all children in one week and to cure all errors of refraction after some months, a year, or longer.

Children with markedly defective vision should be encouraged to read the card more frequently.

Records may be kept as follows:

John Smith, 10, Sept. 15, 1918.
R. V. (vision of the right eye) 20/40.
L. V. (vision of the left eye) 20/20.

John Smith, 11, Jan. 1, 1919.
R. V. 20/30.
L. V. 20/15.

The numerator of the fraction indicates the distance of the test card from the pupil; the denominator denotes the line read, as designated by the figures printed above the middle of each line of the Snellen Test Card.

A certain amount of supervision is absolutely necessary. At least once a year some one who understands the method should visit each classroom for the purpose of answering questions, encouraging the teachers to continue the use of the method, and making a report to the proper authorities.

It is not necessary that either the inspector, the teachers, or the children, should understand anything about the physiology of the eye.

The Fundamental Principle
THE FLASHING CURE

Do you read imperfectly? Can you observe then that when you look at the first word, or the first letter, of a sentence you do not see best where you are looking; that you see other words, or other letters, just as well as or better than the ones you are looking at? Do you observe also that the harder you try to see the worse you see?

Now close your eyes and rest them, remembering some color, like black or white, that you can remember perfectly. Keep them closed until they feel rested, or until the feeling of strain has been completely relieved. Now open them and look at the first word or letter of a sentence for a fraction of a second. If you have been able to relax, partially or completely, you will have a flash of improved or clear vision, and the area seen best will be smaller.

After opening the eyes for this fraction of a second, close them again quickly, still remembering the color, and keep them closed until they again feel rested. Then again open them for a fraction of a second. Continue this alternate resting of the eyes and flashing of the letters for a time, and you may soon find that you can keep your eyes open longer than a fraction of a second without losing the improved vision.

If your trouble is with distant instead of near vision, use the same method with distant letters.

In this way you can demonstrate for yourself the fundamental principles of the cure of imperfect sight by treatment without glasses.

If you fail, ask someone with perfect sight to help you.

THE SWINGING CURE

If you see a letter perfectly, you may note that it appears to pulsate, or move slightly in various directions. If your sight is imperfect, the letter will appear to be stationary. The apparent movement is caused by the unconscious shifting of the eye. The lack of movement is due to the fact that the eye stares, or looks too long at one point. This is an invariable symptom of imperfect sight, and may often be relieved by the following method:

Close your eyes and cover them with the palms of the hands so as to exclude all the light, and shift mentally from one side of a black letter to the other. As you do this, the mental picture of the letter will appear to move back and forth in a direction contrary to the imagined movement of the eye. Just so long as you imagine that the letter is moving, or swinging, you will find that you are able to remember it, and the shorter and more regular the swing, the blacker and more distinct the letter will appear. If you are able to imagine the letter stationary, which may be difficult, you will find that your memory of it will be much less perfect.

Now open your eyes and look first at one side and then at the other of the real letter. If it appears to move in a direction opposite to the movement of the eye, you will find that your vision has improved. If you can imagine the swing of the letter as well with your eyes open as with your eyes closed, as short, as regular and as continuous, your vision will be normal.

THE MEMORY CURE

When the sight is perfect, the memory is also perfect, because the mind is perfectly relaxed. Therefore the sight may be improved by any method that improves the memory. The easiest thing to remember is a small black spot of no particular size and form; but when the sight is imperfect it will be found impossible to remember it with the eyes open and looking at letters, or other objects with definite outlines. It may, however, be remembered for a few seconds or longer, when the eyes are closed and covered, or when looking at a blank surface where there is nothing particular to see. By cultivating the memory under these favorable conditions, it gradually becomes possible to retain it under unfavorable ones, that is, when the eyes are open and the mind conscious of the impressions of sight. By alternately remembering the period with the eyes closed and covered and then looking at the Snellen test card, or other letters or objects; or by remembering it when looking away from the card where there is nothing particular to see, and then looking back; the patient becomes able, in a longer or shorter time, to retain the memory when looking at the card, and thus becomes able to read the letters with normal vision. Many children have been cured very quickly by this method. Adults who have worn glasses have greater difficulty. Even under favorable conditions, the period cannot be remembered for more than a few seconds, unless one shifts from one part of it to another. One can also shift from one period, or other small black object, to another.

THE PALMING CURE

One of the most efficacious methods of relieving eyestrain, and hence of improving the sight, is palming. By this is meant the covering of the closed eyes with the palms of the hands in such a way as to exclude all the light, while avoiding pressure upon the eyeballs. In this way most patients are able to secure some degree of relaxation in a few minutes, and when they open their eyes find their vision temporarily improved.

When relaxation is complete the patient sees, when palming, a black so deep that it is impossible to remember or imagine anything blacker, and such relaxation is always followed by a complete and permanent cure of all errors of refraction (nearsight, farsight, astigmatism and even old sight), as well as by the relief or cure of many other abnormal conditions. In rare cases patients become able to see a perfect black very quickly, even in five, ten or fifteen minutes; but usually this cannot be done without considerable practice, and some never become able to do it until they have been cured by other means. When the patient becomes able after a few trials to see an approximate black, it is worth while to continue with the method; otherwise something else should be tried.

Most patients are helped by the memory of some color, preferably black, and as it is impossible to remember an unchanging object for more than a few seconds, they usually find it necessary to shift consciously from one mental picture to another, or from one part of such a picture to another. In some cases, however, the shifting may be done unconsciously, and the black object may appear to be remembered all alike continuously.

THE IMAGINATION CURE

When the imagination is perfect the mind is always perfectly relaxed, and as it is impossible to relax and imagine a letter perfectly, and at the same time strain and see it imperfectly, it follows that when one imagines that one sees a letter perfectly one actually does see it, as demonstrated by the retinoscope, no matter how great an error of refraction the eye may previously have had. The sight, therefore, may often be improved very quickly by the aid of the imagination. To use this method the patient may proceed as follows:

Look at a letter at the distance at which it is seen best. Close and cover the eyes so as to exclude all the light, and remember it. Do this alternately until the memory is nearly equal to the sight. Next, after remembering the letter with the eyes closed and covered, and while still holding the mental picture of it, look at a blank surface a foot or more to the side of it, at the distance at which you wish to see it. Again close and cover the eyes and remember the letter, and on opening them look a little nearer to it. Gradually reduce the distance between the point of fixation and the letter, until able to look directly at it and imagine it as well as it is remembered with the eyes closed and covered. The letter will then be seen perfectly, and other letters in its neighborhood will come out. If unable to remember the whole letter, you may be able to imagine a black period as forming part of it. If you can do this, the letter will also be seen perfectly.

HALOS

When the eye with normal sight looks at the large letters on the Snellen test card, at any distance from twenty feet to six inches or less, it sees, at the inner and outer edges and in the openings of the round letters, a white more intense than the margin of the card. Similarly, when such an eye reads fine print, the spaces between the lines and the letters and the openings of the letters appear whiter than the margin of the page, while streaks of an even more intense white may be seen along the edges of the lines of letters. These "halos" are sometimes seen so vividly that in order to convince people that they are illusions it is often necessary to cover the letters, when they at once disappear. Patients with imperfect sight also see the halos, though less perfectly, and when they understand that they are imagined, they often become able to imagine them where they had not been seen before, or to increase their vividness, in which case the sight always improves. This can be done by imagining the appearances first with the eyes closed, and then looking at the card, or at fine print, and imagining them there. By alternating these two acts of imagination the sight is often improved rapidly. It is best to begin the practice at the point at which the halos are seen, or can be imagined best. Nearsighted patients are usually able to see them at the near-point, sometimes very vividly. Farsighted people may also see them best at this point, although their sight for form may be best at the distance.

INFLUENZA—A QUICK CURE

When the muscles of the eyes are perfectly relaxed all errors of refraction are not only corrected, but abnormal conditions in other parts of the body are also relieved. It is impossible to relax the muscles of the eyes without relaxing every other muscle in the body. When people have colds or influenza the muscles that control the circulation in the affected parts are under a strain, the arteries are contracted, and the heart is not able to force the normal amount of blood through them. The blood consequently accumulates in the veins and produces inflammation. Hence any treatment which relaxes the muscles of the eyes sufficiently to produce central fixation and normal vision will cure colds and influenza. When one palms perfectly, shifts easily, or has a perfect universal swing, not only the muscles which control the refraction, but the muscles of the arteries which control the circulation of the eyes, nose, lungs, kidneys, etc., are relaxed, and all symptoms of influenza disappear. The nasal discharge ceases as if by magic, the cough is at once relieved, and if the nose has been closed, it opens. Pain, fatigue, fever and chilliness are also relieved. The truth of these statements has been repeatedly demonstrated.

The Editor is very proud of this discovery which is now published for the first time.

Fine Print a Benefit to the Eye

Seven Truths of Normal Sight

1—Normal Sight can always be demonstrated in the normal eye, but only under favorable conditions.
2—Central Fixation: The letter or part of the letter regarded is always seen best.
3—Shifting: The point regarded changes rapidly and continuously.
4—Swinging: When the shifting is slow, the letters appear to move from side to side, or in other directions, with a pendulum-like motion.
5—Memory is perfect. The color and background of the letters, or other objects seen, are remembered perfectly, instantaneously and continuously.
6—Imagination is good. One may even see the white part of letters whiter than it really is, while the black is not altered by distance, illumination, size, or form, of the letters.
7—Rest or relaxation of the eye and mind is perfect and can always be demonstrated.

When one of these seven fundamentals is perfect, all are perfect.

It is impossible to read fine print without relaxing. Therefore the reading of such print, contrary to what is generally believed, is a great benefit to the eyes. Persons who can read perfectly fine print, like the above specimen, are relieved of pain and fatigue while they are doing it, and this relief is often permanent. Persons who cannot read it are benefited by observing its blackness, and remembering it with the eyes open and closed alternately. By bringing the print so near to the eyes that it cannot be read pain is sometimes relieved instantly, because when the patient realizes that there is no possibility of reading it the eyes do not try to do so. In myopia, however, it is sometimes a benefit to strain to read fine print. Persons who can read fine print perfectly imagine that they see between the lines streaks of white whiter than the margin of the page, and persons who cannot read it also see these streaks, but not so well. When the patient becomes able to increase the vividness of these appearances [see *Halos*, February number] the sight always improves.

REST

All methods of curing errors of refraction are simply different ways of obtaining rest.

Different persons do this in different ways. Some patients are able to rest their eyes simply by closing them, and complete cures have been obtained by this means, the closing of the eyes for a longer or shorter period being alternated with looking at the test card for a moment. In other cases patients have strained more when their eyes were shut than when they were open. Some can rest their eyes when all light is excluded from them by covering with the palms of the hands; others cannot, and have to be helped by other means before they can palm. Some become able at once to remember or imagine that the letters they wish to see are perfectly black, and with the accompanying relaxation their vision immediately becomes normal. Others become able to do this only after a considerable time. Shifting is a very simple method of relieving strain, and most patients soon become able to shift from one letter to another, or from one side of a letter to another in such a way that these forms seem to move in a direction opposite to the movement of the eye. A few are unable to do this, but can do it with a mental picture of a letter, after which they become able to do it visually.

Patients who do not succeed with any particular method of obtaining rest for their eyes should abandon it and try something else. The cause of the failure is strain, and it does no good to go on straining.

SUN-GAZING

Light is necessary to the health of the eye, and darkness is injurious to it. Eye shades, dark glasses, darkened rooms, weaken the sight and sooner or later produce inflammations. Persons with normal sight can look directly at the sun, or at the strongest artificial light, without injury or discomfort, and persons with imperfect sight are never permanently injured by such lights, though temporary ill effects, lasting from a few minutes to a few hours, days, weeks, months, or longer, may be produced. In all abnormal conditions of the eyes, light is beneficial. It is rarely sufficient to cure, but is a great help in gaining relaxation by other methods.

The quickest way to get results from the curative power of sunlight is to focus the rays with a burning glass on the white part of the eye when the patient looks far downward, moving the light from side to side to avoid heat. This may be done for part of a minute at frequent intervals.

Looking at the sun, while slower in its results, has often been sufficient to effect permanent cures, sometimes in a very short time. There is a right way and a wrong way to do this. Persons with imperfect sight should never look directly at the sun at first, because, while no permanent harm can come from it, great temporary inconvenience may result. Such persons should begin by looking to one side of the sun, and after becoming accustomed to the strong light, should look a little nearer to its source, and so on until they become able to look directly at the sun without discomfort.

SEE THINGS MOVING

When the sight is perfect the subject is able to observe that all objects regarded appear to be moving. A letter seen at the near point or at the distance appears to move slightly in various directions. The pavement comes toward one in walking, and the houses appear to move in a direction opposite to one's own. In reading the page appears to move in a direction opposite to that of the eye. If one tries to imagine things stationary, the vision is at once lowered and discomfort and pain may be produced, not only in the eyes and head, but in other parts of the body.

This movement is usually so slight that it is seldom noticed till the attention is called to it, but it may be so conspicuous as to be plainly observable even to persons with markedly imperfect sight. If such persons, for instance, hold the hand within six inches of the face and turn the head and eyes rapidly from side to side, the hand will be seen to move in a direction opposite to that of the eyes. If it does not move, it will be found that the patient is straining to see it in the eccentric field. By observing this movement it becomes possible to see or imagine a less conspicuous movement, and thus the patient may gradually become able to observe a slight movement in every object regarded. Some persons with imperfect sight have been cured simply by imagining that they see things moving all day long.

The world moves. Let it move. All objects move if you let them. Do not interfere with this movement, or try to stop it. This cannot be done without an effort which impairs the efficiency of the eye and mind.

THE CURE OF IMPERFECT SIGHT IN SCHOOL CHILDREN

While reading the Snellen test card every day will, in time, cure imperfect sight in all children under twelve who have never worn glasses, the following simple practices will insure more rapid progress:

1. Let the children rest their eyes by closing for a few minutes or longer, and then look at the test card for a few moments only, then rest again, and so on alternately. This cures many children very promptly.

2. Let them close and cover their eyes with the palms of their hands in such a way as to exclude all the light while avoiding pressure on the eyeballs (palming), and proceed as above. This is usually more effective than mere closing.

3. Let them demonstrate that all effort lowers the vision by looking fixedly at a letter on the test card, or at the near-point, and noting that it blurs or disappears in less than a minute. They thus become able, in some way, to avoid unconscious effort.

The method succeeds best when the teachers do not wear glasses.

Supervision is absolutely necessary. At least once a year some person whose sight is normal without glasses and who understands the method should visit the classrooms for the purpose of answering questions, testing the sight of the children, and making a report to the proper authorities.

The Snellen test card is a chart showing letters of graduated sizes, with numbers indicating the distance in feet at which each line should be read by the normal eye. Originally designed by Snellen for the purpose of testing the eye, it is admirably adapted for use in eye education.

MAKE YOUR SIGHT WORSE

Strange as it may seem there is no better way of improving the sight than by making it worse. To see things worse when one is already seeing them badly requires mental control of a degree greater than that required to improve the sight. The importance of these facts is very great. When patients become able to lower their vision by conscious staring, they become better able to avoid unconscious staring. When they demonstrate by increasing their eccentric fixation that trying to see objects not regarded lowers the vision, they may stop trying to do the same thing unconsciously.

What is true of the sight is also true of the imagination and memory. If one's memory and imagination are imperfect, they can be improved by consciously making them worse than they are. Persons with imperfect sight never remember or imagine the letters on the test card as perfectly black and distinct, but to imagine them as grey and cloudy is very difficult, or even impossible, and when a patient has done it, or tried to do it, he may become able to avoid the unconscious strain which has prevented him from forming mental pictures as black and distinct as the reality.

To make imperfect sight worse is always more difficult than to lower normal vision. In other words, to make a letter which already appears grey and indistinct noticeably more cloudy is harder than to blur a letter seen distinctly. To make an imperfect mental picture worse is harder than to blur a perfect one. Both practices require much effort, much hard disagreeable work; but they always, when successful, improve the memory, imagination and vision.

GO TO THE MOVIES

Cinematograph pictures are commonly supposed to be very injurious to the eyes, and it is a fact that they often cause much discomfort and lowering of vision. They can, however, be made a means of improving the sight. When they hurt the eyes it is because the subject strains to see them. If this tendency to strain can be overcome, the vision is always improved, and, if the practice of viewing the pictures is continued long enough, nearsight, astigmatism and other troubles are cured.

If your sight is imperfect, therefore, you will find it an advantage to go to the movies frequently and learn to look at the pictures without strain. If they hurt your eyes, look away to the dark for a while, then look at a corner of the picture; look away again, and then look a little nearer to the center; and so on. In this way you may soon become able to look directly at the picture without discomfort. If this does not help, try palming for five minutes or longer. Dodge the pain, in short, and prevent the eyestrain by constant shifting, or by palming.

If you become able to look at the movies without discomfort, nothing else will bother you.

MAKE YOUR SQUINT WORSE

There is no better way of curing squint than by making it worse, or by producing other kinds of squint. This can be done as follows:

To produce convergent squint, strain to see a point about three inches from the eyes, such as the end of the nose.

To produce divergent squint, fix a point at the distance to one side of any object, and strain to see it as well as when directly regarded.

To produce a vertical squint, look at a point below an object at the distance, and at the same time strain to see the latter.

To produce an oblique divergent squint, look at a point below and to one side of an object at the distance while straining to see the latter.

When successful two images will be seen arranged horizontally, vertically, or obliquely, according to the direction of the strain.

The production of convergent squint is usually easier than that of the other varieties, and most patients succeed better with a light as the object of vision than with a letter, or other non-luminous object.

VOLUNTARY PRODUCTION OF EYE TENSION A SAFEGUARD AGAINST GLAUCOMA

It is a good thing to know how to increase the tension of the eyeball voluntarily, as this enables one to avoid not only the strain that produces glaucoma, but other kinds of strain also. To do this proceed as follows:

Put the fingers on the upper part of the eyeball while looking downward, and note its softness. Then do any one of the following things:

Try to see a letter, or other object, imperfectly, or (with the eyes either closed or open) to imagine it imperfectly.

Try to see a letter, or a number of letters, all alike at one time, or to imagine them in this way.

Try to imagine that a letter, or mental picture of a letter, is stationary.

Try to see a letter, or other object, double, or to imagine it double.

When successful the eyeball will become harder in proportion to the degree of the strain; but, as it is very difficult to see, imagine, or remember, things imperfectly, all may not be able at first to demonstrate the facts.

THE TREATMENT OF CATARACT

From "A Case of Cataract," by Victoria Coolidge, in "Better Eyesight" for June, 1920.

The treatment prescribed was as follows:

Palming six times a day, a half hour or longer at a time.

Reading the Snellen test card at five, ten, and twenty feet.

Reading fine print at six inches, five minutes at a time, especially soon after rising in the morning and just before retiring at night, and reading books and newspapers.

Besides this, he was to subject his eyes, especially the left, to the sunlight whenever an opportunity offered, to drink twelve glasses of water a day, walk five miles a day, and later, when he was in better training, to run half a mile or so every day.

The results of this treatment have been most gratifying. Not only have his eyes improved steadily, but his general health has been so much benefited that at eighty-two he looks, acts and feels better and younger than he did at eighty-one.

THE PREVENTION AND CONTROL OF PAIN BY THE MIND

Anyone who has normal vision can demonstrate in a few moments that when the memory is perfect no pain is felt, and can produce pain by an attempt to keep the attention fixed on a point. To do this proceed as follows:

Look at a black letter, close the eyes and remember it. Look at the letter again and again close the eyes and remember it. Repeat until the memory is equal to the sight. Now press the nail of one finger against the tip of another. If the letter is remembered perfectly, no pain will be felt. With practice it may become possible to remember the letter with the eyes open.

Remember the letter imperfectly, with blurred edges and clouded openings, and again press the nail of one finger against the tip of another. In this case it will be found impossible to continue the pressure for more than a moment on account of the pain.

Try to remember one point of a letter continuously. It will be found impossible to do so, and if the effort is continued long enough pain will be produced.

Try to look continuously at one point of a letter or other object. If the effort is continued long enough, pain will be produced.

HOW TO OBTAIN PERCEPTION OF LIGHT IN BLINDNESS

Two things have always brought perception of light to blind patients. One is palming, and the other is the swing. The swing may take two forms:

1. Let the patient stand with feet apart, and sway the body, including the head and eyes, from side to side, while shifting the weight from one foot to the other.

2. Let him move his hand from one side to the other in front of his face, all the time trying to imagine that he sees it moving. As soon as he becomes able to do this it can be demonstrated that he really does see the movement.

Simple as these measures are they have always, either singly or together, brought relaxation, and with it perception of light, in from fifteen minutes or less to half an hour.

In palming the patient should remember that this does not bring relief unless mental relaxation is obtained, as evidenced by the disappearance of the white, grey and other colors which most blind people see at first with their eyes closed and covered.

HOW TO IMPROVE THE SIGHT BY MEANS OF THE IMAGINATION

Remember the letter *o* in diamond type, with the eyes closed and covered. If you are able to do this, it will appear to have a short, slow swing, less than its own diameter.

Look at an unknown letter on the test card which you can see only as a gray spot, at ten feet or more, and imagine that it has a swing of not more than a quarter of an inch.

Imagine the top of the unknown letter to be straight, still maintaining the swing. If this is in accordance with the fact, the swing will be unchanged. If it is not, the swing will become uneven, or longer, or will be lost.

If the swing is altered, try another guess. If you can't tell the difference between two guesses, it is because the swing is too long. Palm and remember the *o* with its short swing, and you may become able to shorten that of the larger letter.

In this way you can ascertain, without seeing the letter, whether its four sides are straight, curved, or open. You may then be able to imagine the whole letter. This is easiest with the eyes closed and covered. If the swing is modified, you will know that you have made a mistake. In that case repeat from the beginning.

When you get the right letter imagine it alternately with the eyes closed and open, until you are able to imagine it as well when you look at it as when your eyes are closed and covered. In that case you will actually see the letter.

METHODS THAT HAVE SUCCEEDED IN PRESBYOPIA

The cure of presbyopia, as of any other error of refraction, is rest, and many presbyopic patients are able to obtain this rest simply by closing the eyes. They are kept closed until the patient feels relieved, which may be in a few minutes, half an hour, or longer. Then some fine print is regarded for a few seconds. By alternately resting the eyes and looking at fine print many patients quickly become able to read it at eighteen inches, and by continued practice they are able to reduce the distance until it can be read at six inches in a dim light. At first the letters are seen only in flashes. Then they are seen for a longer time, until finally they are seen continuously. When this method fails, palming may be tried, combined with the use of the memory, imagination and swing. Particularly good results have been obtained from the following procedure:

Close the eyes and remember the letter *o* in diamond type, with the open space as white as starch and the outline as black as possible.

When the white center is at the maximum imagine that the letter is moving, and that all objects, no matter how large or small, are moving with it.

Open the eyes and continue to imagine the universal swing,

Alternate the imagination of the swing with the eyes open with its imagination with the eyes closed.

When the imagination is just as good with the eyes open as when they are closed the cure will be complete.

HOW TO DEMONSTRATE THE FUNDAMENTAL PRINCIPLE OF TREATMENT

The object of all the methods used in the treatment of imperfect sight without glasses is to secure rest or relaxation, of the mind first and then of the eyes. Rest always improves the vision. Effort always lowers it. Persons who wish to improve their vision should begin by demonstrating these facts.

Close the eyes and keep them closed for fifteen minutes. Think of nothing particular, or think of something pleasant. When the eyes are opened, it will usually be found that the vision has improved temporarily. If it has not, it will be because, while the eyes were closed, the mind was not at rest.

One symptom of strain is a twitching of the eyelids which can be seen by an observer and felt by the patient with the fingers. This can usually be corrected if the period of rest is long enough.

Many persons fail to secure a temporary improvement of vision by closing their eyes, because they do not keep them closed long enough. Children will seldom do this unless a grown person stands by and encourages them. Many adults also require supervision.

To demonstrate that strain lowers the vision, think of something disagreeable—some physical discomfort, or something seen imperfectly. When the eyes are opened, it will be found that the vision has been lowered. Also stare at one part of a letter on the test card, or try to see the whole letter all alike at one time. This invariably lowers the vision, and may cause the letters to disappear.

HOW NOT TO CONCENTRATE

To remember the letter *o* of diamond type continuously and without effort proceed as follows:

Imagine a little black spot on the right-hand side of the *o* blacker than the rest of the letter; then imagine a similar spot on the left-hand side. Shift the attention from the right-hand period to the left, and observe that every time that you think of the left period the *o* appears to move to the right, and every time you think of the right one it appears to move to the left. This motion, when the shifting is done properly, is very short, less than the width of the letter. Later you may become able to imagine the *o* without conscious shifting and swinging, but whenever the attention is directed to the matter these things will be noticed.

Now do the same with the *a* letter on the test card. If the shifting is normal, it will be noted that the letter can be regarded indefinitely, and that it appears to have a slight motion.

To demonstrate that the attempt to concentrate spoils the memory, or imagination, and the vision:

Try to think continuously of a period on one part of an imagined letter. The period and the whole letter will soon disappear. Or try to imagine two or more periods, or the whole letter, equally black and distinct at one time. This will be found to be even more difficult.

Do the same with a letter on the test card. The results will be the same.

HOW TO IMPROVE THE SIGHT BY MEANS OF THE IMAGINATION: No. 2

In a recent issue directions were given for improving the vision by the aid of the imagination. According to this method the patient ascertains what a letter is by imagining each of the four sides to be straight, curved, or open, and noting the effect of each guess upon the imagined swing of the letter. Another method which has succeeded even better with many patients is to judge the correctness of the guess by observing its effect on the appearance of the letter.

Look at a letter which can be seen only as a gray spot, and imagine the top is straight. If the guess is right, the spot will probably become blacker; if it is wrong, the spot may become fainter or disappear. If no difference is apparent, rest the eyes by looking away, closing, or palming, and try again.

In many cases, when one side has been imagined correctly, the whole letter will come out. If it does not, proceed to imagine the other sides as above directed. If, when all four sides have been imagined correctly, a letter does not come out, palm and repeat.

One can even bring out a letter that one cannot see at all in this way. Look at a line of letters which cannot be seen, and imagine the top of the first letter to be straight. If the guess is correct, the line may become apparent, and by continued practice the letter may come out clearly enough to be distinguished.

CHILDREN MAY IMPROVE THEIR SIGHT BY CONSCIOUSLY DOING THE WRONG THING

Children often make a great effort to see the blackboard and other distant objects in school. It helps them to overcome this habit to have them demonstrate just what the strain to see does.

Tell them to fix their attention on the smallest letter they can see from their seats, to stare at it, to concentrate on it, to partly close their eyelids—in short, to make as great an effort as possible to see it.

The letter will blur, or disappear altogether, and the whole card may become blurred, while discomfort, or pain in the eyes or head, will be produced.

Now direct them to rest their eyes by palming. The pain or discomfort will cease, the letter will come out again, and other letters that they could not see before may come out also.

After a demonstration like this children are less likely to make an effort to see the blackboard, or anything else; but some children have to repeat the experiment many times before the subconscious inclination to strain is corrected.

HOW TO OBTAIN MENTAL PICTURES

Look at a letter on the Snellen test card.

Remember its blackness.

Shift the attention from one part of this spot of black to another. It should appear to move in a direction contrary to the imagined movement.

If it does not, try to imagine it stationary. If you succeed in doing this it will blur, or disappear. Having demonstrated that it is impossible to imagine the spot stationary, it may become possible to imagine it moving.

Having become able to form a mental picture of a black spot with the eyes closed, try to do the same with the eyes open. Alternate till the mental vision with the eyes closed and open is the same.

Having become able to imagine a black spot try to imagine the letter *o* in diamond type with the center as white as snow. Do this alternately with eyes closed and open.

If you cannot hold the picture of a letter or period commit to memory a number of letters on the test card and recite them to yourself while imagining that the card is moving.

If some other color or object is easier to imagine than a black spot it will serve the purpose equally well.

A few exceptional people may get better results with the eyes open than when they are closed.

THE SENSE OF TOUCH AN AID TO VISION

Just as Montessori has found that impressions gained through the sense of touch are very useful in teaching children to read and write, persons with defective sight have found them useful in educating their memory and imagination.

One patient whose visual memory was very imperfect found that if she traced an imaginary black letter on the ball of her thumb with her forefinger, she could follow the imaginary lines with her mind as they were being formed and retain a picture of the letter better than when she gained the impression of it through the sense of sight.

Another patient discovered that when he lost the swing he could get it again by sliding his forefinger back and forth over the ball of his thumb. When he moved his fingers it seemed as if his whole body were moving.

Both these expedients have the advantage of being inconspicuous, and can, therefore, be used anywhere.

The vision was improved in both cases.

THINK RIGHT

"As a man thinketh in his heart so is he," is a saying which is invariably true when the sight is concerned. When a person remembers or imagines an object of sight perfectly the sight is perfect; when he remembers it imperfectly the sight is imperfect. The idea that to do anything well requires effort, ruins the sight of many children and adults; for every thought of effort in the mind produces an error of refraction in the eye. The idea that large objects are easier to see than small ones results in the failure to see small objects. The fear that light will hurt the eyes actually produces sensitiveness to light. To demonstrate the truth of these statements is a great benefit.

Remember a letter or other object perfectly, and note that the sight is improved and pain and fatigue relieved; remember the object imperfectly, and note that the vision is lowered, while pain and fatigue may be produced or increased.

Rest the eyes by closing or palming, and note that the vision is improved, and pain and discomfort relieved; stare at a letter, concentrate upon it, make an effort to see it, and note that it disappears, and that a feeling of discomfort or pain is produced.

Note that a small part of a large object is seen better than the rest of it.

Accustom the eyes to strong light; learn to look at the sun; note that the vision is not lowered but improved, and that the light causes less and less discomfort.

Remember your successes (things seen perfectly); forget your failures (things seen imperfectly); patients who do this are cured quickly.

STOP STARING

It can be demonstrated by tests with the retinoscope that all persons with imperfect sight stare, strain, or try to see. To demonstrate this fact:

Look intently at one part of a large or small letter at the distance or nearpoint. In a few seconds, usually, fatigue and discomfort will be produced, and the letter will blur or disappear. If the effort is continued long enough, pain may be produced.

To break the habit of staring:
(1) Shift consciously from one part to another of all objects regarded, and imagine that these objects move in a direction contrary to the movement of the eye. Do this with letters on the test card, with letters of fine print, if they can be seen, and with other objects.
(2) Close the eyes frequently for a moment or longer. When the strain is considerable, keep the eyes closed for several minutes and open them for a fraction of a second—flashing. When the stare is sufficient to keep the vision down to 2/200 or less, palm for a longer or shorter time; then look at the card for a moment. Later mere closing of the eyes may afford sufficient rest.
(3) Imagine that the white openings and margins of letters are whiter than the rest of the background. Do this with eyes closed and open alternately. It is an interesting fact that this practice prevents staring and improves the vision rapidly.

Test Your Imagination!

WITH the eyes closed remember some letter, as, for example, a small letter o. Imagine the white center to be white as snow with the sun shining on it. Now open the eyes, look at the Snellen Test Card and imagine the white snow as well as you can for a few moments only; without noting so much the clearness of the letters on the card as your ability to imagine the snow white center, alternating as before with the Snellen Card.

Another method: With the eyes closed, remember and imagine as well as you can the first letter, which should be known, on each line of the Snellen Test Card, beginning with the larger letters. Then open your eyes and imagine the same letter for a few moments only, alternating until the known letter is imagined sufficiently well that the second letter is seen without any effort on your part.

Third method: With the eyes closed remember or imagine a small black period for part of a minute or longer. Then with the eyes open, looking at no object in particular and without trying to see, imagine in your mind the black period. Should you believe that your vision is improved, dodge it, look somewhere else. This you can practice at all times, in all places, at your work as well as when sitting quietly in your room practicing with the Snellen Test Card. When the period is imagined perfectly with the eyes open, one cannot dodge perfect sight, which comes without any effort whatsoever.

SEE THINGS MOVING

WHEN riding in a railroad train, travelling rapidly, a passenger looking out a window can imagine more or less vividly that stationary objects, trees, houses, telegraph poles, are moving past in the opposite direction. If one walks along the street, objects to either side appear to be moving. When the eyes move from side to side a long distance with or without the movement of the head or body it is possible to imagine objects not directly regarded to be moving. To see things moving avoid looking directly at them while moving the eyes.

The Long Swing: No matter how great the mental or other strain may be, one can, by moving the eyes a long distance from side to side with the movement of the head and body in the same direction, imagine things moving opposite over a wide area. The eyes or mind are benefitted.

The Short Swing: To imagine things are moving a quarter of an inch or less, gradually shorten the long swing and decrease the speed to a rate of a second or less for each swing. Another method is to remember a small letter perfectly with the eyes closed and noting the short swing. Alternate with the eyes open and closed.

The Universal Swing: Demonstrate that when one imagines or sees one letter on a card at a distance or at a near point that the card moves with the letter and that every other letter or object seen or imagined in turn also swings. This is the universal swing. Practice it all the time because the ability to see or to do other things is benefitted.

Practice the imagination of the swing constantly. If one imagines things are stationary, the vision is always imperfect, and effort is required and one does not feel comfortable. To stare and strain takes time. To let things move is easier. One should plan to practice the swing observed by the eye with normal vision: as short at least as the width of the letter at twenty feet or six inches, as slow as a second to each movement and all done easily, rhythmically, continuously.

RELAXATION FROM FINE PRINT

A BUSINESS card, 3″ x 2″ with fine print on one side is held in front of the eyes as near as possible, the upper part in contact with the eyebrows, the lower part resting lightly on the nose.

The patient looks directly at the fine print without trying to see. Being so close to the eyes most people realize that it is impossible to read the fine print and do not try, in this way they obtain a measure of relaxation which is sufficient to benefit the sight very much.

The patient moves the card from side to side a short distance slowly and sees the card moving provided the movement is not too short or too slow. The shorter the movement and the slower it is, the better.

Some patients, although the card is held very close, note that the white spaces between the lines become whiter and the black letters become blacker and clearer. In some cases one or more words of the fine print will be seen in flashes or even continuously as long as no effort is made to see or to read the fine print.

This movement of the card should be kept up to obtain the best results, for many hours every day. The hand which holds the card may soon become fatigued; one may then use the hands alternately. Some patients vary this by holding the card with both hands at the same time.

The amount of light is not important.

IMPROVE YOUR SIGHT

ALL day long use your eyes right. You have just as much time to use your eyes right as you have to use them wrong. It is easier and more comfortable to have perfect sight than to have imperfect sight.

Practice the long swing. Notice that when your eyes move the great distance rapidly, objects in front of you move in the opposite direction so rapidly that you do not see them clearly. Do not try to see them because that stops the apparent movement.

Rest your eyes continually by blinking, which means to open and close them so rapidly that one appears to see things continuously. Whenever convenient close your eyes for a few minutes and rest them. Cover them with one or both hands to shut out the light and obtain a greater rest.

When the mind is awake it is thinking of many things. One can remember things perfectly or imagine things perfectly, which is a rest to the eyes, mind and the body generally. The memory of imperfect sight should be avoided because it is a strain and lowers the vision.

Read the Snellen Test Card at 20 feet with each eye, separately, twice daily or oftener. Imagine white spaces in letters whiter than the rest of the card. Do this alternately with the eyes closed and opened. Plan to imagine the white spaces in letters just as white, in looking at the Snellen test card, as can be accomplished with the eyes closed.

Remember one letter of the alphabet, or a part of one letter, or a period, continuously and perfectly.

DISCARD GLASSES

EASY to say, something else to do. But it is a fact that no one can be cured without glasses and wear glasses at the same time.

This is a fact that one should keep in mind. It may help to give one backbone sufficient to do the right thing. I know how difficult it is from personal experience. I suppose I have as much originality, if not more, than the average person. It required a year before I was convinced that my eyes could not be cured unless I stopped wearing glasses. I could not wear them even for emergencies without suffering a relapse.

Patients who are really anxious to be cured can discard glasses and obtain benefit almost from the start. Wearing of glasses becomes a fixed habit. The idea of going without them is a shock. The honest determination to do all that is possible to be done for a cure, makes it easy or easier to discard glasses at once. Patients tell me that after they have discarded their glasses for a few days they do not feel as uncomfortable as they expected.

Do not use opera glasses. Do not use a magnifying glass for any purpose.

It is very natural that one should hesitate to discard glasses after he has worn them for many years and obtained what seems considerable benefit. It may help to read what I have published about glasses. Most of the discomforts of the eyes are largely functional or nervous and not due to any real or organic trouble with the eyes. All the symptoms of discomfort are accompanied by a strain which produces a wrong focus of the eyes called myopia, hypermetropia, astigmatism or presbyopia. Glasses may correct the wrong focus produced by the strain, but they do not always, because the eyes are not always strained to fit glasses accurately. While wearing glasses in order to see, one has to strain or, by an effort, squeeze the eye ball out of shape and it is impossible therefore, to obtain relaxation and see with glasses.

If one can understand what I have just stated one can realize the necessity of discarding glasses in order to obtain a cure. I feel that the facts should be emphasized and the patient made to understand the necessity of discarding glasses. This makes it easier for the patient to do without glasses.

Do not argue with yourself about the matter. When you go to a doctor you expect to take his medicine even though you may not know what it is or how it is going to act. When patients come to me for relief I say, "Discard your glasses and you can be cured."

If they are wise they do as I say without any talk.

"PAGE TWO"

ON page two of this magazine are printed each month specific directions for improving the sight in various ways. Too many subscribers read the magazine once and then mislay it. We feel that at least page two should be kept for reference.

When the eyes are neglected the vision may fail. It is so easy to forget how to palm successfully. The long swing always helps but it has to be done right. One may under adverse conditions suffer a tension so great that the ability to remember or imagine perfectly is modified or lost and relaxation is not obtained. The long swing is always available and always brings sufficient relief to practice the short swing, central fixation, the perfect memory and imagination with perfect relief.

Be sure and review page two frequently; not only for your special benefit but also for the benefit of individuals you desire to help!

Persons with imperfect sight often have difficulty in obtaining relaxation by the various methods described in the book and in this magazine. It should be emphasized that persons with good vision are better able to help others than people who have imperfect sight or wear glasses. If you are trying to cure yourself avoid people who wear glasses or do not see well. Those individuals are always under a strain and the strain is manifested in their face, in their voices, in their walk, the way they sit, in short in everything that they do.

Strain is contagious. Teachers in Public Schools who wear glasses are a menace to their pupils' sight. Parents who wear glasses or who have imperfect sight lower the vision of their children. It is always well when treating children or adults to keep them away from people with imperfect sight.

COMPARISONS

IN practicing with the Snellen Test Card, when the vision is imperfect, the blackness of the letters is modified and the white spaces inside the letters are also modified. By comparing the blackness of the large letters with the blackness of the smaller ones it can be demonstrated that the larger letters are imperfectly seen. They really have more of a blur than do the smaller letters which cannot be distinguished.

When one notes the whiteness in the center of a large letter, seen indistinctly, it is usually possible to compare the whiteness seen with the remembered whiteness of something else. By alternately comparing the whiteness in the center of a letter with the memory of a better white, as the snow on the top of a mountain, the whiteness of the letter usually improves. In the same way, comparing the shade of black of a letter with the memory of a darker shade of black of some other object may be also a benefit to the black.

Most persons with myopia are able to read fine print at a near point quite perfectly. They see the blackness and whiteness of the letters much better than they are able to see the blackness of the larger letters on the Snellen Test Card at 15 or 20 feet. Alternately reading the fine print and regarding the Snellen Test Card, comparing the black and white of the small letters with the black and white of the large letters, is often times very beneficial. Some cases of myopia have been cured very promptly by this method.

All persons with imperfect sight for reading are benefitted by comparing the whiteness of the spaces between the lines with the memory of objects which are whiter. Many persons can remember white snow with the eyes closed whiter than the spaces between the lines. By alternately closing the eyes for a minute or longer, remembering white snow, white starch, white paint, white cloud in the sky with the sun shining on it, and flashing the white spaces without trying to read, many persons have materially improved their sight and been cured.

SCHOOL CHILDREN'S EYES

THE cure and prevention of imperfect sight in school children is very simple.

A Snellen Test Card should be placed in the class room where all children can see it from their seats. They should read the card at least once daily with each eye separately, covering the other eye with the palms of the hands, in such a way as to avoid pressing on the eyeball. The time required is less than a minute for both eyes. The card measures the amount of their vision. They will find from time to time that their eyesight varies. Some children are very much disturbed when they cannot see so well on account of the light being dim on a dark or rainy day and although they usually learn the letters by heart they do not always remember or see them. It is well to encourage the children to commit the letters to memory because it is a great help for them to see them. When a child can read the Snellen Test Card with each eye with perfect sight, even although they do know what the letters are, it has been found by numerous observations that their eyes are also normal and not nearsighted, far-sighted nor do they have astigmatism. Many children find that when they have difficulty in reading the writing on the blackboard that they obtain material help after glancing at the Snellen Test Card and reading it with perfect sight.

When the eye is at rest, perfect rest, it always has perfect sight. A great many teachers and others condemn the method unwisely because they say that the children learn, and because they know what the letters are, they recite them without actually seeing them. With my instrument I have observed many thousands of school children reading the Snellen Test Card apparently with perfect sight, the test card that they had committed to memory, and in all cases never did I find anything wrong with their eyes.

About ten years ago I challenged a Doctor, a member of the Board of Education, to prove that the children deceive themselves or others by saying that they see letters when they don't. To me it is very interesting that the most wicked child in school no matter how he may lie about other things with great facility and gets by with it, was never caught lying about his eyesight. I believe that every family should have a Snellen Test Card in the home and the children encouraged to practice reading it for a few minutes or longer a number of times every day. Some children are fond of contests and quite often a child who can demonstrate that his vision was the best of any pupil in the class had a feeling of pride and satisfaction which every one in sporting events can understand.

PRACTICING

A GREAT many people have asked, "How much time should one devote to practicing the methods of central fixation in order to be cured of imperfect sight without glasses?"

The answer is—ALL THE TIME.

One should secure relaxation or rest until one is perfectly comfortable and continue feeling comfortable as long as one is awake.

The feeling of relaxation or comfort can be obtained with the memory of perfect sight. Even if one cannot remember perfect sight one can imagine it. All black objects should be imagined perfectly black. All white objects observed should be imagined perfectly white. All letters observed should be imagined perfectly and everything that is seen should be imagined perfectly.

To imagine anything imperfectly requires a strain, an effort, which is difficult. Choose the easy way. Imagine things perfectly.

If you try to imagine an object as stationary you will strain and your sight become impaired. All day long the eyes are moving from one point to another. Imagine that objects are moving opposite to the movement of the eyes. If one does not notice this one is very apt to strain and imagine things stationary.

One can practice properly for ten minutes and be comfortable. That does not mean that all the rest of the day one can strain and tear one's eyes all to pieces without paying the penalty for breaking the law. If you are under treatment for imperfect sight be sure to keep in mind all day long from the time you wake up in the morning until you go to bed at night the feeling of comfort, of rest, of relaxation, incessantly. It is a great deal better to do that than to feel under a strain and be uncomfortable all day long.

THE VARIABLE SWING

RECENTLY I have been impressed very much by the value of the variable swing. By the variable swing is meant the ability to imagine a near object with a longer swing than one more distant. For example, a patient came to me with conical cornea, which is usually considered incurable. I placed a chair five feet away from her eyes, clearly on a line with the Snellen test card located 15 feet distant. When she looked at the Snellen test card and imagined the letters moving an inch or less she could imagine the chair that she was not looking at moving quite a distance. As is well known the shorter the swing the better the sight. Some persons with unusually good vision have a swing so short that they do not readily recognize it. This patient was able to imagine the chair moving an inch or less and the card on the wall moving a shorter distance. She became able to imagine the chair moving a quarter of an inch and the movement of the Snellen test card at 15 feet was so short that she could not notice it. In the beginning her vision with glasses was poor and without glasses was double, and even the larger letters on the Snellen test card were very much blurred. Now, when she imagined the chair moving a quarter of an inch and the Snellen test card moving so short a distance that she could not recognize it, the conical cornea disappeared from both eyes and her vision became normal. To me it was one of the most remarkable things I have seen in years. I know of no other treatment that has ever brought about so great a benefit in so bad a case.

The variable swing is something that most people can learn how to practise at their first visit. Some people can do it better than others. The improvement depends directly upon their skill in practising the variable swing.

THE EASY SHIFT

SOME time ago a man came to me for treatment of his eyes. Without glasses his vision was about one-half of the normal. This patient could not palm without suffering an agony of pain and depression. He had pain in different parts of his body as well as in his eyes and the pain was usually very severe. The long swing, the short swing tired him exceedingly and made his sight worse. I asked him to tell me what there was that he could remember which caused him no discomfort.

He said, "Everything that I see disturbs me if I make an effort." "I try very hard not to make an effort, but the harder I try the worse do I feel."

When he could not practise palming, swinging or memory successfully I suggested to him that he look from one side of the room to the other, paying no attention to what he saw, but to remember as well as he could a room in his home. For two hours he practised this and was able to move his eyes from one side of the room to the other without paying any attention to the things that were moving or to the things he saw. This was a rest to him, and when his vision was tested, much to my surprise, he read the Snellen Test Card with normal vision at twenty feet. I handed him some diamond type, which he read without difficulty and without his glasses.

Since that time I have had other patients who were unable to remember or imagine things without straining and they usually obtained marked benefit by practising the EASY SHIFT.

No one can obtain perfect sight without constantly shifting, easily, without effort. THE EASY SHIFT is easy because it is done without trying to remember, to imagine or to see. As soon as one makes an effort the shift becomes difficult and no benefit is obtained.

BREATHING

MANY patients with imperfect sight are benefited by breathing. One of the best methods is to separate the teeth while keeping the lips closed, breathe deeply as though one were yawning. When done properly one can feel the air cold as it passes through the nose and down the throat. This method of breathing secures a great amount of relaxation of the nose, throat, the body generally including the eyes and ears.

A man aged sixty-five, had imperfect sight for distance and was unable to read fine print without the aid of strong glasses. After practicing deep breathing in the manner described he became able at once to read diamond type quite perfectly, as close as six inches from the eyes. The benefit was temporary but by repetition the improvement became more permanent.

At one time I experimented with a number of patients, first having them hold their breath and test their vision, which was usually lower when they did not breathe. They became able to demonstrate that holding their breath was a strain and caused imperfect sight, double vision, dizziness and fatigue, while the deep breathing at once gave them relief.

There is a wrong way of breathing in which when the air is drawn into the lungs the nostrils contract. This is quite conspicuous among many cases of tuberculosis.

Some teachers of physical culture in their classes while encouraging deep breathing close their nostrils when drawing in a long breath. This is wrong because it produces a strain and imperfect sight. By consciously doing the wrong thing, breathing with a strain one becomes better able to practice the right way and obtain relaxation and better sight.

The habit of practicing frequently deep breathing one obtains a more permanent relaxation of the eyes with more constant good vision.

THE OPTIMUM SWING

THE optimum swing is the swing which gives the best results under different conditions.

Most readers of the magazine and the book know about the swing. The swing may be spontaneous, that is to say when one remembers a letter perfectly or sees a letter perfectly and continuously without any volition on the part of the patient he is able to imagine that it is a slow, short, easy swing. The speed is about as fast as one would count orally. The width of the swing is not more than the width of the letter, and it is remembered or imagined as easily as it is possible to imagine anything without any effort whatsoever. The normal swing of normal sight brings the greatest amount of relaxation and should be imagined when one is able to succeed when it becomes the optimum swing under favorable conditions. Nearsighted persons have this normal optimum swing usually at the near point when the vision is perfect. At the distance where the vision is imperfect the optimum swing is something else. It is not spontaneous but has to be produced by a conscious movement of the eyes and head from side to side and is usually wider than the width of the letter, faster than the normal swing and not so easily produced.

When one has a headache or a pain in the eyes or in any part of the body the optimum swing is always wider and more difficult to imagine than when one has less strain of the eyes. Under unfavorable conditions the long swing is the optimum swing, but under favorable conditions when the sight is good, the normal swing of the normal eye with normal sight is the optimum swing. The long swing brings a measure of relief when done right and makes it possible to shorten it down to the normal swing of the normal eye.

THE MEMORY SWING

THE memory swing relieves strain and tension as well as does the long or the short swing which has been described at various times. It is done with the eyes closed while one imagines looking over first the right shoulder then over the left shoulder when the eyeballs may be seen through the closed eyelids to move from side to side. When done properly it is just as efficient as the swing which is practiced with the eyes open whether short or long. The memory swing can be shortened by remembering the swing of a small letter, a quarter of an inch or less when the eyes are closed. The memory swing has given relief in many cases of imperfect sight from myopia, astigmatism and inflammations of the outside of the eyeball as well as inflammations of the inside of the eyeball. One advantage is the fact that it can be done without attracting the attention or making one more or less conspicuous to others. It is much easier than the swing practiced with the eyes open and secures a greater amount of relaxation or rest than any other swing. It may be done wrong just as any swing may be done wrong. When done right one does not imagine things are moving necessarily. All that is important is to move the eyes from side to side as far as possible or as far as one can move them when the eyes are open.

> Clarification for the Memory Swing; Do not force, or hold the eyes to the left, right. Imagining looking left and right is done *gently*. The eyes move easy, relaxed left and right under the closed eyelids as you imagine looking over the left and right shoulders. Allow the head to move with the eyes. Imagining seeing the swing of opposite movement (as is taught in this book) when looking left, right is optional.

WATCH YOUR STEP

WHEN you know what is the matter with you it is possible for you to correct it and bring about a cure. If you do not know what is wrong with you the cure of your imperfect sight is delayed. Some persons have been cured quickly when they were able to demonstrate that to see imperfectly required a tremendous effort, an effort which was very difficult. Some persons are cured in one visit and they readily demonstrate that imperfect sight or failure to see is difficult. Others require weeks and months to demonstrate the facts. Perfect sight is quick, comes easy and without any effort whatever. Imperfect sight is slow, difficult. One cannot consciously make the sight worse as readily as it can be done unconsciously. There is no danger in demonstrating the facts.

Look at a small letter on the Snellen test card which can be seen clearly at ten or twenty feet, a letter O for example. When the letter is seen quite perfectly it is usually seen without any apparent effort. However, by looking intently, staring at it and making an effort to improve it the letter blurs. It can always be demonstrated that the effort to see very soon blurs the letter. Now close the eyes and rest them for a part of a minute or longer and then glance at the letter again. It will usually be as clear as it was before. Again by straining, making an effort, the letter becomes blurred. One can readily demonstrate that to make the sight worse requires an effort, a strain.

Many obstinate cases have obtained a permanent cure only after learning how to make the sight worse consciously. In my book are published Seven Truths of Normal Sight. Prove the facts by demonstrating that the sight becomes imperfect when one or all of them is made imperfect by a strain.

Teach Others

MANY teachers have told me that when they taught Arithmetic the one who learned the most was always the teacher. Some ministers have made the remark that the one who profited mostly by the sermon was the man who delivered it.

For many years my patients who have been benefited by treatment without glasses have to a greater or less extent enjoyed the pleasure of helping others. When you think that you understand how to practice the swing with benefit try to teach somebody else how to do it. If you find palming is beneficial find how many of your friends who are also benefited by palming. But when you meet someone who is not benefited by what you tell them to do, you have at this time an opportunity of helping not only your friend but your own eyes as well. It seems a simple matter for you to close your eyes, rest them for a half hour or so and find that your sight is improved by the rest. However, there are some people who are not benefited appreciably by closing their eyes and resting them. One cause of failure is the memory of imperfect sight. Many patients failed to improve because with their eyes closed they think too much of their failure to see. Patients who have improved materially usually can demonstrate that the memory of perfect sight is restful, while the memory of imperfect sight is a strain. If you have a near-sighted friend who can read ordinary print without difficulty at the near point and without glasses, you can spend an hour or two of activity in showing your friend how to demonstrate while regarding fine print that it is impossible to try to concentrate on a point without sooner or later making the sight worse, that it is impossible to remember, imagine or see stationary letters, that it is impossible to maintain normal vision with the eyes kept continuously open without blinking.

Try Dancing

THERE has been repeatedly published in this magazine and in my book that the imagination of stationary objects to be moving is a rest and relaxation and a benefit to the sight. Young children, when one or both eyes turn in or out, are benefitted by having them swing from side to side with a regular rhythmical motion. This motion prevents the stare and the strain and improves the appearance of the eyes. It helps the sight of most children to play puss-in-the-corner or to play hide-and-seek. Children become very much excited and laugh and carry on and have a good time and it certainly is a benefit to their sight. It seems to me that these children would be benefited by going to dancing school. Many of my patients practice the long swing in the office and give strangers the impression that they are practicing steps of a dance. One patient with imperfect sight from detachment of the retina recently told me over the telephone that he went to a dance the night before and although he lost considerable sleep his sight was very much improved on the following morning.

Dancing is certainly a great help to keep things moving or to imagine stationary objects are moving, and is always recommended. Some people have told me that the *memory* of the music, the constant rhythmic motion and the relaxation have improved the vision.

The Short Swing

MANY people with normal sight can demonstrate the short swing readily. They can demonstrate that with normal vision each small letter regarded moves from side to side about a quarter of an inch or less. By an effort they can stop this short swing, and when they are able to demonstrate that, the vision becomes imperfect almost immediately. Practicing the long swing brings a measure of relaxation and makes it possible for those with imperfect sight to see things moving with a shorter swing. It is a good thing to have the help of someone who can practice the short swing successfully. Ask some friend who has perfect sight without glasses, in each eye to practice the variable swing as just described, which is a help to those with imperfect sight who have difficulty in demonstrating the short swing.

Nearsighted patients usually can demonstrate that when the vision is perfect, the diamond type at the reading distance, one letter regarded is seen continuously with a slow, short, easy swing not wider than the diameter of the letter. By staring the swing stops and the vision becomes imperfect. It is more difficult for a nearsighted person to stop the swing of the fine print, letter O, than it is to let it swing. When the sight is very imperfect, it is impossible to obtain the short swing. Many people have difficulty in maintaining mental pictures of any letter or any object. They cannot demonstrate the short swing with their eyes closed until they become able to imagine mental pictures.

The Snellen Test Card

THE Snellen Test Card is used for testing the eyesight. It is usually placed about 20 feet away from the patient. He covers each eye alternately, and reads the card as well as he can. Each line of letters is numbered with a figure which indicates the distance that it should be read with the normal eye. When the vision is recorded it is written in the form of a fraction. The numerator being the distance of the patient from the card, and the denominator denoting the line read. For example:—If a patient at 10 feet can only read the line marked 100 the vision is written 10/100 or 1/10. If the patient at 20 feet can read the line marked 10 the vision is recorded as 20/10 which means that the sight is double that of the average eye. Reading the Snellen Test Card daily helps the sight. Children in a public school with normal eyes under 12 years of age, who have never worn glasses were improved immediately by practicing with the Snellen Test Card. Children with imperfect sight also improved, and with the help of someone with perfect sight in time the vision becomes normal without glasses. School children oftentimes are very much interested in their eyesight and what can be accomplished with the help of the Snellen Test Card. They have contests among themselves to see who can read the card best in a bright light, or on a rainy day when the light is dim. Many of them find out for themselves that straining, makes the sight worse, while palming and swinging improve their vision. Many of them become able to use the Snellen Test Card in such a way as to relieve or prevent nervousness and headaches. Many boards of education hesitate to be responsible for any benefit that may be derived from the Snellen cards in the schools.

Aids to Swinging

IT IS possible for most people to do a very simple thing—to move the finger nail of the thumb from side to side against the finger nail of one finger. This may be done when the patient is in bed or when up and walking around, in the house, in the street or in the presence of other people, and all without attracting attention. With the aid of the movement of the thumb nail which can be felt and its speed regulated one can at the same time regulate the speed of the short swing. The length of the swing can also be regulated because it can be demonstrated that when the body moves a quarter of an inch from side to side that one can move the thumb from side to side. If the long swing is too rapid it can be slowed down with the aid of the thumb nail; when it is too long it can be shortened. At times the short swing may become irregular and then it can be controlled by the movement of the thumb nail. It is very interesting to demonstrate how the short swing is always similar to the movements of the fingernail. One great advantage connected with the short swing is that after a period of time of longer or shorter duration, the swing may stop or it may lengthen. It has been found that the movement of the thumb maintains the short swing of the body, the short swing of the letters or the short swing of any objects which may be seen, remembered or imagined. A letter O with a white center can only be remembered continuously with the eyes closed when it has a slow, short, continuous, regular swing and all without any effort or strain. The imagination may fail at times but the movement of the thumb can be maintained for an indefinite period after a little practice. One can more readily control the movement of the thumb instead of the eye.

Multiple Vision

PERSONS with imperfect sight when they regard one letter of the Snellen Test Card or one letter of fine print instead of seeing just one letter they may see two, three, six or more letters. Sometimes these letters are arranged side by side, sometimes in a vertical line one above the other and in other cases they may be arranged oblique by any angle. Multiple vision can be produced at will by an effort. It can always be corrected by relaxation. One of the best methods is to close the eyes and cover them in such a way as to exclude the light. Do this for five minutes or a half hour or long enough to obtain normal sight. The double vision is then corrected. Practice of the long swing is a great help. When the long swing is done properly the multiple images are always lessened. Do not forget that you can do the long swing in the wrong way and increase the multiple images. One great advantage of the long swing is that it helps you to obtain a slow, short, continuous swing of normal sight. When the vision is normal the letters appear to move from side to side or in some other direction a distance of about a quarter of an inch. The speed is about equal to the time of the moving feet of soldiers on the march. The most important part of the short swing is that it should be maintained easily. Any effort or strain modifies or stops the short swing. Then the eyes begin to stare and the multiple images return. It is a great benefit to learn how to produce multiple images at will because this requires much effort or strain, and is decidedly more difficult than normal single vision which can only be obtained easily without effort.

The Book
Perfect Sight Without Glasses

A GREAT many people have testified that they were cured by the help that they obtained from the book. A large number I believe have failed to be cured with its help although most people have been able to get some benefit from it.

On the first page is described the Fundamental Principle. This should interest most people because if you can follow the directions recommended you will most certainly be cured of imperfect sight from various causes. If you have a serious injury to the eye which destroys some of its essential parts you will find it impossible to carry out the directions. At the bottom of the page is printed: "If you fail ask some one with perfect sight to help you."

It is an interesting fact that only people with perfect sight without glasses can demonstrate the Fundamental Principle. You will read that with your eyes closed you should rest them, which is not possible if you remember things imperfectly. The book recommends that you remember some color that you can remember perfectly because it has been demonstrated that the normal eye is always at rest when it has normal sight. A perfect memory means perfect rest. Should you have perfect rest you have perfect sight. Most people can demonstrate that they can remember some letter or other object or some color better with their eyes closed than with their eyes open. By practice some people become able to remember, imagine and see mental pictures as well with their eyes open as they can with their eyes closed. Then they are cured.

One Thing

BY CENTRAL FIXATION is meant the ability to see one letter or one object regarded in such a way that all other letters or objects are seen worse. Some people have been cured by practicing Central Fixation only, devoting little time to other methods of cure.

SWINGING

When the normal eye has normal sight the small letters of the Snellen Test Card are imagined to be moving from side to side, slow, continuously, not more than the width of the letter. Persons with imperfect sight have become able to imagine this illusion by alternately remembering or imagining the small letter moving from side to side continuously. With their eyes open they may be able to do it for a moment or flash it, at first occasionally, and later more continuously, until they are cured.

IMAGINATION is very efficient in improving the vision. Some persons have told me that when they know what a letter was they could imagine they saw it. By closing their eyes they usually became able to imagine a known letter better than with their eyes open. By alternately imagining a known letter with the eyes open and with the eyes closed, the imagination of the letter often improves to normal when the letter was regarded. The patient who is able to do this is also able to demonstrate that when the imagination is improved for one known letter the vision for unknown letters is also improved. By imagining the first letter of a line perfectly the patient can tell the second letter and other letters which are not known. The imagination cure is curative when other methods of treatment have failed.

Questions

ASKING questions is all too common with patients who have imperfect sight. There are important or necessary questions which the patient should know in order to bring about a cure. The cause of the imperfect sight should be emphasized. In all cases of imperfect sight a strain, an effort, a stare or concentration can be demonstrated. To see imperfectly requires a great deal of trouble. Even the imperfect memory or the memory or imagination of an imperfect letter is an effort. It is so great a strain that the memory or imagination fail if you keep it in mind for any length of time. Perfect sight can only be obtained without an effort, without a strain. It is impossible to remember or imagine things perfectly by an effort.

One may divide questions into (1)—Proper questions; (2)—Improper or useless questions.

It is a waste of time, an injury to the patient, for him to describe the infinite manifestations of imperfect sight. To know its history minutely and its variations require an effort on the part of the patient to describe these things. And this effort increases the imperfect sight. It is absolutely of no help whatever in formulating methods for its cure. Avoid asking questions about the symptoms of imperfect sight or anything connected with imperfect sight. Any question connected with perfect sight may be a good thing for the patient to know. One may ask questions as follows:

How long must one practice a perfect memory, a perfect imagination or study the latest manifestation of perfect sight?

The answer to this question is a benefit to the patient.

The Trinity

THERE are three things which the normal eye practices more or less continuously, which are necessary in order to maintain normal vision.

1—The long swing.
2—The short swing.
3—Blinking or palming.

The long swing has been described repeatedly and most people are able to practice it successfully, especially people whose sight is good. If you have very imperfect sight you may have difficulty in demonstrating the benefit of the long swing. Some patients are indeed difficult to manage. They may be able to practice the long swing when looking out of a window with its light background. By moving the whole body, head and eyes together, a long distance from side to side one becomes able to imagine a cord of the window shade moving in the opposite direction. This makes it possible to imagine the long swing when you turn your back to the window, and look at objects in the room which have a dark background. When the long swing is properly maintained the letters of the Snellen Test Card become darker as long as one does not look directly at the card. Looking above the card or below it is a help in maintaining the long swing of the card when the maximum vision is obtained by the long swing. Never look directly at the card or try to read the letters when practicing the long swing.

By gradually lessening the movement of the body from side to side, the swing of the card becomes shorter and one may soon become able to flash the large letters. The swing of the card can be reduced to an inch or less.

Mental Pictures

MANY patients with imperfect sight complain that when they close their eyes to remember a white card with black letters, they usually fail and remember instead a black card with white letters. The vision of these patients is very much improved when they become able to remember a white card white, with the black letters remembered perfectly black. Imperfect memory, imperfect imagination, imperfect sight are all caused by strain.

One patient could not remember a white pillow, but by first regarding the pillow and seeing one corner best and all the other corners worse and shifting from one corner to another he became able, when closing his eyes, to remember one corner in turn best, and obtained a good mental picture of the whole pillow. One cannot see a pillow perfectly without Central Fixation. To have Central Fixation requires relaxation or rest. One patient who could not remember a large letter C of the Snellen Test Card, with the eyes closed, was able to remember the colors of some flowers, and then he was able to remember a letter C. In order to remember a desired mental picture one should remember perfectly some other things. This is a relaxation which helps to remember the mental picture desired. It is well to keep in mind that one cannot remember one thing perfectly and something else imperfectly at the same time.

In my book is described the case of a woman with imperfect sight who could remember a yellow buttercup with the eyes closed, perfectly, but with her eyes open and regarding the Snellen Card with imperfect sight, she had no memory of the yellow buttercup.

Time to Practice

MANY busy people complain that they have not time to practice my methods. They say that wearing glasses is quicker and much easier. Persons with normal vision or perfect sight without glasses are practicing consciously or unconsciously all the time when they are awake. When one sees a letter or an object perfectly the eyes are at rest. Any effort to improve the sight always makes it worse. The only time the eyes are perfectly at rest is when the vision is perfect. Persons with imperfect sight have to strain in order to see imperfectly. Persons with headaches, pain and other symptoms of discomfort in the eyes or in other parts of the body are under a constant strain to see, which is usually unconscious.

When a patient says he has no time to practice he is mistaken. He has all the time there is to use his eyes in the right way or he can use them in the wrong way. He has just as much time to use his eyes properly as he has to use them improperly. He has the choice and when patients learn the facts, to complain that they have no time to practice is an error.

Some patients object to removing their glasses on the ground that their vision is not sufficiently good for them to attend to their work, and feel that they have to put off the treatment until they have a vacation. Some of my patients have very poor vision and yet find time to practice without their glasses. Some school teachers with 15 diopters of myopia with a vision of less than 10/200 have found time to practice without interfering with their work. In fact practicing without their glasses soon enabled them to do their work much better than before.

Distance of the Snellen Test Card

THE distance of the Snellen Test Card from the patient is a matter of considerable importance. Some patients improve more rapidly when the card is placed fifteen or twenty feet away while others fail to get any benefit with the card at this distance.

In some cases the best results are obtained when the card is as close as one foot. I recall a patient with very poor sight who made no progress whatever, when the card was placed at ten feet or further, but became able to improve the vision very materially with the card at about six inches. After the vision was improved at six inches the patient became able to improve the card at a greater distance until normal sight was obtained at twenty feet. Some cases with poor vision may not improve when the card is placed at ten feet or further, or at one foot or less but do much better when the card is placed at a middle distance, at about eight or ten feet. Other individuals may not improve their vision at all at ten feet, but are able to improve their sight at twenty feet or at one foot. I recall one patient with 20 diopters of myopia whose vision at ten feet was peculiar. The letters at twenty feet and at one foot were apparently all the same normal size, but at ten feet they appeared to be one-fifth of the normal size. Practicing with the card at twenty feet or at one foot helped him greatly, more than practicing with the card at about ten feet. While some patients are benefited by practicing with the card daily always at the same distance, there are others who seem to be benefited when the distance of the card from the patient is changed daily.

Blinking

THE normal eye when it has normal sight rests very frequently by closing the eyes for longer or shorter periods, and when practiced quickly it is called BLINKING. When the normal eye has normal sight and refrains from blinking for some seconds or part of a minute, the vision always becomes imperfect. You can demonstrate that normal vision at the near point or at the distance is impossible without frequent blinking. Most people blink so easily and for such a short period of time that things are seen continuously while the blinking is done unconsciously. In some cases one may blink five times or more in one second. The *frequency* of blinking depends on a number of factors.

The normal eye blinks more frequently or more continuously under adverse conditions as when the illumination is diminished, the distance is increased or the print read is too pale or otherwise imperfect. The distraction of conversation, noise, reflections of light, objects so arranged as to be difficult to see, all increase the frequency of blinking of the normal eye with normal sight. If the frequency of blinking is diminished under adverse conditions or from any cause the vision soon becomes imperfect.

The imperfect eye or the eye with imperfect sight blinks less frequently than the normal eye. Staring stops the blinking. The universal optical swing, the long or short swing when modified or stopped are always accompanied by less frequent blinking.

> Blink in the early morning,
> Blink when the sun sets at night;
> Blink when the sun is dawning,
> But be sure you do it right.

Curable Cases

PATIENTS wearing glasses for the relief of imperfect sight may expect better vision after they are cured than they ever had before with glasses. Adults who have good distant vision but require glasses after middle life, for reading, are also curable without glasses. Such patients, although they may read very well with glasses, complain that, as a rule, they must hold the page at one distance in order to read with the best vision. This reading distance is usually about twelve inches. Some cases require one pair of glasses for reading books or newspapers, but cannot see clearly at a greater distance without another pair of glasses. Musicians especially find that glasses that give them good vision for reading books are useless to them for reading music or for playing the piano. To see closer than twelve inches may require still another pair of glasses. To see more distant objects may require still another pair. Some of my patients have shown me numerous pairs of glasses, each one adapted for certain specific distances. It is a great relief to such cases to be cured, because then they are able, not only to see perfectly at the distance without glasses, but they can read the fine print as well at six inches as they can further off. The eye with normal sight is able to change its focus at will for all distances without any discomfort whatever.

Patients with cataract, glaucoma and other diseases of the eyes may not be able to see even with glasses. When they are cured by my methods they become able to see normally in all kinds of light, in a bright light or in a dim light. Pain, fatigue and other discomforts of the eyes are all relieved.

PERMANENT IMPROVEMENT

MANY patients find that while it is easy for them to obtain a temporary improvement in their sight by palming a sufficient length of time or by other methods, they do not seem to hold it permanently. In this connection it is well to remember that the normal eye with normal sight can only maintain normal sight permanently by consciously or unconsciously practicing the slow, short, easy swing. When the normal eye has imperfect sight it can always be demonstrated that the swing stops from an effort. When the normal eye has normal sight, the eyes are at rest and all the nerves of the body feel comfortable. When the swing stops, one always feels more or less uncomfortable. To have perfect sight can only be obtained easily, without effort. To have imperfect sight always requires a strain or an effort which stops the swing. Near-sighted patients who have normal vision for reading at the near point become able, when their attention is called to it, to demonstrate that they are more comfortable when reading the fine print than they are when they fail to see distant objects perfectly.

One of the great benefits of the drifting swing is the comfortable relaxed feeling it brings. The retinoscope always shows that the eye is not near-sighted when no effort is made. Persons with imperfect sight should imitate the eye with normal sight by practicing a perfect memory, a perfect imagination, a perfect swing, without effort, with perfect comfort all the time that they are awake. As I have said before many times, it is a good thing to know what is the matter with you because it makes it possible to correct it.

The Prevention of Myopia

THE August number of Better Eyesight is a school number devoted almost exclusively to the problem of the cure or prevention of nearsightedness in school children. The great value of the method as a preventive is emphasized by the fact that the vision of all school children has always improved, and when the vision is improved of course imperfect sight is prevented. It is well to remember that my method for the prevention of myopia in school children is the only one that is a success. It has been in continuous use for more than twenty years in the public schools of New York and other cities. Once daily or oftener the children read the card, first with one eye and then with the other, covering each eye alternately with the palm of the hand in such a way as to shut out all the light without any pressure on the eyeball. Teachers who have studied my book or have been patients find it an advantage to have the children palm five minutes three or four times a day. They claim that palming quiets the children and gives them an improved mental efficiency, which is a great help to their memory and imagination as well as their sight. I believe other children should be taught how to palm, swing, blink and improve their vision of the Snellen Test Card. The method is of great value to young children in the kindergarten, children in the high schools, and should be practiced by students and teachers in colleges and universities. In the military school and naval academy the method should be employed for the prevention of imperfect sight.

The Rabbit's Throat

DURING the past ten years a method of breathing has been practiced which has improved the vision of many patients after other methods had failed. It consists of depressing the lower jaw with the lips closed and lowering the tongue and muscles below the chin. At the same time one breathes in through the nose and throat in a manner somewhat similar to snoring and when done properly one can feel a coolness of the air while it passes down into the lungs. This method of breathing is accompanied with the eyelids being more widely open in a natural way without staring. The ear passages, nose, and throat dilate. The tube which goes from the throat to the middle ear becomes more widely open, with improved hearing in chronic deafness which does not respond to any other treatment. If one rests the chin with the thumb below it and the forefinger just below the lower lip, one can feel with the thumb the hardening of the muscles below the jaw accompanied with a decided swelling. By practice, the swelling and hardness increase. This suggested the title of the Rabbit's Throat because of a similar swelling below the rabbit's chin. The tension of the other muscles of the body becomes relaxed. There is a wonderful increase of muscular control.

Music teachers have told me that the singing voice becomes much better because of the relaxation of the muscles of the throat. The involuntary muscles of the digestive tract become relaxed in a striking manner with the relief of many symptoms of discomfort. Redness and inflammation of the mucous membranes of the eye, ear, nose and throat and the rest of the body are relieved in a few minutes with the aid of the Rabbit's Throat.

Eye-Strain During Sleep

Many people complain that when they first wake up in the morning, they are tired, that they have headaches, and that their sight is very imperfect. Later on in the day their eyes feel better, and the vision may become normal.

I have examined with the Ophthalmoscope the eyes of many people during sleep and found much to my surprise, that most people strain much more in their sleep than they ever do when they are awake. Of course, people when unconscious of their acts during sleep, are not aware of this eye-strain.

The prevention of eye-strain during sleep is usually a very difficult matter. Some cases are benefited just before retiring by palming for one-half hour or longer, or until they go to sleep while palming. Others by practicing the long swing for fifteen minutes, have found that the eye-strain becomes less. In some serious cases with imperfect sight, when the eye-strain is not prevented by palming or the swing, they are often materially benefited by shortening their hours of sleep with the help of an alarm clock. One patient had the alarm set for 3 a.m. He would then get out of bed and practice the long swing, alternating with palming for an hour or longer with the result that he slept the rest of the night very comfortably, and awoke the next morning with little or no evidence of eye-strain during sleep.

Some people have told me that they have lessened their eye-strain during sleep materially, by moderate muscular exercises for one-half hour or longer. They find that they obtain the best results when the exercise is continued sufficiently long to produce muscular fatigue.

Suggestions

1. *Imagine things are moving all the time.*

When riding in a railroad train, when one looks out of the car window, telegraph poles and other objects, although they are stationary, appear to be moving. To stop the movement is impossible, and the effort to do so may be very uncomfortable. The greater the effort, the greater the discomfort, and is the cause of heart sickness, headaches and nausea. It can be demonstrated that any movement of the head and eyes produces an apparent movement of stationary objects.

2. *Blink often.*

By blinking is meant, closing and opening both eyes rapidly. When done properly, things are seen continuously and they always move with a quick jump in various directions. Regarding stationary objects without blinking is an effort, a strain which always lowers the vision.

3. *Read the Snellen Test Card at fifteen feet as well as you can, every night and morning.*

School children and others are often cured of imperfect sight by reading a familiar card, first with both eyes and then with each eye separately. It is the only method practiced which prevents Myopia in school children.

4. *Fine Print.*

Read fine print at six inches when possible every night and morning. If not possible, do the best you can. Just regarding the white spaces between the lines of fine print without reading the letters is a benefit.

5. *Palming.*

Palm for five minutes, ten times daily when convenient.

PERFECT SIGHT

If you learn the fundamental principles of perfect sight and will consciously keep them in mind your defective vision will disappear. The following discoveries were made by Dr. Bates and his method is based on them. With it he has cured so-called incurable cases:

1. Many blind people are curable.
2. All errors of refraction are functional, therefore curable.
3. All defective vision is due to strain in some form.
4. Strain is relieved by relaxation.

You can demonstrate to your own satisfaction that strain lowers the vision. When you stare, you strain. Look fixedly at one object for five seconds or longer. What happens? The object blurs and finally disappears. Also, your eyes are made uncomfortable by this experiment. When you rest your eyes for a few moments the vision is improved and the discomfort relieved.

Have some one with perfect sight demonstrate the fundamental principles contained in Dr. Bates' book, "Perfect Sight Without Glasses." If the suggestions and instructions are carried out, and glasses discarded, it is possible to improve the vision without personally consulting a physician.

"Perfect Sight Without Glasses" will be sent C. O. D. on five days' approval. Price, $5.00.

Central Fixation Publishing Company
383 Madison Avenue, New York City

Sun-Gazing
By W. H. Bates, M.D.

It is a well-known fact that the constant protection of the eyes from the sunlight, or from other kinds of light, is followed by weakness or inflammation of the eyes or eyelids. Children living in dark rooms, where the sun seldom enters, acquire an intolerance for the light. Some of them keep their eyes covered with their hands, or bury their faces in a pillow and do all they possibly can to avoid exposure of their eyes to ordinary light. I have seen many hundreds of cases of young children brought to the clinic with ulceration of the cornea, which may become sufficient to cause blindness. Putting these children in a dark room is a blunder. My best results in the cure of these cases were obtained by encouraging the patients to spend a good deal of the time out of doors, with their faces exposed to the direct rays of the sun. In a short time these children became able to play and enjoy themselves a great deal more out of doors, exposed to the sunlight, than when they protected their eyes from the light. Not only is the sun beneficial to children with inflammation of the cornea, but it is also beneficial to adults.

When the patient looks down sufficiently, the white part of the eye can be exposed by gently lifting the upper lid, while the sun's rays strike directly upon this part of the eyeball. In most cases it is possible to focus the strong light of the sun on the white part of the eyeball with the aid of a strong convex glass, being careful to move the light from side to side quite rapidly to avoid the heat. After such a treatment, the patient almost immediately becomes able to open his eyes widely in the light.

The Baby Swing

YOUNG babies suffer very much from eyestrain. The tension of the eye muscles is always associated with the tension of all the other muscles of the body. Their restlessness can be explained by this tension. I was talking with an Italian mother in the clinic one day about restless children, and asked her why it was that her baby was always so quiet and comfortable when she came to the clinic, while many other babies at the same time were very restless and unhappy.

"Oh," she said, "I love my baby. I like to hold her in my arms and rock her until she smiles."

"Yes, I know," I said, "but that mother over there is rocking her baby in her arms, and the child is screaming its head off."

"Yes," exclaimed the Italian mother, "but see how she rocks it."

Then I noticed that the other mother threw the child from side to side in a horizontal direction with a rapid, jerky, irregular motion, and the more she jerked the child from side to side, the more restless did it become.

"Now, doctor," said the Italian mother, "you watch me."

I did watch her. Instead of throwing the child rapidly, irregularly, intermittently from side to side, she handled her baby as though it had much value in her eyes, and moved her not in straight lines from side to side, but continuously in slow, short, easy curves. The Italian mother picked up the other mother's child, and soon quieted it by the same swing.

I learned something that day.

Floating Specks

WHEN a patient stares or strains to see by looking at a light-colored surface he may see, or imagine he sees, floating black specks, strings of black thread or small light-colored globules resembling tears. The floating specks may be apparently a quarter of an inch or more in size and they may be of any shape.

The ability to see or imagine floating specks may occur in children or in adults of any age. Some children have been known to lie on their backs on the ground, look up at light colored clouds and amuse themselves for hours by watching what appeared to be floating specks.

Many nervous people have been made very unhappy, consciously or unconsciously imagining that they see these floating specks.

The cause of floating specks is an imperfect memory of perfect sight. Persons with normal vision who have never been conscious of floating specks can be taught how to imagine them by straining—to imagine letters, colors or other objects imperfectly.

Conversely, patients who are conscious of floating specks are unable to imagine them and perfect sight at the same time.

In the treatment of floating specks it is important to convince the patients thoroughly that they are only imagined and not seen. It helps very much to impress on the patient's mind that to see these floating specks requires a sufficient strain to lose a perfect imagination of all objects seen, remembered or imagined at all times and in all places.

Note.— Floating specks, October, 1919, "Better Eyesight."

Muscae volitantes (floating specks), pages 176 and 236, "Perfect Sight Without Glasses."

The Elliptical Swing

THE normal eye when it has normal sight is always able to imagine stationary objects to be moving from side to side about one quarter of an inch, slowly and without effort. This is called the swing. In order that the swing may be continuous, the movement of the head and eyes should be in the orbit of an ellipse, or in an elongated circular direction.

A patient, aged seventy-seven, with beginning cataract in both eyes had a vision of 3/200 when she looked to one side of the card. When she looked directly at the card or the letters, she complained that she could not see them so well, or at all. She was recommended to practice swaying the body from side to side. Every time she moved to the right or to the left, she stopped at the end of the movement and stared, and that prevented relaxation. With the help of the Elliptical Swing, she obtained at once very marked benefit. Her vision was improved almost immediately when she looked directly at the letters, and her vision became worse when she looked to one side of the card.

A young man, aged sixteen, was treated for progressive myopia for a year or longer. His vision improved for a time, then improvement stopped. Some months later his vision had not become permanently improved. Palming and swinging no longer helped him. I noticed that when he would move his head from side to side, he stopped at the end of the swing and stared. When he practiced the Elliptical Swing, his head and eyes moved continuously, and the staring was prevented. At once there was a decided improvement in his vision, and this improvement continued without any relapse.

Fundamentals

1. Glasses discarded permanently.
2. Favorable conditions: Light may be bright or dim. The distance of the print from the eyes, where seen best, also varies with people.
3. Central Fixation is seeing best where you are looking.
4. Shifting: With normal sight the eyes are moving all the time. This should be practiced continuously and consciously.
5. Swinging: When the eyes move slowly or rapidly from side to side, stationary objects appear to move in the opposite direction.
6. Long Swing: Stand with the feet about one foot apart, turn the body to the right—at the same time lifting the heel of the left foot. Do not move the head or eyes or pay any attention to the apparent movement of stationary objects. Now place the left heel on the floor, turn the body to the left, raising the heel of the right foot. Alternate. This exercise can be practiced just before retiring at night fifty times or more. When done properly, it is a great rest and relieves pain, fatigue, and other symptoms of imperfect sight.
7. Stationary Objects Moving: By moving the head and eyes a short distance from side to side, one can imagine stationary objects to be moving. Since the normal eye is moving all the time, one should imagine all stationary objects to be moving. Never imagine that you see a stationary object stationary.
8. Palming: The closed eyes may be covered with the palm of one or both hands. The patient should rest the eyes and think of something else that is pleasant.
9. Blinking: The normal eye blinks, or closes and opens very frequently. If one does not blink, the vision always becomes worse.

Clarify for #6 - The head and eyes DO MOVE; <u>with the body.</u>

Alternate

IT has always been demonstrated that the continuous memory, imagination, or vision of one thing for any length of time is impossible. To see one letter of the Snellen test card continuously, it is necessary to shift from one part of the letter to another. By alternately moving the eyes from one side of the letter to the other, it is possible to imagine the letter to be moving in the opposite direction to the movement of the eyes. This movement of the letter is called a swing. When it is slow, easy, short, about one-quarter of an inch or less, maximum vision is obtained which continues as long as the swing continues.

As long as we are awake, we are thinking, remembering, or imagining mental pictures, and are comfortable. To go around blind requires a distinct effort which is a strain on all the nerves and is always uncomfortable. The normal mind alternates its attention from one mental picture to another, which is a relaxation or rest. The memory, or imagination, is best when one thing is imagined better than all other things, Central Fixation, but constant shifting is necessary to maintain Central Fixation.

One of the best methods to improve the vision is to regard a letter of the Snellen test card with the eyes open, then close the eyes and remember or imagine the letter better for about ten seconds, open the eyes and regard the letter while testing the imagination of the letter for a moment. By alternately regarding the letter with the eyes open and closed, the imagination of the letter improves in flashes. By continuing to alternate the flashes improve and last longer until the vision becomes continuously improved.

Fear

NEAR-SIGHTED people have frequently been told that it is necessary for them to wear glasses constantly, to prevent their eyes from becoming worse. They are afraid that this statement may be true, and one cannot blame them for hesitating to leave their glasses off permanently.

One of my patients stated that she suffered very much from headaches. They were so severe that they made her ill, and confined her to her bed at least once a week. While wearing her glasses, she still was in pain, but was afraid, if she left them off, the headaches would become worse. By discarding her glasses, practicing palming, swinging, and the memory of perfect sight, her eyes and head improved immediately. When she resumed her glasses again, she at once became uncomfortable, and the pain returned. She decided to leave them off permanently, and her headaches disappeared.

Some years ago an optician consulted me about his headaches. When I examined his glasses, I found that they were plane window glass. He said that when he wore them his headaches were better, but his wife confided to me that this was not true. He was troubled more when he wore them. He was suffering from fear.

I saw him again a year later and learned that he had permanently discarded his glasses, at my suggestion, during all that time, and was free of headaches.

It has been a habit with me, when patients who suffer from fear of the consequences that might happen if they did not wear their glasses, to have them demonstrate the facts. When the truth is known, fear is abolished. It is very easy in most cases to teach patients some of the causes of headaches.

Swaying

IT is a great help in the improving of vision to have the patient demonstrate that staring at one part of a letter at ten feet or further is a difficult thing to do for any length of time without lowering the vision and producing pain, discomfort, or fatigue. With the eyes closed it is impossible to concentrate on the memory or the imagination of a small part of one letter continuously without a temporary or more complete loss of the memory or the imagination.

When an effort is made to think of one part of a letter continuously with the eyes closed, the letter is imagined to be stationary. When the imagination shifts to the right of the letter a short distance and then to the left alternately, every time the attention is directed to the right, the letter is always to the left, and when the attention is directed to the left of the letter, the letter is always to the right. By alternating, the patient becomes able to imagine the letter is moving from side to side, and as long as the movement is maintained the patient is able to remember or imagine the letter. It can be demonstrated that to remember a letter or other object to be stationary always interferes with the perfect memory of the letter. One cannot remember, imagine, or see an object continuously unless it is moving. The movement must be slow, short, and easy.

When patients stare habitually, the eyes become more or less fixed, and are moved with great difficulty. When the patient stands and sways the whole body from side to side, it becomes easier to move the eyes in the same direction as the body moves. No matter how long the staring has been practiced, the sway at once lessens it.

Bates Method Popular with Teachers

THROUGHOUT the past year a group of teachers in one of the city high schools has been much interested in studying the Bates method. One afternoon each week, from three to four, we have a "Bates Class." The number attending has varied, sometimes being as many as fourteen. I feel that the total result has been eminently satisfactory. A great deal of enthusiasm has been aroused and many people helped.

Different individuals have, of course, presented different problems. One woman was beginning to feel that her near vision was blurring. She had never worn glasses. It seemed a very short time—perhaps not more than a month—before her eyes improved so that she could read diamond type. At present she is able to see the microscopic print in the little Bible. A man who had worn glasses many years discarded them last December, and says now he has "forgotten how they feel." Another teacher who took off her glasses two years ago, comes to the class once in a while for a little practice with us when her eyes feel tired.

A certain teacher with three diopters of hyperopia and presbyopia has made great strides. She has a vivid imagination and never-flagging enthusiasm. We both feel that her eyes will be normal some day in the near future.

The teachers who come to the class often look very weary. They always say they feel more rested at the end of the lesson.

Our procedure is the usual one of palming, swinging, sunning and working with the Snellen test card and fine print.

Some of the teachers who understand the method come to help teach the others. A student in the school whom I have trained always assists at the classes, and that makes the handling of the large group much easier.

I am intending to have a similar class next year, and I am sure we are going to accomplish even more.

Optimism

OPTIMISM is a great help in obtaining a cure of imperfect sight. About ten years ago a patient was treated for cataract, complicated with glaucoma. After two weeks of daily treatment the vision improved very much and the patient became able to travel about the streets without a companion to guide her. Her vision at this time had improved from perception of light to 10/200. After palming, swinging, and the memory of perfect sight, her vision was still further improved. She was very much encouraged and returned home full of enthusiasm to carry out the treatment to the very best of her ability.

Soon afterwards things did not go well at home. The patient became very much depressed and stopped her daily practice. Her daughter was very enthusiastic, and realized that her mother had been very materially improved and that further treatment would bring about a complete cure. She talked to her mother for half an hour or more and encouraged her to continue with her practice. The patient responded favorably, got busy, and was able to bring back much of the sight which had been lost. She made further improvement every day.

At times the mother was very pessimistic. She was continually complaining that she knew very well that she would never get her sight back. Then the daughter would start in with her optimism.

One bright, sunshiny morning the mother got up, took a card with diamond type printed on one side, and was greatly surprised to read it without any trouble. In three months her distant vision was normal.

Moving

THE world moves. Let it move. People are moving all day long. It is normal, right, proper that they should move. Just try to keep your head, or one finger, one toe, stationary, or keep your eyes open continuously. If you try to stare at a small letter or a part of it without blinking, note what happens. Most people who have tried it discover that the mind wanders, the vision becomes less, pain and fatigue are produced.

Stand facing a window and note the relative position of a curtain cord to the background. Take a long step to the right. Observe that the background has become different. Now take a long step to the left. The background has changed again. Avoid regarding the curtain cord. While moving from side to side it is possible to imagine the cord moving in the opposite direction. By practice one becomes able to imagine stationary objects not seen to be moving as continuously, as easily, as objects in the field of vision.

Universal Swing: When one becomes able to imagine all objects seen, remembered, or imagined, to be moving with a slow, short, easy swing, this is called the Universal Swing. It is a very desirable thing to have, because when it is imagined with the eyes closed or open, one cannot simultaneously imagine pain, fatigue, or imperfect sight.

The Universal Swing can be obtained without one being conspicuous. With the hand covered, move the thumb from side to side about one-quarter of an inch, and move the eyes with the thumb. Stationary objects can be imagined to be moving.

When walking rapidly forward, the floor or the sidewalk appears to move backward. It is well to be conscious of this imagined movement.

Never imagine stationary objects to be stationary. To do this, is a strain, a strain which lowers the vision.

Read Fine Print

MANY near-sighted patients can read fine print or diamond type at less than ten inches from their eyes easily, perfectly and quickly, by alternately regarding the Snellen test card at different distances, from three feet up to fifteen feet or further. The vision may be improved, at first temporarily, and later, by repetition, a permanent gain usually follows.

It is a valuable fact to know, that when fine print is read perfectly, the near-sightedness or myopia disappears during this period. It can only be maintained at first for a fraction of a second, and later more continuously.

Near-sighted patients and others, with the help of the fine print can usually demonstrate that staring at a small letter always lowers the vision, and that the same fact is true when regarding distant letters or objects.

With the help of the fine print, the near-sighted patient can also demonstrate that one can remember perfectly only what has been seen perfectly; that one imagines perfectly only what is remembered perfectly, and that perfect sight is only a perfect imagination.

A great many people are very suspicious of the imagination, and feel or believe that things imagined are never true. The more ignorant the patient, the less respect do they have for their imagination, or the imagination of other people. It comes to them as a great shock, with a feeling of discomfort, to discover that the perfect imagination of a known letter improves the sight for unknown letters of the Snellen test card, or for other objects.

It is a fact, that one can read fine print perfectly, with perfect relaxation, with great relief to eyestrain, pain fatigue and discomfort, not only of the eyes, but of all other nerves of the body.

Dizziness

DIZZINESS is caused by eyestrain. Some people when standing on the roof of a house looking down, strain their eyes and become dizzy. Usually the dizziness is produced unconsciously. It can be produced consciously, however, by staring or straining to see some distant or near object.

Some persons when riding in an elevator are always dizzy and may suffer from attacks of imperfect sight with headache, nausea, and other nervous discomforts. An old lady, aged sixty, told me that riding in an elevator always made her dizzy, and produced headaches with pain in her eyes and head. I tested her vision and found it to be normal both for distance and for reading without glasses. To obtain some facts, I rode in an elevator with her from the top to the bottom of the building and back again. I watched her eyes closely and found that she was staring at the floors which appeared to be moving opposite to the movement of the elevator. I asked her the question: "Why do you stare at the floors which appear to be moving by?"

She answered: "I do not like to see them move, and I am trying to correct the illusion by making an effort to keep them stationary. The harder I try, the worse I feel."

I suggested to her that she look at one part of the elevator and avoid looking at the floors. Her discomfort was at once relieved, and she was soon cured.

In all cases of dizziness, the stare or strain is always evident. When the stare or strain is relieved or prevented, dizziness does not occur.

With advancing years attacks of dizziness and blindness occur more frequently than in younger individuals. All attacks of dizziness with blindness are quite readily cured by practicing the imagination of the swing, the memory of perfect sight, or by palming.

The Period

THE perfect memory or imagination of a period is a cure for imperfect sight. Only the color needs to be remembered. The size is immaterial, but a small period is remembered with more relaxation than a large one. It it true, however, that with perfect sight, one has the ability to remember all things perfectly.

One cannot remember a period perfectly by any kind of an effort. It usually happens that one may remember a period for a time, and then lose it by an effort. To remember a period stationary, is impossible. One has to shift more or less frequently in order to remember one period perfectly all the time, or one has to imagine the period to be moving, or one has to remember the period by central fixation,—one part best. By shifting, is meant to look away from the period and then back, but to do it so quickly that it is possible to remember the period continuously, although you are not looking at it all the time,— this with the eyes closed. Every time you blink, you shift your eyes. You can blink so rapidly that it is not noticeable. When you close your eyes and remember a period, you cannot remember it unless you are, with your eyes closed, going through the process as though you were blinking, looking away from it and back again, but so quickly that it seems as though you were looking at the period continuously. You cannot remember the whole of the period at once. No matter how small the period is, you cannot see or remember it perfectly, all parts equally well at the same time. You cannot remember the period perfectly by any kind of an effort. When the memory of the period is perfect, the mental and physical efficiency is increased. A perfect memory of the period does not necessarily mean that one should think only of the period.

Demonstrate

1. That an effort to see always lowers the vision. Look at the Snellen test card at a distance of twenty feet. It may be possible for you to see the large letters and read them without any apparent effort, while the smaller letters produce a strain which you can feel. If you consciously increase the effort to see the smaller letters, your vision becomes more imperfect. It is not easy for you to realize that effort is always present when the vision is lowered. Knowing the cause of your imperfect sight is a great help in selecting the remedy.

2. That a stare always lowers the vision. It is a truth that the normal eye blinks very frequently. In order to have normal sight, the eyes must blink. One can demonstrate that, when the patient looks at one letter at the distance with normal sight, or looks at one letter at a near point where it is seen clearly, keeping the eyes continuously open without blinking for a minute or longer, always lowers the vision for the distance or for the near point. This should convince the patient that blinking is absolutely necessary in order to obtain good vision.

3. That palming, when done correctly, improves the vision. When the closed eyes are covered with one or both hands, and all light is excluded, the patient should see nothing at all, or a perfect black. This is a rest to the eyes and always improves the sight at least temporarily. Palming can be done wrong. When it is practiced incorrectly, the field imagined by the patient contains streaks of red, white, blue, or other colors. The eyes are under a strain, and the vision is not materially improved by the wrong method of palming. It can be demonstrated that palming for half an hour or longer is a greater benefit than palming for only a few minutes.

Demonstrate

THAT central fixation improves the vision. The normal eye is always at rest and always has central fixation. Central fixation cannot be obtained through any effort. When an effort is made by the normal eye, central fixation is always lost. In central fixation, one sees best the point regarded while all other points are seen less clearly.

Look at the upper left hand corner of the back of a chair. Note that all other parts of the chair are not seen so well. Look at the top of a letter at a distance at which it can be seen clearly. Then quickly look at the bottom of the letter. Alternate. When the eyes go up, the letter appears to move down. Then the eyes move down, the letter appears to move up. Coincident with this movement, you can observe that you see best the point regarded and all other points less clearly or less distinctly. When you can imagine the letter to be moving, it is possible for you to see best where you are looking.

The size of the letter or object seen, does not matter. Central fixation can be demonstrated with the smallest letters which are printed, or the smallest objects. Close the eyes and remember or imagine how the small letter would look if you imagined one part best. By shifting from one part of the letter to another, central fixation with the eyes closed may be made continuous for one-half minute or longer. Then with the eyes open, it is possible for one second or less to see, remember, or imagine the same small letter or other objects in the same way,—one part best.

Note that when the letters are read easily and clearly, they are always seen by central fixation, and relaxation is felt. Central fixation is a rest to the nerves and when practiced continuously, it relieves strain and improves the vision to normal.

Demonstrate

THAT the optical swing always improves the vision.

Stand before an open window with the feet about one foot apart. Sway the whole body, including the head and eyes, from side to side. When the body moves to the right, the head and eyes also move to the right, while, at the same time, the window and other stationary objects are to the left of where you are looking. When the body sways to the left, the window and other stationary objects are to the right. Be sure that the head and eyes are moving from side to side with the whole body, slowly, without an effort to see. When the swaying is done rapidly, it is possible to imagine stationary objects are moving rapidly in the opposite direction. While the swinging is being practiced, notice that the window and other stationary objects which are nearer, appear to move in the opposite direction to the movement of the body, head and eyes. Objects beyond the window may appear to move in the same direction as the body, head, and eyes move.

Note that when the body is swaying rapidly, the window and other objects are not seen very clearly; but when the swaying is slowed down and shortened, so that parts of the window move one-quarter of an inch or less, the vision is improved for those parts of the window regarded. More distant objects, which move in the same direction as the movement of the body, head, and eyes, are also improved with the slow, short, easy swing.

After you have become able to imagine the window to be moving, practice on other objects. All day long, the head and eyes are moving. Notice that stationary objects are moving in the opposite direction to the movement of the head and eyes. To see stationary objects apparently stationary, is a strain which lowers the vision and may cause pain, fatigue, and other discomforts.

Demonstrate

THAT the long swing not only improves the vision, but also relieves or cures pain, discomfort and fatigue.

Stand with the feet about one foot apart, facing squarely one side of the room. Lift the left heel a short distance from the floor while turning the shoulders, head, and eyes to the right, until the line of the shoulders is parallel with the wall. Now turn the body to the left after placing the left heel upon the floor and raising the right heel. Alternate looking from the right wall to the left wall, being careful to move the head and eyes with the movement of the shouders. When practiced easily, continuously, without effort and without paying any attention to moving objects, one soon becomes conscious that the long swing relaxes the tension of the muscles and nerves.

Stationary objects move with varying degrees of rapidity. Objects located almost directly in front of you appear to move with express train speed and should be very much blurred. It is very important to make no attempt to see clearly objects which seem to be moving very rapidly.

The long swing seems to help patients who suffer from eyestrain during sleep. By practicing the long swing fifty times or more just before retiring and just after rising in the morning, eyestrain during sleep has been prevented or relieved. It is remarkable how quickly the long swing relieves or prevents pain. I know of no other procedure which can compare with it. The long swing has relieved the pain of facial neuralgia after operative measures had failed. Some patients who have suffered from continuous pain in various parts of the body have been relieved by the long swing, at first temporarily, but by repetition the relief has become more permanent. Hay fever, asthma, sea-sickness, palpitation of the heart, coughs, acute and chronic colds are all promptly cured by the long swing.

Demonstrate

1. Demonstrate that when the eyes are stationary, they are under a tremendous strain. Stand before the Snellen test card at a distance of fifteen or twenty feet. Look directly at one small area of a large letter, which can be seen clearly. Stare at that part of the letter without closing the eyes and without shifting the eyes to some other point. The vision becomes worse and the letter blurs. Stare continuously, and note that the longer you stare, the more difficult it is to keep the eyes focused on that one point or part of the letter. Not only does the stare become more difficult, but the eyes become tired; and by making a greater effort, the eyes pain, or a headache is produced. The stare can cause fatigue of the whole body when the effort is sufficiently strong and prolonged.

2. Demonstrate that when the eyes are moving from one point to another, frequently, easily and continuously, the stare, the strain, or the effort to see is prevented and the eyes feel rested. In fact, the eyes are not at rest except when they are moving. Note that when you look at a letter on the Snellen test card and alternately shift from the top to the bottom of it, the vision remains good or is improved. When the letter is seen perfectly, the eyes are shifting; and when seen imperfectly, the shifting stops.

3. Close your eyes and remember your signature. This can usually be done quite perfectly. Try to remember the first and the last letter of your name simultaneously. This is an impossible thing to do and requires a strain. If you shift from one letter to another, you can remember your signature, one letter at a time; but if you make an effort to remember it, the memory and the imagination of your signature disappears.

Demonstrate

I. That the smaller the object regarded, the easier it is to remember. One can, with time and trouble, become able to remember all the words of one page of a book. It is easier to remember one word than all the words of a page. It is still easier to remember one letter of a word better than all the letters. Regard a capital letter. Demonstrate that it is easier to see or remember the top of the letter best, and the bottom of it less clearly than to remember the top and bottom perfectly and simultaneously. Now look directly at the upper right hand corner and imagine one-fourth of the letter best. Then cover the remaining three-quarters of the letter with a piece of paper. It is possible to look directly at the exposed part of the letter and imagine half of it best. Cover the part that is not seen distinctly, and demonstrate that half of the exposed part of the letter can be seen or imagined best, while the rest of it is not seen so clearly. With the aid of the screen, an area as small as an ordinary period, may finally be imagined. Demonstrate that the imagination of a perfectly black small period, forming part of a small letter at fifteen feet, enables one to distinguish that letter.

II. That, with the eyes closed, a small black period can be imagined blacker than one three inches in diameter. If this fact cannot be readily demonstrated with the eyes closed:

1. Stand close to a wall of a room, three feet or less, and regard a small black spot on the wall six feet from the floor. Note that you cannot see a small black spot near the bottom of the wall at the same time.

2. Place your hand on the wall six feet from the floor, and note that you cannot see your hand clearly when you look at the bottom of the wall.

Demonstrate

That vision is always imagination, either perfect or imperfect. What we see is only what we think or imagine we see. The white center of the letter "O", when seen perfectly, appears to be whiter than it really is, or whiter than the rest of the card. That part of the center of the "O" which is in contact with the black appears to be the whitest part of the white center. By covering the black part of the "O" with a screen, which has an opening in the center, the whiteness of the center of the "O" appears to be the same shade of white as the rest of the card. Now, remove the screen, and at the first glance, the center of the "O" appears for a short time to be much whiter than it really is. In other words, one sees something which is not really seen, but only imagined. When some people enter a room which is totally dark, they often imagine that they see a white ghost. They don't really see it; they only imagine it, but their imagination may be so vivid that no amount of argument will convince them that they did not see the ghost.

When one looks at the upper right hand corner of a large letter of the Snellen test card, it is possible to see that point best, and all the rest of the letter not so black. The part seen best appears blacker than it really is. The part seen worse appears less black than it really is. Things seen more perfectly than they really are, are not seen, but imagined. Things seen less perfectly than they really are, are not seen imperfectly, but are imagined imperfectly.

HE WON'T STAY DOWN

This old world is sometimes jealous of the chap who
    means to rise;
    It sneers at what he's doing or it bats him 'twixt
    the eyes;
It trips him when he's careless, and it makes his way
    so hard
    What's left of him is sinew, not a walking tub of
    lard;
But it's only wasting effort, for by George, the guy
    keeps on
    When his hopes have crumbled round him and
    you'd think his faith was gone,
Till the world at last knocks under and it passes him
    a crown:
    Once, twice, thrice it has upset him,
                    but
                      he
                        won't
                          stay
                            down.
What cares he when out he's flattened by the cruel
    blow it deals?
    He has rubber in his shoulders and a mainspring
    in his heels.
Let the world uncork its buffets till he's bruised from
    toe to crown;
    Let it thump him, bump him, dump him, but he
    won't stay down.
                          —ST. CLAIR ADAMS.

Demonstrate

1. That the sway improves the vision because it prevents the stare.

Stand with the feet about one foot apart, facing a Snellen test card about fifteen feet away. Sway the body from side to side, at first with a rapid, wide swing. When the body, head and eyes sway to the right, observe that the Snellen test card is to the left of where you are looking. Then sway the body, head and eyes to the left. The test card is now to the right of where you are looking. Practice this sway for a few minutes and, without looking at the Snellen test card directly, observe that the whiteness of the card becomes whiter and the black spots on the card become a darker shade of black. The test card appears to move in the direction opposite to the movement of the eyes, while objects beyond the card may move in the same direction as the eyes move.

2. That when the forefinger of one hand is held about six inches in front and to one side of the face, the finger appears to move from side to side in the direction opposite to the movement of the head and eyes. Close the eyes and let the hand rest in the lap and remember the swing of the finger. Imagine that the hand, which is fastened to the finger, moves with it. Realize that when the hand moves, the wrist, the arm, the elbow and other parts of the body, being joined together, all move with the finger. Now try to imagine the elbow is stationary, while the finger is moving. It is impossible to do this. When the finger moves, you can imagine not only your body, but also the chair on which you are sitting, the floor on which the chair rests, the walls of the room, the whole building with its foundation, in fact, the universe to be moving with the finger. This is called the universal swing and is possible only when the memory, imagination, or the sight is good.

Demonstrate

1. That a strain to see at the distance produces near-sightedness. Look at a Snellen test card at twenty feet and read it as well as you can. Now strain or make an effort to see it better, and note that instead of becoming better, it becomes worse.

2. That a strain to see at the near point does not increase near-sightedness, but always lessens it.

Look at a card of fine print at six inches from your eyes and read it as well as you can. Now make an effort to see it better, and note that your vision for the near point is lowered, while the ability to read the fine print at a greater distance is improved.

3. That when a mental picture is perfect with the eyes closed for part of a minute or longer, a perfect mental picture can be remembered, imagined, or seen for a second or less with the eyes open.

Remember a black kitten. If your mental picture is gray or an imperfect black with the eyes closed, imagine that you are pouring black ink or black dye over it. Note that the clearness of the mental picture improves.

Look at a page of fine print. Then close your eyes and imagine the white spaces between the lines to be perfectly white. If they appear to be a grayish white, imagine that you are painting the white spaces between the letters, inside the letters, and between the lines, with white paint or whitewash. Then open your eyes for a fraction of a second and note that the white spaces between the lines will appear whiter, if you do not make an effort to see either the black letters or the white spaces.

Demonstrate

That by practicing you can imagine a letter at ten feet as well as you can see it at one foot.

Regard a letter of the Snellen test card at a distance where it cannot be readily distinguished, and appears blurred. Now look at the same letter on a card at the near point, one foot or less, where it can be seen perfectly. Then close your eyes and with your finger draw the same letter in the air as well as you can remember it. Open your eyes and continue to draw the imaginary letter with your finger while looking for only a few seconds at the blurred letter on the card at ten feet. Then close your eyes again and remember the letter well enough to draw the letter perfectly in your imagination with your finger. Alternate drawing the letter at ten feet in your imagination with your eyes open and drawing it with your eyes closed as well as you see it at one foot or nearer. When you can draw the letter as perfectly as you remember it, you see the letter on the distant card in flashes.

By repetition you will become able not only to always imagine the known letter correctly, but to actually see it for a few seconds at a time. You cannot see a letter perfectly unless you see one part best; central fixation. Note that you obtain central fixation while practicing this method, i.e., you see one part best. Drawing the letter with your finger in your imagination enables you to follow the finger in forming the letter, and with the help of your memory, you can imagine each side of the letter best, in turn, as it is formed. By this method the memory and the imagination are improved, and when the imagination becomes perfect, the sight is perfect. You can cure the highest degrees of myopia, hypermetropia, astigmatism, atrophy of the optic nerve, cataract, glaucoma, detachment of the retina and other diseases by this method.

THE USE OF THE SUN GLASS

In using the sun glass, it is well to accustom the eyes of the patient to the strong light by having him sit in the sun with his eyes closed, and at the same time he should slowly move his head from side to side, in order to avoid discomfort from the heat. Enough light shines through the eyelid to cause some people a great deal of discomfort at first, but after a few hours' exposure in this way, they become able to gradually open their eyes to some extent without squeezing the lids. When this stage is reached, one can focus, with the aid of the sun glass, the light on the closed eyelids, which at first is very disagreeable. When the patient becomes able to open the eyes, he is directed to look as far down as possible, and in this way the pupil is protected by the lower lid. Then by gently lifting the upper lid, only the white part of the eye is exposed, while the sun's rays strike directly upon this part of the eyeball. The sun glass may then be used on the white part of the eye. Care should be taken to move the glass from side to side quickly. The length of time devoted to focusing the light on the white part of the eye is never longer than a few seconds. After such a treatment the patient almost immediately becomes able to open his eyes widely in the light.

Demonstrate

*T*HAT it requires an effort or a strain to produce imperfect sight.

Look at the notch at the top of the big "C" of the Snellen test card at fifteen feet. Keep your eyes fixed on the notch. Make an effort to see it and increase that effort as much as you possibly can. Notice that it is difficult to keep your eyes and mind fixed on that one point. Notice also that it is tiresome and makes your eyes pain. If you keep it up long enough, your head begins to ache and all the nerves of your body are strained.

If you look at some of the letters on the lower lines which are much smaller than the big "C", they may appear so blurred that you are not able to distinguish them. Trying to see these small letters blurs them still more.

Now hold the test card in your hand about one foot from your eyes. The big "C" is seen plainly and without any effort. Try to see the top and the bottom of the big "C" perfectly black at the same time. Notice that the "C" becomes blurred and the strain which blurs it also gives much discomfort.

From this evidence, we can conclude that perfect sight comes easily, without any effort or strain, while imperfect sight is always produced by a strain or an effort to see.

Demonstrate

1. That perfect sight is not possible unless one imagines a letter to be moving, and that an effort to imagine a letter stationary always fails. Close your eyes and remember a small letter of the Snellen test card. Imagine that some one is moving the test card a short distance from side to side so that all the letters on the card appear to be moving with the movement of the card. Remember the small letter moving. You can remember it provided you imagine it is moving. Now try to stop this movement by staring at one part of the small letter and imagining that it is stationary. The letter soon becomes blurred.

2. That the circular swing prevents the stare and relieves pain and fatigue.

Hold the forefinger of one hand about six inches in front of one eye and a few inches to the outer side of the face. By moving the head and eyes in a circular or an elliptical orbit, notice that the finger appears to move in the direction opposite to the movement of the head and eyes. Now realize that the hand must move with the finger because the hand and finger are fastened together. When one moves, the other moves in the same direction, up, down, to the right or left. The same fact is true of the arm fastened to the wrist. When the finger moves, the hand, wrist and arm in turn, all move and in the same direction. Likewise when the finger moves, the shoulder moves with it and other parts of the body fastened directly or indirectly to the finger. You may soon become able to imagine the chair on which you are sitting to be fastened indirectly to the finger. When one moves, the other always moves in the same direction. When you become able to imagine all things, one at a time to be moving with the finger, i.e., the universal swing, the stare is prevented and pain and fatigue disappear. The memory, imagination and vision are also improved.

Dizziness

*D*IZZINESS is caused by eyestrain. Some people when standing on the roof of a house looking down, strain their eyes and become dizzy. Usually the dizziness is produced unconsciously. It can be produced consciously, however, by staring or straining to see some distant or near object.

Other people, when riding in an elevator, become dizzy and may suffer from attacks of imperfect sight with headache, nausea, and other nervous discomforts.

An old lady, aged sixty, told me that riding in an elevator always made her dizzy, and produced headaches with pain in her eyes and head. I tested her vision and found it to be normal both for distance and for reading without glasses. To obtain some facts, I rode in an elevator with her from the top to the bottom of the building and back again. I watched her eyes closely and found that she was staring at the floors which appeared to be moving opposite to the movement of the elevator.

I asked her why she stared at the floors which appeared to be moving by. She answered that she did not like to see them move, and was trying to correct the illusion by making an effort to keep them stationary. She said the harder she tried, the worse she felt. I suggested that she look at one part of the elevator and avoid looking at the floors. Her discomfort was at once relieved, and she was soon cured.

In all cases of dizziness, the stare or strain is always evident. When the stare or strain is relieved or prevented, dizziness does not occur. With advancing years attacks of dizziness and blindness occur more frequently than in younger individuals All attacks of dizziness with blindness are quite readily cured by practicing the imagination of the swing, the memory of perfect sight, or by palming.

Demonstrate

That memory and imagination improve the vision.

Look at the large letter at the top of the card and note that it may be more or less blurred. Close the eyes and remember or imagine the same letter perfectly. Then open both eyes and imagine it as well as you can. In a second or less, close your eyes and remember the letter perfectly. When this is accomplished open the eyes and imagine it as well as you can. Close them quickly after a second or less. Practice the slow, short, easy swing and alternately remember the large letter with the eyes closed for part of a minute or longer, and then open the eyes and imagine it as well as you can.

When done properly, you will be able to improve your vision of the large letter until it becomes quite perfect. Then practice in the same way with the first letter of the second line. Improve your imagination of the first letter of the second line in flashes, until it improves sufficiently for you to recognize the next letter without looking at it.

Improve the sight of the first letter of each line by alternately remembering it with the eyes closed for part of a minute and then flashing it for just a moment, a second or less. You should be told what the first letter of each line is. With your eyes closed remember it as perfectly as you can. Then open your eyes and test your imagination for the letter for a very short time, one second or even less. Keep your eyes closed for at least a part of a minute, while remembering the known letter. The flashes of the known letter with the eyes open become more frequent and last longer, until you become able to see, not only the known letter, but other unknown letters on the same line.

Demonstrate

1. That a short, swaying movement improves the vision more than a long sway.

Place the test card at a distance where only the large letter at the top of the card can be distinguished. This may be ten feet, further or nearer. Stand with the feet about one foot apart and sway the body from side to side. When the body sways to the right, look to the right of the card. When the body sways to the left, look to the left of the card. Do not look at the Snellen test card. Sway the body from side to side and look to the right of the Snellen test card, and alternately to the left of it. Note that the test card appears to be moving. Increase the length of the sway and notice that the test card seems to move a longer distance from side to side. Observe the whiteness of the card and the blackness of the letters. Now shorten the sway, which, of course, shortens the movement of the card. The card appears whiter and the letters blacker when the movement of the card is short, than when the movement of the card is long.

2. Demonstrate that when the eyes are stationary, they are under a tremendous strain. Stand before the Snellen test card at a distance of fifteen or twenty feet. Look directly at one small area of a large letter, which can be seen clearly. Stare at that part of the letter without closing the eyes and without shifting the eyes to some other point. The vision becomes worse and the letter blurs. Stare continuously, and note that the longer you stare, the more difficult it is to keep the eyes focused on that one point or part of the letter. Not only does the stare become more difficult, but the eyes become tired; and by making a greater effort, the eyes pain, or a headache is produced. The stare can cause fatigue of the whole body when the effort is sufficiently strong and prolonged.

Demonstrate

1. That palming improves the sight.

When both eyes are closed and covered with one or both hands in such a way as to exclude all light, one does not see red, blue, green or any other color. In short, when the palming is successful one does not see anything but black, and when the eyes are opened, the vision is always improved.

2. That an imperfect memory prevents perfect palming and the vision is lowered.

Remember a letter "O" imperfectly, a letter "O" which has no white center and is covered by a gray cloud. It takes time; the effort is considerable and in spite of all that is done, the memory of the imperfect "O" is lost or forgotten for a time. The whole field is a shade of gray or of some other color, and when the hands are removed from the eyes, the vision is lowered.

3. That when a perfect letter "O" is remembered, palming is practiced properly, continuously and easily and the sight is always benefited.

4. That to fail to improve the sight by palming, or to palm imperfectly is difficult. To fail, requires a stare or a strain and is not easy. When an effort is made the eyes and mind are staring, straining, trying to see. When no effort is made, the palming becomes successful and the vision is benefited. Successful palming is not accomplished by doing things. Palming becomes successful by the things that are not done.

5. That the longer you palm, the greater the benefit to your vision. Palm first for two minutes, then four minutes, six, etc., until you have palmed for fifteen. Notice the improvement gained in 15 minutes has been greater than that in four minutes.

Demonstrate

That the eyes can be used correctly or incorrectly when walking.

Many people have complained that after walking a short distance slowly, easily and without any special effort, they become nervous, tired and their eyes feel the symptoms and consequences of strain. When they were taught the correct way to use their eyes while walking, the symptoms of fatigue or strain disappeared.

The facts can be demonstrated with the aid of a straight line on the floor or the seam in the carpet.

Stand with the right foot to the right of the line and the left foot to the left of the line. Now put your right foot forward and look to the left of the line. Then put your left foot forward and look to the right of the line. When you walk forward, look to the left of the line, when your right foot moves forward. Look to the right of the line when your left foot moves forward. Note that it is difficult to do this longer than a few seconds without uncertainty, discomfort, pain, headache, dizziness or nausea.

Now practice the right method of walking and using the eyes. When the right foot moves forward, look to the right; and when the left foot moves forward, look to the left. Note that the straight line seems to sway in the direction opposite to the movement of the eyes and foot, i.e., when the eyes and foot move to the right, the line seems to move to the left. When the eyes and foot move to the left, the line seems to move to the right. Note that this is done easily, without any hesitation or discomfort.

When you walk, you can imagine that you are looking at the right foot as you step forward with that foot. When you step forward with the left foot, you can imagine that you are looking at your left foot. This can be done in a slow walk or quite rapidly while running straight ahead or in a circle.

Demonstrate

Demonstrate that perfect sight is accomplished when the imagination is good, and that you see only what you imagine you see.

Take a Snellen test card and hold it at a distance from your eyes at which your sight is fairly good. Look at the white center of the large "O" and compare the whiteness of the center of the "O" with the whiteness of the rest of the card. You may do it readily; but if not, use a screen, that is, a card with a small hole in it. With that card, cover over the black part of the letter "O" and note the white center of the letter which is exposed by the opening in the screen. Remove the screen and observe that there is a change in the appearance of the white, which appears to be a whiter white, when the black part of the letter is exposed. When the black part of the letter is covered with a screen, the center of the "O" is of the same whiteness as the rest of the card. It is, therefore, possible to demonstrate that you do not see the white center of the "O" whiter than the rest of the card, because you are seeing something that is not there. When you see something that is not there, you do not really see it, you only imagine it. The whiter you can imagine the center of the "O," the better becomes the vision for the letter "O," and when the vision of the letter "O" improves, the vision of all the letters on the card improves. The perfect imagination of the white center of the "O" means perfect imagination of the black, because you cannot imagine the white perfectly, without imagining the black perfectly. By practice you may become able to imagine the letter "O" much better than it really is, and when this is accomplished, you become able to actually see unknown letters.

Demonstrate

That glasses lower the vision.

Stand fifteen feet from the Snellen test card and test the vision of each eye without glasses. Then test the vision of each eye with glasses on, after having worn them for half an hour or longer. Remove the glasses; test the vision again and compare the results. Note that the vision without glasses becomes better, the longer the glasses are left off.

Test the eyes of a person who is very nearsighted. Remove the glasses and test the sight of each eye at five feet, nearer or farther, until the distance is found at which the vision is best without glasses. Now test the vision for five minutes at this distance, which is the optimum distance, or the distance at which the vision is best. For example, near-sighted people see best when the print is held a foot or nearer to the eyes. If the eyes see best at six inches, the optimum distance is six inches; but if the distance at which the eyes see best is thirty to forty inches, the optimum distance is then thirty or forty inches.

In near-sightedness, glasses always lower the vision at the optimum distance. The same is true in far-sightedness or astigmatism. For example, a near-sighted person may have an optimum distance of six inches. If glasses are worn, the vision is never as good at six inches as it is without them. This demonstrates that glasses lower the vision at six inches, or the optimum distance in this case. In far-sightedness without glasses, the optimum distance, at which objects are seen best, may be ten feet or further. If glasses are worn and the sight is improved at a nearer point, the vision without glasses at the optimum distance becomes worse.

Demonstrate

1. That sun treatment is an immediate benefit to many diseases of the eye.

Before the treatment, take a record of your best vision of the Snellen test card with both eyes together and each eye separately without glasses. Then sit in the sun with your eyes closed, slowly moving your head a short distance from side to side, and allowing the sun to shine directly on your closed eyelids. Forget about your eyes; just think of something pleasant and let your mind drift from one pleasant thought to another. Before opening your eyes, palm for a few minutes. Then test your vision of the test card and note the improvement. Get as much sun treatment as you possibly can, one, two, three or more hours daily.

When the sun is not shining, substitute a strong electric light. A 1,000 watt electric light is preferable, but requires special wiring. However, a 250 watt or 300 watt light can be used with benefit, and does not require special wiring. Sit about six inches from the light, or as near as you can without discomfort from the heat, allowing it to shine on your closed eyelids as in the sun treatment.

2. That the strong light of the sun focussed on the sclera, or white part of the eyeball, with the sun glass, also improves the vision.

After the eyes have become accustomed to the sunlight with the eyes closed, focus the light of the sun on the closed eyelids with the sun glass. Move the glass rapidly from side to side while doing this for a few minutes. Then have the patient open his eyes and look as far down as possible, and in this way, the pupil is protected by the lower lid. Gently lift the upper lid, so that only the white part of the eye is exposed, as the sun's rays fall directly upon this part of the eyeball. The sun glass may now be used on the white part of the eye for a few seconds, moving it quickly from side to side and in various directions. Notice that after the use of the sun glass, the vision is improved.

Demonstrate

1. That the drifting swing improves the sight.

Take a record of your best vision of the Snellen test card with both eyes together and each eye separately without glasses. Now close your eyes and imagine that you are occupying a canoe which is floating down some creek, river or stream. Imagine that the trees, houses and other stationary objects on either side are moving in the direction opposite to the way in which you are moving.

Another way in which to practice the drifting swing is as follows: With the eyes closed, recall a number of familiar objects which can be remembered easily. Sometimes in the course of a few minutes, fifty or one hundred objects may be remembered quickly and then forgotten. Remember each mental picture by central fixation; that is, think of only one part at a time of the object that you are remembering. Just let your mind drift easily from one object to another, without making any effort. Do not try to hold each object as remembered; forget it quickly. Notice that after practicing the above methods for a few minutes the vision for the test card is improved.

2. That the long swing improves the sight, relieves pain, fatigue and many other nervous symptoms.

Take a record of your best vision of the Snellen test card with both eyes together and each eye separately without glasses. Stand, with the feet about one foot apart, facing a blank wall. Turn the body to the left, at the same time raising the heel of the right foot. Now place the heel of the right foot on the floor in its usual position; then turn the body to the right, lifting the heel of the left foot.

The head and eyes move with the body; do not make any effort to see more distinctly stationary objects which are apparently moving. Practice this fifty to one hundred times, easily, without making any effort. Notice that after practicing, the vision for the test card improves.

VOLUNTARY PRODUCTION OF EYE TENSION A SAFEGUARD AGAINST GLAUCOMA

It is a good thing to know how to increase the tension of the eyeball voluntarily, as this enables one to avoid not only the strain that produces glaucoma, but other kinds of strain also. To do this proceed as follows:

Put the fingers on the upper part of the eyeball while looking downward, and note its softness. Then do any one of the following things:

Try to see a letter, or other object, imperfectly, or (with the eyes either closed or open) to imagine it imperfectly.

Try to see a letter, or a number of letters, all alike at one time, or to imagine them in this way.

Try to imagine that a letter, or mental picture of a letter is stationary.

Try to see a letter, or other object, double, or to imagine it double.

When successful, the eyeball will become harder in proportion to the degree of the strain, but, as it is very difficult to see, imagine, or remember, things imperfectly, all may not be able at first to demonstrate the facts.

[*The above article, which appeared in the December, 1920, issue of "Better Eyesight," is reprinted at the request of the editor, in connection with the other articles in this month's issue on "tension."*]

Favorable Conditions

The vision of the human eye is modified in many ways when the conditions are unfavorable to good sight. Unfavorable conditions may prevail when the light is not agreeable to the patient. Some patients require a very bright light and others get along much better in a poor light. Many cases are hypersensitive to the light and suffer from an intolerance for light which has been called photophobia.

While intolerance of light may be manifest in most cases from some diseases of the eyes, there are many cases in which the eye is apparently healthy and in which the photophobia may be extreme. (The cure for this condition is to have the patient sit in the sun with his eyes closed, allowing the sun to shine on his closed eyelids as he moves his head from side to side.)

There are patients with good sight whose vision is materially improved when used in a bright light, as well as those with good sight whose vision improves when the eyes are used in a dim light. The patient should practice with the test card in a bright as well as a dim light to accustom his eyes to all conditions.

The ability to perceive halos, or an increased whiteness, around letters is a favorable condition. By using a screen or a fenestrated card, it is possible for many patients to see an increased whiteness around a letter, which improves their vision for the letter. When a screen is not used, one may be able to imagine a white halo around the inner or outer edge of the black part of the "O." When a screen covers the black part of the letter "O," for instance, the white center becomes of the same whiteness as the rest of the white page, which proves that it is the contrast between the black and the white which enables one to imagine the white halos. The presence of the black improves the white; the presence of the white improves the black.

Eyestrain During Sleep

Many people complain that when they awaken in the morning, they are suffering from pain in their eyes or head. They often feel as weary as though they had been working hard all night long. Many of them do not recover from the pain and fatigue until after they have been up for an hour or longer. Their vision also may be found to be reduced to a very considerable degree. Some complain that they see illusions which are occasionally very slow in disappearing. One patient complained that the tiled floor of a bath room had a very strange appearance; although the tiles were white, to him they appeared blue and red alternately. A feeling of strain was always present and did not subside until the illusion had disappeared. It seemed as though the eyes were under a strain during sleep, because when the eyes were examined with the ophthalmoscope while the patient was asleep, a strain could readily be observed.

Sometimes, as in the case of many children, other parts of the body may be under a strain during sleep. By an unconscious effort, the muscles of the face, arms and limbs may be distorted as may be muscles of different parts of the eyeball. In some cases, the strain produces accommodation or myopia, while in other cases, hypermetropia or astigmatism are produced by this unconscious effort. These eyes frequently were found to be normal during the day.

The treatment to prevent eyestrain during sleep is not always successful. Some patients obtain most relief by practicing the long swing one hundred times or more just before retiring and the same number of times in the morning immediately after awakening. Other patients find that palming for twenty minutes before retiring is a help, and frequently the palms are left in place with benefit after the patients have lost consciousness.

The Thumb Movement

Rest the hand against an immovable surface. Place the ball of the thumb lightly in contact with the forefinger. Now move the end of the thumb in a circle of about one-quarter of an inch in diameter. When the thumb moves in one direction, the forefinger should appear to move in the opposite direction, although in reality it is stationary. In the practice of the universal swing, everything is imagined to be moving in the same direction, except the eyes. With the aid of the thumb movement, however, one can imagine the spine and the head moving opposite to the direction of motion of the thumb, while the eyes, being fastened to the head, also move with the head and hand.

While watching the movement of the thumb, remember imperfect sight. At once, the thumb movement becomes irregular or may stop altogether. Demonstrate that any effort, no matter how slight, to see, remember or imagine, interferes with the movement of the thumb. The thumb is so sensitive to an effort or strain that the slightest effort is at once recorded by the motion.

While watching the movement of the thumb, remember perfect sight. Notice that the movement of the thumb is slow, short, continuous, and restful—with relaxation of all parts of the body.

Many patients have been successfully treated for pain, fatigue, and dizziness with the help of the thumb movement, after other treatment had failed. Some patients with severe pain complain that when they forget to practice the movement of the thumb, the pain comes back.

Not only have patients suffering from pain and symptoms of fatigue been relieved, but an equal number have been relieved of imperfect sight by the correct practice of the thumb movement.

First Visit Cures

The word "cures" is used advisedly. It is a fact that some people have been cured of myopia in one visit, after relaxation of the nerves of the eyes and other parts of the body was obtained.

Suppose the patient is near-sighted and can only see the big letter "C" at fifteen feet, a vision of 15/200. Let the patient walk up close to the card until he can read the bottom line. The distance may be three feet, five feet or farther. The first letter on the bottom line may be the letter "F." With the eyes open, it is possible for the patient to imagine the letter "F" quite perfectly, but with the eyes closed, he is more easily able to remember and imagine he sees the letter "F" much better.

Palming is a great help when remembering or imagining the letter "F" with the eyes closed. By alternately imagining the letter "F" with the eyes open, and remembering or imagining it better with the eyes closed, the memory, the imagination and finally the vision for the letter "F" is very much improved.

If the patient becomes able to see the letter "F" at three feet, or to imagine he sees it quite perfectly, he should be encouraged to walk back and increase the distance between the eyes and the letter "F" about one foot. When the patient becomes able to imagine the letter "F" at four feet, he should go back another foot, alternately imagining it with his eyes open and remembering it much better with his eyes closed. By gradually increasing the distance of the eyes from the letter "F," all patients who practiced this method obtained normal vision temporarily at the first visit.

The length of time required to obtain a permanent cure is variable. Some patients with not more than one or two diopters of myopia may require many weeks or months of daily treatment before they are permanently cured, while others with a higher degree of myopia sometimes obtain a cure in a much shorter time.

Brain Tension

The brain has many nerves. Part of these nerves are called ganglion cells and originate in some particular part of the brain. Each has a function of its own. They are connected with other ganglion cells and with the aid of nerve fibres are connected with others located in various parts of the brain as well as in the spinal cord, the eye, the ear, the nerves of smell, taste, and the nerves of touch. The function of each ganglion cell of the brain is different from that of all others. When the ganglion cells are healthy, they function in a normal manner.

The retina of the eye contains numerous ganglion cells which regulate special things such as normal vision, normal memory, normal imagination and they do this with a control more or less accurate of other ganglion cells of the whole body. The retina has a similar structure to parts of the brain. It is connected to the brain by the optic nerve.

Many nerves from the ganglion cells of the retina carry conscious and unconscious control of other ganglion cells which are connected to other parts of the body.

When the ganglion cells are diseased or at fault, the functions of all parts of the body are not normally maintained. In all cases of imperfect sight, it has been repeatedly demonstrated that the ganglion cells and nerves of the brain are under a strain. When this strain is corrected by treatment, the functions of the ganglion and other cells become normal. The importance of the mental treatment cannot be over-estimated.

A study of the facts has demonstrated that a disease of some ganglion in any part of the body occurs in a similar ganglion in the brain.

Brain tension of one or more nerves always means disease of the nerve ganglia. Treatment of the mind with the aid of the sight, memory and imagination has cured many cases of imperfect sight without other treatment.

Color Blindness

Some people are unable to distinguish red from blue or other colors. Many doctors explain color blindness to be due to something wrong with the retina, optic nerve or brain. They believe that organic changes in the retina are the principal cause. But this is not always true because, in some cases, cures occur without any apparent change in the retina.

I have found that color blindness occurs in a great many cases in an eye apparently normal. There are, however, a number of individuals who can be demonstrated to have color blindness as a result of a disease of the retina caused by mental strain. These cases cannot be cured, however, until the disease of the retina is cured.

Some patients with color blindness are sensitive to a bright light. On the other hand, there are patients with color blindness who are more comfortable in a bright light. These patients are usually relieved by the practice of sun treatment, central fixation, palming, the long swing, or any other method which brings about relaxation.

One patient had a normal perception for colors at three feet and at ten feet. But at a nearer point than three feet she was color blind, the blindness being most marked at three inches. At a distance greater than ten feet the color blindness was evident. After her eyestrain was relieved by relaxation her color blindness disappeared.

People who have been born color blind as well as those who have acquired color blindness have all been cured by the practice of relaxation methods.

Subjective Conjunctivitis

By subjective conjunctivitis is meant that the conjunctiva is inflamed without the evidence of disease. Many people with subjective conjunctivitis will complain of a foreign body in the eye and yet careful search with the use of a good light and a strong magnifying glass will reveal no foreign body present. Some people with subjective conjunctivitis complain that they have granulated lids and that they suffer from time to time from the presence of little pimples on the inside of the eyelids and the pain that they suffer is out of proportion to the cause that they give to it. Among the many symptoms of subjective conjunctivitis may be a flow of tears from very slight irritants. However, the tear ducts, with the aid of which the tears are drained from the eye, are usually open in these cases and they are sufficiently open to receive a solution of boracic acid which may be injected through the tear duct into the nose. This shows that the tear duct is open normally, and therefore can drain the tears from the eyes.

Dr. C. R. Agnew, at one time professor of ophthalmology at Columbia University, gave many lectures on subjective conjunctivitis in 1885 and 1886. The treatment which he advocated was dry massage of the whole body and I can testify that it was an excellent remedy. However, the treatment which I found was the greatest benefit was the aqueous extract of the suprarenal capsule, or adrenalin, the properties of which I discovered, using one drop in each eye three times a day.

Many cases were benefited by the sun treatment, by central fixation and by the practice of the universal swing.

Dark Glasses Are Injurious

He was a very intelligent chauffeur, and very polite and popular with most people. I enjoyed listening to his experiences in driving various types of cars. Nothing seemed to give him so much pleasure as to get into a "jam" and get out without suffering any injury to his own car or without tearing the "enemy" apart. The "enemy," as he explained, were the numerous other cars which were driven by chauffeurs who did not understand their business very well and who enjoyed teasing the inexperienced drivers.

One day we were driving to the seashore. The sun was very bright and the reflection of the light from the sun on the water was very strong and made most of the occupants of the car very uncomfortable. Personally I enjoyed the strong light of the sun. The chauffeur did not wear glasses for the protection of his eyes from the sun or dust and I asked him if he had ever worn them. He very promptly answered me by saying that he had worn them at one time, but discontinued wearing them because he found that after wearing them for a few days, his eyes became more sensitive to the light than they were before. He said he could not understand why it was that when he wore glasses to protect his eyes from the dust he accumulated more foreign bodies in his eyes than ever before. This seemed strange to the people in the car and they asked him to explain. It was decided that when the dust got into the eyes, the glasses prevented the dust from going out.

The eyes need the light of the sun. When the sun's rays are excluded from the eyes by dark glasses, the eyes become very sensitive to the sun when the glasses are removed.

Suggestions

It is recommended by the editor of this magazine that every family should obtain a Snellen test card and place it on the wall of some room where it can be seen and read every day by all the members of the family. Not only does the daily reading of the card help the sight of children, but it is a benefit to the eyes of adults as well.

It is a well known fact that when most people arrive at the age of forty or fifty years, they find that their vision for reading or sewing is lowered. These people believe that they must put on glasses to prevent eyestrain, cataract, glaucoma, et cetera. Daily practice with the Snellen test card, together with the reading of fine print close to the eyes will overcome their difficulty. Reading fine print close to the eyes, contrary to the belief of many ophthalmologists, is a benefit to the eyes of both children and adults.

It has been repeatedly demonstrated, however, that fine print cannot be read clearly or easily when an effort is made. When the eyes look directly at the letters, an effort is required, while looking at the white spaces between the lines is a rest, and by practice in this way, one can become able to see the letters clearly, without looking directly at them. When a patient looks at the white spaces between the lines of ordinary book type, he can read for hours and no fatigue, pain or discomfort is felt. When discomfort and pain in the eyes is felt while reading, it is because the patient is looking directly at the letters.

Eyestrain

The eyes of all people with imperfect sight are under a strain. This is a truth. Most people believe that during sleep the eyes are at rest and that it is impossible to strain the eyes while sound asleep. This, however, is not true. Persons who have good sight in the daytime under favorable conditions may strain their eyes during sleep. Many people awake in the morning suffering pain in the eyes or head. Often the eyes are very much fatigued and have a feeling of discomfort. There may be also a feeling of nervous tension from the eyestrain, or there may be a feeling as of sand in the eyes. At times all parts of the eye may be suffering from inflammation. The vision is sometimes lowered for several hours whereupon it begins to improve until it becomes as good as it was before the person retired the night before. Many people become alarmed and seek the services of some eye doctor. Usually the doctor or doctors consulted prescribe glasses which very rarely give more than imperfect or temporary relief.

There are various methods of correcting eyestrain occurring during sleep. Palming is very helpful even when practiced for a short time. A half an hour is often sufficient to relieve most if not all of the symptoms. In some cases the long swing, practiced before retiring, is sufficient to bring about temporary or permanent benefit. Blinking and shifting are also helpful. Good results have been obtained by practicing a perfect memory or imagination of one small letter of the Snellen test card alternately with the eyes open and closed. A number of patients were benefited and usually cured by remembering pleasant things perfectly.

No Glasses for Quick Results

The first and best thing that all patients should do after their first treatment, or before, is to discard their glasses. It is not always an easy thing to do but it is best for the patient and for the teacher. It is true that at one time I did not encourage patients to learn the treatment unless they discarded their glasses permanently. But since I have studied more about my method and have encouraged some of my clinic patients to wear their glasses at times while under treatment, I find that some of them obtained a cure but it required double the amount of time that was required to cure those who discarded their glasses permanently. During the treatment when the glasses are worn temporarily, even for a short time, the vision sometimes becomes worse and in most cases a relapse is produced. It is much more difficult to regain the lost ground than ever before, and sometimes causes much discomfort.

Glasses for the correction of myopia do not fit the eyes all the time. To obtain good vision with glasses an effort is required to make the eyes change their focus to have the same error of refraction as the glasses correct. When the vision is benefited most perfectly by glasses it is necessary for the eyes to change frequently. To learn the amount of myopia in the eyes by trying different glasses to find the glass which continuously improves the vision best is usually difficult because the amount of the myopia changes so frequently. To change the amount of myopia requires an effort. Some people complain that no glasses fit their eyes permanently. These cases are benefited by discarding their glasses for a longer or a shorter period while being treated. Patients who require good sight to earn a living and find it difficult to discard their glasses while under treatment, have been able to make slow or rapid progress in the cure of their imperfect sight by wearing their glasses only when it was absolutely necessary.

Practice Time

A large number of people have bought the book "Perfect Sight Without Glasses" but do not derive as much benefit from it as they should because they do not know how long they should practice.

Rest: The eyes are rested in various ways. One of the best methods is to close the eyes for half an hour after testing the sight. This usually improves the vision.

Palming: With the eyes closed and covered with the palms of both hands the vision is usually benefited. The patient should do this five minutes hourly.

Shifting: The patient looks from one side of the room to the other, alternately resting the eyes. This may be done three times daily for half an hour at a time. The head should move with the eyes and the patient should blink.

Swinging: When the shifting is slow, stationary objects appear to move from side to side. This should be observed whenever the head and eyes move.

Long Swing: Nearly all persons should practice the long swing one hundred times daily.

Memory: When the vision is perfect, it is impossible for the memory to be imperfect. One can improve the memory by alternately remembering a letter with the eyes open and closed. This should be practiced for half an hour twice daily.

Imagination: It has been frequently demonstrated and published in this magazine that the vision is only what we imagine it to be. Imagination should be practiced whenever the vision is tested. Imagine a known letter with the eyes open and with the eyes closed. This should be practiced for ten minutes twice daily.

Repetition: When one method is found which improves the vision more than any other method, it should be practiced until the vision is continuously improved.

Time For Practice

So many people with imperfect sight say that they have not the time to practice relaxation methods, as their time is taken up at business or in the performance of other duties. I always tell such people, however, that they have just as much time to use their eyes correctly as incorrectly.

They can imagine stationary objects to be moving opposite whenever they move their head and eyes. When the head and eyes move to the left, stationary objects should appear to move to the right, and vice versa.

They can remember to blink their eyes in the same way that the normal eye blinks unconsciously, which is frequently, rapidly, continuously, without any effort or strain, until by conscious practice, it will eventually become an unconscious habit, and one that will be of benefit to the patient.

They can remember to shift or look from one point to another continuously. When practicing shifting, it is well to move the head in the same direction as the eyes move. If the head moves to the right, the eyes should move to the right. If the head moves to the left, the eyes should move to the left. By practicing in this way, relaxation is often obtained very quickly, but if the eyes are moved to the right and at the same time the head is moved to the left, a strain on the nerves of the eyes and the nerves of the body in general is produced.

Practice Methods

Many people have asked for help in choosing the best method of treatment for their particular eye trouble. A woman aged sixty complained that she had never been free of pain; pain was very decided in her eyes and head. She also had continuous pain in nearly all the nerves of the body. The long swing when practiced 100 times gave her great relief from pain. The relief was continuous without any relapse. At the same time a second woman of about the same age complained of a similar pain which, like the first patient, she had had almost continuously. She was also relieved by practicing the long swing. The long swing was practiced by other people with a satisfactory result.

It seemed that the swing was indicated for pain; it seemed to bring about better results than any other treatment. Later on, however, some patients applied for relief from pain which was not benefited by the long swing. Evidently one kind of treatment was not beneficial in every case. A man suffering from tri-facial neuralgia which caused great agony in all parts of the head was not relieved at all by the long swing. Palming seemed to be more successful in bringing about relief. Furthermore, there were patients who did not obtain benefit after half an hour of palming who did obtain complete relief after palming for several hours.

Patients with cataract recovered quite promptly when some special method was tried.

The experience obtained by the use of relaxation methods in the cure of obstinate eye troubles has proved that what was good for one patient was not necessarily a benefit to other patients suffering from the same trouble, and that various methods must be tried in each case in order to determine which is the most beneficial for each particular case.

Correspondence Treatment

Many letters are received from people in various parts of the world who find it impossible to come to New York and who believe that something might be done for them by correspondence treatment. I do not advocate correspondence treatment as a general rule, as the results are uncertain. There is always the possibility that the patient will not practice correctly the things which he is told to do.

If a patient has had one treatment at my office or at the office of one of my representatives, it is possible to treat that patient more intelligently through correspondence.

Some years ago a gentleman living a thousand miles from New York called and asked if anything could be done through correspondence for his wife who was bedridden and suffering with an agony of pain in her eyes. He described all her symptoms to me and gave me her last prescription for glasses. He was told that if he would take the treatment in my office, and so learn how to treat his wife, it would be possible for him to aid her intelligently when he went home. He did this and after taking several treatments, returned. He wrote me later saying that his wife was almost cured.

When my book, "Perfect Sight Without Glasses," is read carefully, those things which are not understood may be cleared up by intelligent questions, which I am always pleased to answer. I do not consider this as regular correspondence treatment.

The Period

Many people have difficulty in obtaining a mental picture of a small black period. They may try to see it by an effort which always fails. They may persist in their efforts to see or remember it, paying little or no attention to their failures or the cause of their failures. As long as they continue to strain by trying to see, they will always fail; the period becomes more indistinct.

A small black period is very readily seen. There is no letter, no figure, no object of any kind which can be obtained more easily. Demonstrate that an effort to see a small black period by staring, concentrating, trying to see, always makes it worse. Rest, relaxation, the swing, shifting, are all a great help. Practice with a large black letter. Imagine that the upper right corner has a small black period. Do the same with other parts of the large letter. This practice will enable you to understand central fixation, seeing best where you are looking. Central fixation can always be demonstrated when the sight is good. When the sight is poor or imperfect, central fixation is absent.

The benefits which can be obtained from the use of the period are very numerous. A perfect memory can only be obtained when the sight is perfect. A perfect imagination can only be obtained when the sight and the memory are perfect. The period is the smallest letter or other object which is perfect or becomes perfect by perfect memory or perfect imagination.

Blinking

Blinking is one of the best methods that may be employed to obtain relaxation or rest. When rest is obtained by blinking, the vision is improved, not only for one letter or part of one letter, but for all the letters of a page, which may be seen some parts best, other parts not so well. This is called central fixation and one cannot see anything clearly without it. In order to maintain central fixation, there should be continuous opening and closing of the eyes by blinking which makes it easier for the vision to improve. When the eye discontinues to blink, it usually stares, strains, and tries to see. Blinking is beneficial only when practiced in the right way.

What is the right way? The question may be answered almost as briefly as it is asked. Blinking when done properly is slow, short, and easy. One may open and close the eyes an innumerable number of times in one second, and do so unconsciously.

Lord Macauley was able to read a page of print in one second, and blinked for every letter. In order to read perfectly, he had to see each side of every letter by central fixation. We know that he acquired or had a perfect memory, because it was only with a perfect memory that he could recite the pages of any book which he had read many years before.

A casual observer would not be able to determine the number of times Lord Macaulay blinked, as it was done so quickly and easily, without any effort on his part. While most of us will not be able to blink without effort as frequently as Lord Macauley did, it is well to practice his methods as well as we can. Those with imperfect sight who do not blink sufficiently should watch someone with normal eyes blink unconsciously and then imitate him.

Shifting

When the normal eye has normal sight it is at rest and when it is at rest it is always moving or shifting. Shifting may be done consciously with improvement in the vision, or it may be done unconsciously with impaired vision.

Shifting can be practiced correctly and incorrectly. A wrong way to shift is to turn the head to the right while the eyes are turned to the left, or to turn the head to the left while the eyes are turned to the right.

To improve imperfect sight by shifting, it is well to move the head and eyes so far away that the first letter or object imagined is too far away to be seen at all clearly. Shifting from small letters to large letters alternately may be a greater benefit than shifting from one small letter to another small letter. Quite frequently the vision is decidedly improved by shifting continuously from one side of a small letter to the other side, while the letter is imagined to be moving in the opposite direction. When the shifting is slow, short, and easy, the best results in the improvement in the vision are obtained. Any attempt to stop the shifting always lowers the vision. The letter or other object which appeared to move is usually shifting a short distance—one half or one quarter of an inch. It is not possible to imagine any particular letter or other object stationary for a longer time than one minute.

While the patient is seated, benefit can be obtained from shifting, but even more benefit can be obtained when the shifting is practiced while the patient is standing and moving the head and shoulders, in fact the whole body, a very short distance from side to side. Shifting the whole body makes it easier to shift a short distance and may explain why this method is best.

Go to the Movies

(Editor's Note.—Recently a great many letters have come from patients and others asking if the movies were injurious to the eyes. For the benefit of these inquirers we are reprinting an article which appeared in this magazine in October, 1920.)

Cinematograph pictures are commonly supposed to be very injurious to the eyes, and it is a fact that they often cause much discomfort and lowering of vision. They can, however, be made a means of improving the sight. When they hurt the eyes it is because the subject strains to see them. If this tendency to strain can be overcome, the vision is always improved, and if the practice of viewing the pictures is continued long enough, nearsight, astigmatism and other troubles are cured.

If your sight is imperfect, therefore, you will find it an advantage to go to the movies frequently and learn to look at the pictures without strain. If they hurt your eyes look away to the dark for a while, then look at a corner of the picture; look away again, and then look a little nearer to the center; and so on. In this way you may soon become able to look directly at the picture without discomfort. If this does not help, try palming for five minutes or longer. Dodge the pain, in short, and prevent the eyestrain by constant shifting, or by palming.

Mental Pictures

With imperfect sight, a mental picture of one known letter of the Snellen test card is seldom or never remembered, imagined, or seen perfectly when regarded with the eyes open. By closing the eyes, the same mental picture may be imagined more perfectly. By alternately imagining the known letter as well as possible with the eyes open and then remembering it better with the eyes closed, the imagination improves the vision and unknown letters are seen with the eyes open.

The improvement of the vision is due to a lessening of the organic changes in the eye. When the imperfect sight is caused by opacities of the cornea, a mental picture imagined clearly lessens or cures the disease of the cornea. A large number of cases of cataract in which the lens is more or less opaque have been benefited or cured by the imagination of mental pictures. Nearly all organic changes in the eyeball which lower the vision have been improved to some extent in a few minutes; by devoting a sufficient amount of time, all organic changes in the eyeball, no matter what the cause may be, are benefited or cured by a perfect imagination of a letter, a tree, a flower, or anything which is remembered perfectly.

I do not know of any method of obtaining relaxation or perfect sight which is as efficient and certain as the imagination of mental pictures. It should be emphasized that a good or perfect imagination of mental pictures has in all cases brought about a measure of improvement which is convincing that the imagination is capable of relieving organic changes in the eye more quickly, more thoroughly, more permanently, than any other method.

The Colon

While the colon is a valuable punctuation mark, it has a very unusual and better use in helping the memory, imagination, and sight. Medium sized or small letters at the distance are improved promptly by the proper use of the colon. While the eyes are closed or open, the top period should be imagined best while the lower period is more or less blurred and not seen so well. In a few moments it is well to shift and imagine the lower period best while the upper period is imagined not so well. Common sense makes it evident that one period cannot be imagined best unless there is some other period or other object which is seen worse. The smallest colon that can be imagined is usually the one that is imagined more readily than a larger colon.

When palming, swinging, et cetera, cannot be practiced sufficiently well to obtain improvement in the eyesight, the memory or imagination of the small colon, one part best, can usually be practiced with benefit. To remember or imagine a colon perfectly requires constant shifting. When the colon is remembered or imagined perfectly, and this cannot be done by any effort or strain, the sight is always improved and the memory and imagination are also improved. It is interesting to note that the smaller the colon, the blacker and better can one remember, imagine, or see one period of it, with benefit to the sight. One may feel that the memory of a very small colon should be more difficult than the memory of a large one, but strange to say it can be demonstrated in most cases that the very small colon is remembered best. If the movement of the colon is absent, the sight is always imperfect. In other words, it requires a stare, strain, and effort to make the colon stop its apparent motion.

Comparisons

In practising with the Snellen test card, when the vision is imperfect, the blackness of the letters is modified and the white spaces inside the letters are also modified. By comparing the blackness of the large letters with the blackness of the smaller ones it can be demonstrated that the larger letters are imperfectly seen.

When one notes the whiteness in the center of a large letter, seen indistinctly, it is usually possible to compare the whiteness seen with the remembered whiteness of something else. By alternately comparing the whiteness in the center of a letter with the memory of a better white, as the snow on the top of a mountain, the whiteness of the letter usually improves. In the same way, comparing the shade of black of a letter with the memory of a darker shade of black of some other object may be also a benefit to the black.

Most persons with myopia are able to read fine print at a near point quite perfectly. They see the blackness and whiteness of the letters much better than they are able to see the blackness of the larger letters on the Snellen test card at 15 or 20 feet. Alternately reading the fine print and regarding the Snellen test card, comparing the black and white of the small letters with the black and white of the large letters, is often times very beneficial. Some cases of myopia have been cured very promptly by this method.

All persons with imperfect sight for reading are benefited by comparing the whiteness of the spaces between the lines with the memory of objects which are whiter. Many persons can remember white snow with the eyes closed whiter than the spaces between the lines. By alternately closing the eyes for a minute or longer, remembering white snow, white starch, white paint, a white cloud in the sky with the sun shining on it, and flashing the white spaces without trying to read, many persons have materially improved their sight and been cured.

The Memory Swing

The memory swing relieves strain and tension as do the long or the short swings which have been described at various times. It is done with the eyes closed while one imagines himself to be looking first over the right shoulder and then over the left shoulder, while the head is moved from side to side. The eyeballs may be seen through the closed eyelids to move from side to side in the same direction as the head is moved. When done properly, the memory swing is just as efficient as the swing which is practiced with the eyes open, whether it be short or long.

The memory swing can be shortened by remembering the swing of a small letter, a quarter of an inch or less, when the eyes are closed.

The memory swing has given relief in many cases of imperfect sight from myopia, astigmatism, and inflammations of the outside of the eyeball as well as inflammations of the inside of the eyeball. It is much easier than the swing practiced with the eyes open and secures a greater amount of relaxation or rest than any other swing. It may be practiced incorrectly, just as any swing may be done wrong, and then no benefit will be obtained.

Improve Your Sight

When convenient, practice the long swing. Stand with the feet about one foot apart, turn the body to the right, at the same time lifting the heel of the left foot. The head and eyes move with the body. Now place the left heel on the floor, turn the body to the left, raising the heel of the right foot. Alternate.

Rest your eyes continually by blinking. The normal eye blinks irregularly but continuously. When convenient, practice blinking in the following way: Count irregularly and blink for each count. By consciously blinking correctly, it will in time become an unconscious habit.

When the mind is awake it is thinking of many things. One can remember things perfectly or imagine things perfectly, which is a rest to the eyes, mind, and the body generally. The memory of imperfect sight should be avoided because it is a strain and lowers the vision.

Read the Snellen test card at 20 feet with each eye, separately, twice daily or oftener when convenient. Imagine the white spaces in letters to be whiter than the rest of the card. Do this alternately with the eyes closed and opened. Plan to imagine the white spaces in letters just as white, in looking at the Snellen test card, as can be accomplished with the eyes closed.

Whenever convenient, close your eyes for a few minutes and rest them.

The Flashing Cure

Do you read imperfectly? Can you observe then that when you look at the first word, or the first letter, of a sentence, you do not see best where you are looking; that you see other words, or other letters, just as well as or better than the ones you are looking at? Do you observe also that the harder you try to see the worse you see?

Now close your eyes and rest them, remembering some color, like black or white, that you can remember perfectly. Keep them closed until they feel rested, or until the feeling of strain has been completely relieved. Now open them and look at the first word or letter of a sentence for a fraction of a second. If you have been able to relax, partially or completely, you will have a flash of improved or clear vision, and the area seen best will be smaller.

After opening the eyes for this fraction of a second, close them again quickly, still remembering the color, and keep them closed until they again feel rested. Then again open them for a fraction of a second. Continue this alternate resting of the eyes and flashing of the letters for a time, and you may soon find that you can keep your eyes open longer than a fraction of a second without losing the improved vision.

If your trouble is with distant instead of near vision, use the same method with distant letters.

In this way you can demonstrate for yourself the fundamental principles of the cure of imperfect sight by treatment without glasses.

If you fail, ask someone with perfect sight to help you.

The Imagination Cure

When the imagination is perfect the mind is always perfectly relaxed, and as it is impossible to relax and imagine a letter perfectly, and at the same time strain and see it imperfectly, it follows that when one imagines that one sees a letter perfectly one actually does see it, as demonstrated by the retinoscope, no matter how great an error of refraction the eye may previously have had. The sight, therefore, may often be improved very quickly by the aid of the imagination. To use this method the patient may proceed as follows:

Look at a letter at the distance at which it is seen best. Close and cover the eyes so as to exclude all the light, and remember it. Do this alternately until the memory is nearly equal to the sight. Next, after remembering the letter with the eyes closed and covered, and while still holding the mental picture of it, look at a blank surface a foot or more to the side of it, at the distance at which you wish to see it. Again close and cover the eyes and remember the letter, and on opening them look a little nearer to it. Gradually reduce the distance between the point of fixation and the letter, until able to look directly at it and imagine it as well as it is remembered with the eyes closed and covered. The letter will then be seen perfectly, and other letters in its neighborhood will come out. If unable to remember the whole letter, you may be able to imagine a black period as forming part of it. If you can do this, the letter will also be seen perfectly.

See Things Moving

When the sight is perfect the subject is able to observe that all objects regarded appear to be moving. A letter seen at the near point or at the distance appears to move slightly in various directions. The pavement comes toward one in walking, and the houses appear to move in a direction opposite to one's own. In reading, the page appears to move in a direction opposite to that of the eye. If one tries to imagine things stationary, the vision is at once lowered and discomfort and pain may be produced, not only in the eyes and head, but in other parts of the body.

This movement is usually so slight that it is seldom noticed till the attention is called to it, but it may be so conspicuous as to be plainly observable even to persons with markedly imperfect sight. If such persons, for instance, hold the hand within six inches of the face and turn the head and eyes rapidly from side to side, the hand will be seen to move in a direction opposite to that of the eyes. If it does not move, it will be found that the patient is straining to see it in the eccentric field. By observing this movement it becomes possible to see or imagine a less conspicuous movement, and thus the patient may gradually become able to observe a slight movement in every object regarded. Some persons with imperfect sight have been cured simply by imagining that they always see things moving.

The world moves. Let it move. All objects move if you let them. Do not interfere with this movement, or try to stop it. This cannot be done without an effort which impairs the efficiency of the eye and mind.

How Not to Concentrate

To remember the letter O of diamond type continuously and within effort proceed as follows:

Imagine a little black spot on the right-hand side of the O blacker than the rest of the letter; then imagine a similar spot on the left-hand side. Shift the attention from the right-hand spot to the left, and observe that every time you think of the left spot the O appears to move to the right, and every time you think of the right one it appears to move to the left. This motion, when the shifting is done properly, is very short, less than the width of the letter. Later you may become able to imagine the O without conscious shifting and swinging, but whenever the attention is directed to the matter these things will be noticed.

Now do the same with a letter on the test card. If the shifting is normal, it will be noted that the letter can be regarded indefinitely, and that it appears to have a slight motion.

To demonstrate that the attempt to concentrate spoils the memory, or imagination, and the vision:

Try to think continuously of a spot on one part of an imagined letter. The spot and the whole letter will soon disappear. Or try to imagine two or more spots, or the whole letter, equally black and distinct at one time. This will be found to be even more difficult.

Do the same with a letter on the test card. The results will be the same.

The Optimum Swing

The optimum swing is the swing which gives the best results under different conditions.

Most readers of this magazine and of "Perfect Sight Without Glasses" know about the swing. The swing may be spontaneous; that is to say, when one remembers a letter perfectly or sees a letter perfectly and continuously without any volition on his part he is able to imagine that it is a slow, short, easy swing. The speed is about as fast as one would count orally. The width of the swing is not more than the width of the letter, and it is remembered or imagined as easily as it is possible to imagine anything without any effort whatsoever. The normal swing of normal sight brings the greatest amount of relaxation and should be imagined. When one is able to succeed then it becomes the optimum swing under favorable conditions. Nearsighted persons have this normal optimum swing usually at the near point when the vision is perfect. At the distance where the vision is imperfect the optimum swing is something else. It is not spontaneous but has to be produced by a conscious movement of the eyes and head from side to side and is usually wider than the width of the letter, faster than the normal swing, and not so easily produced.

When one has a headache or a pain in the eyes or in any part of the body the optimum swing is always wider and more difficult to imagine than when one has less strain of the eyes. Under unfavorable conditions the long swing is the optimum swing, but under favorable conditions when the sight is good, the normal swing of the normal eye with normal sight is the optimum swing. The long swing brings a measure of relief when done right and makes it possible to shorten it down to the normal swing of the normal eye.

Methods that Have Succeeded in Presbyopia

The cure of presbyopia, as of any other error of refraction, is rest, and many presbyopic patients are able to obtain this rest simply by closing the eyes. They are kept closed until the patient feels relieved, which may be in a few minutes, half an hour, or longer. Then some fine print is regarded for a few seconds. By alternately resting the eyes and looking at fine print many patients quickly become able to read it at eighteen inches, and by continued practice they are able to reduce the distance until it can be read at six inches in a dim light. At first the letters are seen only in flashes. Then they are seen for a longer time, until finally they are seen continuously. When this method fails, palming may be tried, combined with the use of the memory, imagination and swing. Particularly good results have been obtained from the following procedure:

Close the eyes and remember the letter o in diamond type, with the open space as white as starch and the outline as black as possible.

When the white center is at the maximum imagine that the letter is moving, and that all objects, no matter how large or small, are moving with it.

Open the eyes and continue to imagine the universal swing.

Alternate the imagination of the swing with the eyes open with its imagination with the eyes closed.

When the imagination is just as good with the eyes open as when they are closed the cure will be complete.

Stop Staring

It can be demonstrated by tests with the retinoscope that all persons with imperfect sight stare, strain, or try to see. To demonstrate this fact:

Look intently at one part of a large or small letter at the distance or nearpoint. In a few seconds, usually, fatigue and discomfort will be produced, and the letter will blur or disappear. If the effort is continued long enough, pain may be produced.

To break the habit of staring:

(1) Shift consciously from one part to another of all objects regarded, and imagine that these objects move in a direction contrary to the movement of the eye. Do this with letters on the test card, with letters of fine print, if they can be seen, and with other objects.

(2) Close the eyes frequently for a moment or longer. When the strain is considerable, keep the eyes closed for several minutes and open them for a fraction of a second—flashing. When the stare is sufficient to keep the vision down to 2/200 or less, palm for a longer or shorter time; then look at the card for a moment. Later mere closing of the eyes may afford sufficient rest.

(3) Imagine that the white openings and margins of letters are whiter than the rest of the background. Do this with eyes closed and open alternately. It is an interesting fact that this practice prevents staring and improves the vision rapidly.

The Late Dr. William H. Bates.
To the Editor of The New York Times:

The press notices upon the death of Dr. William H. Bates failed to give adequate consideration to the truly significant aspects of the career of a man whose unique achievements have not yet been properly understood or generally appreciated.

Meager attention has been given to his priority in the therapeutic application of adrenalin and to his immensely important researches concerning the influence of memory upon vision.

His verification, by every known scientific means, of the fact that the normal fixation of the eye is central, and never stationary, but, on the contrary, constantly unsteady, either swinging or shifting in every direction, and his successful application of this principle to the treatment of eye strain symptoms, should alone be sufficient to merit recognition among his fellow-men.

Here, after all, he but developed practically—that is, through clinical application in the field of ophthalmology—the psychological ideas of Leibnitz and Herbart and the physiological principles of Titchener and Wundt upon the existence of any moment in the consciousness, as in the retina, of a clear point in the centre and a field of increasing vagueness as it departs from that point: the so-called point of apperception.

Of course the technique which he evolved from these fundamental concepts is in direct opposition to the methods ordinarily used for the treatment of errors of refraction and their accompanying symptoms—methods based upon principles still almost universally accepted. It is not to be wondered at, therefore, that the theories and methods of Dr. Bates should have always aroused violent antagonism. But those of us who derived benefit from his new doctrines can testify to the scientific worth of their originator.
R. R. A.
New York, July 12, 1931.

Perfect Sight Without Glasses
By W. H. BATES, M.D.

The author of this book presents evidence that all errors of refraction are caused by strain—and cured by rest and relaxation.

The complete method of treatment is described so clearly that the reader can usually discard his glasses and improve his vision.

For sale at this office and at leading bookstores. Price $3.00 postpaid.

METHODS OF TREATMENT
described in
Stories from the Clinic
By EMILY C. LIERMAN

This book fully explains the author's experience in treating clinic patients and her application of Dr. Bates' method of treatment to each individual case.

"Stories from the Clinic" is a contribution to the practice of Ophthalmology.
Price, $2.00 postpaid

Central Fixation Publishing Company
18 East 48th Street, New York City

Better Eyesight

A MONTHLY MAGAZINE DEVOTED TO THE PREVENTION AND CURE OF IMPERFECT SIGHT WITHOUT GLASSES

Vol. XIV   JUNE, 1930   No. 12

Stop Staring

Imagination Essential to Sight
By W. H. Bates, M.D.

Suggestions
By Emily A. Bates

Questions and Answers

Announcements

$2.00 per year   20 cents per copy   Back numbers 30 cents
Published by the CENTRAL FIXATION PUBLISHING COMPANY
210 MADISON AVENUE   NEW YORK, N. Y.

Announcements

Space does not permit us to print the entire list of Dr. Bates' authorized representatives in the United States, Canada and Europe, which we should like to do for the benefit of our subscribers. The following, however, is a list of those who have taken courses of instruction in the Bates Method within the past few months. Those subscribers who wish to know if there is an authorized representative in their city may obtain this information by writing direct to Dr. Bates at 210 Madison Avenue, New York City.

Miss Clara M. Brewster,
Studio 6, Aquila Court,
Omaha, Nebraska.

Miss Mary E. Wilson,
2538 Channing Way,
Berkeley, Calif.

Dr. Paul J. Dodge,
911 New Industrial Trust Bldg, Providence, R. I.

Mrs. D. L. Corbett,
1712½ Fifth Ave.,
Los Angeles, Calif.

Miss Jane Button,
249 Harvey St.,
Germantown, Pa.

Mr. Fred Baechtold,
572 12th St.,
West New York, N. J.
Tel.—Palisade 6-7735

Mr. Harold E. Ensley,
112 West 104th St.,
New York City.

Dr. Med. E. Schluter,
Hamburg, Mundsburgerdamm 11, Germany.

Mrs. R. Norman Jolliffe,
171 West 71st St.,
New York City.

It has come to our attention that certain parties not connected with Dr. Bates in any way are desirous of publishing a periodical called "Better Eyesight". We wish to say that any such use of this title is not with the permission of Dr. Bates or the Central Fixation Publishing Company and that any magazine issued under this title other than the present one, is not published in the interest of the Bates Method. The title, "Better Eyesight," is protected against illegal usage.

As we have already notified our subscribers, "Better Eyesight" is being discontinued with this issue. This will enable Dr. Bates and Mrs. Bates to devote more time to the writing of new books on treatment alone for which there has been a very great demand. We request that all those who desire to be notified upon the publication of new books kindly send us their names and addresses which will be kept on file.

Bound volumes of "Better Eyesight" containing the issues from July, 1929 to June, 1930, inclusive, will be ready about July 15th. Those subscribers wishing to have their own magazines bound may send them to us before July 10th and they will be bound at the same time our issues are being bound. The price for binding will be $1.00.